Atlas of Postsurgical Neuroradiology

Daniel Thomas Ginat
Per-Lennart A. Westesson

Editors

Atlas of Postsurgical Neuroradiology

Imaging of the Brain, Spine, Head, and Neck

Second Edition

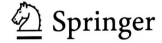 Springer

Editors
Daniel Thomas Ginat
Department of Radiology
University of Chicago
Pritzker School of Medicine
Chicago, IL
USA

Per-Lennart A. Westesson
Division of Diagnostic and
Interventional Neuroradiology
University of Rochester School of
Medicine and Dentistry
Rochester, NY
USA

ISBN 978-3-319-52340-8   ISBN 978-3-319-52341-5   (eBook)
DOI 10.1007/978-3-319-52341-5

Library of Congress Control Number: 2017943020

Printed on acid-free paper

This Springer imprint is published by Springer Nature
The registered company is Springer International Publishing AG
The registered company address is: Gewerbestrasse 11, 6330 Cham, Switzerland

This book is dedicated to my parents, Roselyne and Jonathan.
Daniel Thomas Ginat

This book is dedicated to my wife Ann-Margret and our children Karin, Oscar, and Nils.
Per-Lennart A. Westesson

Foreword

Radiologists and clinicians caring for patients have a plethora of references that provide educational tools for imaging studies illustrating neuroanatomy and many forms of neurological and neurosurgical disease processes. However, even those who are well versed in interpreting imaging examinations often find assessment of imaging studies in the postoperative patient difficult. Information on imaging findings in the postoperative patient is indeed available but, in scattered locations, making ready access for radiologists difficult.

One realm in which radiologists must constantly update their knowledge is that of imaging devices: their composition and appearance, their correct location, and their proper functioning. Such devices are numerous and have many different appearances. Increasingly, radiologists are requested to interpret imaging studies designed to assess the status of devices used in care of patients. These studies are intended to answer questions such as "Is the device properly positioned?" "Is the device intact?" and "Is the device functioning properly?" Resources that can provide information relevant to answering such questions are scarce and cannot generally be found at a single source of information.

Another area in which radiologists need to regularly update their knowledge base is the appearance of the postoperative surgical site. New surgical techniques continually come into use; they may present a baffling appearance to radiologists unfamiliar with their details. As a result, the potential for incorrect reporting of imaging findings is substantial. An up-to-date compendium of normal surgical findings for a given procedure would be of great use. Yet another potential source of consternation for those interpreting postoperative imaging studies is assessing complications of surgical procedures. It is easy to understand how the lack of familiarity of normal and abnormal appearances of postoperative conditions could lead to one being mistaken for the other.

Thus, a need exists for a comprehensive source of information on these topics. In *Atlas of Postsurgical Neuroradiology*, Drs. Ginat and Westesson ably address that need by providing an in-depth and comprehensive explanation of standard postoperative findings as well as a wide array of appearances of therapeutic devices. The assembly of information on these topics in a single reference will, no doubt, prove valuable to radiologists and physicians involved in postsurgical care alike.

Durham, NC, USA   James M. Provenzale, M.D.

Preface

In addition to updating the text according to progress that has occurred in the relevant fields since the 5 years that have ensued since the first edition of Atlas of Postsurgical Neuroradiology, this second edition contains more useful and interesting topics. Indeed, this book includes many new images and sections, such as robot surgery and intraoperative MRI, as well as additional authors.

Chicago, IL, USA   Daniel Thomas Ginat

Acknowledgments

We thank the following individuals for contributing cases, photographs, or insights:

Nishant Agrawal, M.D.
Jene Bohannon
Daniel Cavalcante
Kathryn Colby, M.D.
Joel Curé, M.D.
Shehenaz Ellika, M.D.
Zhen Gooi, M.D.
Melissa Guilbeau
Rajiv Gupta, M.D.
Ryder Gwinn
John W. Henson, M.D.
Justin Hugelier
Gregory Katzman, M.D., M.B.A.
Nina Klionski, M.D.
Patrik Keshishian, D.D.S.
Sarah Paengatelli
Bruno Policeni M.D.
Amy Schneider, Medtronic
Patricia Smith, N.P.
Zimmer Spine (Minneapolis, MN)
Christine Toh, M.D.
Richard White, M.D.
John Wandtke, M.D.
Tina Young Poussaint, M.D.
Jennifer Wulff, ARNP
Fatoumata Yanoga, M.D.
Juan Small, M.D.

We also thank the following companies for providing device images:

Alcon/Novartis
Alphatec Spine
Altomed
Benvenue Medical
Cochlear Corp
Grace Medical
Hoopes Vision
Medtronic
Osmed
Paradigm Spine
Quandary Medical
Synthes

Contents

1   **Imaging of Facial Cosmetic Surgery**   1
    Charles J. Schatz and Daniel Thomas Ginat

2   **Imaging the Postoperative Orbit**   31
    Daniel Thomas Ginat, Gul Moonis, and Suzanne K. Freitag

3   **Imaging the Paranasal Sinuses and Nasal Cavity**   75
    Daniel Thomas Ginat, Mary Elizabeth Cunnane,
    and Robert M. Naclerio

4   **Imaging the Postoperative Scalp and Cranium**   117
    Daniel Thomas Ginat, Ann-Christine Duhaime,
    and Marc Daniel Moisi

5   **Imaging the Intraoperative and Postoperative Brain**   183
    Daniel Thomas Ginat, Pamela W. Schaefer,
    and Marc Daniel Moisi

6   **Imaging of Cerebrospinal Fluid Shunts, Drains, and
    Diversion Techniques**   259
    Daniel Thomas Ginat, Per-Lennart A. Westesson,
    and David Frim

7   **Imaging of the Postoperative Skull Base and
    Cerebellopontine Angle**   311
    Daniel Thomas Ginat, Peleg M. Horowitz, Gul Moonis,
    and Suresh K. Mukherji

8   **Imaging of the Postoperative Ear and Temporal Bone**   351
    Daniel Thomas Ginat, Gul Moonis, Suresh K. Mukherji,
    and Michael B. Gluth

9   **Imaging of Orthognathic, Maxillofacial, and
    Temporomandibular Joint Surgery**   421
    Daniel Thomas Ginat, Per-Lennart A. Westesson,
    and Russell Reid

10 **Imaging the Postoperative Neck**   453
    Daniel Thomas Ginat, Elizabeth Blair, and Hugh D. Curtin

11   Imaging of Postoperative Spine   523
       Daniel Thomas Ginat, Ryan Murtagh, Per-Lennart A. Westesson,
       Marc Daniel Moisi, and Rod J. Oskouian

12   Imaging of Vascular and Endovascular Surgery   627
       Daniel Thomas Ginat, Javier M. Romero,
       and Gregory Christoforidis

Index   697

Contributors

Elizabeth Blair, M.D. Department of Surgery, Section of Otolaryngology-Head and Neck Surgery, University of Chicago, Chicago, IL, USA

Gregory Christoforidis, M.D. Department of Radiology, University of Chicago, Chicago, IL, USA

Mary Elizabeth Cunnane, M.D. Department of Radiology, Harvard Medical School, Massachusetts Eye and Ear Infirmary, Boston, MA, USA

Hugh D. Curtin, M.D. Department of Radiology, Harvard Medical School, Boston, MA, USA

Department of Radiology, Massachusetts Eye and Ear Infirmary, Boston, MA, USA

Ann-Christine Duhaime, M.D. Department of Neurosurgery, Harvard Medical School, Massachusetts General Hospital, Boston, MA, USA

Suzanne K. Freitag, M.D., M.S. Department of Ophthalmology, Harvard Medical School, Massachusetts Eye and Ear Infirmary, Boston, MA, USA

Daniel Thomas Ginat, M.D., M.S. Department of Radiology, University of Chicago, Pritzker School of Medicine, Chicago, IL, USA

Michael B. Gluth, M.D. Department of Surgery, Division of Otolaryngology, University of Chicago, Chicago, IL, USA

Peleg M. Horowitz, M.D., Ph.D. Department of Surgery, University of Chicago, Chicago, IL, USA

Gul Moonis, M.D. Department of Radiology, Columbia University Medical Center, New York City, NY, USA

Suresh K. Mukherji, M.D., FACR Division of Radiology, Michigan State University, East Lansing, MI, USA

Ryan Murtagh, M.D., M.B.A Department of Radiology, Diagnostic Imaging Moffitt Cancer Center, Tampa, FL, USA

Marc D. Moisi, M.D., M.S. Department of Neurosurgery, Swedish Neuroscience Institute, Seattle, WA, USA

Robert M. Naclerio, M.D. Section of Otolaryngology-Head and Neck Surgery, University of Chicago Pritzker School of Medicine, Chicago, IL, USA

Rod J. Oskouian, M.D. Department of Neurosurgery, Swedish Neuroscience Institute, Seattle, WA, USA

Russell Reid, M.D., Ph.D. Department of Surgery, University of Chicago, Chicago, IL, USA

Javier M. Romero, M.D. Department of Radiology, Harvard Medical School, Massachusetts General Hospital, Boston, MA, USA

Pamela W. Schaefer, M.D. Department of Radiology, Harvard Medical School, Massachusetts General Hospital, Boston, MA, USA

Charles J. Schatz, M.D., FACR Beverly Wilshire Tower Advanced Imaging, Beverly Hills, CA, USA

University of Southern California Keck School of Medicine, Los Angeles, CA, USA

Per-Lennart A. Westesson, M.D., Ph.D., DDS Division of Neuroradiology, University of Rochester Medical Center, Rochester, NY, USA

Imaging of Facial Cosmetic Surgery

Charles J. Schatz and Daniel Thomas Ginat

1.1 Overview of Facial Cosmetic Materials and Their Imaging Features

A wide variety of materials have been used to augment facial tissues in the form of implants, grafts, fillers, and injectables (Fig. 1.1). The main types of implant and graft materials (Table 1.1) include solid silicone, polytetrafluoroethylene, high-density porous polyethylene, bone, and fat, while the main types of fillers and injectables (Table 1.2) include hyaluronic acid preparations, calcium hydroxyapatite, collagen, polytetrafluoroethylene, silicone, alkyl-imide gel polymer, and botulinum toxin, among others.

On occasion, CT or MRI will be obtained to evaluate complications, which include foreign body granuloma formation, seroma, infection/fistula/draining sinus, skin atrophy, implant migration and extrusion, change in cosmetic result, functional alteration, vision loss, dysesthesia, ossification, and obstructed breathing, among others, depending on the type of implant or graft. Alternatively, changes related to facial surgery may be encountered incidentally on imaging.

C.J. Schatz, M.D., FACR (✉)
Department of Radiology, Beverly Tower Wilshire,
Advanced Imaging, Beverly Hills, CA, USA

University of Southern California, Keck School of
Medicine, Los Angeles, CA, USA

D.T. Ginat, M.D., M.S.
Department of Radiology, University of Chicago,
Pritzker School of Medicine, Chicago, IL, USA
e-mail: dtg1@uchicago.edu

© Springer International Publishing Switzerland 2017
D.T. Ginat, P.-L.A. Westesson (eds.), *Atlas of Postsurgical Neuroradiology*,
DOI 10.1007/978-3-319-52341-5_1

Fig. 1.1 Photographs
of various facial implants
(**a**, **b**)

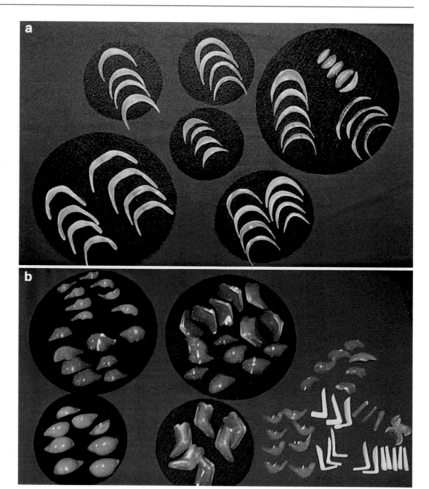

Table 1.1 Implants and grafts

Material	Properties and uses	Imaging appearance
Solid silicone	Rubber elastomer used since 1956	CT: variable attenuation, usually more hyperattenuating than soft tissue, but less hyperattenuating than bone and best discerned using bone windows
	Well-tolerated	MRI: very low signal intensity on T1- and T2-weighted sequences
	Indications: chin, lateral jaw, cheek, and nose augmentation	
Polytetrafluoroethylene	Long-lasting, but can be removed surgically	CT: higher attenuation relative to soft tissues, but lower attenuation than bone
	Indications: lower face-lift, nasal, and forehead augmentation	MRI: hypointense to fat on T1- and T2-weighted sequences
High-density porous polyethylene	Inert and biocompatible	CT: attenuation between fat and water
	Low complication rate	MRI: hypointense to fat on T1- and T2-weighted sequences
	Permanent	Enhancement may occur due to fibrovascular ingrowth
	Indications: lower face and nasal augmentation. Also used for orbital and auricular reconstruction	
Bone	Used more frequently in the past for chin and cheek augmentation, often in the form of "button" implants	CT: same as normal bone elsewhere; cortex and trabecular can be identified unless resorption has occurred
	Bone or osteochondral grafts are sometimes used in rhinoplasty	MRI: same as bone elsewhere
	Harvest sites include the calvarium and rib	

Table 1.2 Fillers and injectables

Filler material	Properties and uses	Imaging appearance
Liquid silicone	Analogous to intraocular silicone injection, but not currently FDA approved for facial cosmesis	CT: variable attenuation, usually similar to soft tissue density
	Permanent agent	MRI: variable signal on T1 and T2 depending on viscosity
	Relatively higher risk of granuloma formation, particularly with non-medical grade formulations	Decrease in signal with fat suppression
		More conspicuous on STIR
Collagen	Naturally occurring protein derived from purified bovine collagen given via a subdermal injection	CT: soft tissue attenuation; subcutaneous fat appears infiltrated
	Indications: wrinkles, scars, and lines Lasts approximately 3–6 months	MRI: same signal intensity as water (hypointense to fat on T1 and hyperintense to fat on T2); occasional minimal peripheral enhancement that can persist up to 2 months
Hyaluronic acid preparations	Injectable gel	CT: water attenuation; subcutaneous fat appears infiltrated
	FDA approved Indications: wrinkles, scars, and lines Lasts about 6 months and can be removed using hyaluronidase injection	MRI: same signal intensity as water (hypointense to fat on T1 and hyperintense to fat on T2); occasional minimal peripheral enhancement that can persist up to 2 months
Polytetrafluoroethylene	Implanted – not injected	CT: higher attenuation relative to soft tissues
	Permanent, threadlike material (not metabolized, but can be removed surgically)	MRI: hypointense to fat on T1- and T2-weighted sequences
	Indications: filler in multiple sites (nasolabial folds, lips, glabella)	
Calcium hydroxyapatite	US FDA approved	CT: high attenuation (generally 280–700 HU) initially; eventually the calcium resorbs, typically incites fibrous tissue formation that may be visible on imaging
	Temporary injectable that lasts up to at least 2 years	MRI: similar to bone (hypointense to muscle on T1- and T2-weighted sequences); no enhancement
	Indications: wrinkles, lines, scars, and HIV lipoatrophy	PET: can lead to hypermetabolic response
Alkyl-imide gel polymer	Injectable, biocompatible, nontoxic, nonallergenic soft tissue filler	CT: water attenuation masses surrounded by thin collagen capsule
	Uses: HIV lipoatrophy and rejuvenation	MRI: same signal intensity as water (hypointense to fat on T1 and hyperintense to fat on T2)
Botulinum toxin	Neurotoxin for the temporary improvement of glabellar lines	CT: nil
	Intramuscular injection (corrugator and procerus muscles; 5 sites – 0.1 ml each)	MRI: nil
	Maximum effect at 30 days. Lasts up to 6 months	

1.2   Forehead Augmentation

1.2.1   Discussion

Forehead augmentation is performed for improving the upper facial contour. A variety of alloplastic implants have been used for this purpose, including polytetrafluoroethylene and silicone. Often, silicone implants have corrugated edges and central perforations in order to optimize fixation and prevent capsular contraction. Fillers, such as calcium hydroxyapatite, also have a role in forehead augmentation. These materials can be inserted in the midline (Figs. 1.2 and 1.3), lateral brow (Fig. 1.4), or both. Botox is another minimally invasive option for reducing lines and wrinkles.

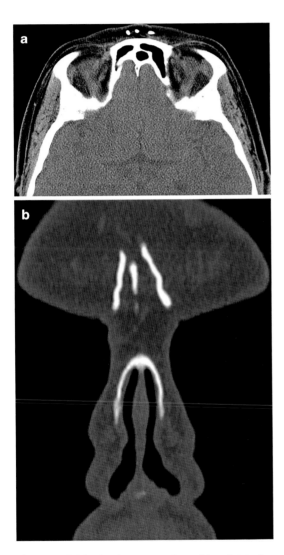

Fig. 1.2 Mid-forehead augmentation with polytetrafluoroethylene. Axial (**a**) and coronal (**b**) CT images demonstrate hyperattenuating linear implants in the glabella

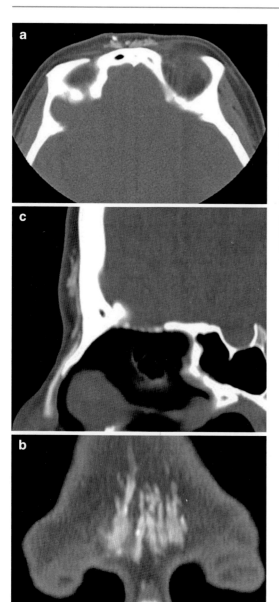

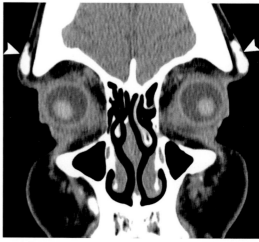

Fig. 1.4 Lateral brow augmentation. Coronal CT image shows collections of calcium hydroxyapatite in the lateral supraorbital areas (*arrowheads*)

Fig. 1.3 Mid-forehead augmentation with calcium hydroxy-apatite. Axial (**a**), coronal (**b**), and sagittal (**c**) CT images demonstrate hyperattenuating linear implants with fuzzy edges, which provide a gentle convex contour to the glabella despite the flat frontal bone. A silicone dorsal nasal implant is also present

1.3 Cheek and Nasolabial Fold Augmentation

1.3.1 Discussion

Cheek augmentation consists of expanding the malar region, submalar region, or a combination of these, often bilaterally. The procedure is performed for soft tissue enhancement or simply for correcting a deficient or atrophic face, including HIV lipoatrophy. A wide variety of materials have been used for these purposes, including coral implants (Fig. 1.5), silicone rubber implants (Fig. 1.6), injectable silicone (Fig. 1.7), injectable calcium hydroxyapatite (Fig. 1.8), polytetrafluoroethylene strips (Fig. 1.9), hyaluronic acid (Fig. 1.10), collagen (Fig. 1.11), alkyl-imide gel polymer (Fig. 1.12), and combination of materials (Fig. 1.13).

Seromas can be present and appear as simple fluid collections surrounding the implants (Fig. 1.14). Seromas typically resolve spontaneously, unless there is superimposed infection. In such cases, the patient may present with fever and purulent drainage. On imaging, stranding of the subcutaneous fat overlying the implant is often evident (Fig. 1.15). Additional manifestations of implant-associated infections include osteomyelitis and draining sinuses (Fig. 1.16). Other complications depend on the type of material used. In particular, liquid silicone can induce extensive inflammation, which appears as stranding or high T2 signal in the subcutaneous tissues (Fig. 1.17). Furthermore, injected nonmedical-grade silicone has a particular propensity to cause scars and granulomas. These complications can develop many years after injection of the filler. Hypertrophic scars can appear as bands of soft tissue within the subcutaneous fat on CT (Fig. 1.18). Granulomas often appear as subcentimeter rounded or oval foci of variable attenuation on CT (Fig. 1.19). Silicone foreign body granulomas can contain microcalcifications or form eggshell calcifications. Implants, such as silicone rubber, can occasionally erode through the bone (Fig. 1.20) and potentially result in sinusitis. Cheek implantation can sometimes induce heterotopic bone formation (Fig. 1.21). Bone grafts can resorb over time, thereby also diminishing cosmetic effect. Migration of fillers or implants can mimic mass lesions and impair vision (Fig. 1.22).

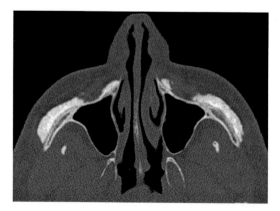

Fig. 1.5 Cheek augmentation with coral implants. Axial CT image shows hyperattenuating *material* overlying the bilateral malar eminences

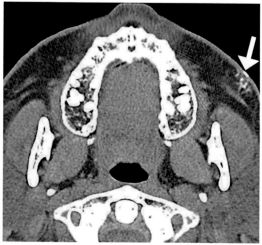

Fig. 1.7 Acne scar treatment with silicone oil filler. Axial CT image shows punctate hyperattenuating foci of the filler material (*arrow*) within the subcutaneous tissues of the left cheek

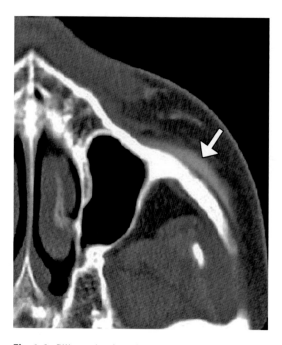

Fig. 1.6 Silicone implant cheek augmentation. Axial CT image shows bilateral crescent-shaped hyperattenuating implants (*arrow*) over the zygomatic and maxillary bones

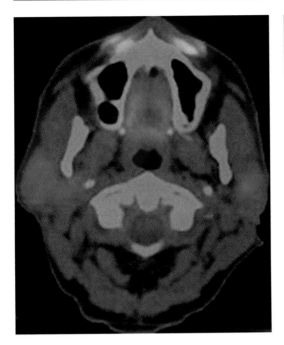

Fig. 1.8 Anterior face and nasolabial fold calcium hydroxyapatite injection. There is hypermetabolism at the site of the nasolabial fold fillers (*arrows*) on 18FDG-PET/CT

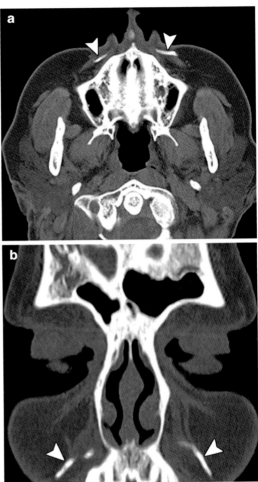

Fig. 1.9 Nasolabial fold polytetrafluoroethylene filler. Axial (**a**) and coronal (**b**) CT image shows thin strips of hyperattenuating material in the bilateral nasolabial folds and subcutaneous tissues (*arrowheads*)

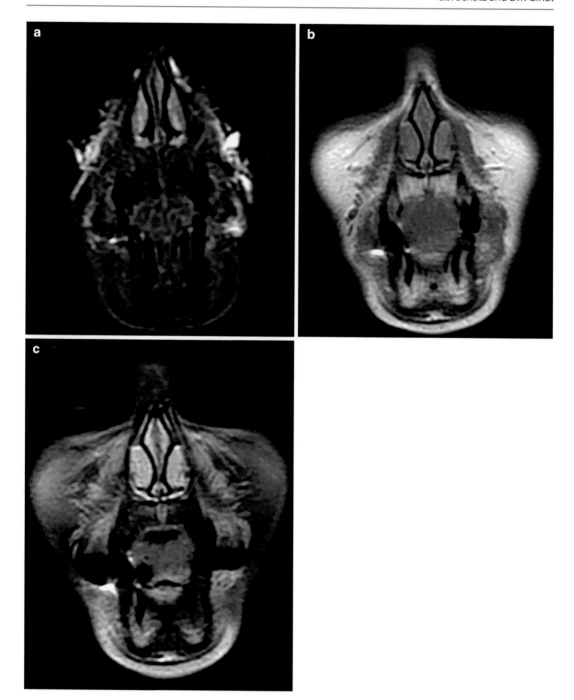

Fig. 1.10 Nasolabial fold hyaluronic acid augmentation. Coronal STIR (**a**), T1-weighted (**b**), and post-contrast fat-suppressed T1-weighted (**c**) MR images demonstrate streaky material with high T2 signal, as well as mild enhancement

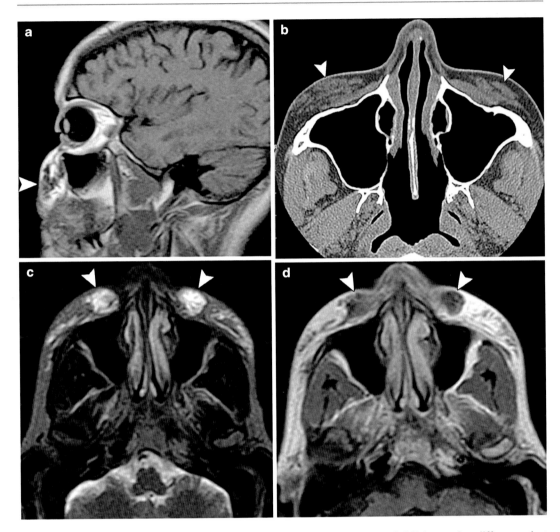

Fig. 1.11 Combined cheek and nasolabial fold collagen injection. Axial CT image (**a**) shows soft tissue attenuation within the bilateral malar fat pads (*arrows*). Axial T2-weighted (**b**), axial post-contrast T1-weighted (**c**), and sagittal T1-weighted (**d**) MR images in a different patient show bilateral globular collections of collagen-based gel filler (*arrows*), which have signal characteristics similar to that of water

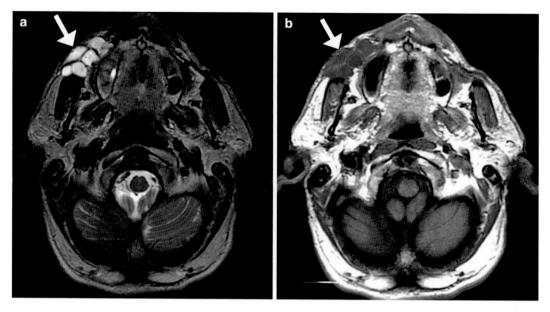

Fig. 1.12 Polyacrylamide gel polymer treatment for HIV lipoatrophy. Axial T2-weighted (**a**) and T1-weighted (**b**) MR images demonstrate encapsulated clusters of material (*arrows*) with similar signal characteristics to water in the right lower cheek. Gel polymer was previously removed from the contralateral side

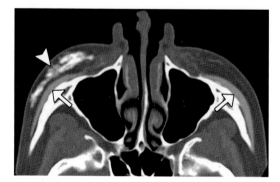

Fig. 1.13 Combined silicone implant and calcium hydroxyapatite cheek augmentation. Axial CT image shows silicone implants bilaterally (*arrows*), as well as calcium hydroxyapatite filler (*arrowheads*) superficial to the right silicone implant

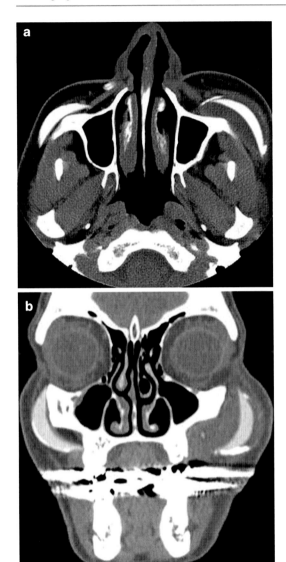

Fig. 1.14 Cheek implant seroma. Axial (**a**) and coronal (**b**) CT images show fluid in the subperiosteal surrounding the displaced left silicone cheek implant

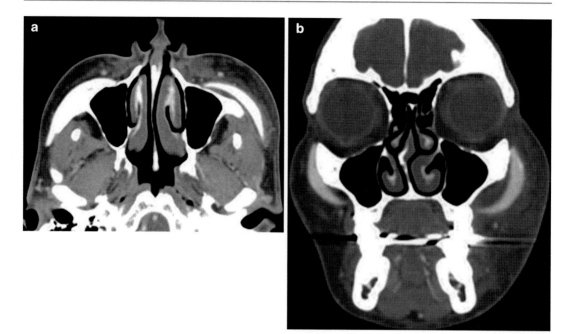

Fig. 1.15 Cheek implant abscess. Axial (**a**) and coronal (**b**) CT images demonstrate left check subcutaneous fat stranding and overlying skin thickening. The left silicone implant is surrounded and displaced by fluid and subcutaneous stranding, while the right silicone implant is unremarkable. Bilateral nasolabial fold fillers are also present

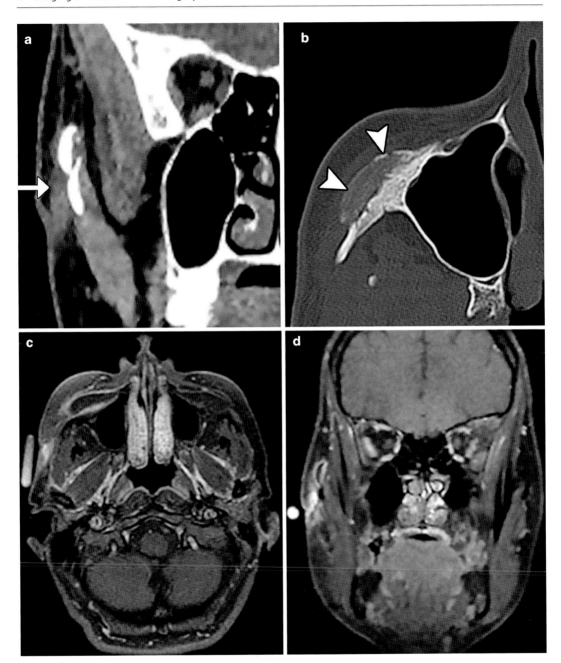

Fig. 1.16 Cheek implant osteomyelitis. Coronal CT image (**a**) shows right cheek skin dimpling overlying a draining sinus (*arrow*) adjacent to a silicone implant. Axial CT (**b**) image in the bone window shows sclerotic thickening of the right anterior maxillary wall and zygoma adjacent to the implant (*arrowheads*). Post-contrast axial (**c**) and coronal (**d**) fat-suppressed T1-weighted MR images show the enhancing draining sinus beneath the external marker

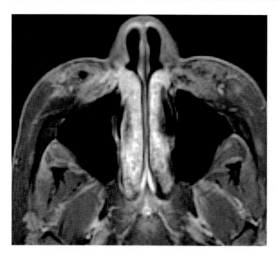

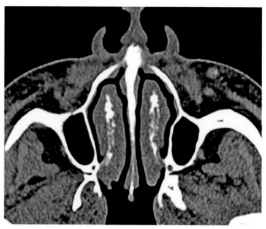

Fig. 1.17 Inflammation. Post-contrast fat-suppressed axial T1-weighted MR image shows diffuse enhancement in the bilateral cheek subcutaneous tissues surrounding the filler material (liquid silicone)

Fig. 1.19 Injectable silicone granulomas. Axial CT image shows several subcentimeter nodular densities in the bilateral nasolabial folds and buccal space fat

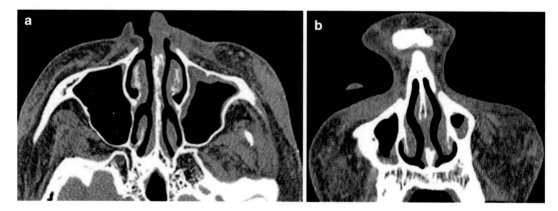

Fig. 1.18 Injectable silicone scars. Axial (**a**) and coronal (**b**) CT images show bilateral confluent bands of soft tissue in the bilateral subcutaneous fat of the anterior face

Fig. 1.20 Cheek implant bone erosion and maxillary sinus penetration. Axial CT image shows medial migration of the right solid silicone implant into the maxillary sinus through a bony defect (*arrow*) caused by long-standing pressure changes from the implant. There is associated mucosal thickening adjacent to the medial tip of the implant

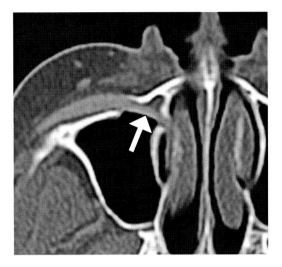

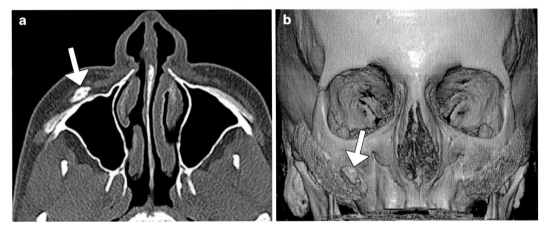

Fig. 1.21 Cheek implant heterotopic ossification. Axial (**a**) and 3D (**b**) CT images show a nodular focus of the bone (*arrows*) adjacent to the right cheek implant. This finding indicates that the surgical procedure is not recent

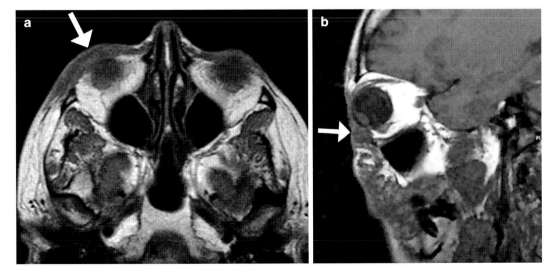

Fig. 1.22 Hyaluronic acid eyelid migration. Axial (**a**) and sagittal (**b**) T1-weighted MRI images demonstrate hyaluronic acid filler in the lower eyelid, resembling a tumor (*arrows*)

1.4   Rhinoplasty

1.4.1   Discussion

Rhinoplasty is performed to restore or enhance the appearance of the nose. There are a wide variety of rhinoplasty techniques, ranging from functional versus aesthetic, open versus closed, augmentation versus reduction, and primary versus secondary. The classic open rhinoplasty features in-fractures of the bilateral nasal processes of the maxilla, which have a characteristic appearance on CT (Fig. 1.23). In addition, different portions of the nose can be altered (i.e., tip, dorsum, nasion, columella, or a combination of these). Both natural and synthetic materials can be used for augmentation rhinoplasty, including cartilage grafts, bone grafts (Figs. 1.24 and 1.25), silicone (Fig. 1.26), polytetrafluoroethyl-

ene (Fig. 1.27), and fillers (Fig. 1.28). The implants are sometimes purposefully positioned such that they appear asymmetric on imaging, but the cosmetic results are considered satisfactory. Kirschner (K) wires may also be used for support when there is total nasal collapse or septal cartilage warping. Although some complications are clinically evident, imaging after rhinoplasty is occasionally requested to evaluate complications related to olfactory dysfunction, retained foreign body (Fig. 1.29), infection (Figs. 1.30 and 1.31), implant extrusion (Fig. 1.32), nerve injury (Fig. 1.33), deformity (Fig. 1.34), and nasal obstruction, which may be due to collapse of the nasal valves and resultant laminar flow (Fig. 1.35). Normally, airflow through the nasal cavity is turbulent (Fig. 1.36). Intracranial complications related to rhinoplasty are very rare.

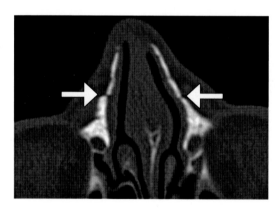

Fig. 1.23 Lateral osteotomy rhinoplasty. Axial CT image shows bilateral in-fractures of the frontal processes of the maxilla, which are characteristic of the procedure (*arrows*)

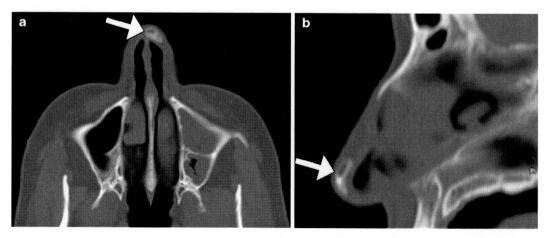

Fig. 1.24 Tip augmentation with the bone. Axial (**a**) and sagittal (**b**) CT images show a bone graft (*arrows*) in the nasal tip

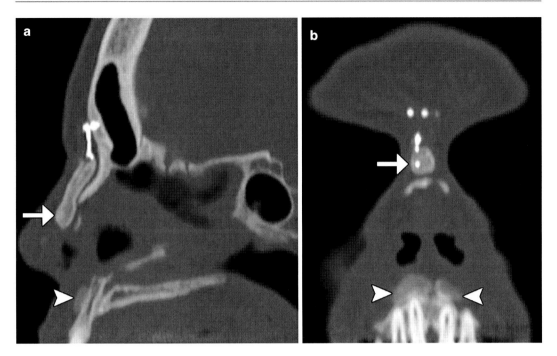

Fig. 1.25 Dorsal augmentation with the bone. Sagittal (**a**) and coronal (**b**) CT images show dorsal bone graft (*arrows*) secured via metallic microfixation plate and screws. Premaxillary augmentation was also performed (*arrowheads*)

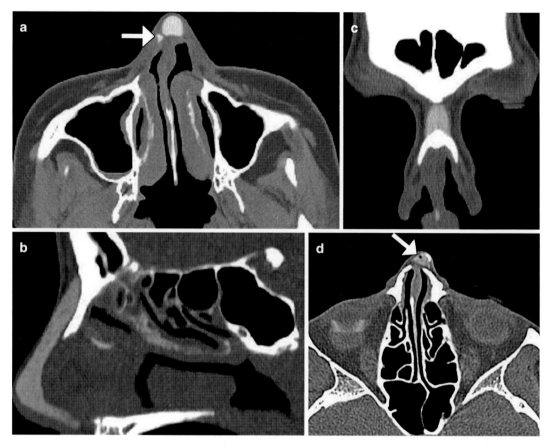

Fig. 1.26 Rhinoplasty with a silicone dorsal tip and columellar nasal implant. Axial (**a**), sagittal (**b**), and coronal (**c**) CT images show an L-shaped silicone implant that provides dorsal, tip, and columella augmentation. A smaller additional piece of silicone is present to the right of the main implant (*arrow*). Axial CT image in another patient (**d**) demonstrates a perforation (*arrow*) in the implant for sutures or to promote tissue ingrowth

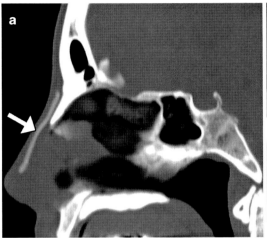

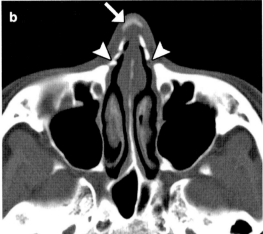

Fig. 1.27 Rhinoplasty with polytetrafluoroethylene implant. Sagittal (**a**) and axial (**b**) CT images show the thin sheet of slightly hyperattenuating implant material used for dorsal augmentation (*arrow*). Bilateral osteotomies of the frontal processes of the maxilla are also present (*arrowheads*)

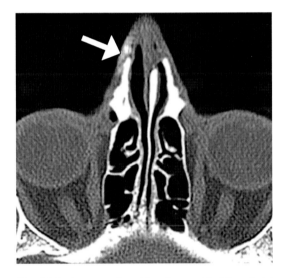

Fig. 1.28 Augmentation rhinoplasty with filler. Axial CT image shows the hyperattenuating hydroxyapatite within the subcutaneous tissues of the right lateral nasal wall and dorsum (*arrow*)

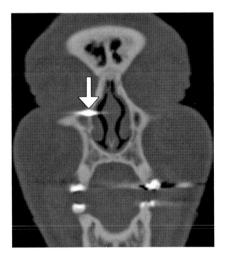

Fig. 1.29 Retained foreign body. The patient presented with swelling at the operative site. Coronal CT image shows a metallic foreign body embedded in the right nasal process of the maxilla (*arrow*). The metallic foreign body was suspected to be a broken osteotome because the other end of the osteotome was discovered in the operating room rhinoplasty kit

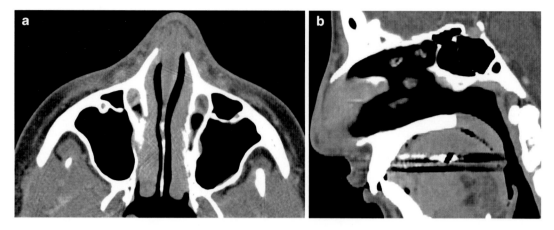

Fig. 1.30 Cellulitis. The patient experienced swelling of the nose after reduction rhinoplasty. Axial (**a**) and sagittal (**b**) CT images demonstrate diffuse inflammatory changes in the subcutaneous tissues of the nose. There is no discrete fluid collection

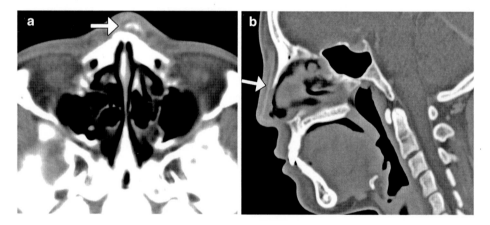

Fig. 1.31 Implant-associated abscess. Axial (**a**) and sagittal (**b**) CT images show inflammatory changes and a small fluid collection (*arrows*) overlying the polytetrafluoroethylene implant

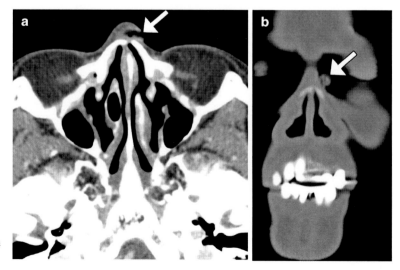

Fig. 1.32 Implant extrusion. Axial (**a**) and coronal (**b**) (**c**) CT images show the low-attenuation implant protruding from the dorsolateral aspect of the nose (*arrows*)

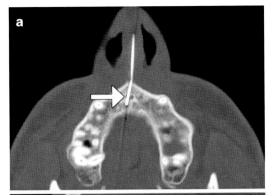

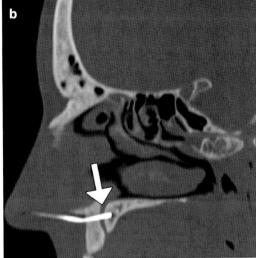

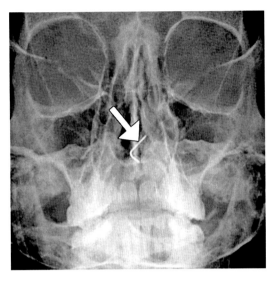

Fig. 1.34 Hardware deformity. Frontal radiograph shows a bend (*arrow*) in the columellar Kirschner wire after trauma

Fig. 1.33 Cranial nerve V2 injury. The patient presented with dysesthesia after rhinoplasty. Axial (**a**) and sagittal (**b**) CT images demonstrate perforation of the incisive canal by the metallic Kirschner wire (*arrows*)

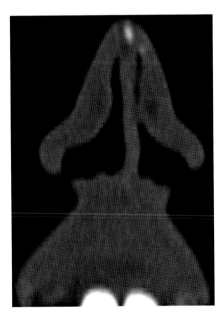

Fig. 1.35 Nasal obstruction after rhinoplasty. Coronal CT image shows collapse of the left external nasal valve and a normal right external nasal valve

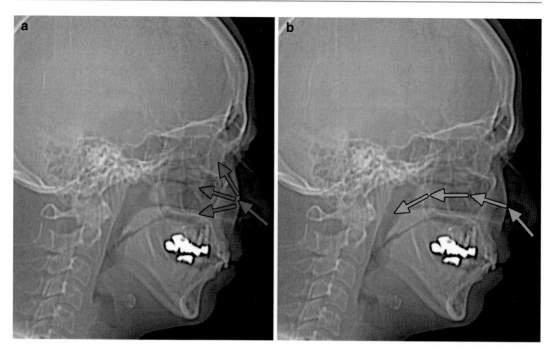

Fig. 1.36 Normally, airflow through the nasal cavity is turbulent (*red arrows*) (**a**). Nasal obstruction results in laminar flow of air in the nasal fossa (*green arrows*) (**b**)

1.5 Lip Augmentation

1.5.1 Discussion

Lip augmentation is performed to achieve the appearance of fuller lips. A wide variety of materials have been used for lip augmentation, including fluid silicone, autologous fat grafts, tissue matrix, polytetrafluoroethylene (Fig. 1.37), and fillers (Fig. 1.38). The implants can be inserted into the upper and/or lower lips via incisions made medial to the oral commissures and threading the implants deep to the submucosal plane. Overcorrection is perhaps the main complication of lip augmentation and is clinically apparent. Conversely, lip atrophy can result, particularly with fat grafts. Other complications, such as implant or filler migration, infection, and extrusion, can also occur.

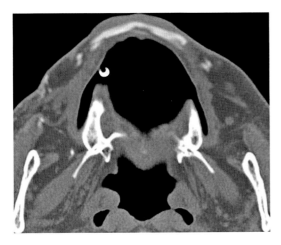

Fig. 1.37 Lip augmentation with polytetrafluoroethylene implants. Axial CT image of the upper lip shows the high-attenuation curvilinear implant within the upper lip (*arrows*)

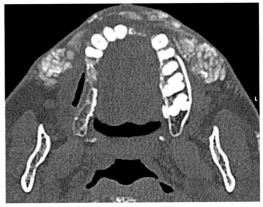

Fig. 1.38 Lip augmentation with calcium hydroxyapatite. Axial CT image shows the hyperattenuating filler within the upper lip

1.6 Chin and Jaw Augmentation

1.6.1 Discussion

Mandible augmentation can be performed with the chin (Figs. 1.39, 1.40, and 1.41), submental (Fig. 1.42), chin/prejowl or prejowl (Fig. 1.42), and lateral/mandibular angle implants (Fig. 1.43), or a combination of these. The implants are typically inserted between the periosteum and cortex of the mandible. Bone graft implants are less commonly used due to the tendency to resorb over time. On the other hand, high-density porous polyethylene and silicone implants molded to the contours of the underlying mandible are popular materials for augmentation. These can be combined with other materials, such as the bone. Screw fixation is occasionally used, particularly for providing stability to combined grafts. Complications include hematoma, infection, seroma, bone erosion, and migration. Seromas may resemble infection on imaging and can alter the intended cosmetic effect, although this may be transient (Fig. 1.44). Mandible implants are sometimes intentionally positioned asymmetrically, but should remain in close approximation to the surface of the mandible. However, pressure-induced bone erosion from the implants is abnormal and can undermine the desired cosmetic

effect (Fig. 1.45). Implant migration can also alter cosmetic result and may be associated with underlying infection. Facial CT can readily characterize implant migration (Fig. 1.46). Bone formation along the periosteum overlying the chin implants is not an uncommon occurrence and is usually thin linear or punctate (Fig. 1.47). Occasionally, the new bone can become large enough to alter the desired cosmetic effects. This phenomenon can be characterized via CT. The bone may be more difficult to discern on MRI, since it may appear as low signal, similar to the silicone implants.

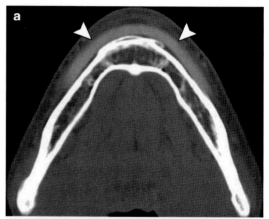

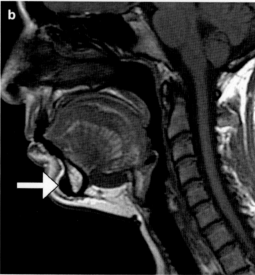

Fig. 1.40 Chin augmentation with silicone implant. Axial CT (**a**) shows a crescent-shaped slightly hyperattenuating implant anterior to the body of the mandible (*arrowheads*). The implant (*arrow*) appears hypointense on the sagittal T1-weighted MRI (**b**)

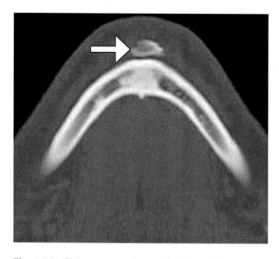

Fig. 1.39 Chin augmentation with "button" bone graft. Axial CT image demonstrates a bone graft anterior to the mandibular symphysis (*arrow*)

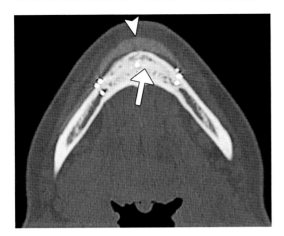

Fig. 1.41 Combined bone and silicone chin implant. Axial CT shows a crescent-shaped bone graft (*arrow*) fused to the mandible. The silicone implant (*arrowhead*) is positioned superficial to the bone graft

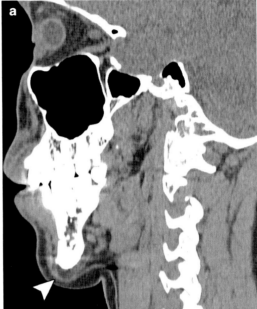

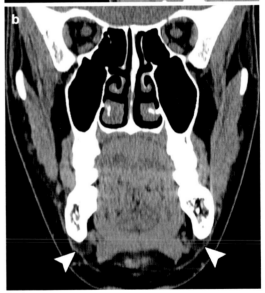

Fig. 1.42 Chin and prejowl porous polyethylene implant. Sagittal (**a**) and coronal (**b**) CT images show implants along the inferior edges of the mandibular body (*arrowheads*). The implants have attenuation intermediate between fat and fluid

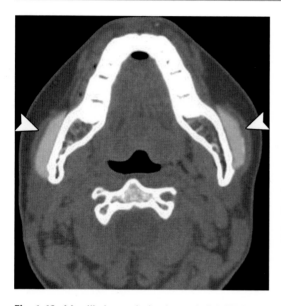

Fig. 1.43 Mandibular angle implants. Axial CT image demonstrates bilateral silicone implants deep to the masseter muscles (*arrowheads*)

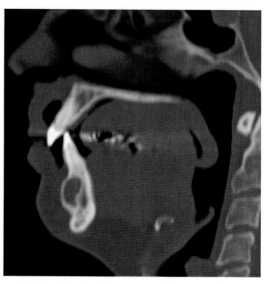

Fig. 1.45 Chin implant bone erosion. Sagittal CT image shows the silicone implant has receded into a smooth defect in the body of the mandible, resulting in diminished cosmetic effect and impingement upon the roots of the teeth

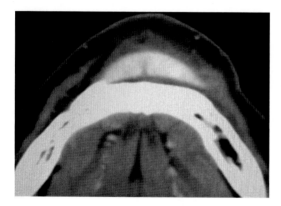

Fig. 1.44 Chin implant seroma. Axial CT image shows fluid surrounding the silicone implant resulting in altered cosmetic effect

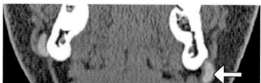

Fig. 1.46 Prejowl implant migration. Coronal CT image shows inferior displacement of the left side of the implant (*arrow*)

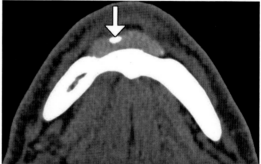

Fig. 1.47 New bone formation. Axial CT image shows hyperattenuating material (*arrow*) superficial to the cleft chin implant along the expected course of the periosteum

Further Reading

Overview of Facial Cosmetic Materials and Their Imaging Features

Chisholm BB (2005) Facial implants: facial augmentation and volume restoration. Oral Maxillofac Surg Clin North Am 17(1):77–84, vi

Lahiri A, Waters R (2007) Experience with Bio-alcamid, a new soft tissue endoprosthesis. J Plast Reconstr Aesthet Surg 60(6):663–667

Schatz CJ, Ginat DT (2013) Imaging of cosmetic facial implants and grafts. AJNR Am J Neuroradiol 34(9):1674–1681

Forehead Augmentation

Maas CS (2006) Botulinum neurotoxins and injectable fillers: minimally invasive management of the aging upper face. Facial Plast Surg Clin North Am 14(3): 241–245

Ousterhout DK, Zlotolow IM (1990) Aesthetic improvement of the forehead utilizing methyl methacrylate onlay implants. Aesthetic Plast Surg 14(4):281–285

Wong JK (2010) Forehead augmentation with alloplastic implants. Facial Plast Surg Clin North Am 18(1): 71–77

Cheek and Nasolabial Fold Augmentation

Constantinides MS, Galli SK, Miller PJ, Adamson PA (2000) Malar, submalar, and midfacial implants. Facial Plast Surg 16(1):35–44

Garner JM, Jordan JR (2008) An unusual complication of malar augmentation. J Plast Reconstr Aesthet Surg 61(4):428–430

Ginat DT, Schatz CJ (2013) Imaging of silastic cheek implant penetration into the maxillary sinus. JAMA Otolaryngol Head Neck Surg 139(2):199–201

Hönig J (2008) Cheek augmentation with Bio-alcamid in facial lipoatrophy in HIV seropositive patients. J Craniofac Surg 19(4):1085–1088

Rhinoplasty

Berghaus A, Stelter K (2006) Alloplastic materials in rhinoplasty. Curr Opin Otolaryngol Head Neck Surg 14(4):270–277

Constantian MB, Clardy RB (1996) The relative importance of septal and nasal valvular surgery in correcting airway obstruction in primary and secondary rhinoplasty. Plast Reconstr Surg 98(1):38–54; discussion 55–58

Fischer H, Gubisch W (2006) Nasal valves–importance and surgical procedures. Facial Plast Surg 22(4):266–280

Gryskiewicz JM, Hatef DA, Bullocks JM, Stal S (2010) Problems in rhinoplasty. Clin Plast Surg 37(2): 389–399

Safian LS (1984) Cosmetic rhinoplasty: radiological features. Head Neck Surg 7(2):139–149

Schatz CJ, Ginat DT (2014) Imaging features of rhinoplasty. AJNR Am J Neuroradiol 35(2):216–222

Lip Augmentation

Ousterhout DK, Zlotolow IM (1990) Aesthetic improvement of the forehead utilizing methyl methacrylate onlay implants. Aesthetic Plast Surg 14(4):281–285

Sarnoff DS, Saini R, Gotkin RH (2008) Comparison of filling agents for lip augmentation. Aesthet Surg J 28(5):556–563

Segall L, Ellis DA (2007) Therapeutic options for lip augmentation. Facial Plast Surg Clin North Am 15(4):485–490, vii

Wong JK (2010) Forehead augmentation with alloplastic implants. Facial Plast Surg Clin North Am 18(1): 71–77

Jaw Augmentation

Bastidas N, Zide BM (2010) The treachery of mandibular angle augmentation. Ann Plast Surg 64(1):4–6

Choe KS, Stucki-McCormick SU (2000) Chin augmentation. Facial Plast Surg 16(1):45–54

Godin M, Costa L, Romo T, Truswell W, Wang T, Williams E (2003) Gore-Tex chin implants: a review of 324 cases. Arch Facial Plast Surg 5(3):224–227

Ousterhout DK (1991) Mandibular angle augmentation and reduction. Clin Plast Surg 18(1):153–161

Romo T 3rd, Baskin JZ, Sclafani AP (2001) Augmentation of the cheeks, chin and pre-jowl sulcus, and nasolabial folds. Facial Plast Surg 17(1):67–78

Semergidis TG, Migliore SA, Sotereanos GC (1996) Alloplastic augmentation of the mandibular angle. J Oral Maxillofac Surg 54(12): 1417–1423

Imaging the Postoperative Orbit

Daniel Thomas Ginat, Gul Moonis, and Suzanne K. Freitag

2.1 Eyelid Weights

2.1.1 Discussion

Facial nerve deficits can lead to keratitis secondary to lagophthalmos and decreased lacrimal gland secretions. Implantable platinum and gold weights are available in various sizes and shapes, including thin profile. Eyelid weights are placed deep to the orbicularis oculi muscle and sutured to the tarsus in the upper eyelid, enabling more complete eyelid closure (Fig. 2.1). The implants generally produce considerable metal streak artifact on CT. Gold and platinum eyelid weights are considered MRI compatible. Complications related to eyelid weight implantation include infection, allergic reaction, migration, and extrusion. Closure of the orbicularis oculi muscle over the implant reduces the risk of extrusion.

D.T. Ginat, M.D., M.S. (✉)
Department of Radiology, University of Chicago,
Pritzker School of Medicine, Chicago, IL, USA
e-mail: dtg1@uchicago.edu

G. Moonis, M.D
Department of Radiology, Columbia Presbyterian,
New York, NY, USA

S.K. Freitag, M.D.
Department of Ophthalmology, Massachusetts Eye
and Ear Infirmary, Harvard Medical School, Boston,
MA, USA

© Springer International Publishing Switzerland 2017
D.T. Ginat, P.-L.A. Westesson (eds.), *Atlas of Postsurgical Neuroradiology*,
DOI 10.1007/978-3-319-52341-5_2

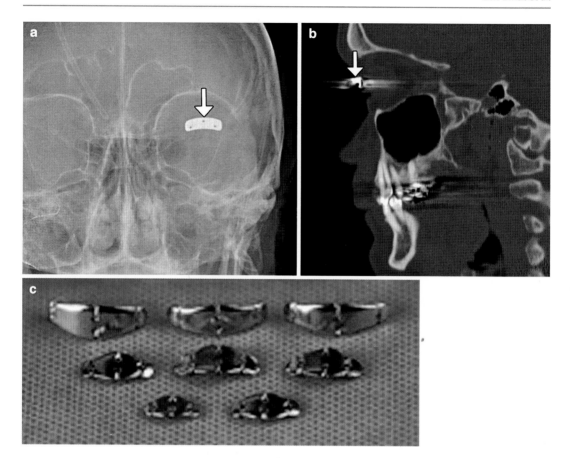

Fig. 2.1 Eyelid weight. The patient has a history of left cranial nerve VII palsy. Frontal radiograph (**a**) shows a left eyelid weight containing three suture holes (*arrows*). Sagittal CT image (**b**) shows a left upper eyelid weight (*arrows*), which produces extensive streak artifact. Photograph of various sizes of gold eyelid weight implants (**c**) (Courtesy of Osmed)

2.2   Palpebral Springs

2.2.1   Discussion

Palpebral springs may rarely be
used to treat patients with lagophthalmos secondary to facial nerve palsy. The device is implanted
via orbitotomy and consists of a palpebral branch
and an orbital branch connected by a spring
mechanism. The positioning and function of the
device can be readily assessed on radiographs
obtained in the open and closed lid positions,
whereby the palpebral branch is expected to
descend with lid closure (Fig. 2.2).

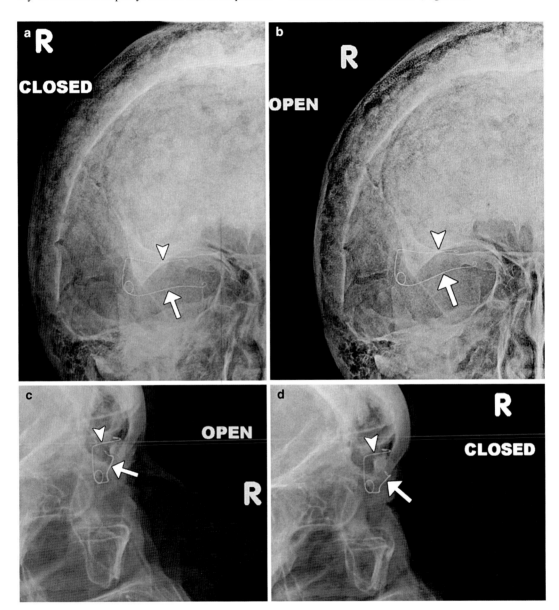

Fig. 2.2 Eyelid spring. Open (**a**) and closed (**b**) lid frontal
and open (**c**) and closed (**d**) lid lateral radiographs show
the spring device to be well seated and functional. The
palpebral branch (*arrows*) is noted to descend with respect
to the orbital branch (*arrowheads*) during lid closure.
There are also stigmata of Paget's disease in the skull.
Axial CT images (**e, f**) in a different patient show the
lower limb (*arrow*) of the spring properly positioned
along the inner surface of the upper eyelid and the upper
limb (*arrowhead*) implanted in the orbital roof

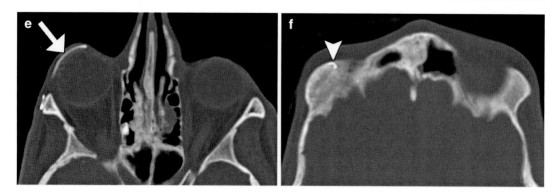

Fig. 2.2 (continued)

2.3   Frontalis Suspension Ptosis Repair

2.3.1   Discussion

Frontalis suspension may be used to elevate severely drooping eyelids in cases where the levator palpebrae superioris muscle is weak. In this procedure, autologous or alloplastic material is used to create a subcutaneous attachment between the eyelid and the frontalis muscle. Expanded polytetrafluoroethylene (ePTFE) strips are visible on CT as hyperattenuating material configured as a sling in the upper eyelid (Fig. 2.3) in order to suspend the eyelid to the frontalis muscle. Potential complications include infection and granuloma formation.

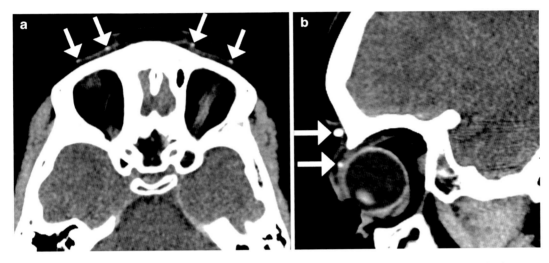

Fig 2.3 Frontalis suspension ptosis repair. The patient is a child with a history of bilateral ptosis due to Marcus Gunn jaw-winking syndrome. Axial (**a**) and sagittal (**b**) CT images show the hyperattenuating sling in the upper eyelids (*arrows*)

2.4 Orbital Wall Reconstruction and Augmentation

2.4.1 Discussion

Traditionally, autologous cartilage or bone (Fig. 2.4), silicone sheet implants (Fig. 2.5), and metal plates or mesh (Fig. 2.6) have been used for orbital wall fracture repair. More recent implant technology, including porous polyethylene materials (Fig. 2.7), has resulted in improved biocompatibility. The porous structure enables rapid ingrowth of vascular structures, soft tissues, and bone. Furthermore, endoscopic transantral approaches are increasingly used in order to avoid eyelid incisions. Wedge implants can be used to augment orbital volume in patients with enophthalmos (Fig. 2.8). Transnasal wires can also be inserted to stabilize the medial canthus in trauma patients (Fig. 2.9). The role of imaging after orbital fracture repair is mainly to asses for complications, which may include infection, hematic cyst formation, implant deformity, and malpositioning, which may be accompanied by mucocele or nasolacrimal duct cyst formation due to obstruction and cerebrospinal fluid (Figs. 2.10, 2.11, 2.12, 2.13, 2.14, 2.15, 2.16, and 2.17). The leaks can be associated with compression of orbital contents, but can resolve spontaneously.

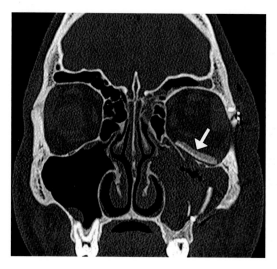

Fig. 2.4 Bone graft. Coronal CT image shows graft (*arrow*) harvested from the iliac bone used to reconstruct the left orbital floor (Courtesy of Gregory Katzman MD, MBA)

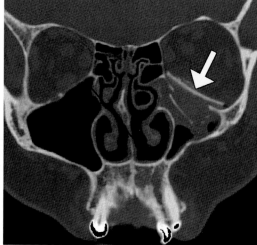

Fig. 2.5 Silicone implant. Coronal CT image shows left orbital floor fracture reconstruction with silicone implant (*arrow*)

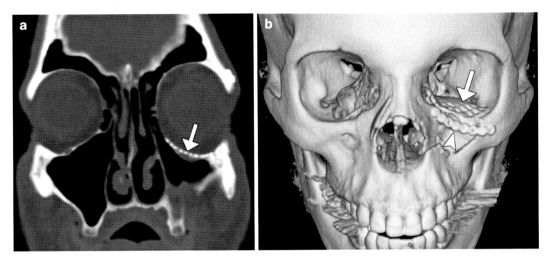

Fig. 2.6 Titanium mesh. Coronal (**a**) and 3D CT (**b**) images show left orbital floor fracture repair with titanium mesh (*arrow*) and inferior orbital rim fracture with malleable titanium plate (*arrowhead*)

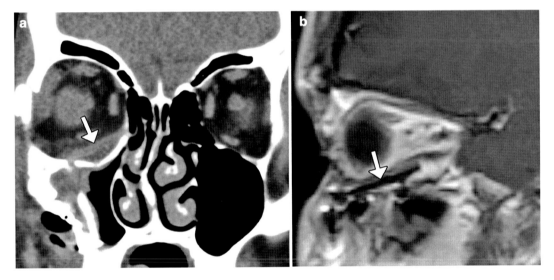

Fig. 2.7 Porous polyethylene implant. Coronal CT image (**a**) shows the intermediate-attenuation sheet implant (*arrow*) positioned along the right orbital floor beneath the inferior rectus muscle. The implant (*arrow*) appears as low signal intensity on the sagittal T1-weighted MRI (**b**)

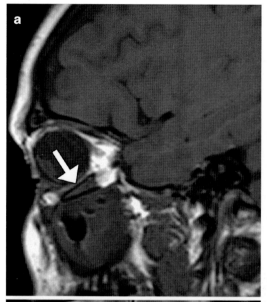

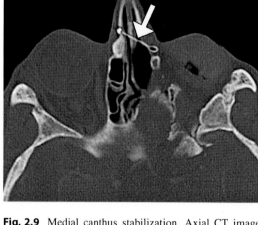

Fig. 2.9 Medial canthus stabilization. Axial CT image shows numerous healed left orbital fractures that involved the medial canthus, which is secured by a transnasal metal wire (*arrow*)

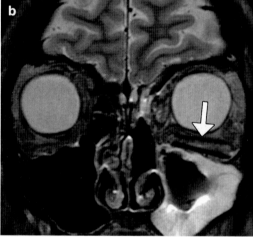

Fig. 2.8 Wedge implants. Sagittal T1-weighted (**a**) and coronal T2-weighted (**b**) MR images show the two low-intensity nearly parallel lines of the implant in the floor of the left orbit (*arrows*)

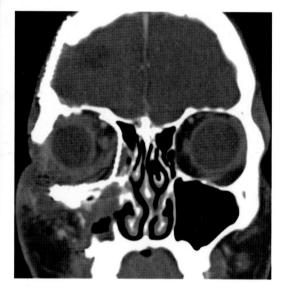

Fig. 2.10 Infection. Coronal post-contrast CT image shows diffuse right pre- and postseptal orbital cellulitis following recent medial and inferior orbital floor fracture repair with titanium mesh

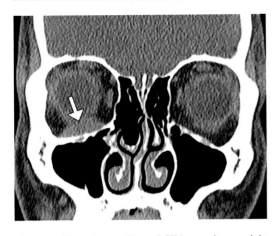

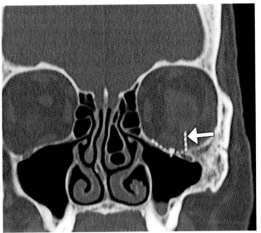

Fig. 2.11 Hematic cyst. Coronal CT image shows a right inferior intraorbital lenticular-shaped fluid collection (*arrow*) along the surface of a silastic plate

Fig. 2.12 Mesh deformity. Coronal CT image shows deformity of the orbital floor titanium mesh implant (*arrow*)

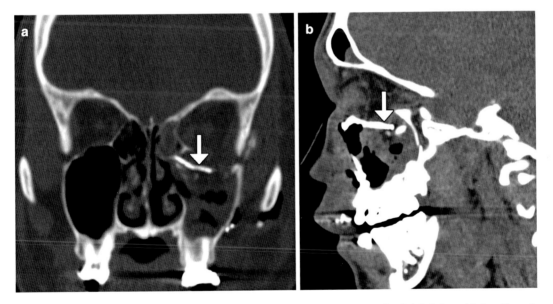

Fig. 2.13 Inferiorly positioned mesh. The patient presented with enophthalmos after left inferior orbital wall repair with titanium mesh. Coronal (**a**) and sagittal (**b**) CT images show inferior displacement of the left orbital mesh (*arrows*)

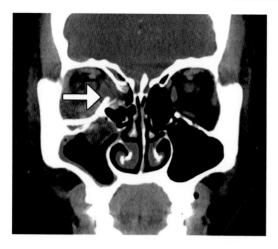

Fig. 2.14 Rectus muscle impingement. Coronal CT image shows lateral right medial orbital wall titanium mesh impinging upon the swollen medial rectus muscle (*arrow*). There is also persistent herniation of right orbital contents

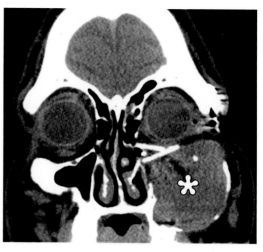

Fig. 2.16 Mucocele secondary to malpositioned implants. Coronal CT image shows an expansile left maxillary opacity (*) and obstruction of the infundibulum by the orbital floor reconstruction plates

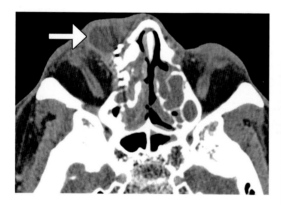

Fig. 2.15 Nasolacrimal duct obstruction. Axial CT image shows dilation of the right lacrimal sac (*arrow*) secondary to obstruction by titanium mesh

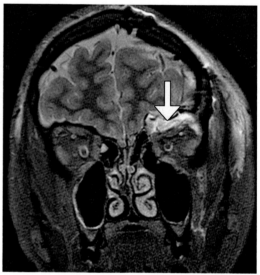

Fig. 2.17 Cerebrospinal fluid leak. The patient underwent biopsy of a suspect orbital roof lesion with mesh reconstruction of the orbital roof. Coronal STIR MR image shows a fluid collection in the superior left orbit (*arrow*), with compression of the orbital contents

2.5   Orbital Decompression and Expansion for Dysthyroid Orbitopathy

2.5.1   Discussion

Orbital decompression for dysthyroid orbitopathy serves to reduce proptosis and intraocular pressure and improve compressive optic neuropathy. Bone from the medial, lateral, or inferior orbital walls may be removed via a variety of endonasal or external approaches (Fig. 2.18). The enlarged orbital fat and rectus muscles can then bulge through these defects, resulting in a decrease in intraorbital pressure. A transnasal endoscopic approach is commonly implemented for inferior and medial wall decompression. As a result, resection of a portion of the paranasal sinuses may also be observed on follow-up imaging. Serious complications related to orbital decompression occur in 3–5% of cases depending on the particular technique and include chronic sinusitis, meningitis, optic neuropathy, orbital cellulitis, hemorrhage, nasolacrimal duct obstruction, and inadequate proptosis reduction. In addition, excess herniation of orbital contents through the surgical defects can result in obstructed paranasal sinus secretions (Fig. 2.19). Diplopia from displacement of orbital contents, including the extraocular muscles occurs in up to 25% of patients.

Another option for treating exophthalmos in patients with dysthyroid orbitopathy is to expand the orbital vault anteriorly, which can be accomplished using augmentation implants attached to the orbital rim (Fig. 2.20).

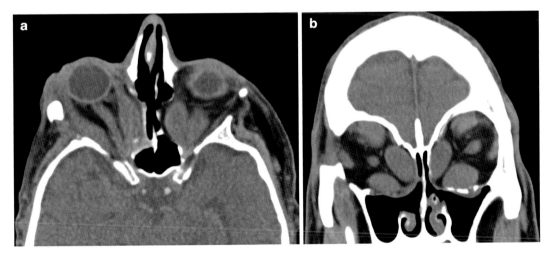

Fig. 2.18   Medial and lateral orbital wall decompression. Axial (**a**) and coronal (**b**) CT images show surgical defects in the bilateral medial, inferior, and lateral bony orbital walls. Note the enlarged rectus muscles

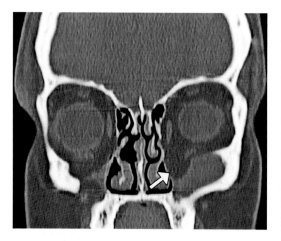

Fig. 2.19 Paranasal sinus obstruction after orbital decompression. The patient presents with left sinus pressure after orbital decompression for dysthyroid orbitopathy. Coronal CT image shows obstructed left maxillary sinus secretions secondary to obstruction by inferior extension of the orbital fat (*arrow*) through the surgical defect

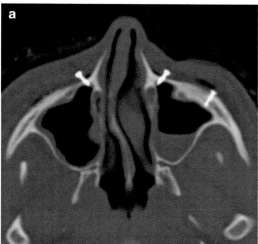

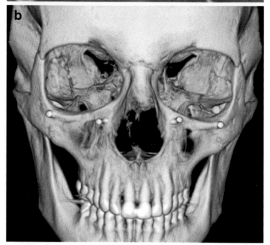

Fig. 2.20 Orbital rim augmentation. Axial (**a**) and 3D (**b**) CT images in a patient with dysthyroid orbitopathy show that hardware below the bilateral inferior orbital rims was used to secure a porous polyethylene implant (not visible on these images)

2.6   Dacryocystorhinostomy and Nasolacrimal Duct Stents

2.6.1   Discussion

Dacryocystorhinostomy (DCR) can be performed to relieve distal lacrimal obstruction at the level of the lacrimal sac or duct. Both external and endonasal approaches can be used to remove bone in the region of the medial canthus in order to create a fistula between the nasolacrimal sac and the medial meatus of the nasal cavity. Silicone tubes are usually temporarily inserted through this fistula to ensure prolonged patency. Postoperative complications occur in about 6% of cases and most commonly include restenosis with recurrent epiphora or dacryocystitis. Patency of the dacryocystorhinostomy can be evaluated via a dacryocystogram (Fig. 2.21). Surgical success rates are high with reports mostly ranging in the 90% and above.

In cases of proximal lacrimal stenosis involving the canaliculi, conjunctivodacryocystorhinostomy (CDCR) can be performed. This procedure involves the placement of a Jones tube, which is a direct bypass from the ocular surface to the middle meatus of the nose (Fig. 2.22). These Pyrex glass tubes are readily depicted on CT, which can be used effectively to assess for complications, such as malposition, migration, or inflammation of surrounding tissues. An uncommon complication of Jones tube placement is pneumo-orbit, which can occur after CPAP use, sneezing, or nose blowing, and can result in proptosis if a significant amount of air is forced through the tube (Fig. 2.23).

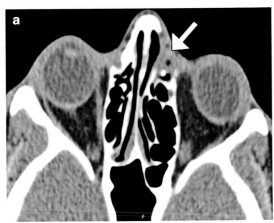
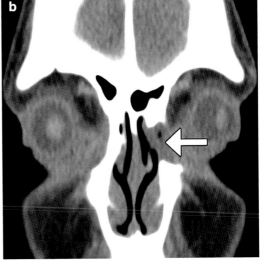

Fig. 2.21 Dacryocystorhinostomy. Axial (**a**) and coronal (**b**) CT images show an osteotomy predominantly through the anterior lacrimal crest of the left maxilla (*arrows*) after external dacryocystorhinostomy. Radiograph (**c**) and axial CT (**d**) images from a left dacryocystogram verify free spillage of contrast into the ethmoid air cells/nasal cavity (*arrowheads*)

0

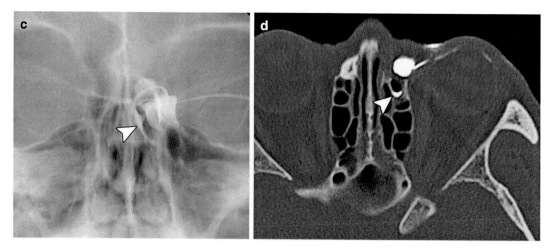

Fig. 2.21 (continued)

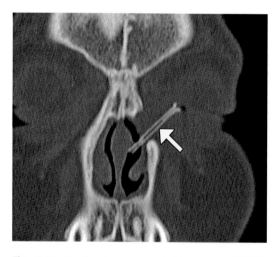

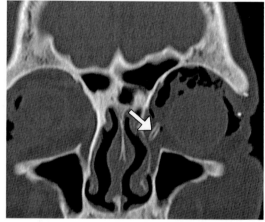

Fig. 2.22 Conjunctivodacryocystorhinostomy (CDCR) with Jones tube. Coronal CT image shows a left CDCR with a Pyrex glass Jones tube in position (*arrow*). The tube connects the ocular surface with the middle meatus of the nose. In this case, it is somewhat medially displaced

Fig. 2.23 Pneumo-orbit with Jones tube. The patient had a history of CDCR with Jones tube placement and presented with proptosis after sneezing. Coronal CT image shows a Jones tube (*arrow*) and extensive air within the left orbit

2.7   Strabismus Surgery

2.7.1   Discussion

Strabismus secondary to cranial nerve palsy can be treated by rectus muscle transposition. Several techniques can be performed, including repositioning portions of the rectus muscle bellies onto the sclera, with or without tenotomy (Fig. 2.24).

The effects of rectus transposition can be appreciated on imaging, including changes in size as morphology of the rectus muscles and signal alterations on MRI. Although improved ocular alignment can also be noted on imaging, this is readily assessed on clinical exam. Nevertheless, imaging can be useful for evaluating postoperative complications, such as rectus muscle rupture (Fig. 2.25) and infection (Fig. 2.26).

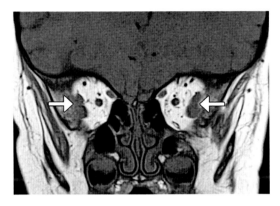

Fig. 2.24 Y splitting of the lateral rectus with medial transposition. Coronal T1-weighted MR image shows splitting and thickening of the bilateral lateral rectus muscle bellies (*arrows*)

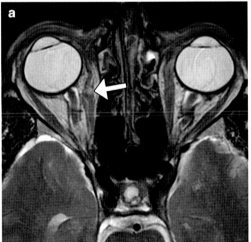
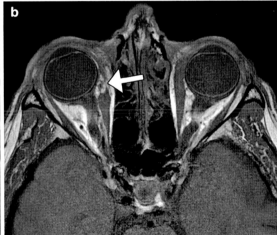

Fig. 2.25 Postoperative rectus muscle rupture. The patient presented with recurrent right exotropia after bilateral medial rectus resections. The right medial rectus muscle was noted to be friable intraoperatively. Axial T2-weighted (**a**) and T1-weighted (**b**) MR images show an abrupt caliber change and signal abnormality in the belly of the right medial rectus muscle (*arrow*). The distal portion of the right medial rectus is lax, and there is lateral rotation of the globe. Bilateral lens implants are also present

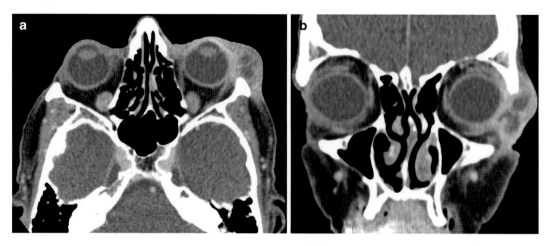

Fig. 2.26 Postoperative abscess. The patient presented with edema and erythema around the left eye after strabismus surgery. Axial (**a**) and coronal (**b**) CT images show a left periorbital rim-enhancing fluid collection

2.8   Glaucoma Surgery

2.8.1   Discussion

Glaucoma shunts and valves are surgically implanted devices that reduce intraocular pressure by decompression of aqueous humor. Several types of implants are commercially available, including the Ahmed, Baerveldt, Krupin, and Molteno. The Molteno and Baerveldt devices are non-valved devices (Fig. 2.27), while the Krupin and Ahmed devices include valves (Fig. 2.28). The basic design of a valved shunt consists of a tube drain, valve, and footplate (Fig. 2.29). The one-way valve closes below a certain intraocular pressure, thereby preventing hypotonia of the globe. End plates with larger surface area have greater ability to dissipate the aqueous humor. The devices are usually implanted superotemporal to the globe, with end plate positioned against the scleral surface and the fine tube drain inserted into the anterior chamber. However, the device can also function in the inferotemporal or superomedial quadrant and can drain into the paranasal sinuses (Fig. 2.30). A fibrous capsule forms around the end plate, eventually forming a reservoir or bleb. The fluid is normally resorbed by the surrounding tissues, such that there is no significant accumulation. Glaucoma valve shunts often contain radiopaque barium-impregnated silicone. Alternatively, these devices can be composed of polypropylene, which is of intermediate attenuation on CT. Glaucoma valve implants are MRI compatible and appear as low signal on both T1- and T2-weighted sequences surrounded by a small amount of fluid in the reservoir. Complications include hypotonia, malposition, tube obstruction, and giant bleb formation (Fig. 2.31), secondary to adhesions between Tenon's capsule and the episcleral space, infection (Fig. 2.32), and choroidal detachment (Fig. 2.33). Newer non-tube implants, such as the Ex-PRESS shunt, do not require iridotomy and result in less postoperative inflammation. The Ex-PRESS shunt is a non-valved stainless steel implant that is inserted under a scleral flap in a paralimbal site (Fig. 2.34).

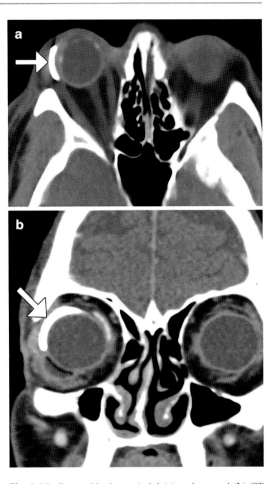

Fig. 2.27   Baerveldt shunt. Axial (**a**) and coronal (**b**) CT images demonstrate the hyperattenuating device (*arrows*) positioned superolateral to the globe. Several radiolucent Ahmed valves are also present within the bilateral orbits

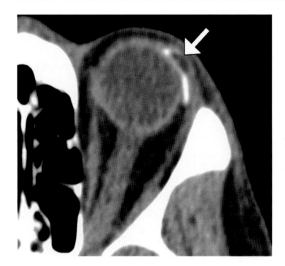

Fig. 2.28 Ahmed valve. Axial CT image shows the valved device (*arrow*) positioned alongside the left globe

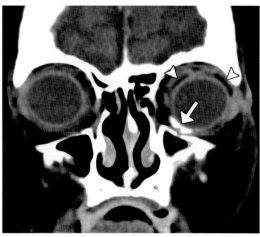

Fig. 2.30 Glaucoma valve drainage into maxillary sinus. Coronal CT image shows a radiopaque Ahmed valve positioned inferior to the left globe (*arrow*), where it drains into the maxillary sinus. There are also superolateral and superomedial radiolucent Ahmed valves (*arrowheads*)

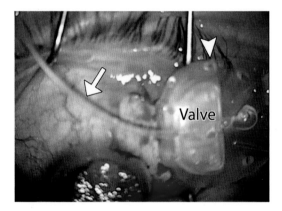

Fig. 2.29 Photo of a glaucoma valve device during surgery. The components include the valve on the footplate (*arrowhead*) and tube (*arrow*) (Courtesy of Fatoumata Yanoga MD)

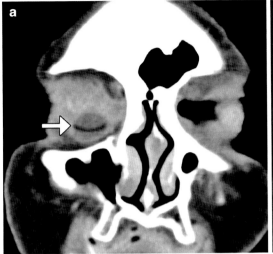

Fig. 2.31 Glaucoma tube shunt-related blebs. Coronal (**a**) CT image shows a large fluid collection (*arrow*) around the radiolucent inferolateral Ahmed valve. Coronal T2-weighted MRI (**b**) shows bilateral linear low-signal Ahmed valves surrounded by minimal fluid on the right and a larger amount fluid on the left (*arrow*), which indents the globe

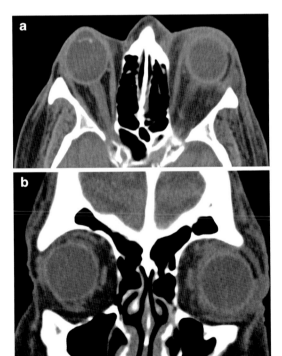

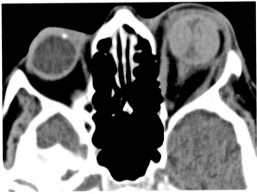

Fig. 2.33 Hemorrhagic suprachoroidal detachments following glaucoma valve implantation. Axial CT image shows a suprachoroidal hemorrhage within the left globe. A radiolucent Ahmed valve is present temporally and there is preseptal edema

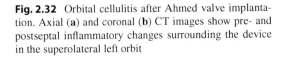

Fig. 2.32 Orbital cellulitis after Ahmed valve implantation. Axial (**a**) and coronal (**b**) CT images show pre- and postseptal inflammatory changes surrounding the device in the superolateral left orbit

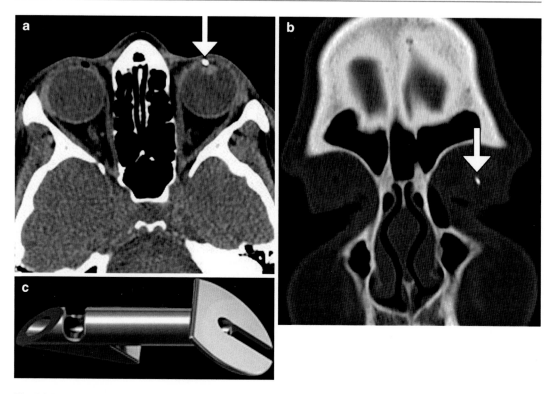

Fig. 2.34 Ex-PRESS glaucoma shunt. Axial (**a**) and coronal (**b**) CT images show a punctate metallic structure in the region of the anterior chamber of the left globe (*arrows*). Photograph of the device (**c**) (Courtesy of Alcon/Novartis)

2.9   Scleral Buckles

2.9.1   Discussion

Scleral buckles partly or completely encircle the globe for the treatment of retinal detachment. The buckles work by exerting pressure in order to appose the layers of the retina together. These devices are composed of either hydrophilic hydrogel polymers or silicone, which in turn are available in the form of solid rubber bands or sponges, or a combination of these (Figs. 2.35, 2.36, and 2.37). On CT, silicone rubber bands are of high density, while the sponges are nearly air attenuation. On MRI, the silicone scleral buckles are of low signal intensity on both T1- and T2-weighted sequences. Mild circumferential indentation of the globe is an expected finding. In the past, small clips composed of tantalum were used to secure the free ends of the buckles (Fig. 2.38). The tantalum clips are MRI compatible. Scleral buckles should not be confused with calcifications, hemorrhage, or masses. The main complication related to scleral buckle implanta-tion that may lead to diagnostic imaging is infec-tion, which can manifest as stranding and enhancement of the orbital fat surrounding the device and thickening of the sclera, with or with-out fluid collections from abscess formation (Fig. 2.39).

Although less stiff and prone to causing scleral erosion than silicone implants, hydrogel (Miragel) scleral buckles are permeable to water and there-fore can gradually swell over years or decades. On MRI, the fluid consistency of the hydrated implant is evident as high T2 signal and low T1 signal (Fig. 2.40). There may be rim enhancement, as a fibrous capsule often forms around these buckles. Dystrophic calcifications can appear as curvilinear or punctate densities along the edges of the implant. Thus, the imaging appearances of this process may mimic an orbital mass or infection. However, available past surgical history, the tubular configu-ration of the implant encircling the globe, and lack of restricted diffusion should lead to the proper diagnosis. Due to brittle nature of the hydrated hydrogel scleral buckles, they have a tendency to fragment and become displaced (Fig. 2.41).

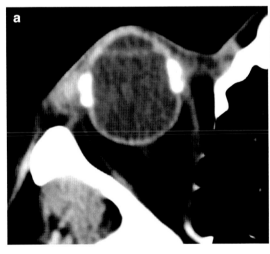
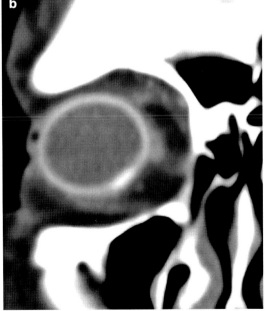

Fig. 2.35 Silicone rubber encircling buckle. Axial (**a**) and coronal (**b**) CT images show a high-attenuation band surrounding the right globe. The scleral band (*arrows*) is of very low signal intensity on MRI (**c**), with expected indentation of the globe

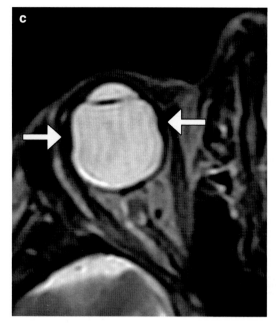

Fig. 2.35 (continued)

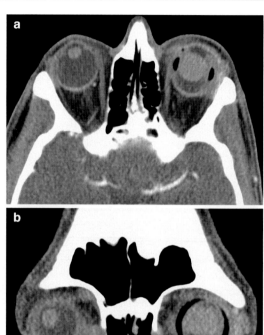

Fig. 2.36 Silicone sponge scleral buckle. Axial (**a**) and coronal (**b**) CT images show a low-attenuation sclera buckle surrounding the left globe. There is also silicone oil in the left globe

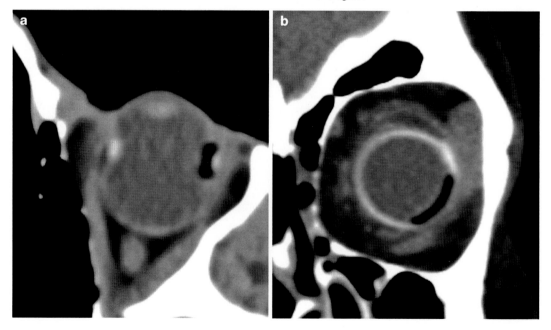

Fig. 2.37 Combined silicone rubber band and sponge. Axial (**a**) and coronal (**b**) CT images show hyperattenuating and hypoattenuating components of the left scleral buckle

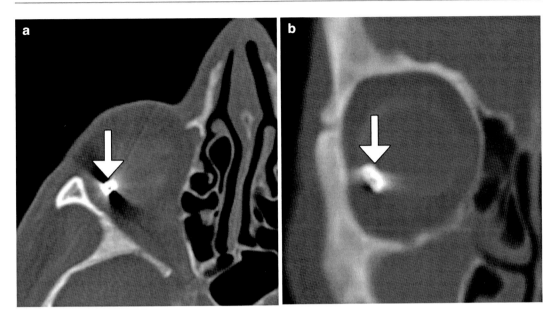

Fig. 2.38 Scleral buckle with tantalum clip. Axial (**a**) and coronal (**b**) CT images show a small metallic clip (*arrows*) adjacent to the globe

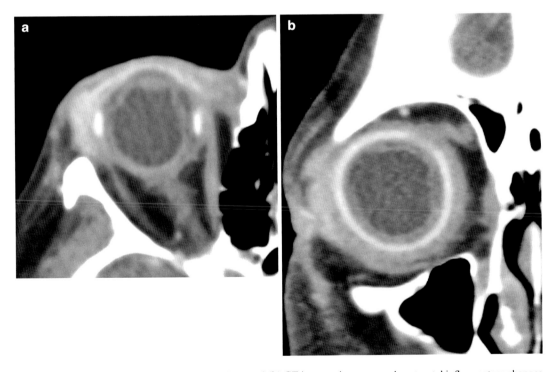

Fig. 2.39 Infected scleral buckle. Axial (**a**) and coronal (**b**) CT images show pre- and postseptal inflammatory changes of the right globe surrounding the scleral buckle. In addition, there is scleritis and a subchoroidal effusion

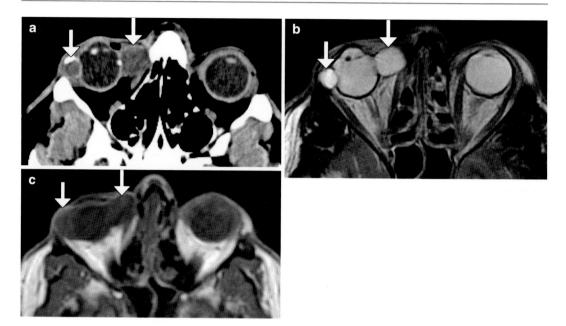

Fig. 2.40 Hydrogel scleral buckle hydration and expansion. Axial CT image (**a**) shows circumferential enlargement of the right hydrogel scleral buckle (*arrows*), which has fluid attenuation. There are also partial rim calcifications. Axial T2-weighted (**b**) and axial T1-weighted (**c**) MRI sequences show that the enlarged right scleral buckle contains fluid signal (*arrows*)

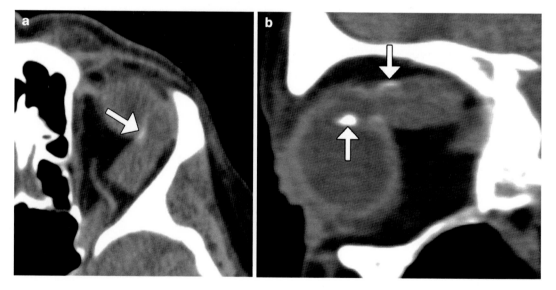

Fig. 2.41 Hydrogel scleral buckle hydration, fragmentation, and migration. Axial (**a**) and sagittal (**b**) CT images show that the unraveled, hydrated, and partially calcified scleral buckle (*arrows*) has migrated into the superotemporal quadrant of the left orbit, where it indents the globe

2.10   Keratoprostheses

2.10.1 Discussion

Keratoprostheses are artificial corneal substitution devices. The Boston keratoprostheses are perhaps the most commonly used and are available in two forms: the type I device is a collar button-shaped device composed of a polymethyl methacrylate (PMMA) front plate and its stem and a PMMA or titanium back plate, while the type II device has an additional anterior nub that allows for through-the-lid implantation (Fig. 2.42). The devices are considered MRI compatible. Complications that can be observed on CT or MRI include inclusion cyst formation and vitreous hemorrhage.

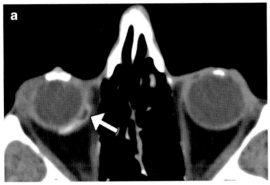
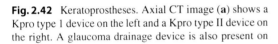
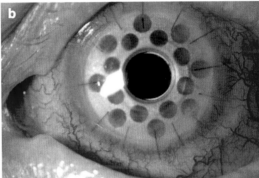

Fig. 2.42 Keratoprostheses. Axial CT image (**a**) shows a Kpro type I device on the left and a Kpro type II device on the right. A glaucoma drainage device is also present on the right side (*arrow*). Photograph of a Kpro device in situ (**b**) (Courtesy of Kathryn Colby MD)

2.11 Intraocular Lens Implants

2.11.1 Discussion

Cataract is a common cause of reversible vision loss and can be treated via cataract extraction and intraocular lens implantation when symptomatic. Intraocular lens implants consist of two main components: the optic and two haptics. These lens implants can be composed of polymethylmethacrylate, silicone, hydrogel, polyethylene, polypropylene, or a combination of these. The lens implants may be positioned posterior or anterior with respect to the plane of the iris. Unlike native lenses, lens prostheses are very thin structures in profile, as seen on an axial image. The optic appears as hyperattenuating on CT and is of low signal intensity on both T1- and T2-weighted MRI sequences (Fig. 2.43). The haptics are not readily visible at 1.5 T or on thin-section CT. Intraocular lens implants do not normally enhance. Complications of cataract surgery with intraocular lens implants include retained lens fragments, implant dislocation, and less commonly dystrophic calcifications. Implant dislocation can result from inadequate capsular or zonular support or following traumatic injury. While some of these complications may be apparent on CT and MRI (Figs. 2.44 and 2.45), ophthalmic ultrasound is generally the modality of choice, but is beyond the scope of this text.

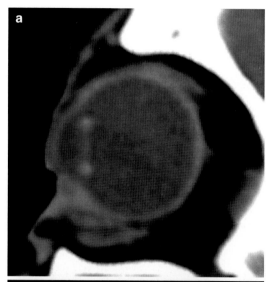

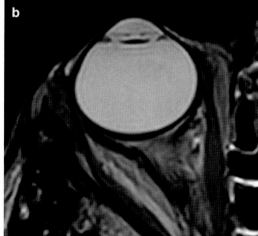

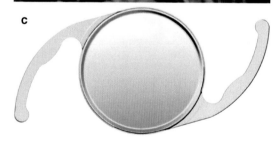

Fig. 2.43 Posterior chamber intraocular lens (IOL) implant following cataract surgery. Sagittal CT (**a**) and T2-weighted MRI (**b**) show a left posterior chamber intraocular lens Photograph of a standard IOL implant (**c**) (Courtesy of Hoopes Vision)

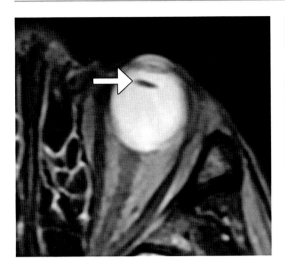

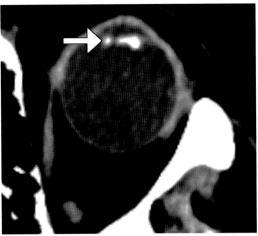

Fig. 2.44 Intraocular lens implant dislocation. Axial T2 MRI shows the posteriorly displaced left lens implant (*arrow*)

Fig. 2.45 Intraocular lens implant dystrophic calcification. Axial CT image shows irregular clumps of calcification deposited on the surface of the left lens implant (*arrow*)

2.12   Surgical Aphakia

2.12.1 Discussion

Historically, cataract surgery was initially performed without placement of an intraocular lens implant. In the modern era, utilizing small incision cataract surgery, a variety of implantable lenses are in common use. However, in certain situations, the implantation of an intraocular lens after cataract surgery is still not undertaken. For example, the placement of intraocular lenses in very small children has been controversial over the years, and some children are left aphakic after surgery. On imaging, there is no apparent separation between the anterior and posterior chambers of the globe (Fig. 2.46).

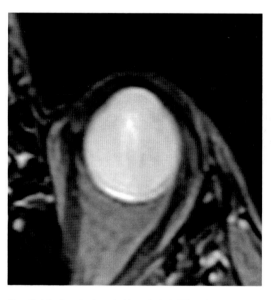

Fig. 2.46 Surgical aphakia. Axial T2-weighted MRI shows absence of the left lens

2.13   Pneumatic Retinopexy

2.13.1 Discussion

Intraocular gas injection is a technique used to tamponade the retina during retinal detachment surgery until chorioretinal adhesions form (pneumatic retinopexy). The procedure is effective for treating retinal detachment in up to 80% of cases. Intraocular gas injection can also be used to restore intraocular volume during scleral buckle surgery. A variety of gases can be used, including air, sulfur hexafluoride, and perfluoropropane. On CT, air lucency is present antidependently in the vitreous body, creating an air-fluid level (Fig. 2.47). Complications of intraocular air injection include secondary glaucoma, subretinal gas or anterior chamber migration, vitreous hemorrhage, new retinal breaks, endophthalmitis, and delayed reabsorption of subretinal fluid.

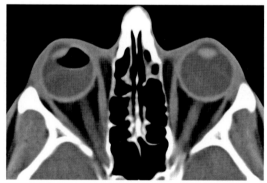

Fig. 2.47 Pneumatic retinopexy. Axial CT image demonstrates intravitreal gas on the right side

2.14   Intraocular Silicone Oil

2.14.1 Discussion

Intravitreal silicone oil placement is sometimes used in cases of intractable retinal detachment. The silicone oil is visible on CT and MR imaging (Fig. 2.48). On CT, silicone oil is hyperattenuating, measuring up to 120 HU, but floats. On MRI, silicone oil tends to be hyperintense to water on T1-weighted sequences and hypointense to water on T2-weighted sequences. Chemical shift artifact at the interface between the silicone oil and fluid can be used to distinguish the two entities.

Fat saturation pulses can also cause some degree of signal suppression, also differentiating it from hemorrhage. The silicone oil used for tamponade is often surgically removed after placement, but may remain permanently, depending on the risk of recurrent detachment. Complications of silicone oil retinopexy include choroidal detachment, retinal re-detachment, glaucoma, migration to the anterior chamber with corneal endothelial damage, and cataract formation. In very rare instances, intracranial migration of silicone oil can occur via the optic nerve and into the ventricular system via the subarachnoid space in optic nerve sheath (Fig. 2.49).

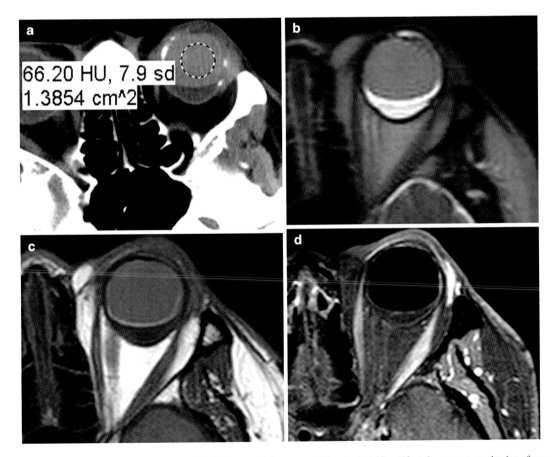

Fig. 2.48 Intraocular silicone oil. Axial CT image (**a**) shows globular high-attenuation material floating within the posterior chamber of the left globe. T2-weighted MRI (**b**) and T1-weighted MRI (**c**) showing the intraocular sili-cone. Chemical shift artifact is present at the interface between the silicone and the vitreous and loses signal with fat suppression (**d**)

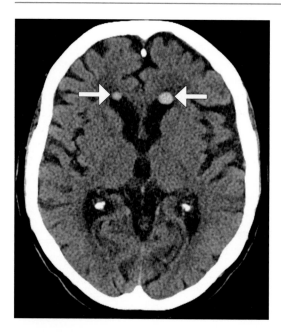

Fig. 2.49 Intraventricular silicone oil migration. Axial CT image shows the hyperattenuating silicone oil floating within the bilateral frontal horns of the lateral ventricles (*arrows*) (Courtesy of Bruno Policeni MD)

2.15   Evisceration, Enucleation, and Globe Prostheses

2.15.1   Discussion

Evisceration consists of removing the globe contents while preserving the sclera and extraocular muscles, while enucleation consists of removing the globe entirely along with the anterior portion of the optic nerve. These procedures are mainly performed for intraocular malignancies and irreparable globe rupture. Following enucleation, globe implants are often used to provide orbital volume and cosmetic effect. Although a wide variety of globe implant designs are available, the typical globe implant has two components: a deep spherical orbital implant, which can be placed within the remaining sclera, and an anterior scleral cover shell prosthesis, somewhat analogous to a large contact lens in terms of shape and location. In the past, a wide variety of metallic implants were used in globe prostheses,

including hollow glass spheres (Fig. 2.50). Currently, hydroxyapatite, solid silicone, and porous polyethylene prostheses are most commonly used. These prostheses have distinct features on imaging (Figs. 2.51, 2.52, and 2.53). Diffuse linear enhancement surrounding the implant components is frequently present on MRI and is of no clinical significance. Occasionally, the scleral cover shell prosthesis is used alone if orbital volume is adequate (Fig. 2.54). Since the orbital implant volumes are virtually always smaller than the normal globe, various materials have been used as support materials for the orbital prosthesis, including silicone blocks and glass beads (Figs. 2.55 and 2.56), and are generally located in the extraconal space. Complications related to orbital implants are uncommon, but include rotation, infection, inflammation, and exposure (Figs. 2.57 and 2.58). Imaging is complimentary to physical examination for evaluating some of these complications.

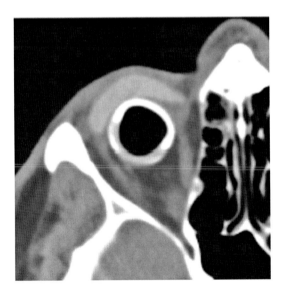

Fig. 2.50 Hollow glass globe implant. Axial CT image (**a**) shows an air-filled right orbital implant

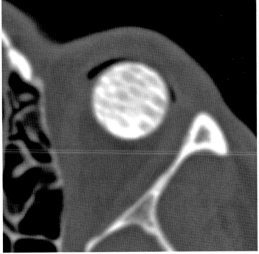

Fig. 2.51 Hydroxyapatite implant. Axial CT image shows a hyperattenuating left globe implant with a characteristic cobblestone pattern

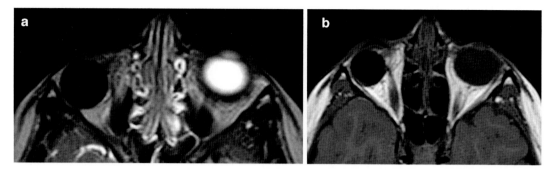

Fig. 2.52 Silicone implant. Axial T2-weighted (**a**) and T1-weighted (**b**) MR images show a markedly hypointense implant in the right orbit

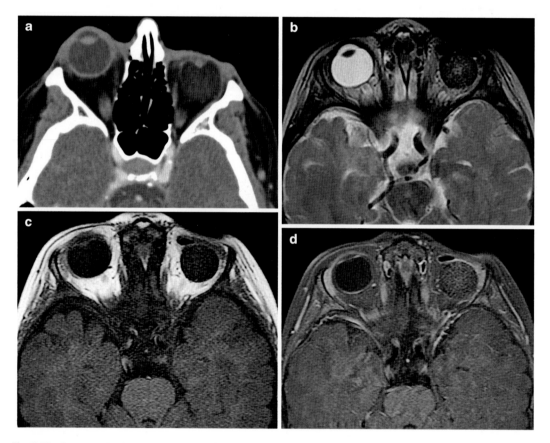

Fig. 2.53 Porous polyethylene implant. Axial CT image (**a**) shows that the left globe implant has a density between that of fluid and fat. Axial T2-weighted (**b**), T1-weighted (**c**), and post-contrast T1-weighted (**d**) MR images in a different patient show that the left globe implant has relatively low T1 and T2 signal, but enhances due to fibrovascular ingrowth

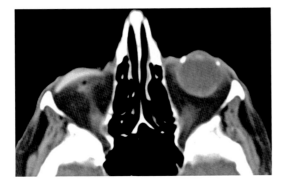

Fig. 2.54 Scleral cover shell prosthesis. Axial CT image shows a right scleral cover shell prosthesis used without orbital augmentation following enucleation

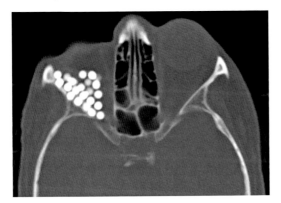

Fig. 2.55 Orbital augmentation beads. Axial CT image shows multiple hyperattenuating beads in the right orbit, where enucleation has been performed

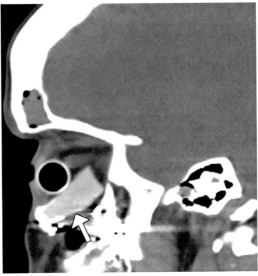

Fig. 2.56 Orbital augmentation with silicone implant. Sagittal CT image shows a hyperattenuating silicone implant (*arrow*) beneath a hollow prosthesis

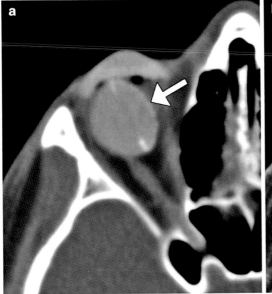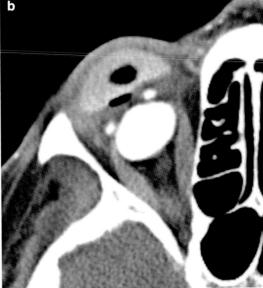

Fig. 2.57 Globe implant rotation. Axial CT image (**a**) shows a gap between the rectus muscles and the implant, which is rotated 90°, such that the metal mesh (*arrow*) is oriented medially, compared with the normal configuration of the implant in a different patient (**b**)

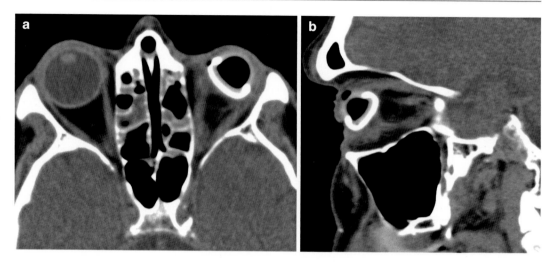

Fig. 2.58 Globe implant exposure. The patient had a history of enucleation approximately 40 years prior to presentation with discomfort and discharge from the left orbit. Physical examination revealed an extruding orbital implant, but no evidence of infection. Axial (**a**) and sagittal (**b**) CT images show infiltration of the left orbital fat and soft tissue surrounding the prosthesis, which proved to be granulation and scar tissue at subsequent surgery. The inferior portion of the implant is angled anteriorly, and the scleral cover shell prosthesis is absent

2.16   Orbital Tissue Expanders

2.16.1 Discussion

Orbital tissue expanders are implanted devices used for enlarging the orbital cavity in patients with congenital anophthalmia and microphthalmia and can obviate surgery. The main types of orbital expanders include hydrophilic osmotic hydrogel devices or inflatable saline globes. The placement and volume of the expanders can be evaluated via CT or MRI. Hydrogel expanders appear as either spherical or hemispherical structures with nearly fluid attenuation on CT and low T1 and high T2 MRI signal intensity and do not enhance (Fig. 2.59). Saline expanders appear as spherical fluid-density structures on CT adjacent to the metal-density T-plate. The saline expanders have similar imaging characteristics as the aqueous on CT and MRI and are attached to metallic T-plate.

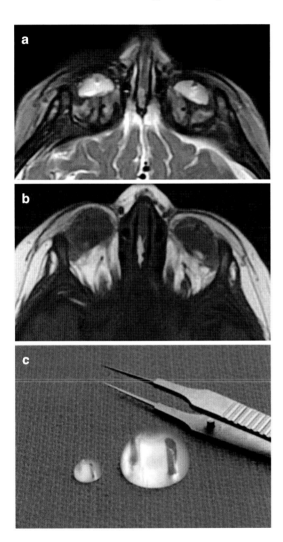

Fig. 2.59 Hemispheric hydrogel expander. Axial T2-weighted (**a**) and T1-weighted (**b**) MR images show bilateral orbital implants with similar signal characteristics as fluid. Photograph of the hydrogel hemispheric implants when dry and hydrated (**c**) (Courtesy of Osmed)

2.17   Orbital Exenteration

2.17.1   Discussion

Orbital exenteration is performed for treatment of primary orbital malignancies and periorbital malignancies that invade the orbit. Several types of orbital exenteration procedures can be performed with various degrees of dissection, ranging from extended enucleation, subtotal exenteration with sparing of the eyelid, total exenteration with removal of the eyelid in addition to orbital contents, and radical exenteration with removal of structures surrounding the orbit, such as paranasal sinuses and skull base (Figs. 2.60, 2.61, 2.62, and 2.63). The socket created by more extensive exenteration procedures can either heal by granulation or lined with skin graft or tissue flap. Since patients who undergo exenterations for malignant neoplasms typically receive radiation therapy, complications may include necrosis (Fig. 2.64), infection, tumor recurrence (Fig. 2.65), and radiation-induced neoplasms (Fig. 2.66), which can occur many years after treatment.

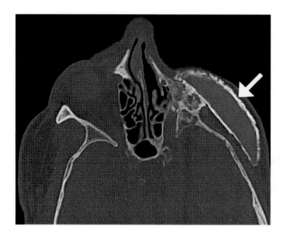

Fig. 2.60 Orbital exenteration and facial implant. The patient had a remote history of advanced retinoblastoma treated with orbital exenteration and radiation. Axial CT image shows resection of the left orbit and reconstruction via silicone implant (*arrow*), with surrounding dystrophic calcifications

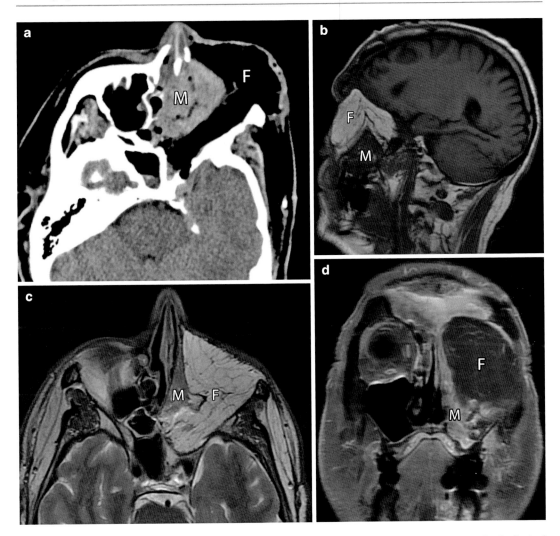

Fig. 2.61 Orbital exenteration with maxillectomy and flap reconstruction. The patient has a history of recurrent stage IV left face squamous cell carcinoma treated with radical exenteration with myocutaneous flap reconstruction in addition to chemoradiation. Axial CT image (**a**) shows the normal-appearing muscle (*M*) and fat (*F*) components of the myocutaneous thigh flap within the left orbit and maxillectomy defect. The vascular supply to the graft is derived from the left facial artery and vein. Sagittal (**b**) T1-weighted, axial T2-weighted (**c**), and fat-suppressed coronal contrast-enhanced T1-weighted (**d**) MRI sequences show the subcutaneous fat (*F*) portion of the graft, which loses signal with fat suppression. There is normal enhancement of the muscle component of the graft (*M*), which suggests viability

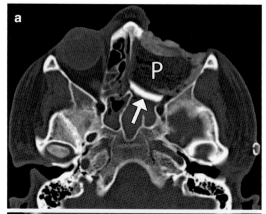

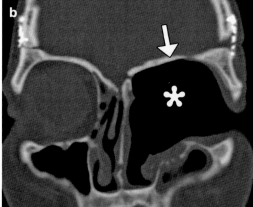

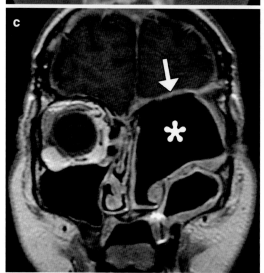

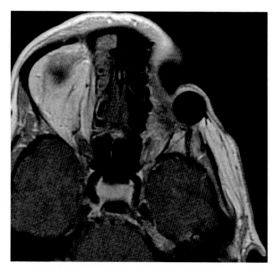

Fig. 2.63 Orbital exenteration with implant. The patient has a history of left ocular melanoma with extrascleral extension. Axial contrast-enhanced T1-weightwed MR images demonstrate a left orbital exenteration and reconstruction using an orbital implant

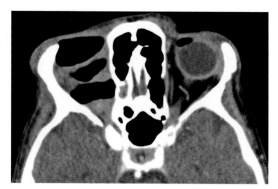

Fig. 2.64 Graft necrosis. Axial CT image shows right orbital exenteration. Sheets of air are present within the shrunken myocutaneous flap

Fig. 2.62 Radical orbital exenteration. The patient has a history of squamous cell carcinoma involving the left orbit and treated with radical orbital exenteration. Recent postoperative axial CT image (**a**) shows left radical orbital exenteration with bone flap reconstruction of the orbital floor and surgical packing (*P*). Coronal CT (**b**) and post-contrast T1-weighted MRI (**c**) shows bifrontal craniotomies, an air-filled left orbit that communicates with the nasal cavity (*), and a denuded orbital roof (*arrows*), which was allowed to heal via granulation

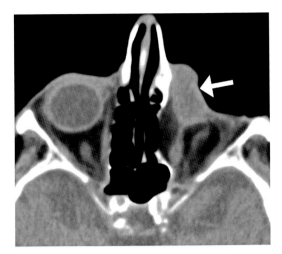

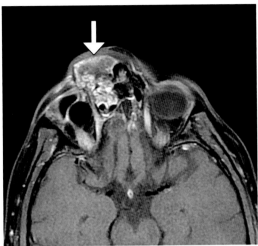

Fig. 2.65 Tumor recurrence. The patient has a history of exenteration of the left orbit for squamous cell carcinoma. Axial CT image shows a nodular lesion in the medial aspect of the left orbit (*arrow*)

Fig. 2.66 Radiation-induced osteosarcoma. Axial fat-suppressed post-contrast T1-weighted MRI shows a heterogeneously enhancing mass (*arrow*) arising medal to the right orbit, which contains an ocular implant and prosthesis

2.18 Orbital Radiation Therapy Fiducial Markers

2.18.1 Discussion

Stereotactic radiosurgery can be used to treat a variety of ocular tumors. Small tantalum ring orbital radiation therapy fiducial markers are initially surgically sutured to the globe for tumor localization during treatment. The markers may be incidentally encountered on CT as tiny metallic structures along the surface of the globe (Fig. 2.67) and are compatible with MRI at 1.5 T.

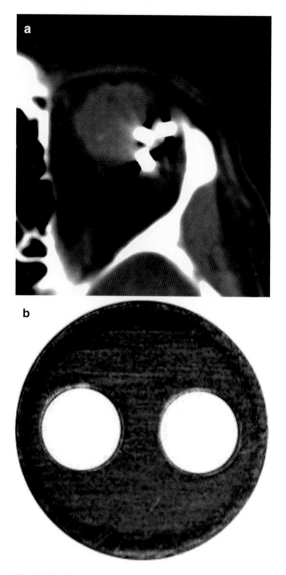

Fig. 2.67 Tantalum rings. Axial (**a**) CT image shows three metallic markers along the surface of the left globe. Photograph of a tantalum ring (**b**) (Courtesy of Altomed)

Further Reading

Eyelid Weights

Caesar RH, Friebel J, McNab AA (2004) Upper lid loading with gold weights in paralytic lagophthalmos: a modified technique to maximize the long-term functional and cosmetic success. Orbit 23(1):27–32

Jayashankar N, Morwani KP, Shaan MJ, Bhatia SR, Patil KT (2008) Customized gold weight eyelid implantation in paralytic lagophthalmos. J Laryngol Otol 122(10):1088–1091

Kartush JM, Linstrom CJ, McCann PM, Graham MD (1990) Early gold weight eyelid implantation for facial paralysis. Otolaryngol Head Neck Surg 103(6):1016–1023

Marra S, Leonetti JP, Konior RJ, Raslan W (1995) Effect of magnetic resonance imaging on implantable eyelid weights. Ann Otol Rhinol Laryngol 104(6):448–452

Palpebral Spring

Bergeron CM, Moe KS (2008) The evaluation and treatment of upper eyelid paralysis. Facial Plast Surg 24(2):220–230

Demirci H, Frueh BR (2009) Palpebral spring in the management of lagophthalmos and exposure keratopathy secondary to facial nerve palsy. Ophthal Plast Reconstr Surg 25(4):270–275

Terzis JK, Kyere SA (2008) Experience with the gold weight and palpebral spring in the management of paralytic lagophthalmos. Plast Reconstr Surg 121(3):806–815

Frontalis Suspension Ptosis Repair

Nakauchi K, Mito H, Mimura O (2013) Frontal suspension for congenital ptosis using an expanded polytetrafluoroethylene (Gore-Tex(®)) sheet: one-year follow-up. Clin Ophthalmol 7:131–136

Kokubo K, Katori N, Hayashi K, Kasai K, Kamisasanuki T, Sueoka K, Maegawa J (2016) Frontalis suspension with an expanded polytetrafluoroethylene sheet for congenital ptosis repair. J Plast Reconstr Aesthet Surg 69:673–678

Orbital Wall Reconstruction and Augmentation

Badilla J, Dolman PJ (2007) Cerebrospinal fluid leaks complicating orbital or oculoplastic surgery. Arch Ophthalmol 125(12):1631–1634

Jordan DR, St Onge P, Anderson RL, Patrinely JR, Nerad JA (1992) Complications associated with alloplastic implants used in orbital fracture repair. Ophthalmology 99(10):1600–1608

Lelli GJ Jr, Milite J, Maher E (2007) Orbital floor fractures: evaluation, indications, approach, and pearls from an ophthalmologist's perspective. Facial Plast Surg 23(3):190–199

Liss J, Stefko ST, Chung WL (2010) Orbital surgery: state of the art. Oral Maxillofac Surg Clin North Am 22(1):59–71

Mauriello JA Jr (1987) Complications of orbital trauma surgery. Adv Ophthalmic Plast Reconstr Surg 7:99–115

Orbital Decompression for Dysthyroid Orbitopathy

Hu WD, Annunziata CC, Chokthaweesak W, Korn BS, Levi L, Granet DB, Kikkawa DO (2010) Radiographic analysis of extraocular muscle volumetric changes in thyroid-related orbitopathy following orbital decompression. Ophthal Plast Reconstr Surg 26(1): 1–6

Leong SC, White PS (2010) Outcomes following surgical decompression for dysthyroid orbitopathy (Graves' disease). Curr Opin Otolaryngol Head Neck Surg 18(1):37–43

Dacryocystorhinostomy and Nasolacrimal Duct Stents

Bartley GB, Gustafson RO (1990) Complications of malpositioned Jones tubes. Am J Ophthalmol 109(1):66–69

Ginat DT, Freitag SK. Orbital emphysema complicating jones tube placement in a patient treated with continuous positive airway pressure. Ophthal Plast Reconstr Surg 2015;31(1):e25

Leong SC, Macewen CJ, White PS (2010) A systematic review of outcomes after dacryocystorhinostomy in adults. Am J Rhinol Allergy 24(1):81–90

Onerci M (2002) Dacryocystorhinostomy. Diagnosis and treatment of nasolacrimal canal obstructions. Rhinology 40(2):49–65

Pinto IT, Paul L, Grande C (1998) Nasolacrimal polyurethane stent: complications with CT correlation. Cardiovasc Intervent Radiol 21(6):450–453

Yazici Z, Yazici B, Parlak M, Tuncel E, Ertürk H (2002) Treatment of nasolacrimal duct obstruction with polyurethane stent placement: long-term results. AJR Am J Roentgenol 179(2):491–494

Strabismus Surgery

Mehendale RA, Dagi LR, Wu C, Ledoux D, Johnston S, Hunter DG (2012) Superior rectus transposition and medial rectus recession for Duane syndrome and sixth nerve palsy. Arch Ophthalmol 130(2):195–201

Nishida Y, Inatomi A, Aoki Y, Hayashi O, Iwami T, Oda S, Nakamura J, Kani K (2003) A muscle transposition procedure for abducens palsy, in which the halves of the vertical rectus muscle bellies are sutured onto the sclera. Jpn J Ophthalmol 47(3):281–286

Yurdakul NS, Ugurlu S, Maden A (2011) Surgical management of chronic complete sixth nerve palsy. Ophthalmic Surg Lasers Imaging 42(1):72–77

Glaucoma Surgery

Ceballos EM, Parrish RK 2nd (2002) Plain film imaging of Baerveldt glaucoma drainage implants. AJNR Am J Neuroradiol 23(6):935–937

Dugel PU, Heuer DK, Thach AB, Baerveldt G, Lee PP, Lloyd MA, Minckler DS, Green RL (1997) Annular peripheral choroidal detachment simulating aqueous misdirection after glaucoma surgery. Ophthalmology 104(3):439–444

Freedman J (2010) What is new after 40 years of glaucoma implants. J Glaucoma 19(8):504–508

Jeon TY, Kim HJ, Kim ST, Chung TY, Kee C (2007) MR imaging features of giant reservoir formation in the orbit: an unusual complication of Ahmed glaucoma valve implantation. AJNR Am J Neuroradiol 28(8):1565–1566

Lachkar Y, Hamard P (2002) Nonpenetrating filtering surgery. Curr Opin Ophthalmol 13(2):110–115

Patel S, Pasquale LR (2010) Glaucoma drainage devices: a review of the past, present, and future. Semin Ophthalmol 25(5–6):265–270

Pirouzian A, Scher C, O'Halloran H, Jockin Y (2006) Ahmed glaucoma valve implants in the pediatric population: the use of magnetic resonance imaging findings for surgical approach to reoperation. J AAPOS 10(4):340–344

Scleral Buckles

Bernardino CR, Mihora LD, Fay AM, Rubin PA (2006) Orbital complications of hydrogel scleral buckles. Ophthal Plast Reconstr Surg 22(3):206–208

Bhagat N, Khanna A, Langer PD (2005) Hydrated scleral buckle: a late complication of MAI explants. Br J Ophthalmol 89(10):1380

Lane JI, Randall JG, Campeau NG, Overland PK, McCannel CA, Matsko TA (2001) Imaging of hydrogel episcleral buckle fragmentation as a late complication after retinal reattachment surgery. AJNR Am J Neuroradiol 22(6):1199–1202

Lane JI, Watson RE Jr, Witte RJ, McCannel CA (2003) Retinal detachment: imaging of surgical treatments and complications. Radiographics 23(4):983–994

Ginat DT, Singh AD, Moonis G. (2012) Multimodality imaging of hydrogel scleral buckles. Retina. 32:1449–1452

Keratoprostheses

Colby KA, Koo EB (2011) Expanding indications for the Boston keratoimplant. Curr Opin Ophthalmol 22(4):267–273

Garcia JP Jr, de la Cruz J, Rosen RB, Buxton DF (2008) Imaging implanted keratoprostheses with anterior-segment optical coherence tomography and ultrasound biomicroscopy. Cornea 27(2):180–188

Gomaa A, Comyn O, Liu C (2010) Keratoprostheses in clinical practice – a review. Clin Experiment Ophthalmol 38(2):211–224

Robert MC, Harissi-Dagher M (2011) Boston type 1 keratoimplant: the CHUM experience. Can J Ophthalmol 46(2):164–168

Intraocular Lens Implants

Aksoy FG, Gomori JM, Halpert M (1999) CT and MR imaging of contact lenses and intraocular lens implants. Comput Med Imaging Graph 23(4):205–208

Bucher PJ, Büchi ER, Daicker BC (1995) Dystrophic calcification of an implanted hydroxyethylmethacrylate intraocular lens. Arch Ophthalmol 113(11):1431–1435

Kuo MD, Hayman LA, Lee AG, Mayo GL, Diaz-Marchan PJ (1998) In vivo CT and MR appearance of prosthetic intraocular lens. AJNR Am J Neuroradiol 19(4):749–753

Rofagha S, Bhisitkul RB (2011) Management of retained lens fragments in complicated cataract surgery. Curr Opin Ophthalmol 22(2):137–140

Sourdille P (1997) Lensectomy-vitrectomy indications and techniques in cataract surgery. Curr Opin Ophthalmol 8(1):56–59

Yong JL, Lertsumitkul S, Killingsworth MC, Filipic M (2004) Calcification of intraocular hydrogel lens: evidence of dystrophic calcification. Clin Experiment Ophthalmol 32(5):492–500

Surgical Aphakia

Sourdille P (1997) Lensectomy-vitrectomy indications and techniques in cataract surgery. Curr Opin Ophthalmol 8(1):56–59

Pneumatic Retinopexy

Berrod JP, Rozot P, Raspiller A, Thiery D (1994–1995) Fluid air exchange in vitreo retinal surgery. Int Ophthalmol 18(4):237–241

Chan CK, Lin SG, Nuthi AS, Salib DM (2008) Pneumatic retinopexy for the repair of retinal detachments: a comprehensive review (1986–2007). Surv Ophthalmol 53(5):443–448

Krzystolik MG, D'Amico DJ (2000) Complications of intraocular tamponade: silicone oil versus intraocular gas. Int Ophthalmol Clin 40(1):187–200

Wirostko WJ, Han DP, Perkins SL (2000) Complications of pneumatic retinopexy. Curr Opin Ophthalmol 11(3): 195–200

Intraocular Silicone Oil

Eller AW, Friberg TR, Mah F (2000) Migration of silicone oil into the brain: a complication of intraocular silicone oil for retinal tamponade. Am J Ophthalmol 129: 685–688

Fangtian D, Rongping D, Lin Z, Weihong Y (2005) Migration of intraocular silicone into the cerebral ventricles. Am J Ophthalmol 140:156–158

Herrick RC, Hayinan LA, Maturi RK, Diaz-Marchan PJ, Tang RA, Lambert HM (1998) Optimal imaging protocol after intraocular silicone oil tamponade. AJNR Am J Neuroradiol 19:101–108

Lane JI, Watson RE, Witte RJ, McCannel CA (2003) Retinal detachment: imaging of surgical treatments and complications. Radiographics 23:983–994

Mathews VP, Elster AD, Barker PB, Buff BL, Haller JA, Greven CM (1994) Intraocular silicone oil: in vitro and in vivo MR and CT characteristics. AJNR Am J Neuroradiol 15:343–347

Evisceration, Enucleation, and Globe Prostheses

Christmas NJ, Gordon CD, Murray TG, Tse D, Johnson T, Garonzik S, O'Brien JM (1998) Intraorbital implants after enucleation and their complications: a 10-year review. Arch Ophthalmol 116(9):1199–1203

LeBedis CA, Sakai O (2008) Nontraumatic orbital conditions: diagnosis with CT and MR imaging in the emergent setting. Radiographics 28(6):1741–1753

Orbital Tissue Expanders

Mazzoli RA, Raymond WR 4th, Ainbinder DJ, Hansen EA (2004) Use of self-expanding, hydrophilic osmotic expanders (hydrogel) in the reconstruction of congenital clinical anophthalmos. Curr Opin Ophthalmol 15(5):426–431

Tse DT, Abdulhafez M, Orozco MA, Tse JD, Azab AO, Pinchuk L (2011) Evaluation of an integrated orbital tissue expander in congenital anophthalmos: report of preliminary clinical experience. Am J Ophthalmol 151(3):470–82.e1

Orbital Exenteration

Nassab RS, Thomas SS, Murray D (2007) Orbital exenteration for advanced periorbital skin cancers: 20 years experience. J Plast Reconstr Aesthet Surg 60(10): 1103–1109

Tyers AG (2006) Orbital exenteration for invasive skin tumours. Eye (Lond) 20(10):1165–1170

Orbital Radiation Therapy Fiducial Markers

Ahn YC, Lee KC, Kim DY, Huh SJ, Yeo IH, Lim DH, Kim MK, Shin KH, Park S, Chang SH (2000) Fractionated stereotactic radiation therapy for extracranial head and neck tumors. Int J Radiat Oncol Biol Phys 48(2): 501–505

Daftari IK, Aghaian E, O'Brien JM, Dillon W, Phillips TL (2005) 3D MRI-based tumor delineation of ocular melanoma and its comparison with conventional techniques. Med Phys 32(11):3355–3362

Imaging the Paranasal Sinuses and Nasal Cavity

3

Daniel Thomas Ginat, Mary Elizabeth Cunnane, and Robert M. Naclerio

3.1 Nasal Fracture Reconstruction (Posttraumatic Rhinoplasty)

3.1.1 Discussion

The aim of posttraumatic rhinoplasty surgery is to restore the pretraumatic state and normal function and appearance of the nose. The surgical technique depends on the degree of comminution, associated septal fracture, and presence of other facial fractures. Internal and external fixation approaches can be implemented. Bone grafting can be used to reconstruct substantial defects (Fig. 3.1). Low-profile mesh material provides fracture fixation with good cosmetic results (Fig. 3.2). Likewise, temporary external plates and transcutaneous wire can help restore satisfactory alignment. Nasal stents are sometimes inserted to maintain patent nasal passages, while the fracture and associated soft tissue injury heal. CT is generally the imaging modality of choice for postoperative traumatic rhinoplasty assessment. Low-radiation dose techniques are typically adequate. Cosmetic rhinoplasty is otherwise discussed in Chap. 1.

D.T. Ginat, M.D., M.S. (✉)
Department of Radiology, University of Chicago
Pritzker School of Medicine, Chicago, IL, USA
e-mail: dtg1@uchicago.edu

M.E. Cunnane, M.D.
Department of Radiology, Harvard Medical School,
Massachusetts Eye and Ear Infirmary,
Boston, MA, USA

R.M. Naclerio, M.D.
Section of Otolaryngology-Head and Neck Surgery,
University of Chicago Pritzker School of Medicine,
Chicago, IL, USA

© Springer International Publishing Switzerland 2017
D.T. Ginat, P.-L.A. Westesson (eds.), *Atlas of Postsurgical Neuroradiology*,
DOI 10.1007/978-3-319-52341-5_3

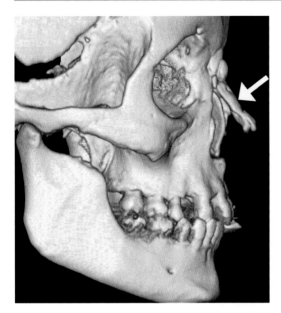

Fig. 3.1 Cortical bone reconstruction. 3D CT image shows cortical bone graft positioned along the expected site of the nasal dorsum (*arrow*) and absence of the native nasal bones and frontal processes of the maxilla

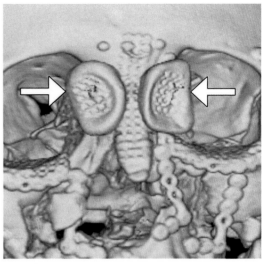

Fig. 3.2 Nasal fracture reconstruction with low-profile mesh. 3D CT image shows a mesh positioned along the nasal dorsum secured via low-profile screws. There are also bilateral molded polyvinyl siloxane plates (*arrows*) fit over the nasal soft tissue in the medial canthal area and secured via transcutaneous wires

3.2   Septoplasty

3.2.1   Discussion

Septoplasty is performed to treat a deviated nasal septum and can be performed in conjunction with rhinoplasty (septorhinoplasty). Classic septoplasty consists of creating a mucoperichondrial flap in order to remove the offending portion of the nasal septum via sharp dissection (Fig. 3.3). Silastic sheets or stents are often inserted along both sides of the nasal septum to prevent the formation of adhesions (Fig. 3.4). These are later removed once the surgical site heals. The postoperative imaging appearance often consists of a straightened and thinned nasal septum with widened nasal passages, which can be subtle. Complications are uncommon and include hemorrhage, cerebrospinal fluid leak, infection, septal hematoma or abscess, overcorrected septum, septal perforation (Fig. 3.5), adhesions, and sensory disturbances.

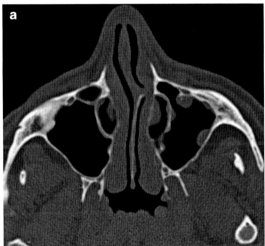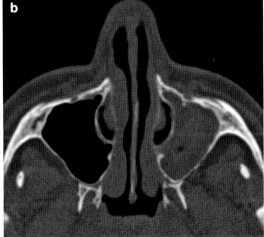

Fig. 3.3 Septoplasty. The patient has a history of a deviated nasal septum with spur causing nasal obstruction. Preoperative axial CT image (**a**) shows leftward deviation of the nasal septum with a spur. Axial CT image obtained 1 year after surgery (**b**) shows interval removal of the spur and straightening of the nasal septum. There is also increased opacification of the left maxillary sinus

3.3 Nasal Septal Button Prosthesis

3.3.1 Discussion

Nasal septal perforation may present with various symptoms: epistaxis, crusting, secondary infection, whistling, and nasal obstruction. Perforation can be treated by conservative pharmacological treatment or by surgical closure. Alternatively, a nasal septal button, often composed of silicone, can be inserted transnasally to span the perforation (Fig. 3.6).

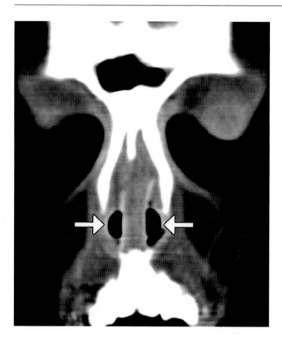

Fig. 3.4 Nasal stents. The patient has a history of nasal septal deviation and adhesions treated via septoplasty and lysis of adhesions. Coronal CT image shows a straight, midline septum flanked by bilateral nasal stents (*arrows*)

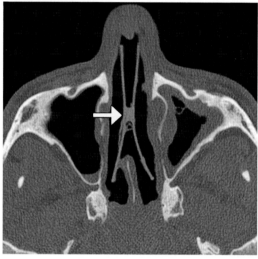

Fig. 3.6 Nasal septal button prosthesis. Axial CT image shows the two discs connected to one another across the nasal septal defect (*arrow*)

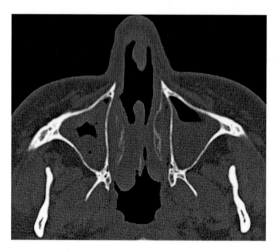

Fig. 3.5 Septoplasty perforation. Axial CT image shows a defect in the anterior nasal septum. The septum is otherwise straight. However, there is acute sinusitis

3.4   Inferior Turbinate Outfracture and Reduction

3.4.1   Discussion

Inferior turbinate outfracture and reduction are treatment options for nasal obstruction related to inferior turbinate hypertrophy. Outfracture consists of laterally displacing the inferior turbinates, while radio-frequency treatment coagulates the inferior turbinate submucosa. This results in a widened nasal airway passage. The procedures are often performed in conjunction with septoplasty. Lateral displacement of the anterior, middle, and posterior portions is usually apparent on postoperative sinus CT (Fig. 3.7). Alternatively, turbinate reduction surgery typically results in a truncated appearance of the inferior turbinates and enlargement of the nasal passages (Fig. 3.8).

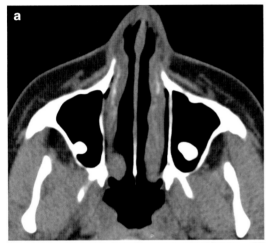

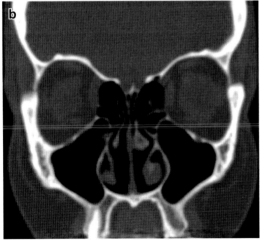

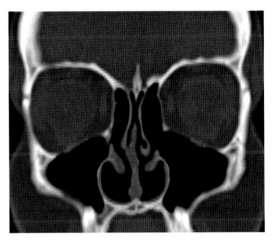

Fig 3.8 Inferior turbinate reduction. Coronal CT image shows truncation of the inferior portions of the bilateral inferior turbinates. Findings related to endoscopic sinus surgery are also apparent

Fig. 3.7 Inferior turbinate outfracture. Axial (**a**) and coronal (**b**) CT images show lateral deviation of the bilateral inferior turbinates with reduced mucosa and evidence of septoplasty, which result in a widened nasal passage

3.5   Nasal Packing Material

3.5.1   Discussion

Nasal packs are routinely used in sinonasal surgery in order to apply pressure, fill preformed spaces, create moist environments to facilitate physiological processes, function as a barrier, and induce physiological hemostatic and reparative processes. Nasal packings, including Merocel and MeroGel packs, and alginate strips have a tendency to imbibe blood products in the early perioperative period, which is reflected in the appearance on imaging (Fig. 3.9). Bismuth and iodoform paraffin paste using some packing material displays high CT attenuation that results in severe image degradation. Aqueous Betadine gauze also displays high attenuation on CT. Myospherulosis, a foreign body-type granulomatous reaction to lipid-containing material, has a characteristic fat-attenuation appearance on CT.

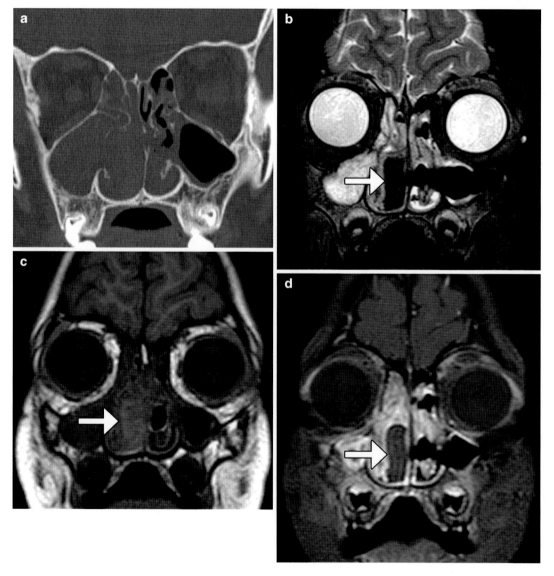

Fig. 3.9 Nasal packing. Coronal CT image (**a**) shows opacification of the right nasal cavity and paranasal sinuses. Coronal T1-weighted MRI (**b**) shows that the nasal packing material is very hypointense (*arrow*). The T1-weighted (**c**) and fat-suppressed post-contrast T1-weighted (**d**) MR images show that the nasal packing (*arrows*) is mildly T1 hyperintense and does not enhance, unlike the surrounding mucosa

3.6   Rhinectomy

3.6.1   Discussion

Rhinectomy is an oncological procedure that involves resecting part or all of the external nose when involved by high-risk nasal malignancies.

Prosthetic rehabilitation can be an alternative to flap reconstruction, particularly in those patients unsuitable for major reconstruction. Customized prostheses can be created via computer-aided design based on preoperative virtual laser scanning or CT of the affected site adapted to the postoperative laser-scanned surface or CT (Fig. 3.10).

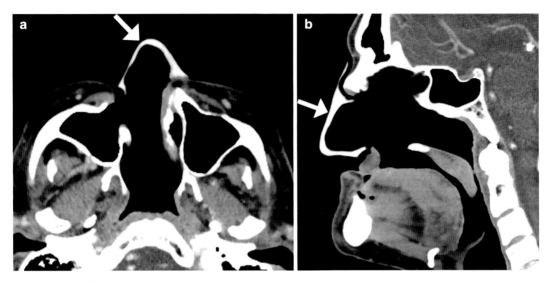

Fig. 3.10 Total rhinectomy with nose prosthesis. The patient had a history of nasal squamous cell carcinoma. Axial (**a**) and sagittal (**b**) CT images show a total rhinectomy defect that was reconstructed using a custom-made silicone prosthesis (*arrows*)

3.7 Sinus Lift Procedure

3.7.1 Discussion

The sinus lift or augmentation procedure is performed to build up a deficient maxillary alveolus for subsequent osseointegrated dental implant insertion. The procedure involves accessing the maxillary sinus and elevating the mucous membrane at the inferior aspect of the maxillary to create a space in the floor of the sinus where bone graft material is inserted, typically with a

dome-shaped configuration on coronal images (Fig. 3.11). The bone graft initially has a porous appearance but consolidates with a more uniformly hyperattenuating appearance on CT as osseointegration and osteogenesis ensure after 6–8 months. Disruption of the sinus mucosa may result in sinusitis, graft infection, or formation of oroantral fistula, which is best depicted on coronal plane CT images (Fig. 3.12). Furthermore, graft material scattered in the sinus may also indicate surgical failure.

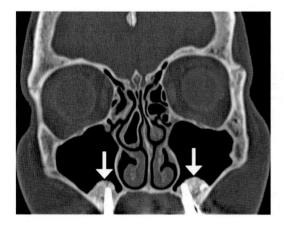

Fig. 3.11 Sinus lift procedure. Coronal CT image shows bone graft material (*arrows*) within the inferior maxillary sinuses adjacent to the alveolar ridge. There are bilateral osseointegrated implants

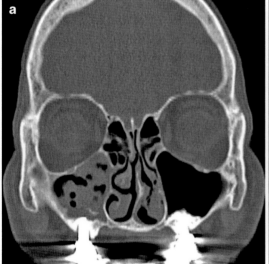
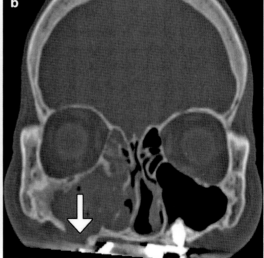

Fig. 3.12 Sinusitis and oroantral fistula after sinus lift procedure. Coronal CT image (**a**) shows bilateral sinus lift procedures with osseointegrated implants and opacification of the right maxillary sinus. Follow-up CT image (**b**) shows a defect in the maxillary sinus floor (*arrow*) and persistent right-sided sinus opacification

3.8 Caldwell-Luc Procedure

3.8.1 Discussion

The Caldwell-Luc procedure was described by Caldwell in 1893, Spicer in 1894, and Luc in 1897 for the treatment of maxillary sinusitis. The technique originally consisted of creating a defect in the inferior aspect of the anterior maxillary wall via a canine fossa approach and removing diseased mucosa from the maxillary sinus, combined with inferior or middle meatus antrostomy, in order to facilitate gravitational intranasal counterdrainage and antral lavage (Fig. 3.13).

Historically, the Caldwell-Luc procedure was the primary sinus surgery until it was largely supplanted by functional endoscopic sinus surgery. The Caldwell-Luc procedure has fallen out of favor since it interrupts the ciliary clearance mechanism of the maxillary sinus mucosa. As a result, the procedure often exacerbates the conditions that it is intended to treat. Indeed, on postoperative imaging, inflammatory sinus disease, sinus collapse, and sinus wall sclerosis (osteitis) are found in over 80%, over 90%, and up to 100% of cases, respectively (Fig. 3.14). Currently, modification of the Caldwell-Luc procedure is mainly reserved as an approach for resection of selected maxillary sinus tumors and antrochoanal polyps.

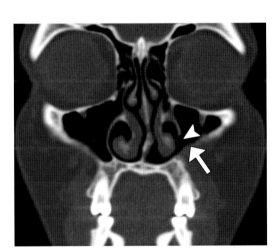

Fig. 3.13 Caldwell-Luc surgery. Coronal CT image shows a defect in the left anterior maxillary sinus wall (*arrowhead*) and nasoantral wall (*arrow*)

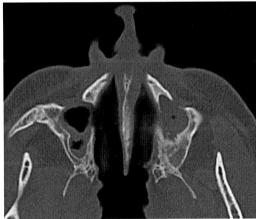

Fig. 3.14 Chronic recurrent sinusitis after bilateral Caldwell-Luc surgery. Axial CT shows the bilateral postoperative changes with mucosal thickening and hyperostosis of the remaining maxillary sinus walls

3.9   External Ethmoidectomy

3.9.1   Discussion

In the past, before the advent of functional endoscopic surgery techniques, resection of the ethmoid labyrinth was commonly performed for the
treatment of sinusitis via a transorbital approach.
The lamina can also be removed endoscopically
for tumors such as inverted papillomas. The surgery involves resection of the ipsilateral lamina
papyracea through which the paranasal sinuses
can be visualized and accessed. The resulting
defect in the lamina papyracea can be substantial
(Fig. 3.15). Although external ethmoidectomy
has been largely supplanted by FESS for treating
rhinosinusitis, the approach may still be implemented for resecting certain sinonasal tumors.

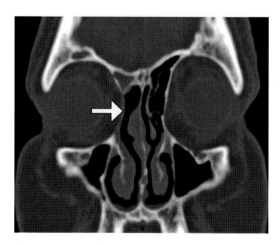

Fig. 3.15 External ethmoidectomy. Coronal CT image
shows a defect in the right lamina papyracea (*arrow*),
through which the right ethmoid air cells were resected.
There is also right frontal blockage, which can be a complication of this approach

3.10   Functional Endoscopic Sinus Surgery

3.10.1   Discussion

Functional endoscopic sinus surgery (FESS) is
used to treat chronic sinusitis and is occasionally
performed as part of tumor resection. The objec-
tive of FESS is to relieve obstruction of mucus
drainage while preserving the mucociliary clearance mechanism. The procedure consists of
resecting various portions of the paranasal
sinuses using an intranasal endoscope depending
on the extent of disease and whether the anterior
or posterior drainage routes are predominantly
affected. The resulting changes are not necessarily symmetric from right to left or reproducible
from one patient to another. Nevertheless, certain
fundamental strategies are generally implemented, which are based on the major mucosal
drainage pathways. CT with multiplanar
reformatted images is the first-line modality for
evaluating the paranasal sinuses and surrounding
structures following FESS.

Turbinoplasty or partial anterior middle turbinectomy is sometimes performed in order to
increase the exposure of the paranasal sinuses.
The middle turbinate can be completely resected
if it is responsible for obstructing the middle
meatus (Fig. 3.16).

Uncinectomy is essentially performed during all types of FESS when the ostiomeatal
complex is affected by rhinosinusitis, along
with resection of variable amounts of the anterior ethmoid air cells. Since the anterior ethmoid air cells normally comprise two-thirds to
three-quarters of the ethmoid air cells, the
resection cavity can extend rather far

posteriorly. Typically, anterior ethmoidectomies and uncinectomies are performed together in order to optimally decompress the ostiomeatal complex and access the maxillary sinuses (Fig. 3.17).

Disease of the posterior drainage system can be treated via ethmoidectomy alone or in combination with sphenoidotomy, which consists of enlarging the sphenoid sinus ostium (Figs. 3.18 and 3.19). This is often performed in conjunction with decompression of the ostiomeatal complex.

Disease that affects the frontoethmoid drainage pathway can be addressed via frontal recess sinusotomy. Frontal recess sinusotomy approaches have been traditionally classified as

Draf type I through III based on the extent of agger nasi and frontal air cells resected (Figs. 3.19, 3.20, 3.21, and 3.22). The Draf type III (modified Lothrop) procedure is the most radical form of frontal sinusotomy and involves resection of the upper internasal septum in addition to the frontal air cells.

Occasionally, a defect is created in the medial maxillary sinus wall (antrostomy or nasoantral window), although this is not considered a standard part of FESS (Fig. 3.23). Another twist that is sometimes performed during FESS is Bolgerization, which consists of stripping away part of the mucosa of the nasal septum in order to secure a loose middle turbinate and prevent lateralization.

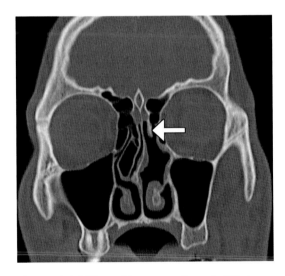

Fig. 3.16 Middle turbinectomy. Coronal CT image shows resection of the left middle turbinate, leaving behind a portion of the left vertical lamella (*arrow*). There is a concha bullosa on right side

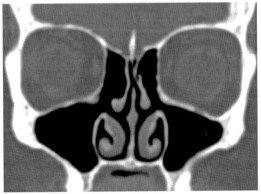

Fig. 3.17 Typical pattern of ostiomeatal unit FESS. Coronal CT image shows the absence of the bilateral anterior ethmoid air cells and uncinate processes, resulting in widely patent anterior drainage pathways and clear sinuses

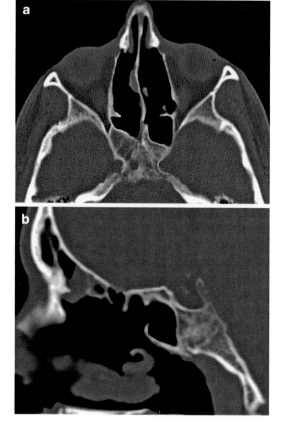

Fig. 3.18 Posterior drainage pathway FESS. Axial (**a**) and sagittal (**b**) CT images show bilateral enlarged sphenoid ostia (*arrows*). Bilateral total ethmoidectomies and middle turbinectomies were also performed

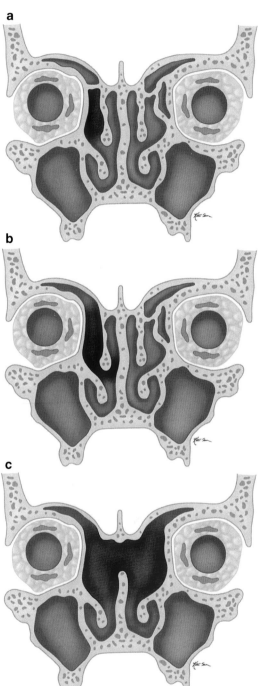

Fig. 3.19 Illustration of the types of frontal sinusotomy. Draf type I (**a**), Draf type II (**b**), and Draf type III (**c**)

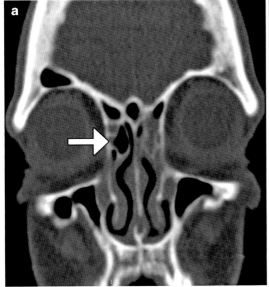
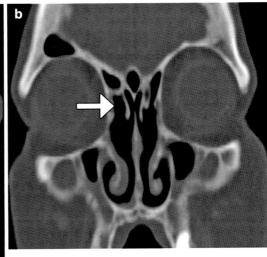

Fig. 3.20 Draf type I frontal sinusotomy. Preoperative coronal CT image (**a**) shows a partially opacified right agger nasi cell (*arrow*). Postoperative coronal CT image (**b**) shows a defect in the inferior aspect of the right agger nasi cell (*arrow*)

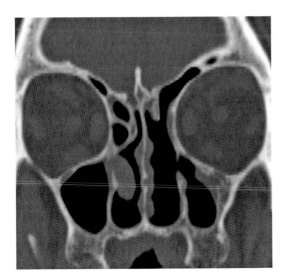

Fig. 3.21 Draf type II frontal sinusotomy. Coronal CT image shows a complete absence of the air cells in the left frontoethmoidal sinus drainage pathway, as compared to the intact contralateral side. Turbinate resection was also performed

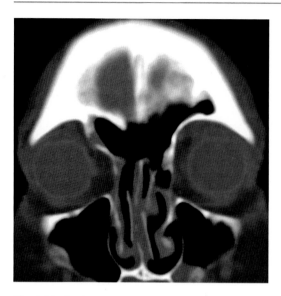

Fig. 3.22 Draf type III frontal sinusotomy (modified Lothrop). Coronal CT image shows contiguous bilateral enlargement of the frontal sinus floors and resection of the interfrontal sinus septum and superior nasal septum. Septoplasty was also performed with Silastic plates in position

3.11 FESS Complications

3.11.1 Discussion

Surgical packing material, such as gauze, may sometimes be left temporarily in the sinuses after functional endoscopic surgery for hemostasis. In the early postoperative period, the gauze can appear as heterogeneous material often containing foci of trapped air, but over time the retained gauze resembles a soft tissue mass with an attenuation of approximately 50 HU on CT (Fig. 3.24). Not all types of gauze packing contain radioattenuating markers. Furthermore, the retained packing may not show enhancement on CT or MRI. Occasionally, patients may not return for postsurgical follow-up, and the packing may remain for long periods of time, resulting in a gossypiboma. This may cause recurrence of sinus symptoms and may even predispose to infection. However, resorbable packing materials have also been developed that do not require removal.

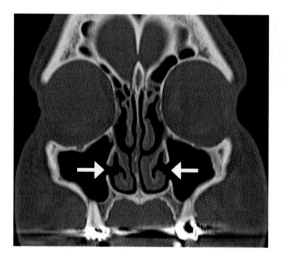

Fig. 3.23 Nasoantral window. Coronal CT image shows surgical defects in the bilateral medial maxillary antrum walls (*arrows*) in addition to bilateral partial ethmoidectomies

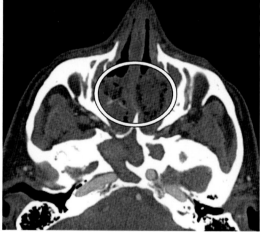

Fig. 3.24 Retained surgical packing (gossypiboma). The patient presents with headache after functional endoscopic sinus surgery a couple of weeks before and neglected to attend the routine postoperative appointment to have the packing removed. Axial CT image shows changes related to FESS and non-enhancing material that contains foci of air filling the ethmoid sinuses (*encircled*)

3.11.2 Discussion

Cephaloceles and cerebrospinal fluid leaks are serious complications of endoscopic sinus surgery that can result from inadvertently creating defects in the floor of the anterior cranial fossa. On CT, the presence of pneumocephalus is a helpful indicator that there is indeed intracranial penetration and cerebrospinal fluid leak (Fig. 3.25). High-resolution CT with multiplanar reconstructions is useful for evaluating the presence of bony dehiscence. However, the presence of sinus opacification contiguous with the intracranial compartment is suggestive, but not specific for encephalocele or meningocele. Rather, MRI is better suited for diagnosing meningoceles, encephaloceles, and associated soft tissue injury (Fig. 3.26). Radionuclide cisternographic studies do not adequately localize and characterize skull base defects well enough to be the sole diagnostic examination. Rather, radionuclide cisternography is reserved for complex cases when the diagnosis is in uncertain.

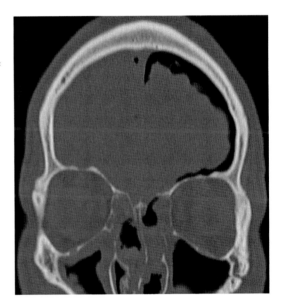

Fig. 3.25 Cerebrospinal fluid leak. The patient presented with headache and rhinorrhea after FESS. Coronal CT image shows left-sided pneumocephalus and a defect in the left cribriform plate

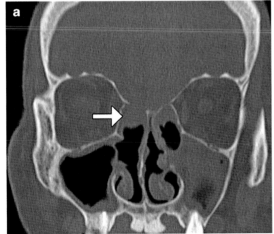

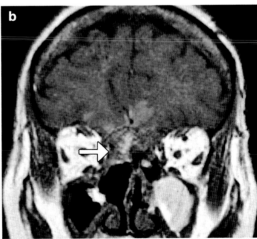

Fig. 3.26 Encephalocele and intraparenchymal hemorrhage. Coronal CT image (**a**) shows internal ethmoidectomies and dehiscence of the right ethmoid roof (*arrow*). There is nonspecific opacification inferior to the dehiscence. Coronal (**b**) T1-weighted MRI shows herniation of brain tissue through the defect in the ethmoid roof. In addition, there is high signal intensity in a linear distribution (*arrows*), which corresponds to hemorrhage along the path of the misdirected surgical instrument

3.11.3 Discussion

Intraorbital complications related to FESS include herniation of intraorbital contents through iatrogenic defects in the lamina papyracea, orbital hemorrhage, optic nerve transection (Fig. 3.27), and orbital cellulitis. Intraorbital hemorrhage can result from direct injury to orbital vessels, ethmoid arteries, or extension into the orbit through a medial wall defect and may cause an acute rise in orbital pressure with rapid onset of proptosis and loss of vision. Orbital CT and MRI are both suitable modalities for evaluating orbital trauma related to FESS.

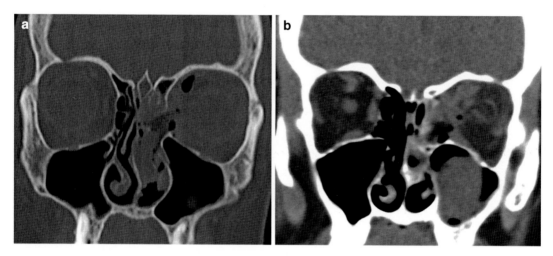

Fig. 3.27 Orbital injury. The patient presented with left vision loss after FESS. Coronal CT images in the bone (**a**) and soft tissue (**b**) windows show a large defect in the left lamina papyracea, abundant pneumo-orbit, retrobulbar hemorrhage, and deformity of the optic nerve on the left side

3.11.4 Discussion

Both extracranial and intracranial vessels can be injured during FESS. The anterior ethmoidal arteries are particularly susceptible to laceration. Although this can be treated by clipping during the procedure (Fig. 3.28), the artery can potentially retract into the orbit, resulting in intraorbital hemorrhage. High-resolution CT can accurately detect the site of entry, which is usually via the fovea ethmoidalis or roof of the ethmoid sinus. Cerebral angiography is recommended to locate an associated pseudoaneurysm, which can often be treated endovascularly (Fig. 3.29).

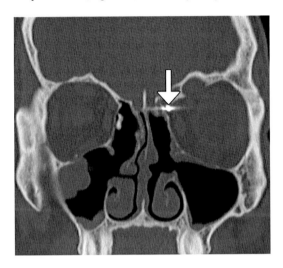

Fig. 3.28 Ethmoid artery injury. Coronal CT image shows a vascular clip (*arrow*) in the region of the left anterior ethmoid artery groove, which was applied to stop bleeding from the injury artery. There is evidence of left-sided internal ethmoidectomy with the presence of bony defect within the left lamina papyracea

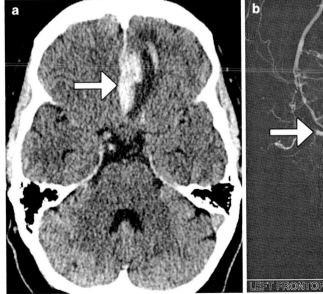
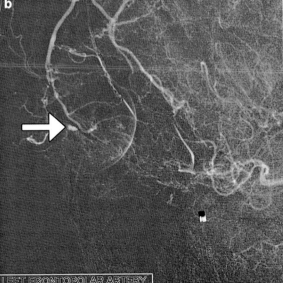

Fig. 3.29 Anterior cerebral artery pseudoaneurysm. The patient presented with sudden-onset mental status changes and headache a few days after undergoing polyp ypectomy. Axial CT image (**a**) shows left gyrus rectus intraparenchymal hemorrhage with a flame-shaped configuration (*arrow*). Digital subtraction cerebral angiogram (**b**) reveals a pseudoaneurysm (*arrow*)

3.11.5 Discussion

Medial bowing of the lamina papyracea can occur following internal ethmoidectomy perhaps due to the loss of internal structural support and forces of contracture during the postoperative healing period (Fig. 3.30). On average, the interorbital distance decreases by about 1 mm after surgery and mild enophthalmos results. These changes are usually subclinical.

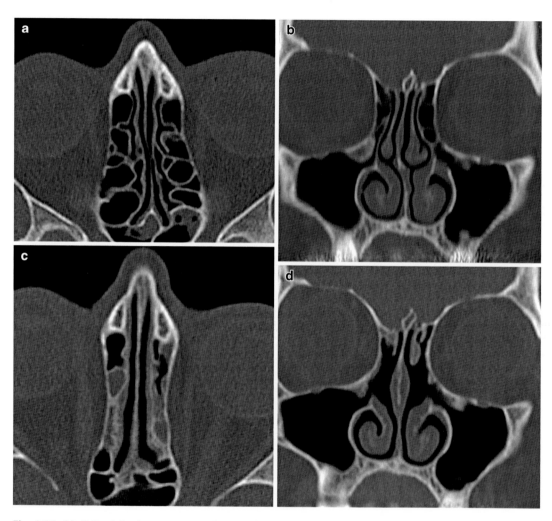

Fig. 3.30 Medialized lamina papyracea. Preoperative axial (**a**) and coronal (**b**) CT images show normal alignment of the bilateral lamina papyracea. Postoperative axial (**c**) and coronal (**d**) CT images show bilateral internal ethmoidectomies and middle turbinate with medial bowing of the laminae papyracea. There is also new opacification of the ethmoid sinuses

3.11.6 Discussion

Mucosal inflammatory disease is common after FESS (Fig. 3.31). Mucosal thickening up to 3 mm is considered normal. However, the degree of mucosal thickening demonstrated on imaging does not necessarily correlate with recurrent symptoms. Mucosal inflammation and synechiae are often indistinguishable on imaging and may certainly coexist. However, synechiae can appear as thin bands of soft tissue within or adjacent to the operative sinonasal cavity. These are most common after frontal sinusotomy.

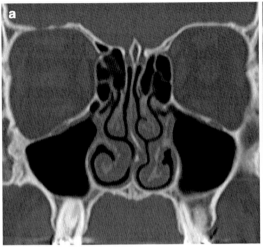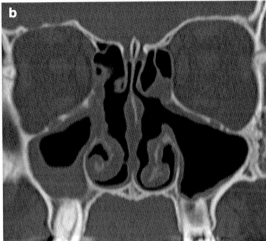

Fig. 3.31 Mucosal inflammation. Preoperative coronal CT image (**a**) shows mild mucosal thickening. Postoperative CT image (**b**) shows diffusely increased mucosal thickening, particularly in the right maxillary sinus after bilateral uncinectomy, as well as correction of septal deviation

3.11.7 Discussion

Mucoceles can form in previously operated sinuses due to blockage by the bone and/or scar tissue. Mucoceles are characterized by expansion of the sinus (Fig. 3.32). Although the absence of air within the affected sinus is sine qua non for mucoceles in nonoperated patients, this is not necessarily the case for postoperative mucoceles. Postoperative scar tissue may isolate a portion of the sinus, forming a compartment where the mucocele can form. This is sometimes termed "surgical ciliated cyst."

3.11.8 Discussion

Recurrent polyposis after surgery may require revision surgery. The frequency varies with comorbidities like ASA sensitivity and asthma. This complication is particularly predisposed by a history of cystic fibrosis, aspirin-exaggerated respiratory disease (AERD), and allergic fungal sinusitis. These patients are also prone to developing inspissated secretions. Polyposis is recognized by the presence of soft tissue attenuation material with smooth, convex margins on CT (Fig. 3.33).

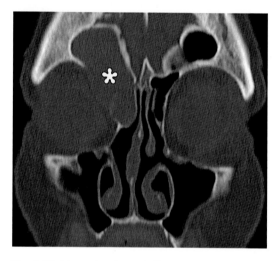

Fig. 3.32 Mucocele. Coronal CT image shows a right frontoethmoid mucocele (*) following frontal sinusotomy

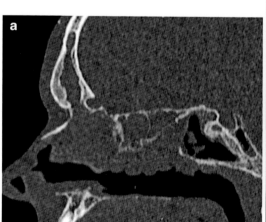
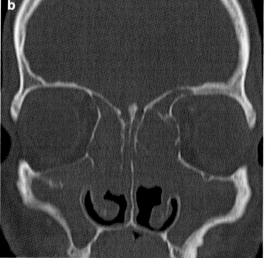

Fig. 3.33 Recurrent polyposis. Sagittal (**a**) and coronal (**b**) CT images demonstrate extensive opacification of the bilateral paranasal sinuses and nasal cavity with convex borders

3.11.9 Discussion

A laterally displaced remnant of the middle turbinate can obstruct the frontal recess after FESS. This can happen due to inadvertent loosening of the middle turbinate during surgery, whereby the turbinate can become adherent to the lamina papyracea. The altered anatomy and obstructed secretions are best depicted on coronal CT image (Fig. 3.34).

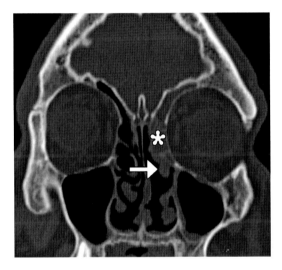

Fig. 3.34 Lateralized middle turbinate. Coronal CT image shows marked lateral deviation of the left middle turbinate (*arrow*) with resultant obstruction of the frontal and ethmoid sinuses, which are opacified (*)

3.11.10 Discussion

Osteoneogenesis is a form of osteitis or hyperostosis that can result from iatrogenic mucosal disruption. There may also be superimposed chronic inflammation or infection. On CT, osteoneogenesis appears as high-attenuation thickening of the sinus walls and septa (Fig. 3.35). The thickened bone may be patchy and irregular. There may also be accompanying mucosal thickening and scarring. The significance of osteoneogenesis is that it can predispose to restenosis of the involved sinus.

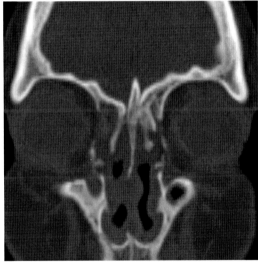

Fig. 3.35 Osteoneogenesis. Coronal CT image demonstrates areas of new bone formation in the left frontoethmoid recess region

3.11.11 Discussion

Performing inferior turbinectomy as part of FESS is a somewhat controversial treatment of nasal obstruction or snoring. Most patients experience improved nasal breathing and some have resolution of anosmia. However, when extensive turbinectomy is combined with resection of other nasal and paranasal structures, empty nose syndrome is a potential complication (Fig. 3.36). This is an uncommon iatrogenic condition that results from inadequate nasal tissue and presents with persistent symptoms due to increased laminar airflow. Nevertheless, patients experience symptoms due to loss of normal turbulent flow through the nasal cavity and the lack of the ability to humidify air.

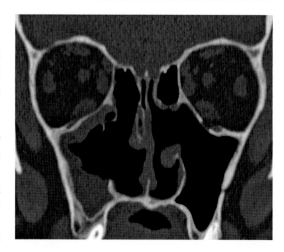

Fig. 3.36 Empty nose syndrome. The patient presents with persistent sensation of nasal obstruction following extensive FESS. Coronal CT image shows the results of septoplasty and extensive resection of the bilateral middle and inferior turbinates, with only a residual portion of the left inferior turbinate. There is right maxillary sinus mucosal thickening

3.12   Osteoplastic Flap with Frontal Sinus Obliteration

3.12.1   Discussion

The osteoplastic flap is an option for treating chronic frontal sinusitis refractory to endoscopic surgery, mucopyocele, extensive fractures that obstruct the drainage pathways, and following resection of large tumors in the frontal recess region. The procedure consists of performing an osteotomy in the coronal plane to open the frontal sinus (Fig. 3.37). Typically, the sinus mucosa is removed and the frontal recess is packed with fat graft or other material, and the bone flap is then returned to its original position. Complications of the osteoplastic flap frontal sinus obliteration include retained secretions (Fig. 3.38); mucoceles (Fig. 3.39), which can result in mass effect upon the brain or orbital contents; extrusion of packing material (Fig. 3.40); and hardware complications (Fig. 3.41). While CT is useful for delineating the condition of the osteoplastic flap and associated hardware, MRI is useful for further characteriz-ing the contents of the appearance of the surgical bed on MRI varies based on the contents as follows:

Central

High T2-weighted signal intensity, no enhancement: Secretions or fat

High T2-weighted signal intensity, enhancement: Granulation tissue or inflammation

Low T2-weighted signal intensity, no enhancement: Fibrosis or secretions

Low T2-weighted signal intensity, enhancement: Granulation or scar tissue

Peripheral

High T2-weighted signal intensity, no enhancement: Mucosa or fluid

High T2-weighted signal intensity, enhancement: Mucosa or granulation tissue

Low T2-weighted signal intensity, no enhancement: Fibrosis

Low T2-weighted signal intensity, enhancement: Granulation tissue and neovascularity

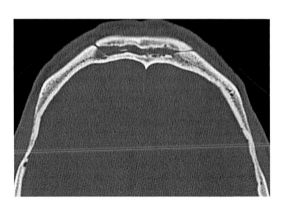

Fig. 3.37 Osteoplastic flap expected appearance. Axial CT image shows bilateral frontal bone osteotomies and obliteration of the frontal sinuses

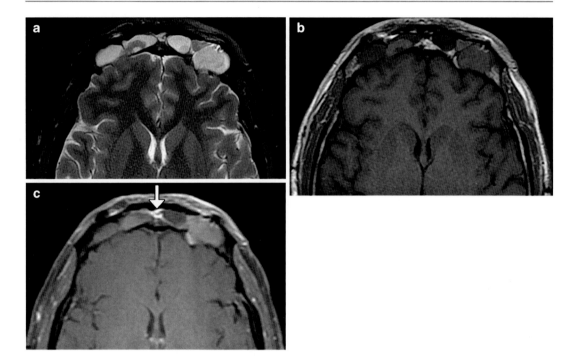

Fig. 3.38 Osteoplastic flap with retained secretions. Axial fat-suppressed T2-weighted (**a**), T1-weighted (**b**), and fat-suppressed post-contrast T1-weighted (**c**) MRI images show extensive non-enhancing material within the frontal sinuses beneath the osteoplastic flap, as well as enhancing mucosa (*arrow*)

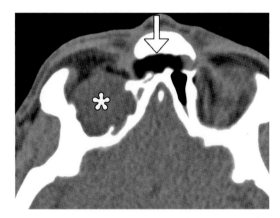

Fig. 3.39 Mucocele associated with frontal sinus obliteration. Axial CT image shows a mucocele with intraorbital extension (*) that resulted from obstruction of a supraorbital ethmoid cell by the osteoplastic flap fat packing material (*arrow*)

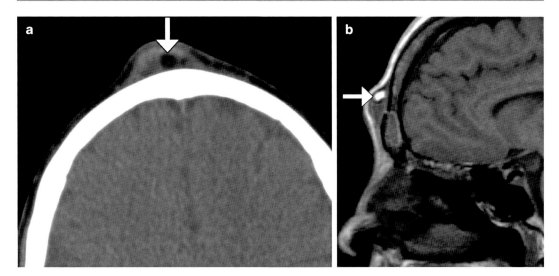

Fig. 3.40 Extruded packing material and inflammatory debris. The patient presented with forehead swelling after osteoplastic flap surgery. Axial CT image (**a**) shows a fragment of fat packing in the frontal subgaleal space (*arrow*) surrounded by soft tissue material. Sagittal T1-weighted MRI (**b**) shows that the soft tissue (*arrow*) in the subgaleal space indeed communicates with the residual frontal sinus through the osteotomy. The soft tissue represents a mucocele with chronic inflammatory debris

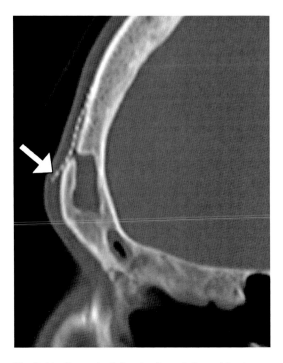

Fig. 3.41 Cosmetic deformity from deformed hardware. Sagittal CT image demonstrates a kink in the osteoplastic flap titanium mesh, which projects into the subcutaneous tissues (*arrow*). The patient subsequently underwent hardware removal

3.13   Frontal Sinus Cranialization

3.13.1 Discussion

Cranialization of the frontal sinuses is performed when there is disruption of the posterior wall of the frontal sinus, which can be secondary to mucoceles, trauma, arteriovenous malformations, or infection, and serves to incorporate the frontal sinus into the intracranial compartment. The procedure involves mucosal exenteration, irrigation, cranialization, and packing of the residual frontal sinus cavity and frontonasal drainage pathway using various materials (Fig. 3.42).

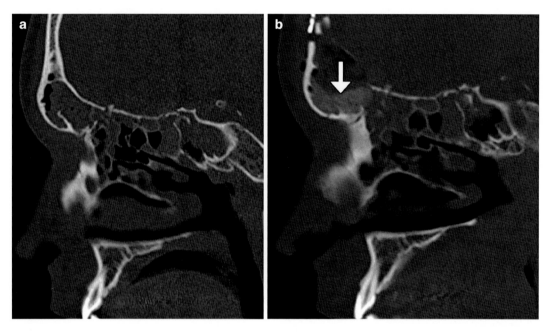

Fig. 3.42 Frontal sinus cranialization. The patient incurred facial fractures, which involved the frontal sinuses, which is shown to be opacified on the preoperative sagittal CT image (**a**). Postoperative sagittal CT image (**b**) shows interval frontobasal craniotomy for removal of the inner table of the frontal sinus and insertion of bone paste (*arrow*) to eliminate the connection with the rest of the sinonasal cavities

3.14   Paranasal Sinus Stents

3.14.1 Discussion

Paranasal sinus stents can be used to improve intranasal drainage and to maintain patency and drainage after sinus surgery, particularly when the neo-ostium measures less than 5 mm. Most stents are self-retaining and can be inserted endoscopically. The stents are usually a temporary measure, but occasionally remain for over 1 year. Potential complications include dislodgment and obstruction, especially for long-term stents. In particular, stents can predispose to scarring. Sinus stents are hollow tubular structures with a relatively wide flange or "mushroom" at one end in order to secure the device in position. CT is useful for evaluating the position of the stent and associated complications, if needed (Fig. 3.43).

3.15   Frontal Sinus Trephination

3.15.1 Discussion

Frontal sinus trephination consists of creating a defect in the sinus and is performed to provide access for drainage or culture of infected material, particularly if there is intracranial involvement. The procedure can also be performed in conjunction with functional endoscopic sinus surgery for enhanced visualization and irrigation of the frontal sinus and for resection of type IV frontal cells, which cannot be attained from an endonasal approach. The trephination defect is usually located approximately 1 cm lateral to the midline, and an external drainage catheter can be left in position (Fig. 3.44).

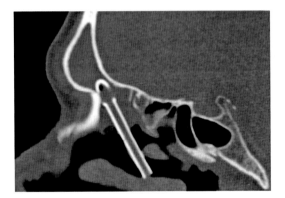

Fig. 3.43 Sinus stent. The patient was treated for frontal sinus obstruction secondary to a mass lesion. Sagittal CT image demonstrates a right frontal sinus stent that is actually positioned too far inferiorly

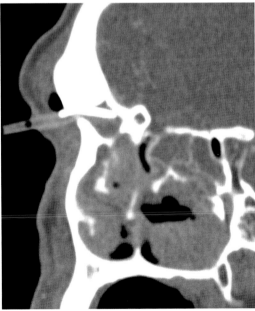

Fig. 3.44 Frontal sinus trephination with catheter. Sagittal CT image shows a catheter that exits through the skin from the opacified right frontal sinus via a window in the outer table of the inferior sinus projecting through the skin

3.16   Decompression, Enucleation, and Ostectomy

3.16.1   Discussion

Ostectomy and drainage can be used to treat cystic lesions that involve maxillary sinuses. This involves creating a Caldwell-Luc-type defect in the maxillary antrum and inserting a drainage tube in order to decompress the lesion (Fig. 3.45). Alternatively, surgical enucleation can be used to treat keratocystic odontogenic tumors, which originate in the maxillary alveolus and extend into the maxillary sinus. In order to minimize the recurrence rate, adjunctive measures such as ostectomy or en bloc resection can be performed. Furthermore, cryotherapy and instillation of the cyst cavity with Carnoy's solution or balsam of Peru after enucleation can be used to ablate residual tissue (Fig. 3.46). Recurrent odontogenic cysts manifest as gradual scalloping of the maxillary bone at the resection site on follow-up imaging (Fig. 3.47).

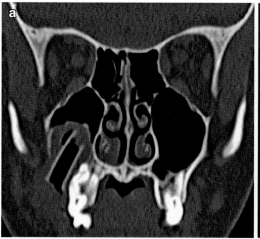
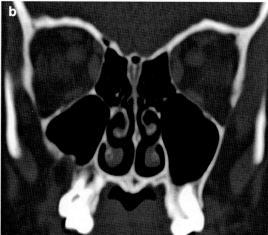
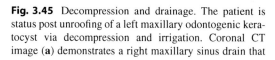

Fig. 3.45 Decompression and drainage. The patient is status post unroofing of a left maxillary odontogenic keratocyst via decompression and irrigation. Coronal CT image (**a**) demonstrates a right maxillary sinus drain that passes across a wide antrostomy. Coronal CT (**b**) image obtained 1 year later demonstrates interval removal of the drain and resolution of the lesion

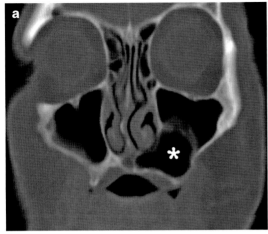
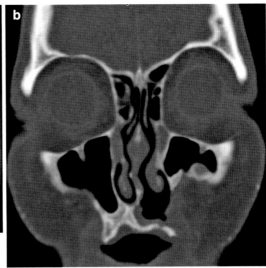

Fig. 3.46 Enucleation and ostectomy. Preoperative coronal CT image (**a**) shows an odontogenic keratocyst (*) projecting into the left maxillary sinus. The cyst is air filled due to prior spontaneous drainage into the oral cavity. Postoperative coronal CT image (**b**) obtained 1 year following enucleation and packing with balsam of Peru shows soft tissue filling the space previously occupied by the cyst (*arrow*)

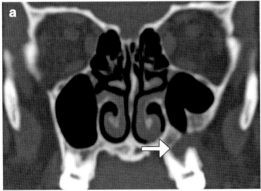
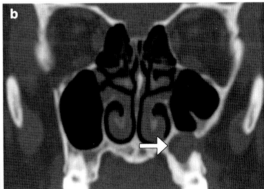

Fig. 3.47 Residual/recurrent lesion. The patient is status post enucleation and ostectomy for a left maxillary odontogenic keratocyst. Initial postoperative coronal CT image (**a**) shows the left maxillary sinus ostectomy site (*arrow*). Follow-up CT at 1 year (**b**) demonstrates interval scalloping of the maxillary bone (*arrow*)

3.17 Maxillectomy and Palatectomy

3.17.1 Discussion

Maxillectomy consists of removing at least a portion of the maxillary sinus. The degree of resection ranges from partial/lateral maxillectomy, total maxillectomy, maxillectomy with palatectomy, and pterygoid plate resection to craniofacial resection, depending on the extent of disease (Figs. 3.48 and 3.49). Obturators are often used to occlude the oronasal communication that results from palatectomy (Fig. 3.50). Many of these devices contain metal parts and should be removed prior to imaging in order to minimize artifact. Obturators otherwise have variable appearances on CT, ranging from hyperattenuating to heterogeneous to air-filled components. Bone and soft tissue flaps can also be used to reconstruct the surgical resection defects (Figs. 3.51 and 3.52). In addition, titanium mesh, plates and screws, and plastic slings are often used to support the constructs. Both CT and MRI with contrast are useful for follow-up, particularly to asses for recurrent tumor. With extensive resections, the pterygopalatine fossa becomes altered by scar tissue (Fig. 3.53), which should not be confused with tumor recurrence on imaging, since these can feature enhancing soft tissue on imaging. Recurrent tumors can have variable appearances, but most commonly appear as growing mass lesions located at the surgical margins (Fig. 3.54). Comparison with prior studies, short-term follow-up, PET-CT, or biopsy should be considered in ambiguous cases. Of note, synthetic materials, such as polytetrafluoroethylene, that are sometimes used as slings in reconstruction of the soft tissues overlying the maxillectomy can produce foreign body granulomas, which can mimic tumor recurrence (Fig. 3.55). Similarly, dacryocystoceles in patients treated for sinonasal cancer can mimic recurrent tumor. However, these lesions characteristically appear as fluid-filled structures in the anteromedial orbit (Fig. 3.56). Dacryocystoceles may form secondary to obstruction by recurrent tumor, ablative surgery, radiation therapy, or certain chemotherapeutic agents. Finally, infected maxillectomy sites may be treated with implantation of antibiotic impregnated methyl methacrylate beads, which appear as hyperattenuating on CT (Fig. 3.57).

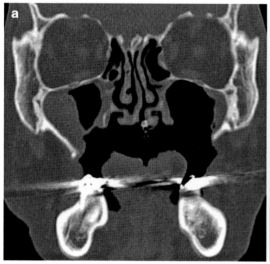
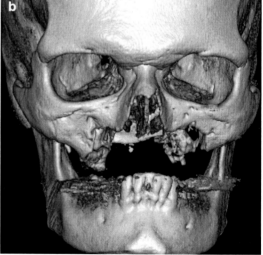

Fig. 3.48 Partial maxillectomy and total palatectomy. The patient has a history of leukemia status post bone marrow transplant with graft-versus-host disease invasive fungal infection involving the hard palate and maxillary sinuses. Bilateral partial maxillectomy was performed. Coronal (**a**) and 3D CT (**b**) images show resection of the bilateral medial maxillary sinus walls and the hard palate, resulting in continuity between the oral cavity, maxillary sinuses, and nasal cavity. There are mandibular dental amalgam artifacts that should not be confused for a prosthesis related to the surgery

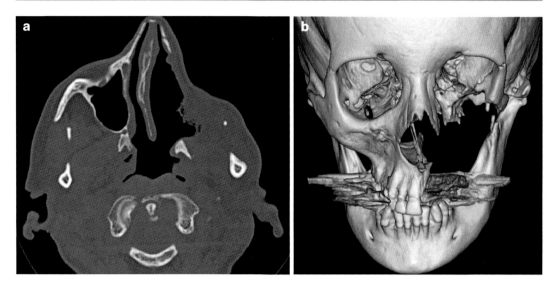

Fig. 3.49 Total maxillectomy. Axial (**a**) and 3D (**b**) CT images show the absence of the vast majority of the left maxillary bone, leaving the pterygoid plate intact, but sclerotic

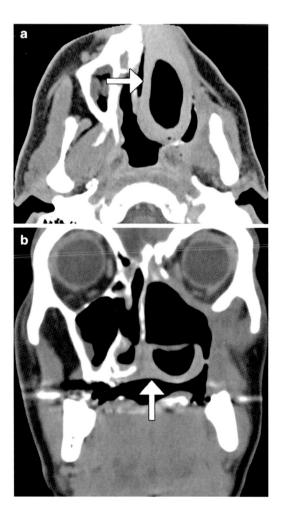

Fig. 3.50 Total maxillectomy and palatectomy with obturator. Axial (**a**) and coronal (**b**) CT images show complete resection of the left maxillary sinus, including the orbital floor, and left hemipalatectomy. An obturator device is present (*arrows*)

Fig. 3.51 Palatectomy with radial forearm free flap reconstruction. Coronal (**a**) and sagittal (**b**) CT images show resection of the hard and soft palate. The defect is closed using a soft tissue graft (*arrows*)

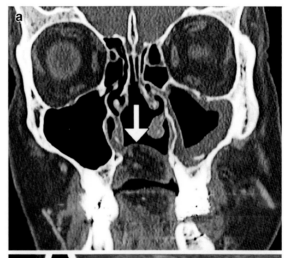

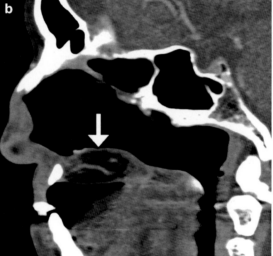

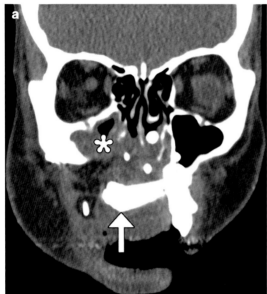
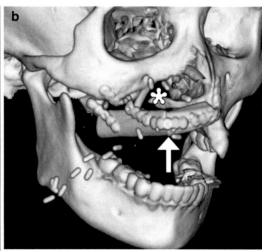

Fig. 3.52 Palatectomy and maxillectomy with osteomyocutaneous flap reconstruction. The patient has a history of desmoplastic ameloblastoma extending into the right maxillary sinus. Coronal (**a**) and 3D (**b**) CT images show right partial maxillectomy and palatectomy. Fibular graft (*arrows*) has been used to reconstruct the contours of the maxillary alveolus, and the myocutaneous portion of the graft forms the floor of the maxillary sinus and nasal cavity, creating a neoantrum (*)

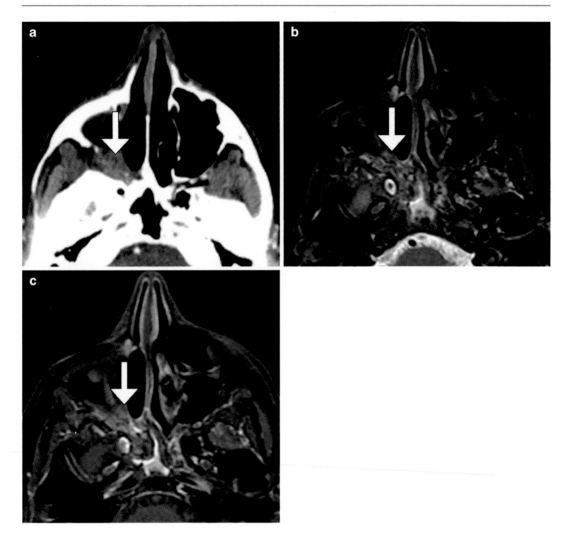

Fig. 3.53 Postoperative pterygopalatine fossa. The patient underwent maxillectomy for breast cancer metastasis. Axial CT image (**a**) shows amorphous fibrovascular tissue at the posterior margin of the left partial maxillec-tomy (*arrows*). Axial T2-weighted (**b**) and post-contrast T1-weighted (**c**) MR images show that this tissue has low T1 and T2 signal, but enhances (*arrows*)

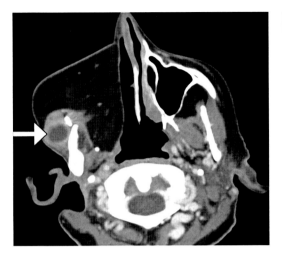

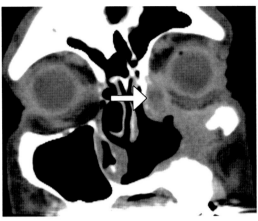

Fig. 3.56 Postoperative dacryocystocele. Coronal CT image shows postoperative findings related to left sinonasal surgery, with dilatation of the lacrimal sac (*arrow*)

Fig. 3.54 Flap reconstruction with tumor recurrence. The patient has a history of squamous cell carcinoma and is status post right total maxillectomy with flap reconstruction. Axial CT image shows a necrotic mass (*arrow*) at the reconstruction flap margin

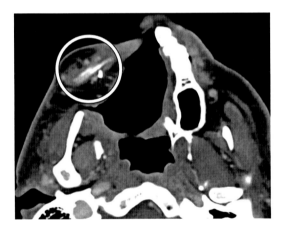

Fig. 3.55 Foreign body reaction. Axial CT image shows soft tissue surrounding a polytetrafluoroethylene sling (*encircled*)

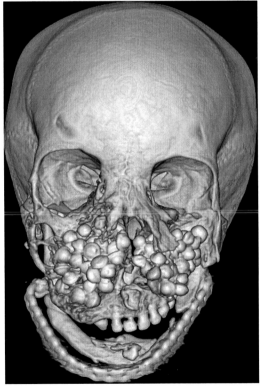

Fig. 3.57 Antibiotic-impregnated beads. 3D CT image shows numerous hyperattenuating beads in the bilateral maxillectomy cavities in a patient who underwent prior odontogenic myxoma debulking with superimposed infection of the surgical bed

3.18 Maxillary Swing

3.18.1 Discussion

The maxillary swing approach is sometimes used to resect nasopharyngeal and pterygopalatine fossa tumors. The technique includes several osteotomies through and around the maxillary sinus in order to free the structure and rotate it laterally and expose the underlying lesions (Fig. 3.58). The infraorbital nerve is often sacrificed during the procedure. Recurrent tumors can spread through the osteotomy sites (Figs. 3.58 and 3.59).

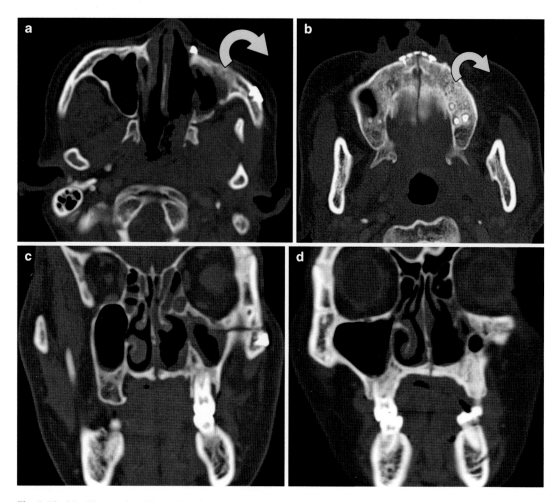

Fig. 3.58 Maxillary swing. The patient has a history of nasopharyngeal carcinoma, which was resected via the maxillary swing approach. Axial (**a**, **b**) and coronal (**c**, **d**) CT images show multiple osteotomy sites, most of which are secured by microfixation plates, including the left nasal process of the maxillary bone, the posterior maxillary wall, the zygomatic process, and the midline hard palate, in order to allow the maxillary sinus to rotate laterally (*curved yellow arrows*). The left infraorbital nerve was sacrificed by the osteotomy

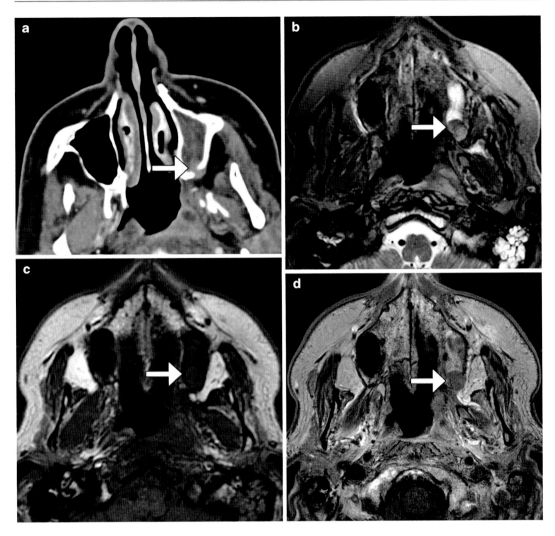

Fig. 3.59 Recurrent tumor. The patient has a history of nasopharyngeal carcinoma resected via a maxillary swing approach. Axial CT image (**a**) demonstrates a nodular lesion (*arrows*) that insinuates across the left posterior maxillary wall osteotomy defect. The corresponding axial T2-weighted (**b**), T1-weighted (**c**), and post-contrast T1-weighted (**d**) MR images show that the intermediate T2 signal lesion enhances (*arrows*)

Further Reading

Nasal Fracture Reconstruction (Posttraumatic Rhinoplasty)

Cox AJ 3rd (2000) Nasal fractures – the details. Facial Plast Surg 16(2):87–94

Frodel JL Jr (1995) Management of the nasal dorsum in central facial injuries. Indications for calvarial bone grafting. Arch Otolaryngol Head Neck Surg 121(3):307–312

Mondin V, Rinaldo A, Ferlito A (2005) Management of nasal bone fractures. Am J Otolaryngol 26(3):181–185

Ziccardi VB, Braidy H (2009) Management of nasal fractures. Oral Maxillofac Surg Clin North Am 21(2):203–208, vi

Septoplasty

Bloom JD, Kaplan SE, Bleier BS, Goldstein SA (2009) Septoplasty complications: avoidance and management. Otolaryngol Clin North Am 42(3):463–481

Dobratz EJ, Park SS (2009) Septoplasty pearls. Otolaryngol Clin North Am 42(3):527–537

Fettman N, Sanford T, Sindwani R (2009) Surgical management of the deviated septum: techniques in septoplasty. Otolaryngol Clin North Am 42(2):241–252, viii

Nasal Septal Button Prosthesis

Blind A, Hulterström A, Berggren D (2009) Treatment of nasal septal perforations with a custom-made prosthesis. Eur Arch Otorhinolaryngol 266(1):65–69

Mullace M, Gorini E, Sbrocca M, Artesi L, Mevio N (2006) Management of nasal septal perforation using silicone nasal septal button. Acta Otorhinolaryngol Ital 26(4):216–218

Inferior Turbinate Outfracture and Reduction

Min JY, Dhong HJ, Cho HJ, Chung SK, Kim HY. Evaluation of inferior turbinate outfracture outcomes using computed tomography. Rhinology. 2013;51(3):275–9

Nease CJ, Krempl GA (2004) Radiofrequency treatment of turbinate hypertrophy: a randomized, blinded, placebo-controlled clinical trial. Otolaryngol Head Neck Surg 130(3):291–299

Nurse LA, Duncavage JA (2009) Surgery of the inferior and middle turbinates. Otolaryngol Clin North Am 42(2):295–309. ix

Porter MW, Hales NW, Nease CJ, Krempl GA (2006) Long-term results of inferior turbinate hypertrophy with radiofrequency treatment: a new standard of care? Laryngoscope 116(4):554–557

Nasal Packing Material

Coulier B, Desgain O, Gielen I (2012) Sinonasal myospherulosis and paraffin retention cysts suggested by CT: report of a case. Head Neck Pathol 6(2):270–274

Hartley C, Ng KL, Jackson A (1995) CT and MR appearance of otolaryngologic packing materials. AJNR Am J Neuroradiol 16(8):1697–1702

Sindwani R, Cohen JT, Pilch BZ, Metson RB (2003) Myospherulosis following sinus surgery: pathological curiosity or important clinical entity? Laryngoscope 113(7):1123–1127

Weber RK (2009) Nasal packing and stenting. GMS Curr Top Otorhinolaryngol Head Neck Surg 8:Doc02

Rhinectomy

Chipp E, Prinsloo D, Rayatt S (2011) Rhinectomy for the management of nasal malignancies. J Laryngol Otol 125(10):1033–1037

Ciocca L, Bacci G, Mingucci R, Scotti R (2009) CAD-CAM construction of a provisional nasal prosthesis after ablative tumour surgery of the nose: a pilot case report. Eur J Cancer Care (Engl) 18(1):97–101

Sinus Lift

Abrahams JJ, Hayt MW, Rock R (2000) Sinus lift procedure of the maxilla in patients with inadequate bone for dental implants: radiographic appearance. AJR Am J Roentgenol 174(5):1289–1292

Ozyuvaci H, Aktas I, Yerit K, Aydin K, Firatli E (2005) Radiological evaluation of sinus lift operation: what the general radiologist needs to know. Dentomaxillofac Radiol 34(4):199–204

Caldwell-Luc Procedure

Barzilai G, Greenberg E, Uri N (2005) Indications for the Caldwell-Luc approach in the endoscopic era. Otolaryngol Head Neck Surg 132(2):219–220

Han JK, Smith TL, Loehrl TA, Fong KJ, Hwang PH (2005) Surgical revision of the post-Caldwell-Luc maxillary sinus. Am J Rhinol 19(5):478–482

Nemec SF, Peloschek P, Koelblinger C, Mehrain S, Krestan CR, Czerny C (2009) Sinonasal imaging after

Caldwell-Luc surgery: MDCT findings of an abandoned procedure in times of functional endoscopic sinus surgery. Eur J Radiol 70(1):31–34

Peleg M, Chaushu G, Mazor Z, Ardekian L, Bakoon M (1999) Radiological findings of the post-sinus lift maxillary sinus: a computerized tomography follow-up. J Periodontol 70(12):1564–1573

External Ethmoidectomy

Neal GD (1985) External ethmoidectomy. Otolaryngol Clin North Am 18(1):55–60

Functional Endoscopic Sinus Surgery

Archer S (2003) Functional endoscopic sinus surgery. Atlas Oral Maxillofac Surg Clin North Am 11(2):157–167

Ginat DT (2015) Posttreatment imaging of the paranasal sinuses following endoscopic sinus surgery. Neuroimaging Clin N Am 25(4):653–665

Kennedy DW, Zinreich SJ, Rosenbaum AE, Johns ME (1985) Functional endoscopic sinus surgery. Theory and diagnostic evaluation. Arch Otolaryngol 111(9):576–582

Levine HL (1990) Functional endoscopic sinus surgery: evaluation, surgery, and follow-up of 250 patients. Laryngoscope 100(1):79–84

FESS Complications

Bhatti MT, Schmalfuss IM, Mancuso AA (2005) Orbital complications of functional endoscopic sinus surgery: MR and CT findings. Clin Radiol 60(8):894–904

Bonfils P, Tavernier L, Abdel Rahman H, Mimoun M, Malinvaud D (2008) Evaluation of combined medical and surgical treatment in nasal polyposis – III. Correlation between symptoms and CT scores before and after surgery for nasal polyposis. Acta Otolaryngol 128(3):318–323

Chhabra N, Houser SM (2009) The diagnosis and management of empty nose syndrome. Otolaryngol Clin North Am 42(2):311–330. ix

Cunnane ME, Platt M, Caruso PA, Metson R, Curtin HD (2009) Medialization of the lamina papyracea after endoscopic ethmoidectomy: comparison of preprocedure and postprocedure computed tomographic scans. J Comput Assist Tomogr 33(1):79–81

DelGaudio JM, Hudgins PA, Venkatraman G, Beningfield A (2005) Multiplanar computed tomographic analysis of frontal recess cells: effect on frontal isthmus size and frontal sinusitis. Arch Otolaryngol Head Neck Surg 131(3):230–235

Friedman M, Bliznikas D, Vidyasagar R, Joseph NJ, Landsberg R (2006) Long-term results after endo-

scopic sinus surgery involving frontal recess dissection. Laryngoscope 116(4):573–579

Gotwald TF, Sprinzl GM, Fischer H, Rettenbacher T (2001) Retained packing gauze in the ethmoidal sinuses after endonasal sinus surgery: CT and surgical appearances. AJR Am J Roentgenol 177(6):1487–1489

Hol MK, Huizing EH (2000) Treatment of inferior turbinate pathology: a review and critical evaluation of the different techniques. Rhinology 38(4):157–166

Huang BY, Lloyd KM, DelGaudio JM, Jablonowski E, Hudgins PA (2009) Failed endoscopic sinus surgery: spectrum of CT findings in the frontal recess. Radiographics 29(1):177–195

Hudgins PA, Browning DG, Gallups J, Gussack GS, Peterman SB, Davis PC, Silverstein AM, Beckett WW, Hoffman JC Jr (1992) Endoscopic paranasal sinus surgery: radiographic evaluation of severe complications. AJNR Am J Neuroradiol 13(4):1161–1167

Kennedy DW (1992) Prognostic factors, outcomes, and staging in ethmoid sinus surgery. Laryngoscope 102(12 pt 2 suppl 57):1–18

Lee JT, Kennedy DW, Palmer JN, Feldman M, Chiu AG (2006) The incidence of concurrent osteitis in patients with chronic rhinosinusitis: a clinicopathological study. Am J Rhinol 20(3):278–282

Maskell S, Eze N, Patel P, Hosni A (2007) Laser inferior turbinectomy under local anaesthetic: a well tolerated out-patient procedure. J Laryngol Otol 121(10):957–961

May M, Levine HL, Mester SJ, Schaitkin B (1994) Complications of endoscopic sinus surgery: analysis of 2108 patients – incidence and prevention. Laryngoscope 104(9):1080–1083

McDonald SE, Robinson PJ, Nunez DA (2008) Radiological anatomy of the anterior ethmoidal artery for functional endoscopic sinus surgery. J Laryngol Otol 122(3):264–267

Musy PY, Kountakis SE (2004) Anatomic findings in patients undergoing revision endoscopic sinus surgery. Am J Otolaryngol 25(6):418–422

Ophir D, Shapira A, Marshak G (1985) Total inferior turbinectomy for nasal airway obstruction. Arch Otolaryngol 111(2):93–95

Otto KJ, DelGaudio JM (2010) Operative findings in the frontal recess at time of revision surgery. Am J Otolaryngol 31(3):175–180

Payne SC (2009) Empty nose syndrome: what are we really talking about? Otolaryngol Clin North Am 42(2):331–337. ix–x

Platt MP, Cunnane ME, Curtin HD, Metson R (2008) Anatomical changes of the ethmoid cavity after endoscopic sinus surgery. Laryngoscope 118(12):2240–2244

Rene C, Rose GE, Lenthall R, Moseley I (2001) Major orbital complications of endoscopic sinus surgery. Br J Ophthalmol 85(5):598–603

Schaitkin B, May M, Shapiro A, Fucci M, Mester SJ (1993) Endoscopic sinus surgery: 4-year follow-up on the first 100 patients. Laryngoscope 103(10):1117–1120

Thacker NM, Velez FG, Demer JL, Rosenbaum AL (2004) Strabismic complications following endoscopic sinus surgery: diagnosis and surgical management. J AAPOS 8(5):488–494

Yang BT, Liu YJ, Wang YZ, Wang XY, Wang ZC (2012) CT and MR imaging findings of periorbital lipogranuloma developing after endoscopic sinus surgery. AJNR Am J Neuroradiol 33(11):2140–2143

Osteoplastic Flap with Frontal Sinus Obliteration

Isa AY, Mennie J, McGarry GW (2011) The frontal osteoplastic flap: does it still have a place in rhinological surgery? J Laryngol Otol 125(2):162–168

Lee JM, Palmer JN (2011) Indications for the osteoplastic flap in the endoscopic era. Curr Opin Otolaryngol Head Neck Surg 19(1):11–15

Loevner LA, Yousem DM, Lanza DC, Kennedy DW, Goldberg AN (1995) MR evaluation of frontal sinus osteoplastic flaps with autogenous fat grafts. AJNR Am J Neuroradiol 16(8):1721–1726

Frontal Sinus Cranialization

Donath A, Sindwani R (2006) Frontal sinus cranialization using the pericranial flap: an added layer of protection. Laryngoscope 116(9):1585–1588

Rodriguez ED, Stanwix MG, Nam AJ, St Hilaire H, Simmons OP, Manson PN (2009) Definitive treatment of persistent frontal sinus infections: elimination of dead space and sinonasal communication. Plast Reconstr Surg 123(3):957–967

Rontal ML (2008) State of the art in craniomaxillofacial trauma: frontal sinus. Curr Opin Otolaryngol Head Neck Surg 16(4):381–386

van Dijk JM, Wagemakers M, Korsten-Meijer AG, Kees Buiter CT, van der Laan BF, Mooij JJ (2012) Cranialization of the frontal sinus--the final remedy for refractory chronic frontal sinusitis. J Neurosurg 116(3):531–535

Paranasal Sinus Stents

Lin D, Witterick IJ (2008) Frontal sinus stents: how long can they be kept in? J Otolaryngol Head Neck Surg 37(1):119–123

Rains BM 3rd (2001) Frontal sinus stenting. Otolaryngol Clin North Am 34(1):101–110

Frontal Sinus Trephination

Batra PS, Citardi MJ, Lanza DC (2005) Combined endoscopic trephination and endoscopic frontal sinusotomy for management of complex frontal sinus pathology. Am J Rhinol 19(5):435–441

Hahn S, Palmer JN, Purkey MT, Kennedy DW, Chiu AG (2009) Indications for external frontal sinus procedures for inflammatory sinus disease. Am J Rhinol Allergy 23(3):342–347

Lee AS, Schaitkin BM, Gillman GS (2010) Evaluating the safety of frontal sinus trephination. Laryngoscope 120(3):639–642

Decompression, Enucleation, and Ostectomy

Brown JS, Rogers SN, McNally DN, Boyle M (2000) A modified classification for the maxillectomy defect. Head Neck 22(1):17–26

Parrish NC, Warden PJ (2010) A review of oro-antral communications. Gen Dent 58(4):312–317

Sharif FNJ, Oliver R, Sweet C, Sharif MO (2010) Interventions for the treatment of keratocystic odontogenic tumours (KCOT, odontogenic keratocysts (OKC)). Cochrane Database Syst Rev (9):CD008464

Maxillectomy and Palatectomy

Bridger AG, Smee D, Baldwin MA, Kwok B, Bridger GP (2005) Experience with mucosal melanoma of the nose and paranasal sinuses. ANZ J Surg 75(4):192–197

Chan LL, Chong J, Gillenwater AM, Ginsberg LE (2000) The pterygopalatine fossa: postoperative MR imaging appearance. AJNR Am J Neuroradiol 21(7):1315–1319

Debnam JM, Esmaeli B, Ginsberg LE (2007) Imaging characteristics of dacryocystocele diagnosed after surgery for sinonasal cancer. AJNR Am J Neuroradiol 28(10):1872–1875

Huang SF, Liao CT, Kan CR, Chen IH (2007) Primary mucosal melanoma of the nasal cavity and paranasal sinuses: 12 years of experience. J Otolaryngol 36(2):124–129

Moreno MA, Roberts DB, Kupferman ME, DeMonte F, El-Naggar AK, Williams M, Rosenthal DS, Hanna EY (2010) Mucosal melanoma of the nose and paranasal sinuses, a contemporary experience from the M.D. Anderson Cancer Center. Cancer 116(9):2215–2223

Maxillary Swing

Bendor-Samuel R, Chen YR, Chen PK (1995) Unusual complications of the Le Fort I osteotomy. Plast Reconstr Surg 96(6):1289–1296

Bhaskaran AA, Courtney DJ, Anand P, Harding SA (2010) A complication of Le Fort I osteotomy. Int J Oral Maxillofac Surg 39(3):292–294

Brown DH (1989) The Le Fort I maxillary osteotomy approach to surgery of the skull base. J Otolaryngol 18(6):289–292

Honda K, Asato R, Tanaka S, Endo T, Nishimura K, Ito J (2008) Vidian nerve schwannoma with middle cranial fossa extension resected via a maxillary swing approach. Head Neck 30(10):1389–1393

Wei WI, Ho CM, Yuen PW, Fung CF, Sham JS, Lam KH (1995) Maxillary swing approach for resection of tumors in and around the nasopharynx. Arch Otolaryngol Head Neck Surg 121(6):638–642

Imaging the Postoperative Scalp and Cranium

4

Daniel Thomas Ginat, Ann-Christine Duhaime, and Marc Daniel Moisi

4.1 Occipital Nerve Stimulator

4.1.1 Discussion

Occipital neuralgia that does not respond to conservative management is sometimes responsive to occipital nerve stimulation. Unilateral or bilateral electrodes are implanted in the posterior scalp subcutaneous tissues in contact with the occipital nerves. The device is connected to a generator that is typically located subcutaneously in the chest. The main complications of this technique include electrode dislodgment and infection. Radiographs can depict the course of the leads, which is a nearly horizontal orientation in the occipital subcutaneous tissues, perpendicular to the course of the greater occipital nerves (Fig. 4.1). CT or MRI can be used to evaluate the extent of clinically suspected infection and other soft tissue complications.

D.T. Ginat, M.D., M.S. (✉)
Department of Radiology,
University of Chicago, Chicago, IL, USA
e-mail: dtg1@uchicago.edu

A.-C. Duhaime, M.D.
Harvard Medical School,
Massachusetts General Hospital, Boston, MA, USA

M.D. Moisi, M.D., M.S.
Swedish Neuroscience Institute, Seattle, WA, USA

© Springer International Publishing Switzerland 2017
D.T. Ginat, P.-L.A. Westesson (eds.), *Atlas of Postsurgical Neuroradiology*,
DOI 10.1007/978-3-319-52341-5_4

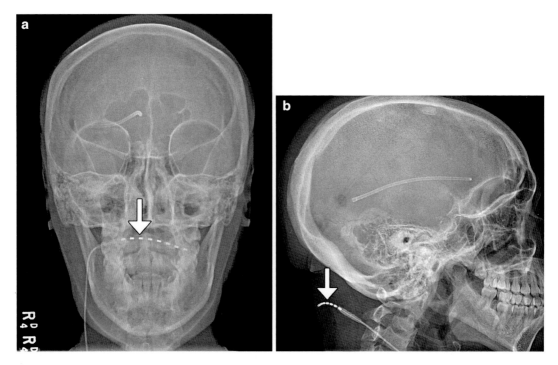

Fig. 4.1 Occipital nerve stimulator. The patient has a history of intractable migraine headaches. Frontal (**a**) and lateral (**b**) radiographs of the skull show the electrodes situated in the bilateral occipital subcutaneous tissues (*arrows*)

4.2   Tissue Expander

4.2.1   Discussion

Tissue expanders are used to stretch the skin for later use in various reconstructive procedures, such as to correct burn alopecia. These devices are essentially fluid-filled silicone sacs, connected to an infusion port. The conventional expander requires serial filling over a period of several months. Osmotic self-filling expanders are also available. On CT, the expander appears as a fluid-filled sac within the scalp (Fig. 4.2). A radial fold may project into the lumen of the expander. These can attain relatively large sizes. Identification of an infusion port helps distinguish the device from an abscess. Many of the infusion ports have magnetic components that are not MRI compatible. Complications related to tissue expanders include extrusion and rupture. The presence of a radial fold is a normal feature of certain tissue expanders and should not be mistaken for rupture.

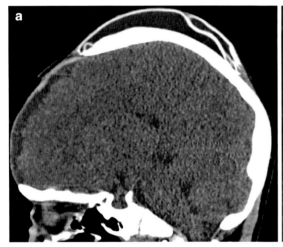
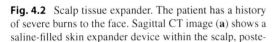
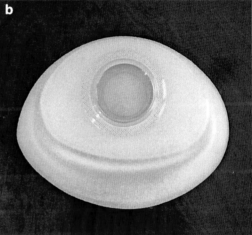

Fig. 4.2 Scalp tissue expander. The patient has a history of severe burns to the face. Sagittal CT image (**a**) shows a saline-filled skin expander device within the scalp, posterior to the craniectomy defect. Photograph of an unfilled expander (**b**) (Courtesy of Melissa Guilbeau)

4.3   Temporal Fossa Implants

4.3.1   Discussion

Soft tissue deficiency in the temporal fossa can produce cosmetic impairment and can result from the transposition of temporalis myofascial flaps and tumor debulking procedures, among other surgeries. The contours of the temporal fossa can be augmented using implants, such as prefabricated porous high-density polyethylene (Fig. 4.3), silicone (Fig. 4.4), and methyl methacrylate (Fig. 4.5). The implants are usually inserted via a hemicoronal approach and can be secured using titanium screws to the underlying bone.

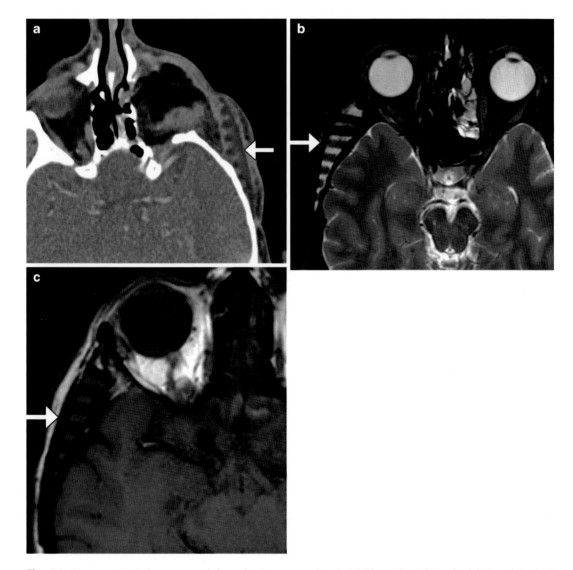

Fig. 4.3 Porous polyethylene temporal fossa implant. Axial CT image (**a**) shows a low-attenuation polyethylene implant with inner ridged surface positioned in the left temporal fossa (*arrows*). There is also left orbital exenteration. Axial T2-weighted (**b**) *and* axial T1-weighted (**c**) MR images in a different patient show a polyethylene implant in the right temporal fossa (*arrows*) with near-anatomic contours of the overlying scalp

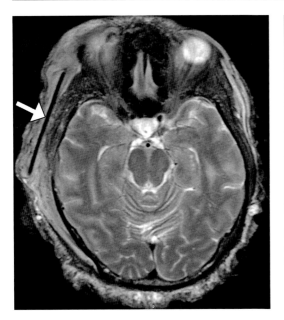

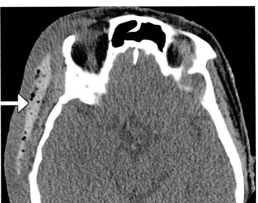

Fig. 4.5 Methyl methacrylate temporal fossa implant. Axial CT image shows a heterogeneous plate implanted in the right temporal scalp soft tissues (*arrow*)

Fig. 4.4 Silicone temporal fossa implant. The patient has a history of neurofibromatosis and is status post tumor debulking. Axial T2-weighted MRI shows a low-intensity plate in the right temporal scalp subcutaneous tissues (*arrow*)

4.4   Mohs Micrographic Surgery and Skin Grafting

4.4.1   Discussion

Mohs micrographic surgery is a technique that enables skin neoplasms to be fully resected while maximizing preservation of normal tissues. Mohs surgery consists of removing the tumor via sequential thin sections, which are concurrently examined under the microscope. The process is repeated until no remaining tumor is identified microscopically. When discernible on imaging, the defects characteristically appear as well-defined cavities in the skin and underlying soft tissues (Fig. 4.6). Large defects can be reconstructed using split-thickness skin grafts (Fig. 4.7), flaps, or synthetic materials such as AlloDerm.

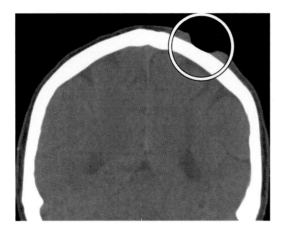

Fig. 4.6 Mohs micrographic surgery. The patient has a history of basal-cell carcinoma of the scalp. Coronal CT image shows a well-defined defect in the left scalp (*encircled*)

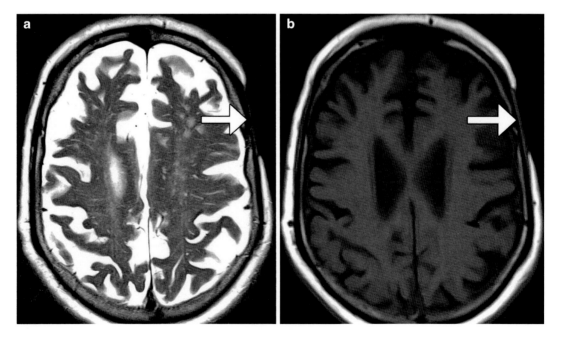

Fig. 4.7   Split-thickness skin graft. Axial T2-weighted (**a**) and T1-weighted (**b**) MR images show that the skin graft (*arrows*) is thinner than the adjacent normal scalp

4.5   Rotational Galeal Flap Scalp Reconstruction

4.5.1   Discussion

Galeal flaps, such as the retroauricular rotation flap, can be used to cover scalp defects as large as 60% of the scalp surface area. Galeal flaps are comprised of fascia, subcutaneous tissue, and vascular components. In the early postoperative period, a remote donor site defect can be apparent, such as with "flip-flop" flaps (Fig. 4.8). Galeal flaps can incur essentially the same complications as other types of flaps, including infection, tumor recurrence, and necrosis, as well as dehiscence and alopecia.

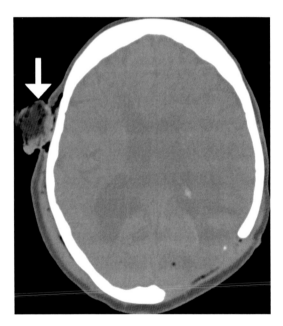

Fig. 4.8 Galeal flap, early postoperative period. The patient has a history of infected hardware, necrotic bone, and open scalp wound. A rotational scalp flap was advanced to cover the defect after wound debridement. Axial CT image shows a left parietal skull defect covered by a rotational fasciocutaneous flap. There is surgical packing material (*arrow*) in the contralateral donor site

4.6   Free Flap Reconstruction of Complex Scalp Defects

4.6.1   Discussion

Free flap transfer is used for repairing complex scalp defects in order to provide functional, cosmetic, and structural support when the use of skin grafts, locoregional flaps, and tissue expanders is not feasible. The latissimus dorsi myocutaneous flap is particularly useful for subtotal and total skull reconstruction, in which there is considerable dead space (Fig. 4.9). Latissimus dorsi flaps can be harvested with ribs (myo-osseocutaneous) or combined with titanium mesh for added support. Omental flaps are another option for closing large scalp and cranium defects (Fig. 4.10). These contain mostly adipose tissues and are covered by skin grafts. Other donor tissues for free flap transfer include rectus abdominis muscle flaps, scapular flap, radial forearm flap, and anterolateral thigh flap. Vascular supply is typically obtained via anastomosis to the superficial temporal artery and vein or at times the occipital artery. Complications include delayed flap failure, which requires secondary reconstruction, neck hematoma, venous thrombosis, skull base infection, large wound dehiscence, small wound dehiscence, donor site hematoma and seroma, and cerebrospinal fluid leak.

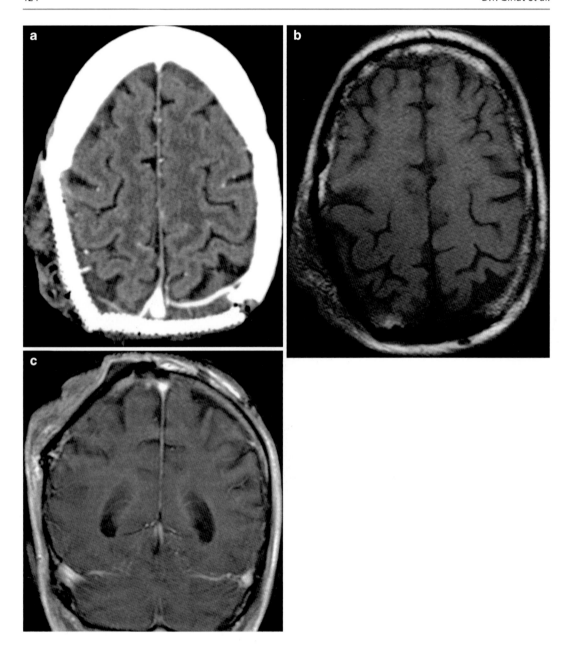

Fig. 4.9 Latissimus dorsi muscle flap. The patient has a history of extensive squamous cell carcinoma of the scalp, with invasion of the calvarium. Axial CT image (**a**) shows titanium cranioplasty of the right occipital and parietal regions and an overlying muscle flap. Characteristic muscle fibers are apparent in the flap on the axial T1-weighted MRI (**b**). Axial post-contrast T1-weighted MRI (**c**) shows enhancement of at least some of the muscle fibers

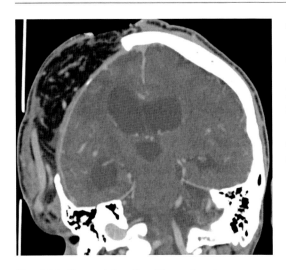

Fig. 4.10 Omental free flap. The patient is status post motorcycle accident during which loss of cranial bone occurred. Coronal CT image shows the flap overlying the right hemicraniectomy site contains fat and omental vessels and is covered by skin graft

4.7   Scalp Tumor Recurrence

4.7.1   Discussion

Most recurrent tumors manifest within the first 2 years following resection and are most common in the tumor bed near the anastomosis. Imaging can detect both locoregional recurrence and the extent of intracranial extension of recurrent tumors (Fig. 4.11). Postoperative imaging can also help in distinguishing tumor recurrence from fibrosis related to the surgery or radiation therapy. Recurrent tumors typically appear as nodular foci of enhancement and have higher T2-weighted signal intensity on MRI than fibrosis.

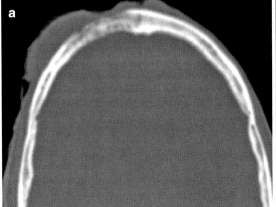
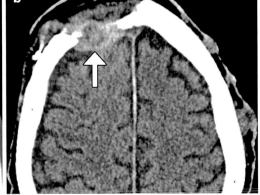

Fig. 4.11 Skin tumor recurrence. The patient has a history of locally invasive squamous cell carcinoma, presenting as a large fungating scalp lesion. Axial preoperative CT image (**a**) shows a right frontal scalp mass that invades the underlying skull. CT images obtained 14 months after surgery (**b**) show an enhancing mass (*arrow*) deep to the myocutaneous free flap. There are also several metastatic nodules in the left scalp

4.8 Burr Holes

4.8.1 Discussion

Burr hole craniostomy is a commonly performed maneuver as part of creating craniotomy flaps, stereotactic biopsy, hematoma decompression, ventricular endoscopic procedures, insertion of ventricular catheters, drains, and electrode insertion. Burr holes are surgical defects that traverse the full thickness of the calvarium created using various drills and can be packed with a variety of materials, such as bone wax and methyl methacrylate and may be covered with a plate (Fig. 4.12). Linear enhancement along the edges of burr holes is commonly observed as vascular granulation tissue forms, thereby potentially mimicking abscesses or neoplasms (Fig. 4.13).

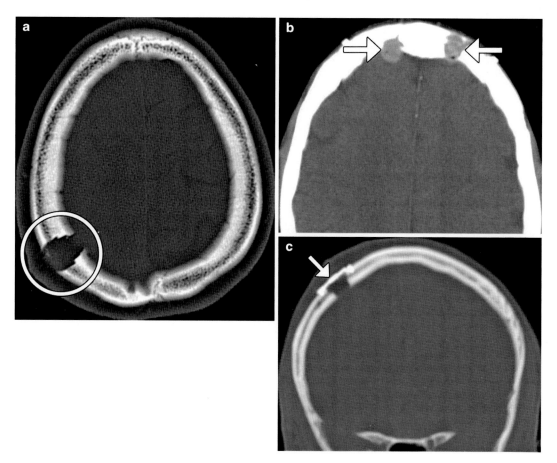

Fig. 4.12 Burr holes. Axial CT image (**a**) shows a right parietal calvarium defect that matches the contours of the drill (*encircled*). Axial CT image (**b**) shows methyl meth- acrylate filling the bifrontal burr holes (*arrows*). Axial CT image (**c**) shows a metallic burr hole cover (*arrow*)

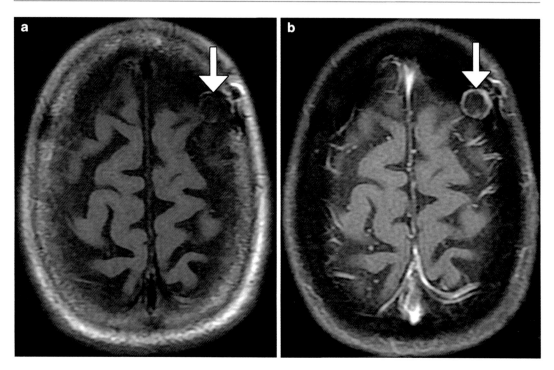

Fig. 4.13 Burr hole neovascularization. Axial T1-weighted (**a**) and post-contrast fat-suppressed T1-weighted (**b**) MR images show a left frontal burr hole with marginal enhancement (*arrows*)

4.9   Craniotomy

4.9.1   Discussion

Craniotomy consists of opening the cranial vault by removing a bone flap during the course of surgery and replacing it at the completion of the procedure, as opposed to craniectomy in which the bone is removed and not replaced. Once the skull is exposed by raising the overlying scalp and pericranial flap, burr holes are drilled, from which the bone flap is created using a saw or drill. The bone flap is set aside during the procedure and replaced upon completion of the surgery. Some of the standard types of craniotomy include the following:

- Pterional
- Orbitozygomatic
- Modified orbitozygomatic
- Frontal or bifrontal
- Parietal or biparietal
- Subtemporal
- Anterior parasagittal
- Posterior parasagittal
- Suboccipital
- Retrosigmoid
- Pre-sigmoid
- Far lateral
- Hemicraniotomy

Skin staples are often used to close the scalp flap after surgery and can be present on imaging during the early postoperative period (Fig. 4.14). A variety of devices and methods are available to secure cranial bone flaps following craniotomy. The most commonly used are microfixation plates or clamps (Fig. 4.15). Microfixation plates are often composed of titanium, which produces minimal streak or susceptibility artifact. Complications related to the presence of microfixation plates and screws, such as transcranial migration, are uncommon, except in young children, where absorbable hardware or suture may be used. Stainless steel wires threaded across the craniotomy margin to the bone plates is no longer performed in developed countries, but may still be encountered on imaging (Fig. 4.16).

Hinge craniotomy is an alternative to traditional decompressive craniectomy and allows swollen brain parenchyma to expand extracranially while avoiding some of the complications associated with cranial revision. The bone flap is left attached on one side to the scalp soft tissues, usually the temporalis muscle. This results in the appearance of an outwardly displaced bone flap on CT (Fig. 4.17).

The normal imaging appearance of the craniotomy site can evolve over time. In the early postoperative period, the bone flap margins are sharp and should align precisely with the rest of the skull, unless a craniectomy was done to provide more surgical accessibility. The extent of dural enhancement that normally occurs after craniotomy ranges considerably. Dural enhancement is present in the majority of patients following cranial surgery and can be seen within the first postoperative day (Fig. 4.18). The presence and degree of enhancement are largely dependent on the time elapsed since the time of surgery and the types of substitutes used during closure, which in some cases can persist indefinitely. Dural enhancement tends to be apparent earlier and lasts longer with gadolinium-based contrast than with iodine-based contrast. Granulation tissue also normally forms along the edges of the bone flap, which manifests as linear enhancement that is often visible on MRI and often accompanies dural enhancement. This type of enhancement usually persists up to 1 year following craniotomy.

Pneumocephalus is the presence of intracranial air and is an expected finding after recent cranial surgery. Indeed, virtually all patients exhibit some degree of pneumocephalus during the immediate postoperative period. Pneumocephalus can be identified by air attenuation on CT and signal voids on MRI (Fig. 4.19). Regardless of the location, pneumocephalus normally resolves within 3 weeks of surgery.

During the early postoperative period, typical changes also occur in the soft tissues overlying the craniotomy site, including temporalis muscle swelling (Fig. 4.20), which likely represents edema due to manipulation during surgery.

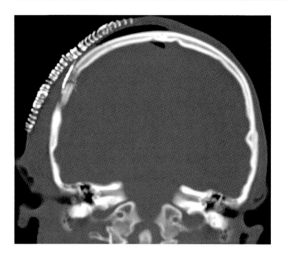

Fig. 4.14 Skin staples. Coronal CT image shows numerous staples (*arrows*) used to close the skin flap after craniotomy

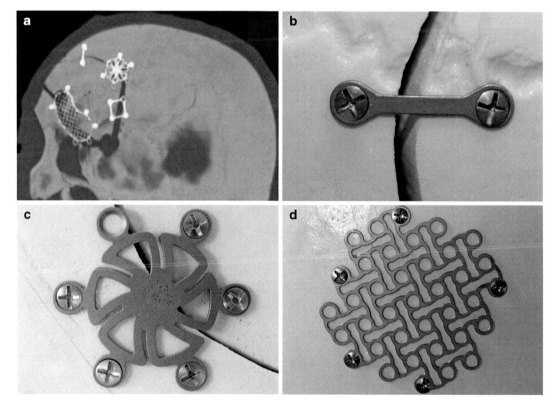

Fig. 4.15 Microfixation plates. 3D CT image (**a**) shows a variety of titanium microfixation plates securing the bone flap. Photographs of a variety of low-profile fixation plates (**b**–**d**) (Courtesy of Patricia Smith and Sarah Paengatelli)

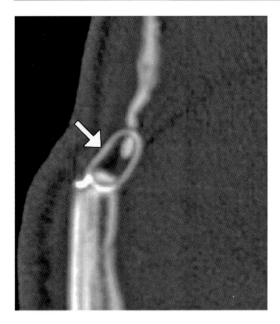

Fig. 4.16 Fixation wire. Axial CT image shows a stainless steel wire that secures the bone flap (*arrow*)

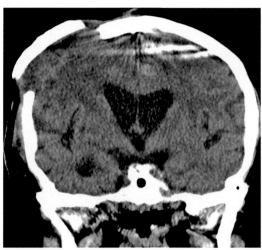

Fig. 4.17 Hinge craniotomy. Coronal CT image shows that the right parasagittal bone flap is not secured to the adjacent calvarium in order to allow the edematous brain to expand freely across the craniotomy defect

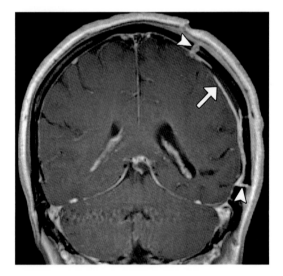

Fig. 4.18 Expected dural enhancement after craniotomy. Coronal post-contrast T1-weighted MRI shows linear dural enhancement deep to the craniotomy flap (*arrow*). There is also enhancement along the edges of the bone flap (*arrowheads*)

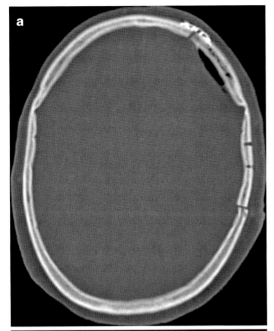

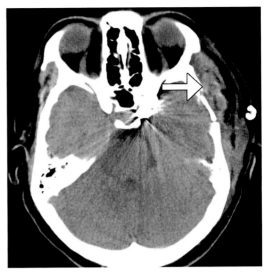

Fig. 4.20 Temporalis muscle swelling. Axial CT image obtained after recent left pterional craniotomy shows diffuse enlargement of the left temporalis muscle (*arrow*)

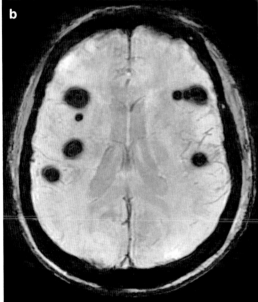

Fig. 4.19 Postoperative pneumocephalus. Axial CT image (**a**) shows and small amount of left frontal convexity extra-axial pneumocephalus. Axial SWI image in another patient (**b**) shows scattered foci of supratentorial signal voids from subarachnoid pneumocephalus after posterior fossa surgery

4.10 Cranioplasty

4.10.1 Discussion

Intraoperatively fashioned acrylic cranioplasty is composed of methyl methacrylate resin that can be molded to a desired shape on the surgical field. The material tends to appear heterogeneous on CT and low signal on MRI (Fig. 4.21). The material often contains multiple foci of air due to the exothermic reaction that occurs when formed. The trapped bubbles should not be confused with infection. The methyl methacrylate at times can migrate prior to hardening, the appearance of which can potentially mimic hemorrhage on CT.

Preformed acrylic methyl methacrylate plates are specially molded to fit individual craniectomy defects using a computer-aided design system and 3D CT data. These flaps are usually secured to the adjacent calvarium using titanium plates and are thus continuous with the calvarium. On CT, preformed acrylic plates demonstrate homogeneous intermediate attenuation, around 100 HU (Fig. 4.22). Unlike the acrylic plates prepared intraoperatively, the preformed plates do not contain air bubbles. However, the preformed acrylic plates contain holes that are drilled to promote tissue ingrowth and leave a pathway to prevent accumulation of fluid in the epidural space.

Hydroxyapatite cement paste is sometimes used to close off small gaps in the calvarium. It can be molded to match the particular anatomy and can be applied in conjunction with other materials, such as titanium mesh. The cement appears as homogeneously hyperattenuating on CT, similar in attenuation as natural bone (Fig. 4.23). On MRI, the hydroxyapatite appears as a signal void.

Titanium mesh is commonly used as a cranioplasty material. These plates generally produce good cosmetic results and minimal discomfort. Titanium produces minimal streak artifact on CT (Fig. 4.24). Solid titanium plates are now infrequently used but may be observed on follow-up imaging (Fig. 4.25).

Porous polyethylene implants are also suitable for covering cranial defects. This type of implant is also custom created for each patient using a computer-aided design system and 3D CT data. The material enables soft tissue and bone ingrowth and displays low attenuation on CT and low signal intensity on T2- and T1-weighted MRI sequences (Fig. 4.26).

Synthetic bone grafts that are biocompatible have been developed for cranioplasty. For example, Bioplant HTR Synthetic Bone is a microporous composite of poly(methyl methacrylate) (PMMA), polyhydroxyethylmethacrylate (PHEMA), and calcium hydroxide. On CT, the HTR cranioplasty appears as heterogeneous with an overall attenuation that is greater than soft tissue but lower than bone (Fig. 4.27).

Autologous bone grafts can also be used for cranioplasty. These are often used in the form of split calvarial grafts in which the inner table is separated from the outer table in order to increase surface area for maximal coverage of a craniectomy defect (Fig. 4.28).

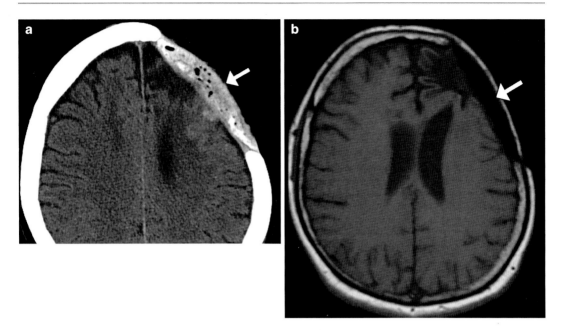

Fig. 4.21 Intraoperatively fashioned acrylic cranioplasty. Axial CT image (**a**) shows an acrylic cranioplasty flap containing low-attenuation bubbles (*arrow*). The cranio- plasty plate (*arrow*) has low signal on the corresponding T1-weighted MRI (**b**)

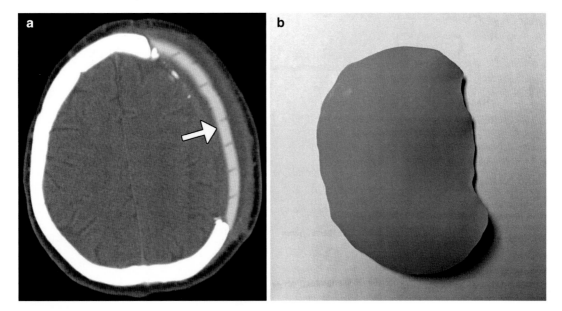

Fig. 4.22 Preformed acrylic cranioplasty. Axial CT image (**a**) demonstrates a high-attenuation left frontal acrylic cranioplasty (*arrow*), conforming to the natural contours of the calvarium. The plate is traversed by numerous holes to allow tissue ingrowth. Photograph of customized acrylic cranioplasty flap without holes (**b**)

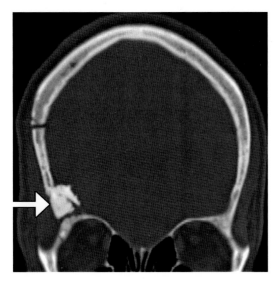

Fig. 4.23 Hydroxyapatite cement. Coronal CT image shows the hyperattenuating material (*arrow*) filling a gap between the craniotomy flap and the adjacent skull

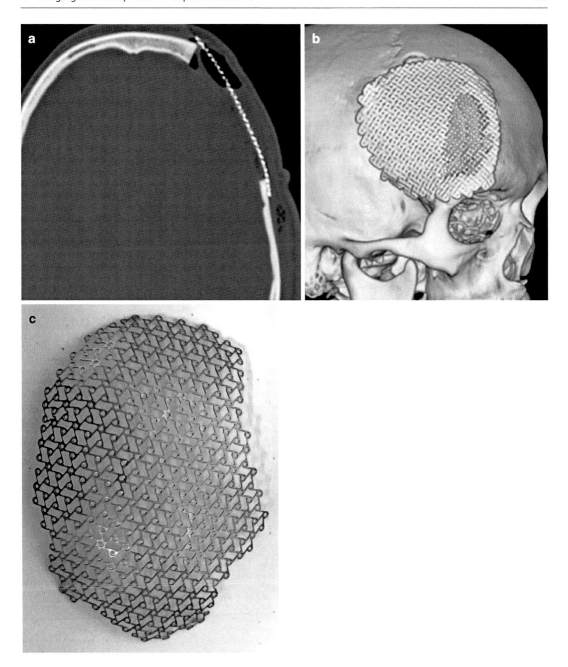

Fig. 4.24 Titanium mesh cranioplasty. Axial (**a**) and 3D surface rendered (**b**) CT images show a titanium mesh that spans a left frontal craniectomy defect. Photograph (**c**) of a titanium mesh (Courtesy of Caroline Dufault, RN)

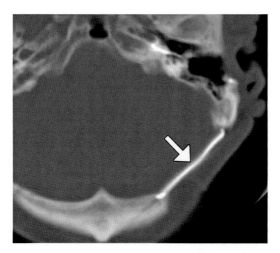

Fig. 4.25 Titanium plate. Axial CT image shows the metal attenuation plate (*arrow*) that spans the left retrosigmoid craniectomy, which was performed in the 1980s

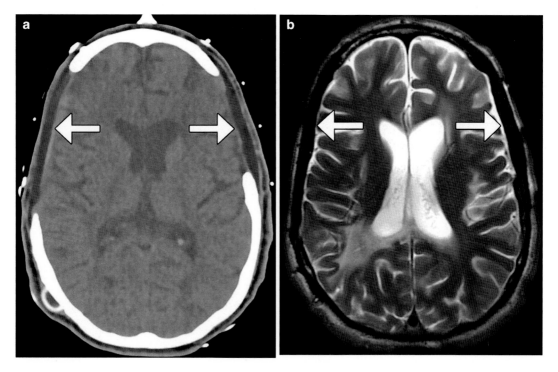

Fig. 4.26 Porex (porous polyethylene) cranioplasty. Axial CT image (**a**) shows bilateral low-attenuation implants (*arrow*). The cranioplasty material also displays low signal on T2-weighted (**b**) and T1-weighted (**c**) MR images

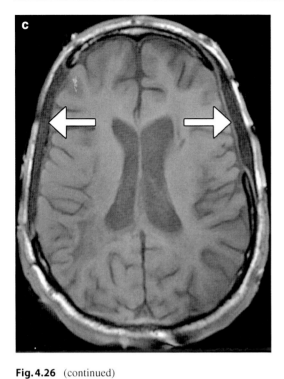

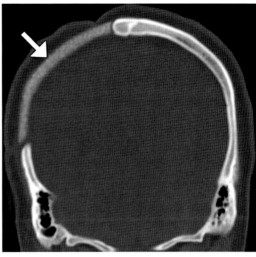

Fig. 4.27 Synthetic (HTR) bone graft cranioplasty. Coronal CT image shows right hemicraniectomy with heterogeneously hyperattenuating cranioplasty material (*arrow*)

Fig. 4.26 (continued)

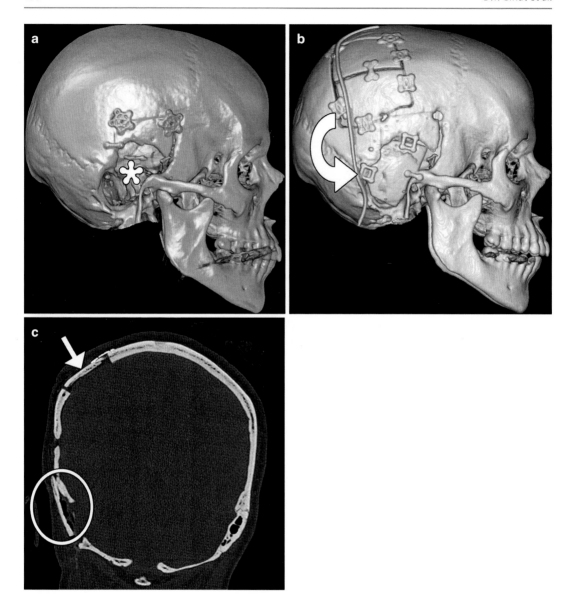

Fig. 4.28 Split-thickness bone graft cranioplasty. Initial 3D CT image (**a**) shows a right temporal skull defect (*). 3D CT image after cranioplasty (**b**) shows interval harvesting of bone from the right parietal calvarium and repositioning it into the temporal skull defect (*curved arrow*). Corresponding coronal CT image (**c**) shows the split calvarium at the donor site (*arrow*) and the repositioned split calvarial graft in the right temporal region (*encircled*)

4.11   Autocranioplasty

4.11.1   Discussion

Several options are available for storing autologous bone flaps after decompressive craniectomy for delayed autocranioplasty. Often, bone flaps are stored in a sterile freezer. This approach preserves the bone flap very well, providing good cosmetic results. An alternative is subcutaneous storage, which allows the bone flap to stay with the patient and may decrease the risk of devitalization and/or infection of the flap. Bone flaps can be kept fresh by implanting them into subcutaneous pockets in the abdomen and may be encountered on imaging (Fig. 4.29). Bone grafts stored in this manner tend to undergo remodeling.

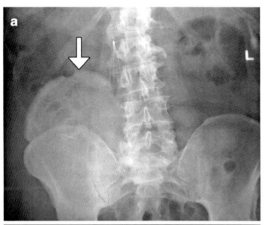
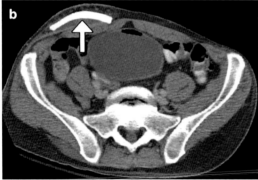

Fig. 4.29 Autocranioplasty. Frontal radiograph (**a**) and axial CT image (**b**) show a skull flap (*arrows*) embedded within the right lower quadrant subcutaneous tissues

4.12 Craniectomy, the Meningogaleal Complex, and Suboccipital Craniectomy

4.12.1 Discussion

Decompressive craniectomy is performed in order to decrease intracranial pressure when medical management alone is insufficient and is most commonly used in the setting of traumatic brain injury, subarachnoid hemorrhage, intraparenchymal hemorrhage, and cerebral infarction. The procedure consists of removal of portions of the skull, which is not replaced during the procedure. Hemicraniectomy is performed when one side of the brain is affected and usually entails removal of bone in the frontoparietotemporal region. On the other hand, bilateral (bifrontal) craniectomy is performed when both sides of the brain are affected and consists of removing the calvarium of the anterior cranial fossa to the coronal sutures.

Decompressive craniectomy has characteristic imaging findings. Following craniectomy, the galea aponeurotica becomes juxtaposed against the dura. Scar tissue then forms between these two layers, which creates the meningogaleal complex beneath the subcutaneous tissues. Normally, this complex measures between 2 and 6 mm in thickness. On CT, the meningogaleal complex is slightly hyperattenuating, while the appearance on MRI is variable depending on the degree of hypervascular tissue that is incorporated (Fig. 4.30). Smooth, uniform enhancement is expected on CT and MRI.

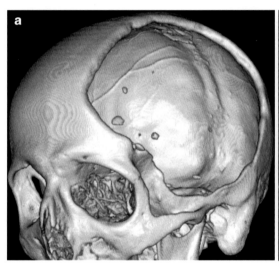
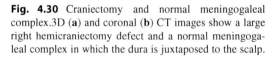
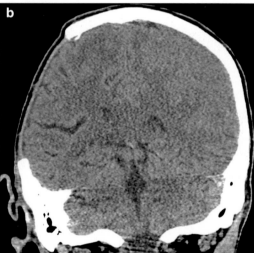

Fig. 4.30 Craniectomy and normal meningogaleal complex.3D (**a**) and coronal (**b**) CT images show a large right hemicraniectomy defect and a normal meningogaleal complex in which the dura is juxtaposed to the scalp.

Axial T2-weighted (**c**), T1-weighted (**d**), and post-contrast T1-weighted (**e**) MRI sequences in a different patient show enhancement of the left hemicraniectomy meningogaleal complex (*arrows*)

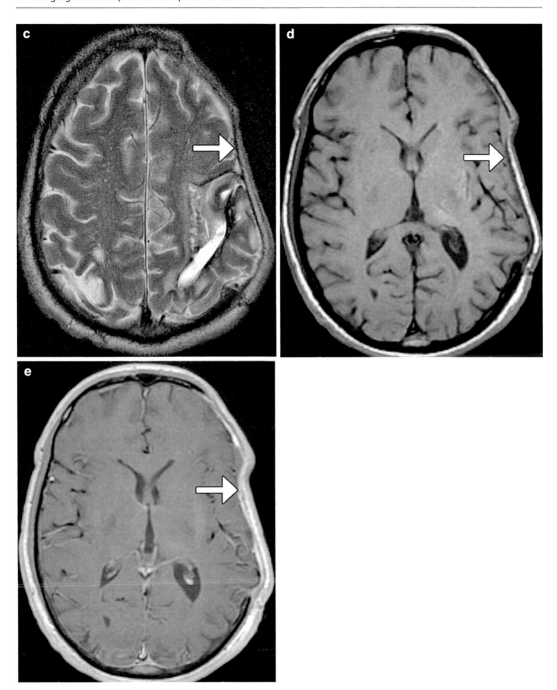

Fig. 4.30 (continued)

4.13 Cranial Vault Surgical Remodeling for Craniosynostosis

Sagittal synostosis is a relatively common type of craniosynostosis that results from premature fusion of the sagittal suture. Surgery is performed for relieving associated elevated intracranial pressure and for cosmesis. There are several approaches to correcting the deformity including bone removal and reshaping with barrel stave osteotomies (Fig. 4.31), endoscopic craniectomy with adjuvant use of a remodeling helmet, and placement of distraction devices. Follow-up imaging may be obtained for planning additional surgical reconstruction or if complications are suspected.

Correction cranioplasty and orbitofrontal advancement is a treatment option for trigonocephaly. This procedure generally entails take down of a bifrontal bone flap, removal of the orbital bandeau, followed by cranial vault reconstruction and advancement (Fig. 4.32). The use of reabsorbable fixation plate and screws yields superior cosmetic results and can appear as tiny bone defects without discernible radio-attenuating components otherwise on CT. The orbitofrontal advancement procedure can be augmented using onlay cements (Fig. 4.33). The incidence of complications is about 2%, and there is a 12% reoperation rate. Residual hypotelorism usually autocorrects, while bitemporal depressions may develop over time. High-resolution craniofacial CTs with 3D reformatted images are particularly useful for postoperative assessment and planning additional surgical intervention, if needed.

Management of raised intracranial pressure in syndromic multi-suture craniosynostosis by cranial vault expansion can be achieved by posterior calvarial vault expansion using distraction osteogenesis (Fig. 4.34).

Endoscopic craniosynostosis repair is a minimally invasive treatment option available to patients under 6 months of age. The technique consists of performing a strip craniectomy, whereby the affected suture is resected (suturectomy). This results in a linear gap along the course of the suture and allows the calvarium to be remodeled with postoperative helmet therapy (Fig. 4.35). Endoscopic-assisted wide-vertex craniectomy and barrel stave osteotomies can also be performed.

Calcium phosphate cement has been used to fill bony defects created during cranial remodeling surgery for craniosynostosis repair in the pediatric population and is intended to be osteoconductive. The bone cement initially has a putty-like consistency and can be applied in an inlay or onlay fashion. The material can undergo bioresorption and generally does not impede the actively growing calvarium. On CT, calcium phosphate cement appears as hyperattenuating with respect to bone (Fig. 4.36). The appearance of the junction between the native bone and the bone cement is variable, ranging from a sharp interface to a lucent gap when resorption occurs. The bone cement tends to be brittle and can also fragment. The presence of bone cement fragmentation does not necessarily imply palpable motility and is not particularly problematic if fragmentation occurs as an onlay.

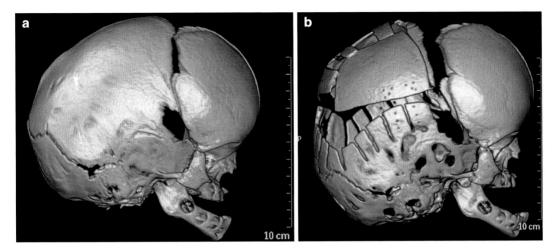

Fig. 4.31 Barrel stave osteotomies and cranial remodeling for scaphocephaly. Preoperative 3D CT image (**a**) shows dolichocephaly. Postoperative 3D CT image (**b**) demonstrates multiple parietal barrel stave osteotomies, resulting in improved skull morphology

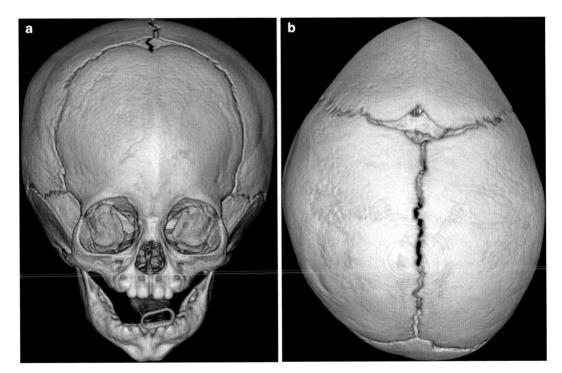

Fig. 4.32 Correction cranioplasty and orbitofrontal advancement. The patient has a history of nonsyndromic trigonocephaly. Preoperative frontal (**a**) and top view 3D CT (**b**) images show fusion of the metopic suture, with prominent frontal beaking. Postoperative frontal (**c**) and top view 3D CT (**d**) images show osteotomies along the orbital bandeau (*arrowheads*). The multiple tiny holes in the calvarium correspond to the attachment sites of the absorbable plates, which are otherwise not visible

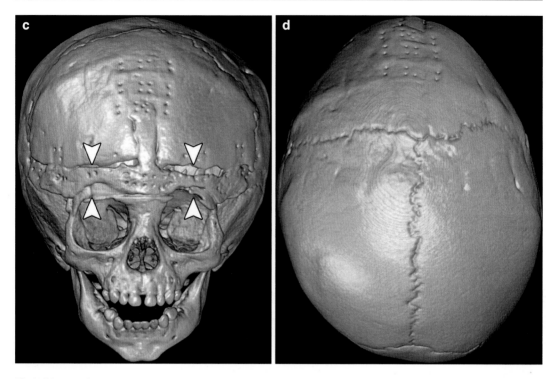

Fig. 4.32 (continued)

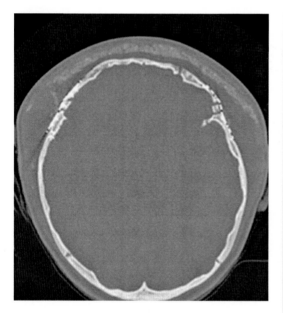

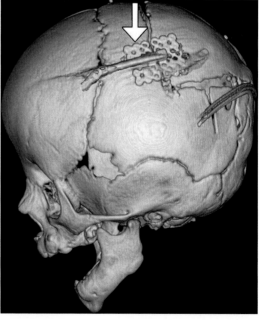

Fig. 4.33 Orbitofrontal advancement surgery with onlay cement. Axial CT image shows the hyperattenuating artificial bone cement superficial to the reconstructed frontal bone. The presence of seroma displaces the cement away from the surface of the calvarium and bifrontal craniotomies

Fig. 4.34 Posterior cranial vault distraction. Lateral 3D CT image of the skull shows parietal osteotomies with a distraction device in position (*arrow*)

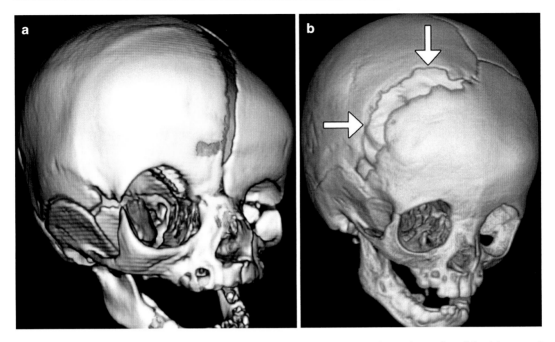

Fig. 4.35 Endoscopic strip craniectomy. Preoperative 3D CT image (**a**) shows asymmetric right coronal synostosis, resulting in deformity of the calvarium. Postoperative 3D CT image (**b**) shows interval resection of the right coronal suture (*arrows*), resulting in improved contours of the skull

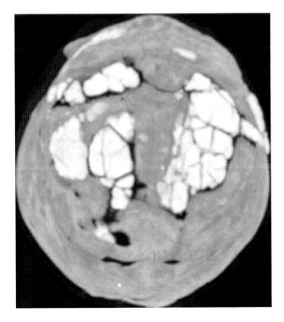

Fig. 4.36 Calcium phosphate cement for craniosynostosis repair. 3D CT image shows several areas of the hyperattenuating cement used to fill the craniectomy defects

4.14 Cranial Vault Encephalocele Repair

4.14.1 Discussion

Traditional management of encephaloceles consists of resecting the abnormal herniated brain tissue and closing the wound via primary intention if there is sufficient skin available (Fig. 4.37), with the goal of avoiding new deficits related to extended surgery. Cranioplasty can be performed at the same time as the primary surgery or at a later time, using materials such as methyl methacrylate, hydroxyapatite bone cement, demineralized bone matrix, and autologous grafts, which can be harvested from the adjacent calvarium, for example (Fig. 4.38). If a substantial amount of functional brain tissue has herniated through the encephalocele sac, expansile cranioplasty can be performed. This technique consists of reconstructing the calvarial defect with autologous bone graft harvested from the adjacent parietal region. This approach effectively enlarges or extends the intracranial cavity to encompass the herniated brain tissue.

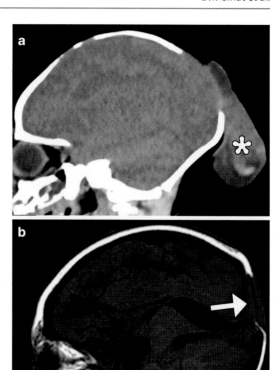

Fig. 4.37 Occipital encephalocele resection and primary closure. Preoperative sagittal CT image (**a**) shows herniation of dysplastic brain tissue (*) through a posterior calvarial defect. Postoperative sagittal T1-weighted MRI (**b**) shows interval resection of the herniated brain tissue and closure of the defect via duraplasty and skin (*arrow*)

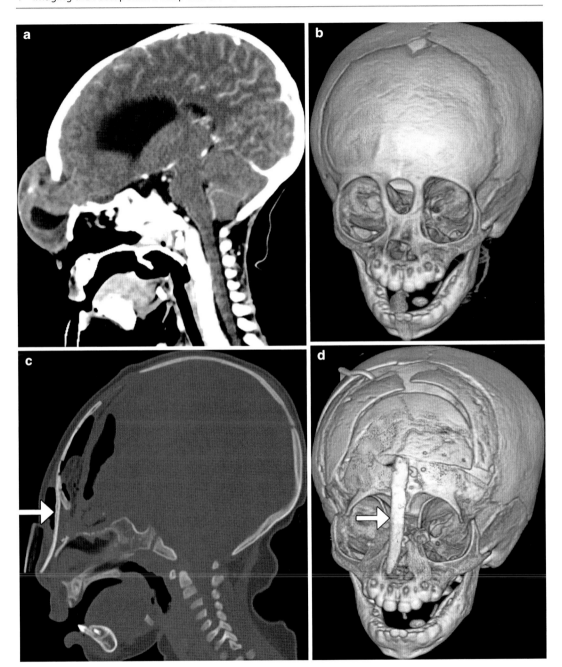

Fig. 4.38 Frontonasal encephalocele repair. Preoperative sagittal (**a**) and 3D (**b**) CT images show a frontonasal encephalocele herniating through a midline skull defect. Postoperative sagittal (**c**) and 3D (**d**) CT images show interval resection of the encephalocele and repair of the defect using calvarial bone graft (*arrows*)

4.15   Box Osteotomy

Hypertelorism can be corrected by performing box osteotomy, which involves creating a frontal bone flap to help remove excess interorbital bone and to mobilize the orbits. Once the orbits are repositioned closer to one another, they can be secured with plates and screws (Fig. 4.39).

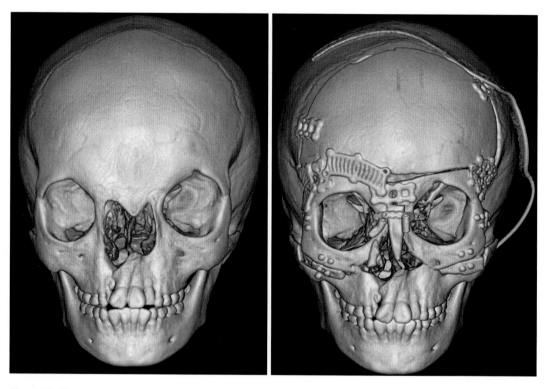

Fig. 4.39 Box osteomtomy. Preoperative 3D CT image (**a**) shows craniofacial dysplasia with hypertelorism. Postoperative 3D CT image (**b**) shows interval medial repositioning of the orbits and reconstruction of the nose with bone graft

4.16 Absorbable Hemostatic Agents

4.16.1 Discussion

Several types of topical absorbable hemostatic agents are available for neurosurgical procedures, including cellulose-, gelatin-, and collagen-based agents and thrombin and fibrin glue.

Oxidized regenerated cellulose, such as Surgicel, is available in the form of a fabric that can be used to line the margins of resection cavities or packed tightly to control a more focal source of bleeding. Implanted oxidized cellulose has been reported to mimic abscesses and masses on postoperative imaging. On CT, oxidized cellulose often displays low attenuation, and on MRI, it usually shows low signal on T2, but variable T1 signal (Fig. 4.40). Sometimes, the presence of high T1 signal can potentially mimic residual tumor on contrast-enhanced images. The hemostatic agent ultimately resorbs over the course of months.

Gelatin hemostatic agents, such as Surgifoam and Gelfoam, are available in powder or sponge form. On CT, the sponge usually displays air attenuation during the early postoperative period, but becomes higher attenuation as it absorbs cerebrospinal fluid/blood, resulting in high T2 and low T1 signal on MRI (Fig. 4.41), for example. Eventually, the sponge resorbs and is no longer apparent on imaging. Although gelatin foam hemostasis may incite varying degrees of granulomatous reaction, complications related to the use of these agents are unusual.

Gelatin-thrombin matrix (Floseal) functions as a sealant that acts at the end stage of the coagulation cascade. The material has a rather characteristic appearance of a pseudomass with relatively low signal speckles in a background of hyperintensity on T2-weighted MRI (Fig. 4.42), when clusters have formed with fluid absorbed by the granules and retained in the matrix. These microbubbles and clot formation in the matrix cause magnetic field inhomogeneity with T2* effects evident by blooming susceptibility of the gelatin-thrombin matrix in the surgical cavity.

Neurosurgical procedures can involve a great degree of complexity and occur over extended periods of time, and the contents of the surgical cavity can be obscured by blood products. These circumstances can make it difficult for the neurosurgeon to visually identify surgical paraphernalia left within the surgical field. However, radiopaque markers can help to localize a retained sponge or instrument with imaging when the surgical count is not reached. For example, cottonoids are compressed rayon cotton pledgets or strips used for hemostasis, soft tissue protection, and tissue dissection that contain radiographically detectable markers (Fig. 4.43). Typically, cottonoids are not thrown off the field into a kick bucket when soiled as are other larger sponges. Rather, they are kept on the sterile field or discarded in a separate area to prevent them from being picked up with larger sponges leading to incorrect counts. Radiographs with at least two orthogonal views are usually sufficient for localizing retained surgical paraphernalia. Nevertheless, when other metallic implants are intentionally present, the task can be more difficult, and CT may be useful.

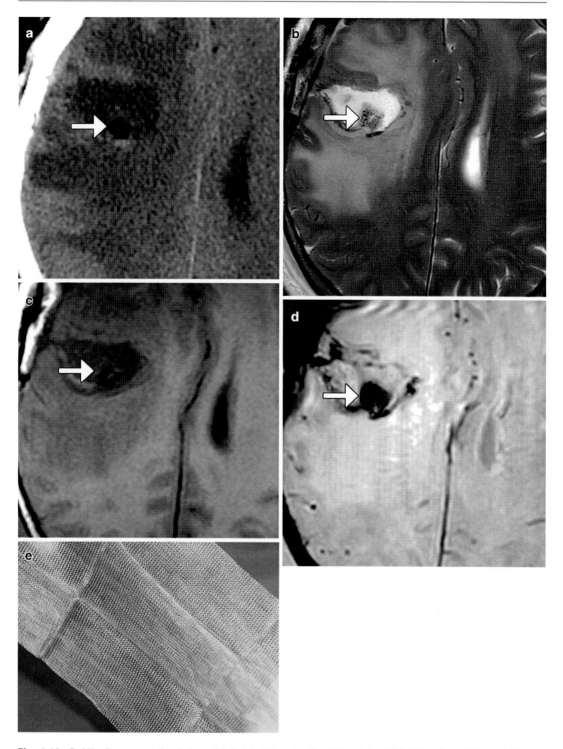

Fig. 4.40 Oxidized regenerated cellulose. (**a**) Axial CT image obtained after recent surgery shows globular low-attenuation material with the right frontal lobe surgical cavity (*arrow*). The Surgicel (*arrows*) has relatively low signal on T2-weighted (**b**), T1-weighted (**c**), and SWI (**d**) sequences. Photograph of Surgicel (**e**) (Courtesy of Patricia Smith and Sarah Paengatelli)

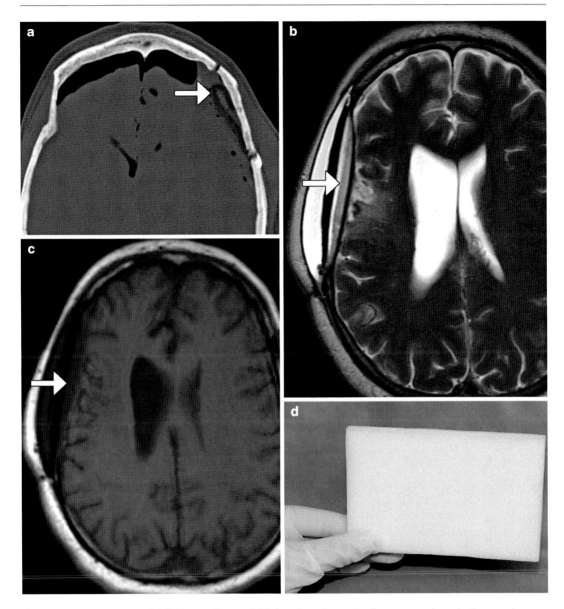

Fig. 4.41 Gelatin foam. Axial CT image shows a folded sheet of Gelfoam (*arrow*) deep to the craniotomy, which has higher attenuation than the surrounding pneumocephalus but lower attenuation than the surrounding fluid. Axial T2-weighted (**b**) and T1-weighted (**c**) MR images about 1 month after surgery show the hemostatic agent between the duraplasty and cranioplasty (*arrows*). Photograph of Surgifoam (**d**) (Courtesy of Patricia Smith and Sarah Paengatelli)

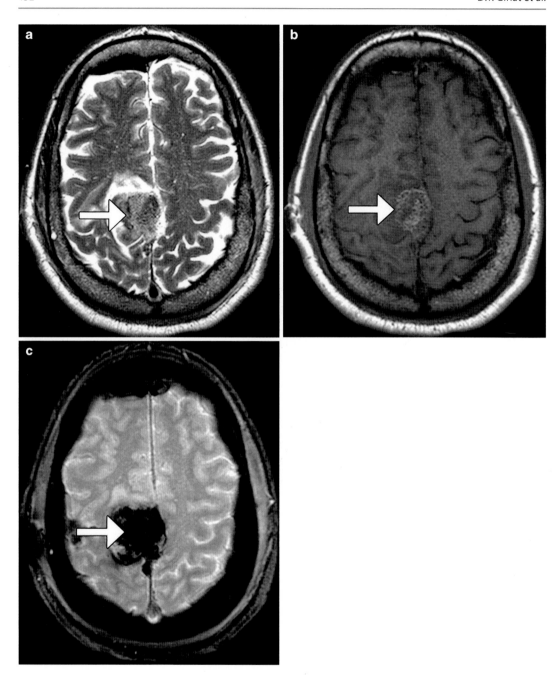

Fig. 4.42 Gelatin-thrombin matrix. Axial T2-weighed (**a**), T1-weighted (**b**), and SWI (**c**) MR images show a somewhat foamy appearance of the clustered hemostatic agent within the deep right cerebral (*arrows*), which has developed blood clots

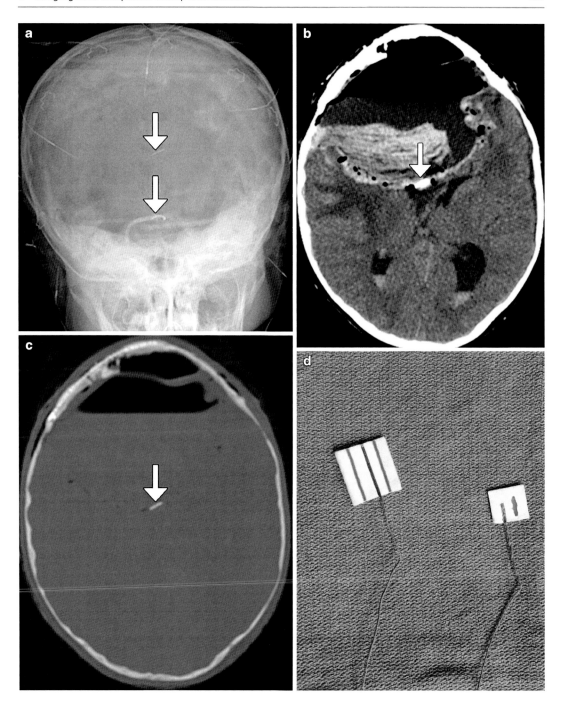

Fig. 4.43 Retained cottonoid. Immediately follow-ing resection of a large frontal meningioma, the neuro-surgeons informed the radiologist that cottonoids were left behind. Postoperative frontal radiograph (**a**) and CT in soft tissue (**b**) and bone (**c**) windows show the linear metallic structures associated with the cottonoids left the surgical bed (*arrows*) (Courtesy of Shehanaz Ellika MD). Photograph of cottonoids (**d**) (Courtesy Jene Bohannon)

4.17 Duraplasty and Sealant Agents

4.17.1 Discussion

Duraplasty consists of reconstructing the dura following cranial surgery in order to minimize cerebrospinal fluid leakage. Several dural substitutes and sealant agents are commercially available, including bovine pericardium, elastin-fibrin, biosynthetic cellulose, polytetrafluoroethylene, and collagen matrix sheets, among others.

Some formulations of collagen matrix duraplasty have a spongelike consistency, while others are more flat and compressed. These materials appear as a low attenuation on CT and often of low-to-intermediate signal intensity on both T1-weighted and T2-weighted MRI sequences (Fig. 4.44). Associated dural enhancement can be seen in over 10% of cases. The dural regenerative matrix intentionally resorbs at a similar rate as the new tissue that forms, thus preventing encapsulation. Specifically, the collagen matrix typically resorbs within 1–6 months, depending on the particular type.

Polytetrafluoroethylene (Gore-Tex) sheets appear as high attenuation on CT and very low signal on T1-weighted and T2-weighted MRI sequences (Fig. 4.45). Small collections of cerebrospinal fluid form adjacent to the duraplasty in 15% of cases. Often, thin membranes of granulation tissue form between the duraplasty and the surface of the brain. In general, complications related to duraplasty procedures are infrequent and include graft failure with pseudomeningocele formation, epidural fibrosis, and infection.

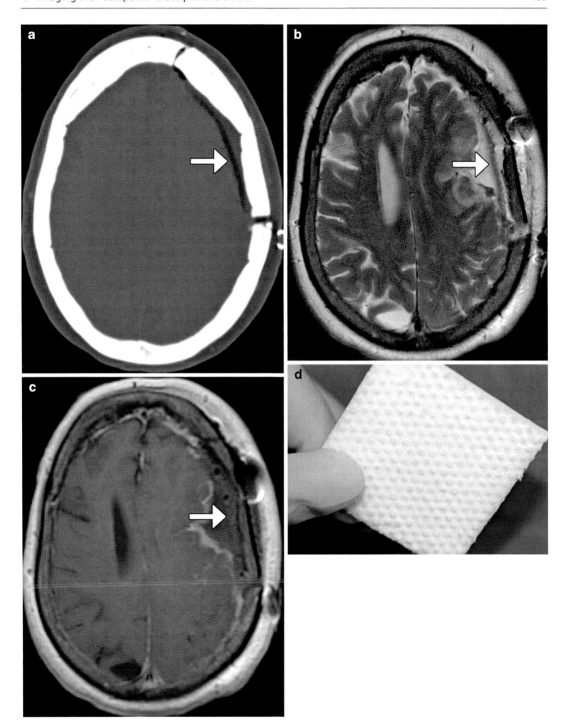

Fig. 4.44 Collagen matrix duraplasty. The patient has a history of a large left frontal meningioma status post resection and duraplasty using DuraGen. CT image (**a**) shows the sheetlike low-attenuation duraplasty material (*arrows*) in the left frontal region. T2-weighted (**b**) and post-contrast T1-weighted (**c**) MRI sequences show that the duraplasty material (*arrows*) displays low T2 and intermediate T1 signal. Photograph of suturable DuraGen (**d**) (Courtesy of Patricia Smith and Sarah Paengatelli)

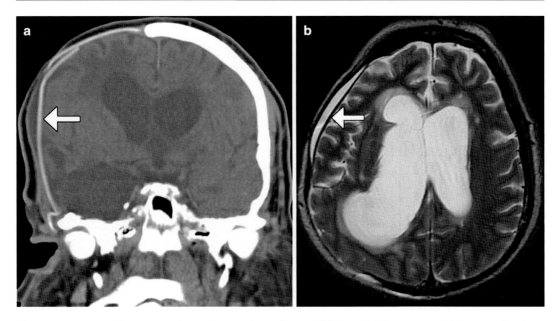

Fig. 4.45 Polytetrafluoroethylene (Gore-Tex) duraplasty. Coronal CT image (**a**) demonstrates high-attenuation dura-plasty (*arrow*) after hemicraniectomy. On the T2-weighted MRI (**b**), the material (*arrow*) displays low signal

4.18   Intracranial Pressure Monitors

4.18.1   Discussion

Conditions associated with raised intracranial pressure, such as hemorrhage, cerebral infarcts, or trauma, can compromise cerebral blood flow. A variety of intracranial pressure monitors are available, including fiber optic monitors. The filamentous fiber optic monitor enters the intracranial cavity through a bolt that is introduced into a burr hole (Fig. 4.46). Other devices for measuring intracranial pressure include diaphragm-type monitors and ventricular catheters with pressure sensors. Pressure monitors can be placed in the subarachnoid or subdural space, brain parenchyma, or ventricle. The components of the monitors are readily apparent on CT, allowing the precise position to be determined.

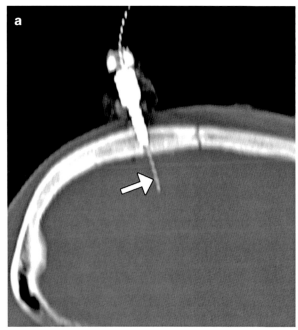
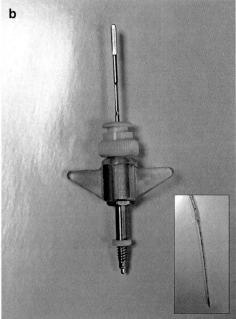

Fig. 4.46 Intraparenchymal pressure monitor. The patient has a history of severe traumatic brain injury resulting in a left subdural hematoma and intraparenchymal contusions. Sagittal CT image (**a**) shows the pressure bolt monitor seated in the burr hole through which a fiber optic monitor enters the brain parenchyma (*arrow*). Photograph of a Camino Bolt and pressure monitor and fiber optic (*inset*) (Codman Neuro New Brunswick NJ) (**b**) (Courtesy of Justin Hugelier)

4.19   Subdural Drainage Catheters

4.19.1 Discussion

Chronic subdural hematomas can be treated via burr hole evacuation. The use of drainage catheters that extend through the burr holes from the subdural collections to the skin surface can reduce incidence of recurrence. Imaging can be used to confirm the position of catheters and assess changes in size of the hematomas. The hyperattenuating catheters are readily apparent on CT (Fig. 4.47).

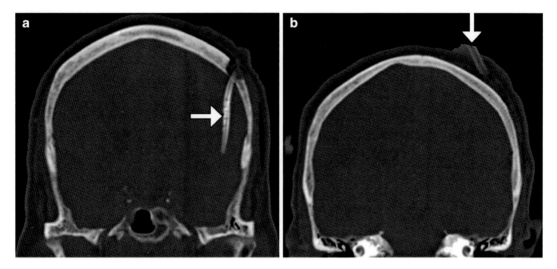

Fig. 4.47 Subdural drainage catheter. Coronal CT images (**a, b**) show a catheter (*arrows*) extending from the subdural space to an opening in the scalp

4.20   Cranial Surgery Complications

4.20.1 Tension Pneumocephalus

Tension pneumocephalus following neurosurgery is an uncommon but emergent condition. Indeed, tension pneumocephalus can be life-threatening since it can cause brainstem herniation. Possible risk factors include posterior fossa craniotomy, the use of nitrogen oxide for anesthesia, lumbar drainage, and cerebrospinal fluid leakage, with dural defects that function as one-way valves.

A characteristic axial CT feature of tension pneumocephalus is the "peaking" sign, in which the lateral aspects of the bilateral frontal lobes are compressed together by the pressurized intracranial air. Another related appearance is the "Mount Fuji" sign, which describes the combination of compressed and separated frontal lobes with widened interhemispheric space (Fig. 4.48). This sign is fairly specific for tension pneumocephalus.

Ultimately, the diagnosis of tension pneumocephalus requires accompanying decline in clinical status manifesting as lethargy, a hissing noise during release of the pneumocephalus, and resolution of symptoms thereafter. Treatment consists of one or more of the following: 100% oxygen supplementation, repair of dural defect, and burr hole decompression.

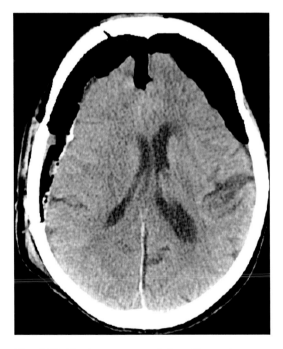

Fig. 4.48 Tension pneumocephalus. The patient presented with lethargy on postoperative day #3. Axial CT image obtained after craniotomy shows extensive pneumocephalus that compresses the bilateral frontal lobes and lateral ventricles. There is separation of the frontal lobes and a pointed appearance of the bilateral anterior frontal lobes

4.20.2 Entered Frontal Sinus, Entered Orbit, and Air Leak

The frontal sinus and orbits are entered in about 30% of craniotomies in adults, particularly via the pterional or orbitozygomatic approach. However, these are usually noted during surgery and repair using fat graft and mesh (Figs. 4.49 and 4.50). Superimposed complications are uncommon and include mucoceles, cerebrospinal fluid leak, and air leak with frontal sinus entry and orbital hematomas and rectus muscle injury with orbital entry. The presence of persistent pneumocephalus or pneumo-orbit on serial CT exams raises the suspicion of air leaks (Fig. 4.51). High-resolution CT with multiplanar reconstructions is the first-line modality recommended for assessing suspected cerebrospinal fluid leaks.

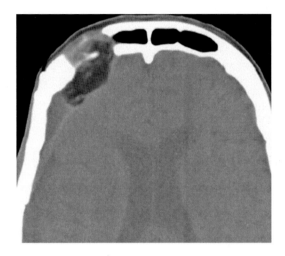

Fig. 4.49 Entered frontal sinus. Axial CT image demonstrates a right frontal craniotomy that extended through the right frontal sinus, which was obliterated with fat graft

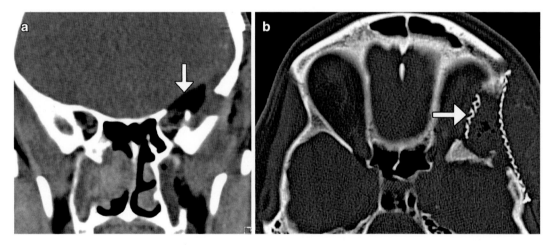

Fig. 4.50 Entered orbit. Coronal CT image (**a**) shows a defect in the left posterior orbital roof closed with fat graft (*arrow*). Axial CT image (**b**) in a different patient shows entry of the left lateral orbit repaired with mesh (*arrow*)

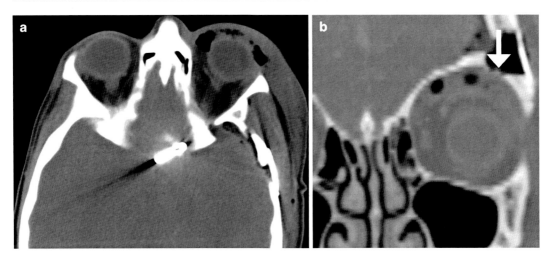

Fig. 4.51 Air leak. Axial (**a**) and coronal (**b**) CT images show left intraorbital air and proptosis after aneurysm clipping. There is a defect in the superior orbital roof (*arrow*)

4.20.3 Postoperative Hemorrhage and Hematomas

Small, asymptomatic hematomas are common and can be considered an expected consequence of craniotomy and cranioplasty. Subgaleal hematomas are ubiquitous in the early postoperative period and are usually self-limited. Occasionally, subgaleal hematomas can be voluminous and exert mass effect (Fig. 4.52). Similarly, postoperative intracranial hematomas can occasionally cause symptoms such as altered mental status, neurological deficits, and seizures, which may require surgical evacuation. The variety of postoperative hematomas includes epidural (33%), subdural (5%), parenchymal (43%), or a combination of these (8%) and can be further classified as regional, adjacent, or remote (Figs. 4.53, 4.54, 4.55, and 4.56). Acute hematomas tend to be hyperattenuating on CT, while chronic hematomas evolve toward fluid attenuation.

- Regional hematomas are the most common and occur directly beneath the bone flaps.
- Adjacent extradural hematomas are more commonly posterior rather than anterior to the craniotomy site and may be caused by separation of the dura at the craniotomy margin, sudden collapse of the brain, or inferior extension of regional hemorrhage.
- Remote intracranial hemorrhage is a relatively uncommon complication of intracranial surgery, comprising about 6% of extradural hematomas. This type of hemorrhage may be related to cerebrospinal fluid volume depletion and decreased intracranial pressure and has a predilection for the cerebellum. Remote cerebellar hemorrhage characteristically appears as curvilinear high attenuation in the cerebellar sulci and folia on CT, which has been termed the "zebra sign." Remote cerebral hemorrhages most commonly occur in the frontal and then followed by the temporal lobe. These are most commonly related to the use of intraoperative retractors creating venous congestion leading to a hemorrhagic venous infarct. Hemorrhagic venous infarcts can also be due to sacrificing crucial venous structures.
- Abdominal wall hematomas may result from storage of calvarial bone flaps for autocranioplasty (Fig. 4.57).

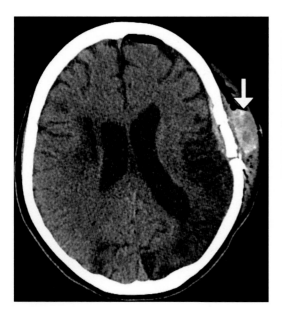

Fig. 4.52 Subgaleal hematoma. Axial CT image shows a hyperattenuation mass-like collection in the left scalp overlying the craniotomy flap (*arrow*). There is also a small amount of underlying extra-axial hemorrhage and multiple cerebral infarcts

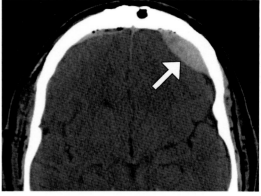

Fig. 4.53 Adjacent epidural hematoma. Axial CT image shows lentiform high-attenuation extradural hematoma (*arrow*) along the posterior margin of the craniotomy

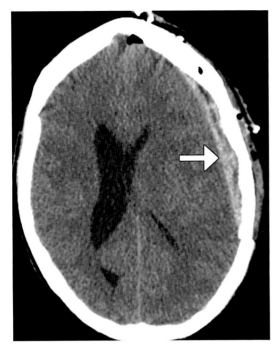

Fig. 4.54 Regional subdural hematoma. Axial CT image shows a heterogeneous left subdural hematoma (*arrow*) deep to the craniotomy flap

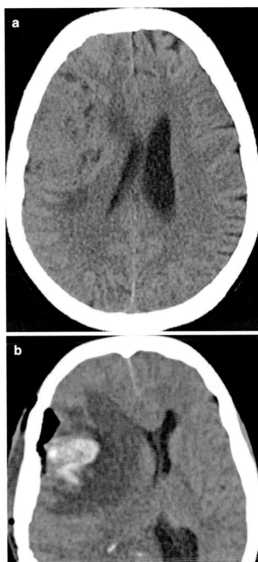

Fig. 4.55 Adjacent intraparenchymal hematoma. Preoperative CT image (**a**) shows a large right frontal convexity meningioma. Immediate postoperative CT image (**b**) shows a large hyperattenuating hematoma subjacent to the resection cavity. There is also extensive surrounding vasogenic edema

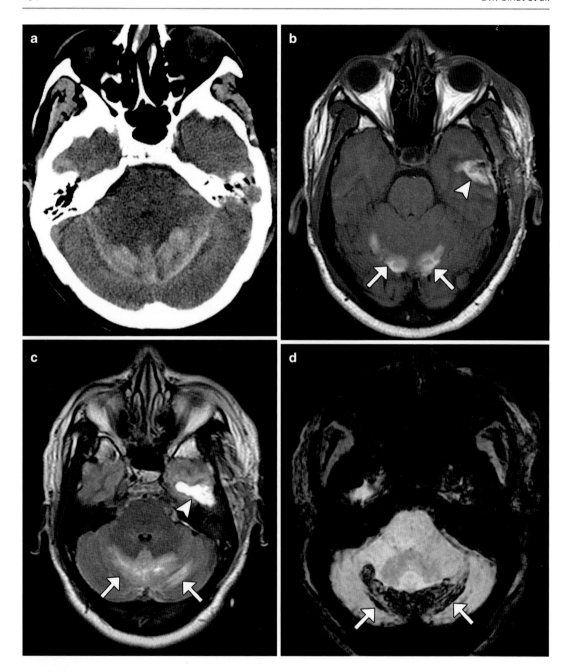

Fig. 4.56 Remote cerebellar hemorrhage. Axial CT image (**a**) in a patient who underwent supratentorial craniotomy shows crescentic hemorrhage in the bilateral cerebellar hemispheres. Axial T1-weighted (**b**), axial T2-weighted (**c**) and axial susceptibility-weighted (**d**) MRI images in a different patient demonstrate curvilinear areas of subacute hemorrhage and edema in the bilateral cerebellar hemisphere (*arrows*) following left temporal lobe tumor resection (*arrowheads*)

Fig. 4.57 Axial CT image shows a large hematoma (*) subjacent to the skull flap within the subcutaneous tissues

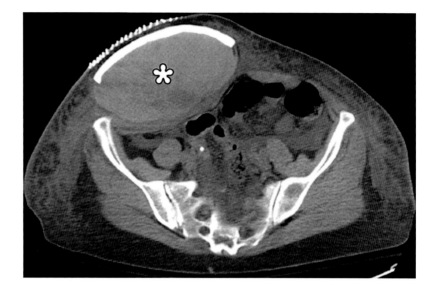

4.20.4 Postoperative Hygromas and Effusions

Hygromas develop in up to 60% of cases following craniectomy, particularly decompressive craniectomy for intracranial hypertension related to head trauma. Up to 90% of subdural hygromas are ipsilateral to the craniectomy site. Interhemispheric fissure subdural hygromas are uncommon, as are subarachnoid hygromas. Hygromas can also occur after craniotomy and cranioplasty.

Hygromas usually appear after 1 week of surgery, reach a maximum volume at 3–4 weeks, and resolve over several months. On CT and MRI, hygromas appear as simple fluid collections (Fig. 4.58). However, nearly 8% convert to subdural hematomas by 2 months, resulting in higher attenuation. Most hygromas are of little clinical significance, although some of these may be associated with mass effect that may require additional decompressive surgery.

A particular complication related to posterior fossa tumor resection in pediatric patients is the formation of spinal subdural effusions. These fluid collections result from sudden postoperative normalization of the excessive intraspinal pressure caused by spinal sequestration by tonsillar herniation. On MRI, the effusions display T1 and T2 cerebrospinal fluid signal characteristics, but can also enhance (Fig. 4.59). The collections also tend to have wavy margins and can compress the spinal canal contents, thereby interfering with workup for metastatic disease. Otherwise, the collections are generally clinically silent and resolve within 1 month.

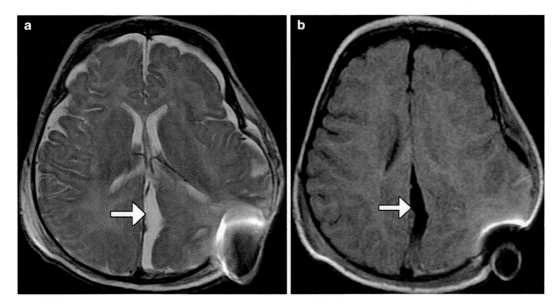

Fig. 4.58 Subdural hygroma. Axial T2 (**a**) and T1 (**b**) MR images in a different patient show a cerebrospinal fluid intensity collection along the left falx cerebri (*arrows*)

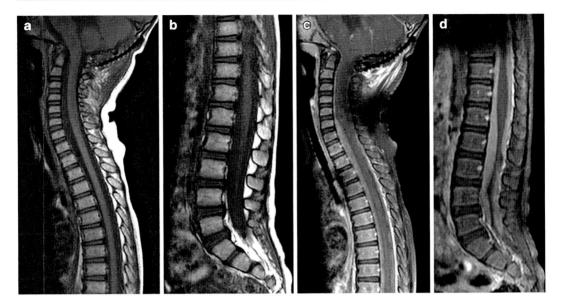

Fig. 4.59 Postoperative intraspinal subdural effusions. This pediatric patient underwent recent resection of a posterior fossa medulloblastoma. Sagittal T1-weighted (**a**, **b**) and fat-suppressed post-contrast T1-weighted (**c**, **d**) MR images show postoperative findings related to suboccipital cranioplasty and diffuse, but somewhat wavy, enhancing subdural collections that compress the spinal canal contents

4.20.5 Pseudomeningoceles

Pseudomeningoceles represent contained cerebrospinal fluid leakage or herniation of the subarachnoid space through a defect in the dura. Pseudomeningoceles are common postsurgical complications, especially in the suboccipital region. On imaging, pseudomeningoceles appear as simple fluid collections that bulge into the scalp or posterior cervical soft tissues and communicate with the intracranial space (Fig. 4.60).

Pseudomeningoceles often resolve spontaneously as the dura seals over time and cerebrospinal fluid absorption returns to normal. However, when these are persistent or the suture line is under excess tension, exploration, repair, and/or cerebrospinal fluid diversion can be considered. Persistent or enlarging cerebrospinal fluid collections near burr holes can sometimes reflect impairments in cerebrospinal fluid absorption, except in infants, where cerebrospinal fluid can be extruded while crying and can get trapped extracranially.

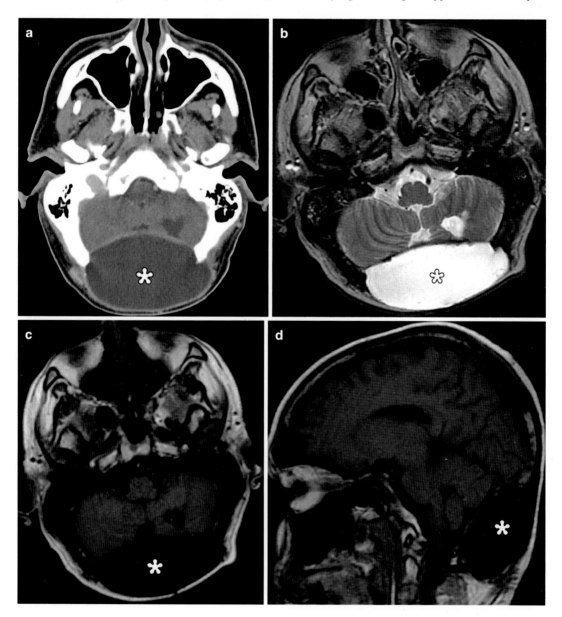

Fig. 4.60 Suboccipital craniectomy pseudomeningocele. Axial CT image (**a**) shows a large fluid collection at the suboccipital craniectomy site (*). Axial T2–weighted (**b**) and axial (**c**) and sagittal (**d**) T1-weighted MRI sequences show a fluid collection that follows cerebrospinal fluid signal intensity (*) at the suboccipital craniectomy site

4.20.6 Pseudoaneurysm

Significant arterial injury resulting from retrosigmoid craniotomy is an uncommon incident. Significant injury of the scalp arteries from cranial surgery is uncommon, but can lead to pseudoaneurysms. Patients can present with a pulsatile mass that appears as a hyperattenuating collection in the scalp on CT (Fig. 4.61). Angiography is recommended to ascertain the presence of a pseudoaneurysm, which appears as an ovoid structure that enhances in parallel with the arteries. Pseudoaneurysms can resolve spontaneously but may be amenable to endovascular therapy.

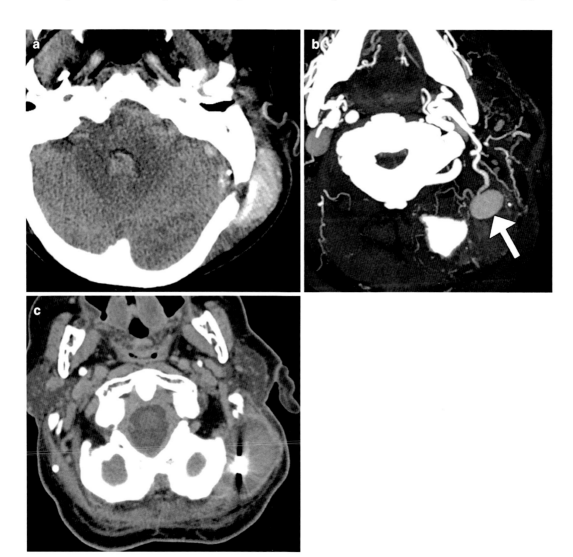

Fig. 4.61 Postoperative occipital artery pseudoaneurysm. Axial CT image (**a**) shows hemorrhage overlying the left retrosigmoid craniotomy site. CTA MIP image (**b**) shows a large left occipital artery pseudoaneurysm (*arrow*). The pseudoaneurysm was subsequently coiled, as shown on a follow-up CT (**c**)

4.20.7 Postoperative Infection

Infection is a serious complication of craniotomy, craniectomy, and cranioplasty that can occur in the subgaleal, extradural, or subdural spaces within the bone flap and surrounding the cranioplasty (Figs. 4.62 and 4.63). The incidence is generally 4.5–6%, but varies depending upon the type of material used. *Staphylococcus aureus* is the most common responsible organism. The appearance on CT is that of a fluid collection with peripheral enhancement. MRI may show restricted diffusion in the abscess. In addition, MR spectroscopy may show elevated lactate. Although systemic signs of infection can be mild, management consists of wound debridement, antibiotics, and removal of the cranioplasty. Progressive increase in size of the collection over time is a particularly suspicious finding. Osteomyelitis of bone flaps comprises over 40% of all infectious complications following craniotomy. The vast majority of these cases are due to infection by *Staphylococcus aureus*. Infected bone flaps may either demonstrate areas of lucency or sclerosis on CT. These findings are not specific for osteomyelitis and can be seen in normal bone flaps. However, the presence of secondary changes, such as overlying sinus tracts, skin thickening, fat stranding, and adjacent fluid collections, should raise the suspicion of an infected bone flap. MRI can demonstrate increased T2 signal and decreased T1 signal intensity within the infected bone flap marrow. In addition, predisposing factors include communication with the sinuses, multiple surgeries, long intraoperative times, and surgery for preexisting intracranial infection. Treatment of bone flap osteomyelitis ranges from conservative management to bone flap removal.

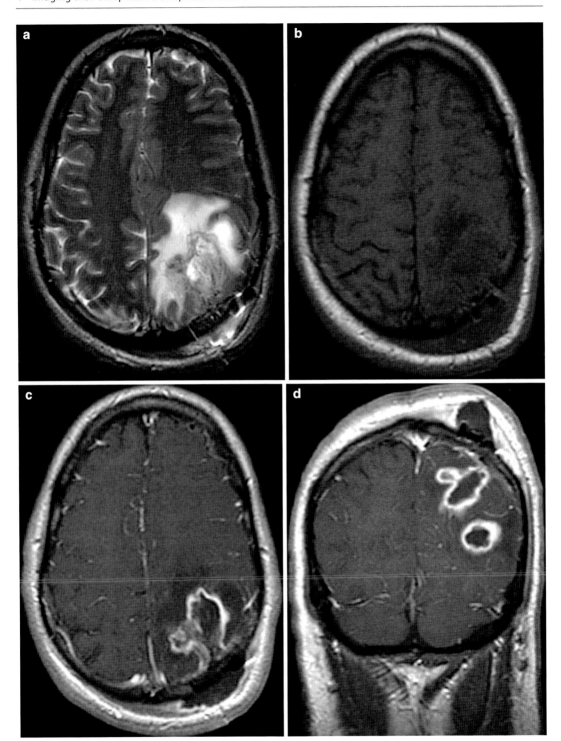

Fig. 4.62 Infected craniotomy bed. Axial T2 (**a**), axial T1 (**b**), post-contrast axial (**c**), and coronal (**d**) T1 show irregular fluid collections with rim enhancement in the left parietal lobe and scalp overlying the craniotomy. There is restricted diffusion within the intraparenchymal abscess on DWI (**e**) and ADC map (**f**) and abnormal signal in the craniotomy flap due to osteomyelitis

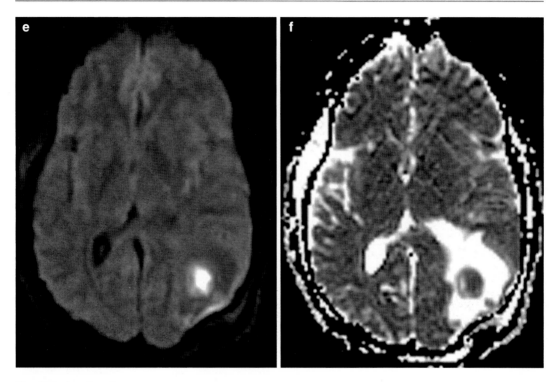

Fig. 4.62 (continued)

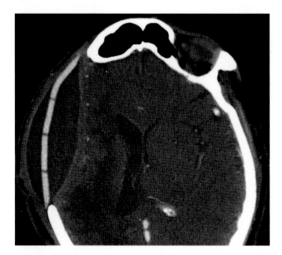

Fig. 4.63 Infected cranioplasty prosthesis. The patient presented with fever and pain at surgical site several months after acrylic cranioplasty. Axial contrast-enhanced CT image obtained 1 week later shows a biconvex fluid collection surrounding the cranioplasty plate. Cultures grew *Staphylococcus aureus*, and the cranioplasty material was subsequently removed

4.20.8 Textiloma

Resorbable and nonresorbable hemostatic agents can incite foreign body reactions that appear mass-like and can mimic neoplasm or abscess. Various terms are used to describe this granulomatous reaction, such as textilomas, gossypibomas, gau-zomas, surgicelomas, and muslinomas. While each agent exhibits distinctive morphologic features that often permit specific identification, these typically consist of a core of degenerating hemostatic agent surrounded by an inflammatory reaction, which can demonstrate enhancement on imaging (Fig. 4.64). The presence of hemostatic material at the site of the lesion on baseline imaging, if available, can be a helpful clue.

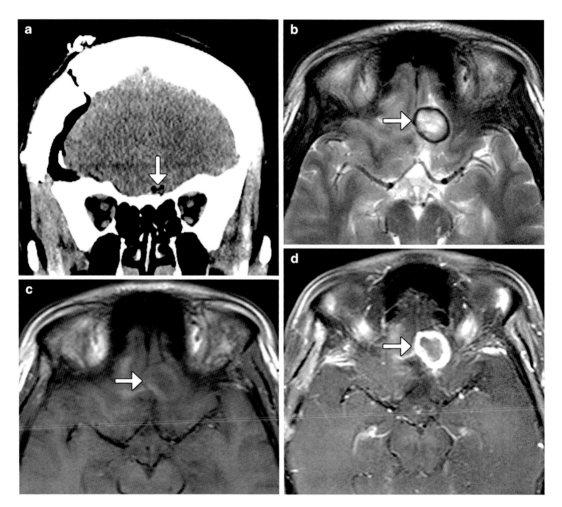

Fig. 4.64 Textiloma. Initial postoperative CT image (**a**) shows the hemostatic agent along the left planum sphenoi-dale (*arrow*). Follow-up axial T2-weighted (**b**), T1-weighted (**c**), and post-contrast T1-weighted (**d**) MR images show a well-defined lesion with peripheral enhancement (*arrows*)

4.20.9 Sunken Skin Flap Syndrome

Sunken skin flap syndrome (syndrome of the trephined) is an uncommon, late complication of
craniectomy, usually occurring 1 month after surgery. This complication consists of depression of
the scalp flap and brain deformity at the site of
craniectomy (Fig. 4.65). The cause is presumed to
be atmospheric pressure that exceeds intracranial

pressure. Large craniectomy defects predispose to
the development of sunken skin flap syndrome,
and brain atrophy accentuates the degree of concavity. This condition is certainly not cosmeti-
cally pleasing and may even compromise cerebral
blood flow. Furthermore, along with headache,
fatigue, and seizure, sunken skin flaps may be a
manifestation of trephine syndrome. These outcomes often improve following cranioplasty.

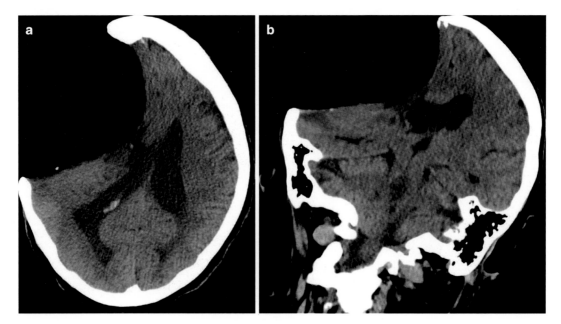

Fig. 4.65 Sunken flap syndrome. Axial (**a**) and coronal (**b**) CT images show severe concavity of the scalp contours at
the craniectomy site. There is no associated brain herniation

4.20.10 External Brain Herniation

Following craniectomy for cerebral edema, extra-cranial herniation of the brain occurs in over 25% of cases. Although some degree of brain expansion is expected after craniectomy, extension of brain tissue beyond 1.5 cm measured at the center of the osseous defect with respect to the outer table of the calvarium is generally considered abnormal. Extracranial cerebral herniation is more likely to occur with small craniectomy defects. This can produce a characteristic "mushroom cap" appearance of the deformed brain tissue (Fig. 4.66). The herniated brain tissue is particularly susceptible to trauma. Extracranial herniation can also lead to venous infarcts secondary to cortical vein compression. This risk of substantial external brain herniation is lower with larger craniectomies.

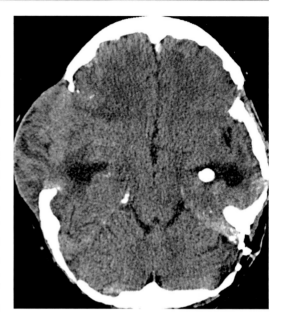

Fig. 4.66 External brain herniation. Axial CT shows substantial herniation of the intracranial contents through the left craniectomy defect with a "mushroom cap" appearance posteriorly

4.20.11 Bone Flap Resorption

Although mild remodeling of the bone flap edges over time is expected and of no consequence, severe bone flap resorption can be problematic. This is a delayed complication that occurs in 6–12% of cases. As resorption progresses, the bone flap becomes detached from the securing plates, and sunken scalp syndrome may ensue. Alternatively, intracranial contents can herniate through the defects. On CT, bone flap resorption appears as tapered edges and wide gaps between the calvarium (Fig. 4.67). These patients can benefit from artificial cranioplasty, and high-resolution 3D CT is particularly helpful for surgical planning subsequent repair.

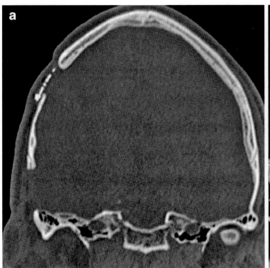 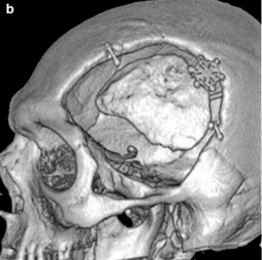

Fig. 4.67 Bone flap resorption. Coronal CT (**a**) and 3D CT (**b**) images demonstrate thinning of the right frontal bone flap edges with wide gaps between the craniotomy flap and the rest of the calvarium. Consequently, some of the cranial plates are not fully anchored to bone

Further Reading

Occipital Nerve Stimulator

Kapural L, Mekhail N, Hayek SM, Stanton-Hicks M, Malak O (2005) Occipital nerve electrical stimulation via the midline approach and subcutaneous surgical leads for treatment of severe occipital neuralgia: a pilot study. Anesth Analg 101(1):171–174, table of contents

Slavin KV, Nersesyan H, Wess C (2006) Peripheral neurostimulation for treatment of intractable occipital neuralgia. Neurosurgery 58(1):112–119; discussion 112–119

Tissue Expander

Ortega MT, McCauley RL, Robson MC (1990) Salvage of an avulsed expanded scalp flap to correct burn alopecia. South Med J 83(2):220–223

Sharony Z, Rissin Y, Ullmann Y (2009) Postburn scalp reconstruction using a self-filling osmotic tissue expander. J Burn Care Res 30(4):744–746

Temporal Fossa Implant

Baj A, Spotti S, Marelli S, Beltramini GA, Gianni AB (2009) Use of porous polyethylene for correcting defects of temporal region following transposition of temporalis myofascial flap. Acta Otorhinolaryngol Ital 29(5):265–269

Rapidis AD, Day TA (2006) The use of temporal polyethylene implant after temporalis myofascial flap transposition: clinical and radiographic results from its use in 21 patients. J Oral Maxillofac Surg 64(1):12–22

Mohs Micrographic Surgery and Skin Grafting

Chun YS, Verma K (2011) Single-stage full-thickness scalp reconstruction using acellular dermal matrix and skin graft. Eplasty 11:e4

Cumberland L, Dana A, Liegeois N (2009) Mohs micrographic surgery for the management of nonmelanoma skin cancers. Facial Plast Surg Clin North Am 17(3):325–335

Lesesne CB, Rosenthal R (1986) A review of scalp split-thickness skin grafts and potential complications. Plast Reconstr Surg 77(5):757–758

Stone JL (1993) Mohs micrographic surgery: a synopsis. Hawaii Med J 52(5):134–139

Vuyk HD, Lohuis PJ (2001) Mohs micrographic surgery for facial skin cancer. Clin Otolaryngol Allied Sci 26(4):265–273

Rotational Galeal Flap Scalp Reconstruction

Chang KP, Lai CH, Chang CH, Lin CL, Lai CS, Lin SD (2010) Free flap options for reconstruction of complicated scalp and calvarial defects: report of a series of cases and literature review. Microsurgery 30(1):13–18

Guerrissi JO (1999) Reconstruction of large defects in the scalp with fasciocutaneous flaps. Scand J Plast Reconstr Surg Hand Surg 33(2):217–224

Talmi YP, Liokumovitch P, Wolf M, Horowitz Z, Kopolovitch J, Kronenberg J (1997) Anatomy of the postauricular island "revolving door" flap ("flip-flop" flap). Ann Plast Surg 39(6):603–607

Free Flap Reconstruction of Complex Scalp Defects

Angelos PC, Downs BW (2009) Options for the management of forehead and scalp defects. Facial Plast Surg Clin North Am 17(3):379–393

Chang KP, Lai CH, Chang CH, Lin CL, Lai CS, Lin SD (2010) Free flap options for reconstruction of complicated scalp and calvarial defects: report of a series of cases and literature review. Microsurgery 30(1):13–18

Chong J, Chan LL, Langstein HN, Ginsberg LE (2001) MR imaging of the muscular component of myocutaneous flaps in the head and neck. AJNR Am J Neuroradiol 22(1):170–174

Hierner R, van Loon J, Goffin J, van Calenbergh F (2007) Free latissimus dorsi flap transfer for subtotal scalp and cranium defect reconstruction: report of 7 cases. Microsurgery 27(5):425–428

O'Connell DA, Teng MS, Mendez E, Futran ND (2011) Microvascular free tissue transfer in the reconstruction of scalp and lateral temporal bone defects. J Craniomaxillofac Surg 22(3):801–804

Oh SJ, Lee J, Cha J, Jeon MK, Koh SH, Chung CH (2011) Free-flap reconstruction of the scalp: donor selection and outcome. J Craniomaxillofac Surg 22(3):974–977

Seitz IA, Adler N, Odessey E, Reid RR, Gottlieb LJ (2009) Latissimus dorsi/rib intercostal perforator myoosseocutaneous free flap reconstruction in composite defects of the scalp: case series and review of literature. J Reconstr Microsurg 25(9):559–567

Scalp Tumor Recurrence

Chong J, Chan LL, Langstein HN, Ginsberg LE (2001) MR imaging of the muscular component of myocutaneous flaps in the head and neck. AJNR Am J Neuroradiol 22(1):170–174

Hudgins PA, Burson JG, Gussack GS, Grist WJ (1994) CT and MR appearance of recurrent malignant head and neck neoplasms after resection and flap reconstruction. AJNR Am J Neuroradiol 15(9):1689–1694

Tomura N, Watanabe O, Hirano Y, Kato K, Takahashi S, Watarai J (2002) MR imaging of recurrent head and neck tumours following flap reconstructive surgery. Clin Radiol 57(2):109–113

Box Osteotomy

Breakey W, Abela C, Evans R, Jeelani O, Britto J, Hayward R, Dunaway D (2015) Hypertelorism correction with facial bipartition and box osteotomy: does soft tissue translation correlate with bony movement? J Craniofac Surg 26(1):196–200

Absorbable Hemostatic Agents

Barbolt TA, Odin M, Leger M, Kangas L (2001) Pre-clinical subdural tissue reaction and absorption study of absorbable hemostatic devices. Neurol Res 23(5):537–542

Ferroli P, Broggi M, Franzini A, Maccagnano E, Lamperti M, Boiardi A, Broggi G (2006) Surgifoam and mitoxantrone in the glioblastoma multiforme postresection cavity: the first step of locoregional chemotherapy through an ad hoc-placed catheter: technical note. Neurosurgery 59(2):433–434; discussion E433–E4334

Learned KO, Mohan S, Hyder IZ, Bagley LJ, Wang S, Lee JY (2014) Imaging features of a gelatin-thrombin matrix hemostatic agent in the intracranial surgical bed: a unique space-occupying pseudomass. AJNR Am J Neuroradiol 35(4):686–690.

Oto A, Remer EM, O'Malley CM, Tkach JA, Gill IS (1999) MR characteristics of oxidized cellulose (surgicel). AJR Am J Roentgenol 172(6):1481–1484

Spiller M, Tenner MS, Couldwell WT (2001) Effect of absorbable topical hemostatic agents on the relaxation time of blood: an in vitro study with implications for postoperative magnetic resonance imaging. J Neurosurg 95(4):687–693

Young ST, Paulson EK, McCann RL, Baker ME (1993) Appearance of oxidized cellulose (surgicel) on postoperative CT scans: similarity to postoperative abscess. AJR Am J Roentgenol 160(2):275–277

Duraplasty and Sealant Agents

Berjano R, Vinas FC, Dujovny M (1999) A review of dural substitutes used in neurosurgery. Crit Rev Neurosurg 9(4):217–222

Filippi R, Schwarz M, Voth D, Reisch R, Grunert P, Perneczky A (2001) Bovine pericardium for duraplasty: clinical results in 32 patients. Neurosurg Rev 24(2–3):103–107

Narotam PK, Jose S, Nathoo N, Taylon C, Vora Y (2004) Collagen matrix (DuraGen) in dural repair: analysis of a new modified technique. Spine (Phila Pa 1976) 29(24):2861–2867; discussion 2868–2869

Narotam PK, Reddy K, Fewer D, Qiao F, Nathoo N (2007) Collagen matrix duraplasty for cranial and spinal surgery: a clinical and imaging study. J Neurosurg 106(1):45–51

Zerris VA, James KS, Roberts JB, Bell E, Heilman CB (2007) Repair of the dura mater with processed collagen devices. J Biomed Mater Res B Appl Biomater 83(2):580–588

Burr Holes

Sinclair AG, Scoffings DJ (2010) Imaging of the postoperative cranium. Radiographics 30(2):461–482

Vogel TW, Dlouhy BJ, Howard MA 3rd (2011) Don't take the plunge: avoiding adverse events with cranial perforators. J Neurosurg 115(3):570–575

Craniotomy

Duke BJ, Mouchantat RA, Ketch LL, Winston KR (1996) Transcranial migration of microfixation plates and screws. Case report. Pediatr Neurosurg 25(1):31–34; discussion 35

Schmidt JH 3rd, Reyes BJ, Fischer R, Flaherty SK (2007) Use of hinge craniotomy for cerebral decompression. Technical note. J Neurosurg 107(3):678–682

Sinclair AG, Scoffings DJ (2010) Imaging of the postoperative cranium. Radiographics 30(2):461–482

Winston KR, Wang MC (2003) Cranial bone fixation: review of the literature and description of a new procedure. J Neurosurg 99(3):484–488

Cranioplasty

Benzel EC, Thammavaram K, Kesterson L (1990) The diagnosis of infections associated with acrylic cranioplasties. Neuroradiology 32(2):151–153

Cabraja M, Klein M, Lehmann TN (2009) Long-term results following titanium cranioplasty of large skull defects. Neurosurg Focus 26(6):E10

Chandler CL, Uttley D, Archer DJ, MacVicar D (1994) Imaging after titanium cranioplasty. Br J Neurosurg 8(4):409–414

Couldwell WT, Chen TC, Weiss MH, Fukushima T, Dougherty W (1994) Cranioplasty with the Medpor porous polyethylene flexblock implant. Technical note. J Neurosurg 81(3):483–486

Dean D, Min KJ, Bond A (2003) Computer aided design of large-format prefabricated cranial plates. J Craniomaxillofac Surg 14(6):819–832

Eufinger H, Wehmöller M, Harders A, Heuser L (1995) Prefabricated prostheses for the reconstruction of skull defects. Int J Oral Maxillofac Surg 24(1 Pt 2):104–110

Malis LI (1989) Titanium mesh and acrylic cranioplasty. Neurosurgery 25(3):351–355

Martin MP, Olson S (2009) Post-operative complications with titanium mesh. J Clin Neurosci 16(8):1080–1081

Mason TO, Rose BS, Goodman JH (1986) Gas bubbles in polymethylmethacrylate cranioplasty simulating abscesses: CT appearance. AJNR Am J Neuroradiol 7(5):829–831

Rogers GF, Greene AK, Mulliken JB, Proctor MR, Ridgway EB (2011) Exchange cranioplasty using autologous calvarial particulate bone graft effectively repairs large cranial defects. Plast Reconstr Surg 127(4):1631–1642

Weissman JL, Snyderman CH, Hirsch BE (1996) Hydroxyapatite cement to repair skull base defects: radiologic appearance. AJNR Am J Neuroradiol 17(8):1569-1574.

Autocranioplasty

Shoakazemi A, Flannery T, McConnell RS (2009) Long-term outcome of subcutaneously preserved autologous cranioplasty. Neurosurgery 65(3):505–510; discussion 510

Sinclair AG, Scoffings DJ (2010) Imaging of the postoperative cranium. Radiographics 30(2):461–482

Craniectomy and the Meningogaleal Complex

Holland M, Nakaji P (2004) Craniectomy: surgical indications and technique. Oper Tech Neurosurg 7(1):10–15

Lanzieri CF, Som PM, Sacher M, Solodnik P, Moore F (1986) The postcraniectomy site: CT appearance. Radiology 159(1):165–170

Cranial Vault Reconstruction for Craniosynostosis

Boyle CM, Rosenblum JD (1997) Three-dimensional CT for pre- and postsurgical imaging of patients with craniosynostosis: correlation of operative procedure and radiologic imaging. AJR Am J Roentgenol 169(4):1173–1177

Derderian CA, Wink JD, McGrath JL, Collinsworth A, Bartlett SP, Taylor JA (2015) Volumetric changes in cranial vault expansion: comparison of fronto-orbital advancement and posterior cranial vault distraction osteogenesis. Plast Reconstr Surg 135(6):1665–1672.

Eppley BL, Sadove AM (1994) Surgical correction of metopic suture synostosis. Clin Plast Surg 21(4):555–562

Greenberg BM, Schneider SJ (2006) Trigonocephaly: surgical considerations and long term evaluation. J Craniomaxillofac Surg 17(3):528–535

Jimenez DF, Barone CM (2010) Endoscopic techniques for craniosynostosis. Atlas Oral Maxillofac Surg Clin North Am 18(2):93–107

Kirschner RE, Karmacharya J, Ong G, Gordon AD, Hunenko O, Losee JE, Gannon FH, Bartlett SP (2002) Repair of the immature craniofacial skeleton with a calcium phosphate cement: quantitative assessment of craniofacial growth. Ann Plast Surg 49(1):33–38; discussion 38

Losee JE, Karmacharya J, Gannon FH, Slemp AE, Ong G, Hunenko O, Gorden AD, Bartlett SP, Kirschner RE (2003) Reconstruction of the immature craniofacial skeleton with a carbonated calcium phosphate bone cement: interaction with bioresorbable mesh. J Craniomaxillofac Surg 14(1):117–124

Mehta VA, Bettegowda C, Jallo GI, Ahn ES (2010) The evolution of surgical management for craniosynostosis. Neurosurg Focus 29(6):E5

Murad GJ, Clayman M, Seagle MB, White S, Perkins LA, Pincus DW (2005) Endoscopic-assisted repair of craniosynostosis. Neurosurg Focus 19(6):E6

Posnick JC, Lin KY, Chen P, Armstrong D (1993) Sagittal synostosis: quantitative assessment of presenting deformity and surgical results based on CT scans. Plast Reconstr Surg 92(6):1015–1024; discussion 1225–1226

Smartt JM Jr, Karmacharya J, Gannon FH, Ong G, Jackson O, Bartlett SP, Poser RD, Kirschner RE (2005) Repair of the immature and mature craniofacial skeleton with a carbonated calcium phosphate cement: assessment of biocompatibility, osteoconductivity, and remodeling capacity. Plast Reconstr Surg 115(6):1642–1650

van der Meulen JJ, Nazir PR, Mathijssen IM, van Adrichem LN, Ongkosuwito E, Stolk-Liefferink SA, Vaandrager MJ (2008) Bitemporal depressions after cranioplasty for trigonocephaly: a long-term evaluation of (supra) orbital growth in 92 patients. J Craniomaxillofac Surg 19(1):72–79

White N, Evans M, Dover MS, Noons P, Solanki G, Nishikawa H (2009) Posterior calvarial vault expansion using distraction osteogenesis. Childs Nerv Syst 25(2):231–236.

Ylikontiola LP, Sándor GK, Salokorpi N, Serlo WS. (2012) Experience with craniosynostosis treatment using posterior cranial vault distraction osteogenesis. Ann Maxillofac Surg 2(1):4–7.

Cranial Vault Encephalocele Repair

Bozinov O, Tirakotai W, Sure U, Bertalanffy H (2005) Surgical closure and reconstruction of a large occipital encephalocele without parenchymal excision. Childs Nerv Syst 21(2):144–147

Ginat DT, Reid R, Frim DM (2016) Imaging assessment of re-exploratory repair of an occipital bone defect-associated tectocerebellar dysraphism via hybrid cranioplasty. Pediatr Neurosurg 51(3):164–166

Hockley AD, Goldin JH, Wake MJ (1990) Management of anterior encephalocele. Childs Nerv Syst 6(8): 444–446

Mohanty A, Biswas A, Reddy M, Kolluri S (2006) Expansile cranioplasty for massive occipital encephalocele. Childs Nerv Syst 22(9):1170–1176

Satyarthee GD, Mahapatra AK (2002) Craniofacial surgery for giant frontonasal encephalocele in a neonate. J Clin Neurosci 9(5):593–595

Subdural Drainage Catheters

Santarius T, Kirkpatrick PJ, Ganesan D, Chia HL, Jalloh I, Smielewski P, Richards HK, Marcus H, Parker RA, Price SJ, Kirollos RW, Pickard JD, Hutchinson PJ (2009) Use of drains versus no drains after burr-hole evacuation of chronic subdural haematoma: a randomised controlled trial. Lancet 374(9695):1067–1073.

Peng D, Zhu Y (2016) External drains versus no drains after burr-hole evacuation for the treatment of chronic subdural haematoma in adults. Cochrane Database Syst Rev. (8):CD011402

Intracranial Pressure Monitor

Stefini R, Rasulo FA (2008) Intracranial pressure monitoring. Eur J Anaesthesiol Suppl 42:192–195

Steiner LA, Andrews PJ (2006) Monitoring the injured brain: ICP and CBF. Br J Anaesth 97(1):26–38

Cranial Surgery Complications

Aarabi B, Hesdorffer DC, Ahn ES, Aresco C, Scalea TM, Eisenberg HM (2006) Outcome following decompressive craniectomy for malignant swelling due to severe head injury. J Neurosurg 104:469–479

Aarabi B, Chesler D, Maulucci C, Blacklock T, Alexander M (2009) Dynamics of subdural hygroma following decompressive craniectomy: a comparative study. Neurosurg Focus 26(6):E8

Akins PT, Guppy KH (2008a) Sinking skin flaps, paradoxical herniation, and external brain tamponade: a review of decompressive craniectomy management. Neurocrit Care 9(2):269–276

Akins PT, Guppy KH (2008b) Sinking skin flaps, paradoxical herniation, and external brain tamponade: a review of decompressive craniectomy management. Neurocrit Care 9(2):269–276

Brisman MH, Bederson JB, Sen CN, Germano IM, Moore F, Post KD (1996) Intracerebral hemorrhage occurring remote from the craniotomy site. Neurosurgery 39(6):1114–1121; discussion 1121–1122

Browning CJ, Harland SP, Burnet NG (2000) Gas in the cranium: an unusual case of delayed pneumocephalus following craniotomy. Clin Oncol (R Coll Radiol) 12(2):118–120

Caroli E, Rocchi G, D'Andrea G, Delfini R (2004) Management of the entered frontal sinus. Neurosurg Rev 27(4):286–288

Cheng YK, Weng HH, Yang JT, Lee MH, Wang TC, Chang CN (2008) Factors affecting graft infection after cranioplasty. J Clin Neurosci 15(10):1115–1119

Dashti SR, Baharvahdat H, Spetzler RF et al. (2008) Operative intracranial infection following craniotomy. Neurosurg Focus 24(6):E10

Friedman JA, Piepgras DG, Duke DA, McClelland RL, Bechtle PS, Maher CO, Morita A, Perkins WJ, Parisi JE, Brown RD Jr (2001) Remote cerebellar hemorrhage after supratentorial surgery. Neurosurgery 49(6):1327–1340

Gnanalingham KK, Lafuente J, Thompson D, Harkness W, Hayward R (2002) Surgical procedures for posterior fossa tumors in children: does craniotomy lead to fewer complications than craniectomy? J Neurosurg 97(4):821–826

Harreld JH, Mohammed N, Goldsberry G, Li X, Li Y, Boop F, Patay Z (2015) Postoperative intraspinal subdural collections after pediatric posterior fossa tumor resection: incidence, imaging, and clinical features. AJNR Am J Neuroradiol 36(5):993–999.

Honeybul S, Ho KM (2011) Long-term complications of decompressive craniectomy for head injury. J Neurotrauma 28(6):929–935

Joseph V, Reilly P (2009) Syndrome of the trephined. J Neurosurg 111(4):650–652

Kothbauer KF, Jallo GI, Siffert J, Jimenez E, Allen JC, Epstein FJ. (2001). Foreign body reaction to hemostatic materials mimicking recurrent brain tumor. Report of three cases. J Neurosurg 95(3):503-506.

Michel SJ (2004) The Mount Fuji sign. Radiology 232(2):449–450

Mori K, Nakajima M, Maeda M (2003) Simple reconstruction of frontal sinus opened during craniotomy using small autogenous bone piece: technical note. Surg Neurol 60(4):326–328; discussion 328

Paízek J, Mericka P, Nemecek S, Nemecková J, Spacek J, Suba P, Sercl M (1998) Posterior cranial fossa surgery in 454 children. Comparison of results obtained in pre-CT and CT era and after various types of management of dura mater. Childs Nerv Syst 14(9):426–438; discussion 439

Palmer JD, Sparrow OC, Iannotti F (1994) Postoperative hematoma: a 5-year survey and identification of avoidable risk factors. Neurosurgery 35(6):1061–1064; discussion 1064–1065

Patel RS, Yousem DM, Maldjian JA, Zager EL (2000) Incidence and clinical significance of frontal sinus or orbital entry during pterional (frontotemporal) craniotomy. AJNR Am J Neuroradiol 21(7):1327–1330

Polin RS, Shaffrey ME, Bogaev CA, Tisdale N, Germanson T, Bocchicchio B et al. (1997) Decompressive bifrontal craniectomy in the treatment of severe refractory posttraumatic cerebral edema. Neurosurgery 41:84–92

Ribalta T, McCutcheon IE, Neto AG, Gupta D, Kumar AJ, Biddle DA, Langford LA, Bruner JM, Leeds NE, Fuller GN (2004) Textiloma (gossypiboma) mimicking recurrent intracranial tumor. Arch Pathol Lab Med 128(7):749–758.

Sinclair AG, Scoffings DJ (2010) Imaging of the postoperative cranium. Radiographics 30(2):461–482

Stiver SI (2009) Complications of decompressive craniectomy for traumatic brain injury. Neurosurg Focus 26(6):E7

Su FW, Ho JT, Wang HC (2008) Acute contralateral subdural hygroma following craniectomy. J Clin Neurosci 15(3):305–307

Tokoro K, Chiba Y, Tsubone K (1989) Late infection after cranioplasty-review of 14 cases. Neurol Med Chir (Tokyo) 29(3):196–201

Webber-Jones JE (2005) Tension pneumocephalus. J Neurosurg Nurs 37(5):272–276

Imaging the Intraoperative and Postoperative Brain

5

Daniel Thomas Ginat, Pamela W. Schaefer, and Marc Daniel Moisi

5.1 Intraoperative MRI

5.1.1 Discussion

The main goal of using MRI during brain tumor resection is to safely maximize the extent of tumor resection. In particular, imaging during surgery can also help compensate for the brain shift, which represents surgically induced volumetric deformation of the intracranial contents attributable to resection of the tumor, as well as intracranial pressure changes that result from craniotomy and cerebrospinal fluid (Fig. 5.1). Intraoperative MRI is also useful for identifying complications during surgery that might require intervention, such as hyperacute intracranial hemorrhage. Hyperacute intraparenchymal hemorrhage typically appears as isointense to the surrounding parenchyma on T1-weighted sequences, but hyperintense on T2-weighted sequences due to the presence of oxyhemoglobin. On susceptibility-weighted sequences, hyperacute intraparenchymal hematomas tend to appear hyperintense centrally with a thin rim of dark signal. Extraparenchymal hyperacute hemorrhage tends to be of intermediate signal on T1-weighted sequences, but conspicuously hyperintense on T2-FLAIR MRI (Fig. 5.2). Hemostatic agents can mimic hemorrhage or residual enhancing tumor due to the rapid T1 shortening effect on blood products. Serial postcontrast T1-weighted images can be useful for depicting residual enhancing tumor. A potential confounder is the presence of contrast leakage at the margins of the resection cavity, which tends to appear more diffuse than nodular (Fig. 5.3).

Laser interstitial thermal therapy comprises various minimally invasive procedures that are increasingly used to treat selected brain tumors, neuropsychiatric disorders, and epileptogenic foci. MRI is also useful for real-time monitoring of these thermal ablation procedures. In particular, MR thermography, which can exploit phase shifts of protons at different temperatures, can provide a temperature map during ablation and from which an irreversible damage model can be derived based on the treatment duration (Fig. 5.4). Besides coagulative necrosis, a small amount of hemorrhage and transient swelling commonly result from thermal ablation (Fig. 5.5). However, an increase in lesion size, heterogeneity, peripheral nodular enhancement, restricted diffusion, elevated blood volume,

D.T. Ginat, M.D., M.S. (✉)
University of Chicago, Pritzker School of Medicine, Chicago, IL, USA
e-mail: dtg1@uchicago.edu

P.W. Schaefer, M.D.
Department of Neuroradiology, Harvard Medical School, Massachusetts General Hospital, Boston, MA, USA

M.D. Moisi, M.D., M.S.
Department of Neurosurgery, Swedish Neuroscience Institute, Seattle, WA, USA

© Springer International Publishing Switzerland 2017
D.T. Ginat, P.-L.A. Westesson (eds.), *Atlas of Postsurgical Neuroradiology*,
DOI 10.1007/978-3-319-52341-5_5

and surrounding edema that persists or develops after one or 2 months following treatment should raise the suspicion for tumor recurrence (Fig. 5.6). Otherwise, thermal ablation results in a predictable progression of signal changes on MRI. In particular, MRI of recently thermally ablated lesions displays a marginal zone with low T1 and high T2 signal due to edema with rim enhancement, which eventually transforms into gliosis; a peripheral zone with low T1 and high T2 signal due to additional edema, which ultimately resolves; and a central zone surrounding the probe tract with high T1 and low T2 signal due to the presence of blood products and coagulative necrosis, which persists amidst encephalomalacia. Some of these findings are exemplified in subsequent sections of this chapter.

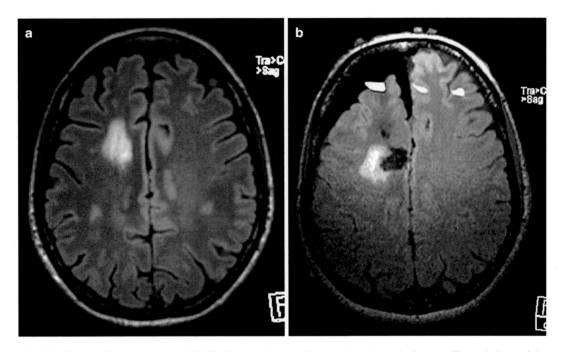

Fig. 5.1 Brain shift. Preoperative FLAIR image (**a**) shows a hyperintense lesion in the right frontal lobe. Intraoperative FLAIR image (**b**) shows partial resection of the lesion and a change in the overall morphology of the surrounding right frontal lobe parenchyma

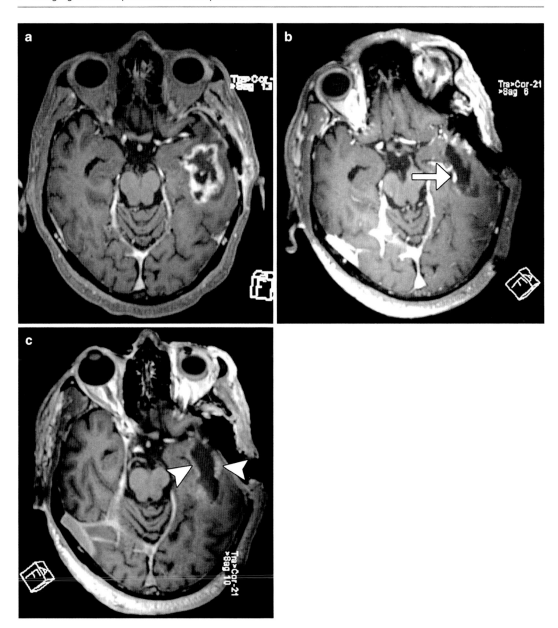

Fig. 5.2 Enhancing tumor resection and contrast leakage. Initial axial post-contrast T1-weighted image (**a**) shows a peripherally enhancing left temporal lobe glioblastoma. Axial post-contrast T1-weigthted MRI (**b**) obtained after the first resection attempt shows a punctate focus of nodular enhancement in the medial resection bed (*arrow*), which represented residual tumor. Axial post-contrast T1-weigthted MRI (**c**) obtained after further resection shows that there are no longer residual enhancing tumor components. Faint enhancement along the margins of the resection cavity represents contrast leakage (*arrowheads*)

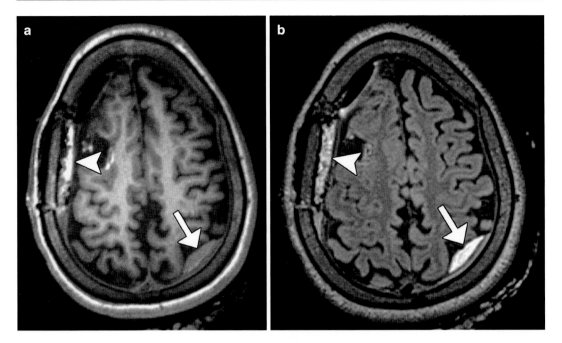

Fig. 5.3 Hyperacute hemorrhage and hemostatic material. Axial T1- (**a**) and T2-FLAIR (**b**) intraoperative MR images obtained at the end of right frontal lobe tumor resection show a small left parietal convexity subdural hematoma with intermediate T1 and high T2 signal (*arrows*). The hemostatic agent in the extradural space along the right frontal convexity surgical bed displays high T1 and T2 signal (*arrowheads*)

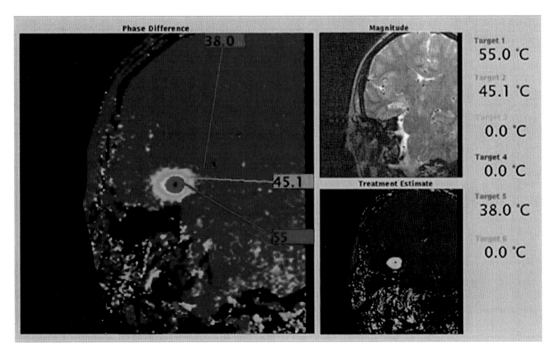

Fig. 5.4 Laser ablation. MR thermography performed during ablation of the right hippocampus shows real-time temperature monitoring and irreversible damage model (Courtesy of Amy Schneider, Medtronic)

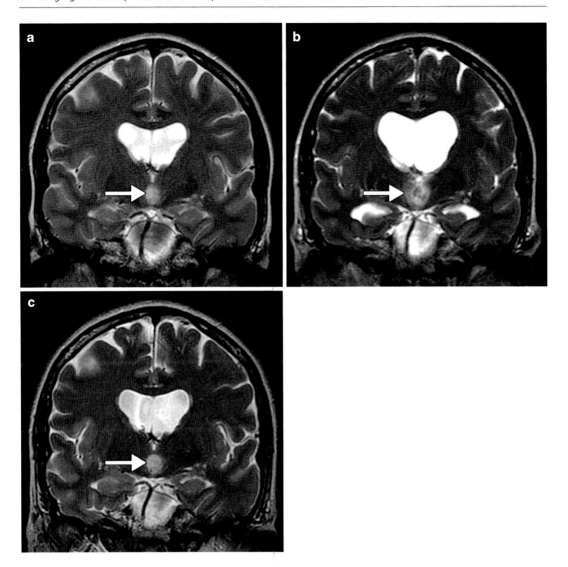

Fig. 5.5 Transient tumor swelling after laser ablation. Preoperative coronal T2-weighted MRI (**a**) shows a hyperintense hypothalamic tumor, which proved to be a pilocytic astrocytoma (*arrow*). The coronal T2-weighted MRI (**b**) obtained 1 week after laser ablation of the tumor when the patient developed memory formation difficulties shows increase in size of the tumor (*arrows*) and lateral ventricles. Follow-up coronal T2-weighted MRI (**c**) after steroid taper shows interval decrease in size of the tumor (*arrow*) and lateral ventricles

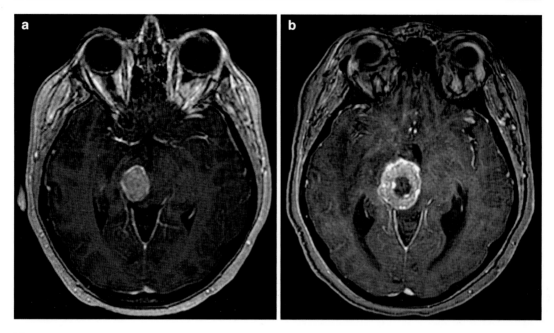

Fig. 5.6 Tumor progression after laser ablation. Preoperative axial T1-weighted MRI (**a**) shows a homogeneously enhancing right midbrain tumor. Axial T1-weighted MRI (**b**) obtained over 1 month after laser ablation shows central necrosis, but overall increase in size of the enhancing tumor

5.2 Brain Tumor Surgery and Treatment Accessories

5.2.1 Stereotactic Biopsy

5.2.1.1 Discussion

Stereotactic biopsy is an image-guided procedure that is commonly performed to obtain tissue samples of intracranial lesions. Hemorrhage is one of the most common findings after stereotactic brain biopsy, occurring in up to 9% of cases. Hemorrhage along the biopsy trajectory has a characteristic linear configuration. Small amounts of blood products along the path of the biopsy that may only be discernible on T2* GRE or SWI sequences are usually of no clinical concern and resolve spontaneously. Rather, such findings serve to delineate the path of the biopsy needle and can help account for new neurological deficits (Fig. 5.7). In addition, the blood products left along the biopsy path that are apparent on MRI can also serve as a useful indicator of whether the lesion was appropriately sampled. Nevertheless, some operators prefer to insert a metal marker in the biopsy cavity as a reliable indicator that is visible on imaging (Fig. 5.8). Although off-target biopsy can yield tumor cells if the lesion is an infiltrative tumor, the grade may be underestimated. Ideally, biopsy of the enhancing portion of the tumor with the highest cerebral blood volume (CBV) on perfusion-weighted MRI should be performed. Another uncommon, but notable complication of stereotactic biopsy is tumor seeding (Fig. 5.9). Otherwise, a mild degree of enhancement in the brain parenchyma along the biopsy path is often encountered on early postoperative imaging as an incidental finding that typically resolves within a couple of months (Fig. 5.10).

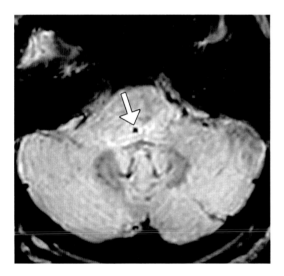

Fig. 5.7 Blood products along the path of biopsy. The patient experienced new right-sided abducens palsy after right transfrontal biopsy of a medulla lesion. Axial SWI shows susceptibility effect along the expected location of the right abducens nucleus/nerve (*arrow*)

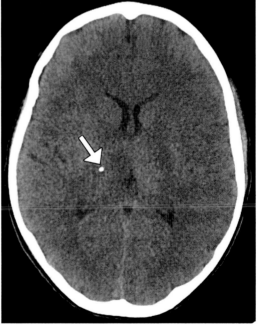

Fig. 5.8 Biopsy cavity marker. Axial CT image shows a titanium clip (*arrow*) deposited in the right thalamocapsular junction biopsy site, not to be mistaken for hemorrhage or an unintended foreign body

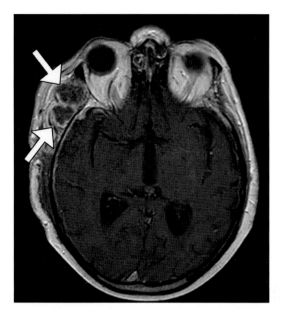

Fig. 5.9 Tumor seeding. Axial post-contrast T1-weighted MRI shows necrotic tumors (*arrows*) in the right temporal fossa, near the surgical approach in a patient with renal cell carcinoma that had metastasized to the brain

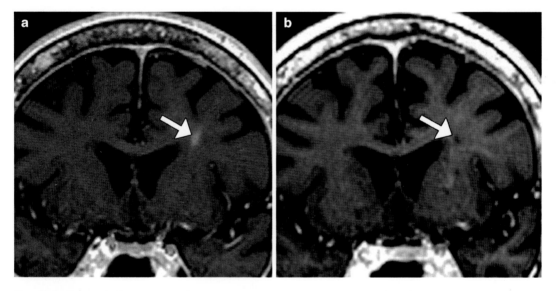

Fig. 5.10 Expected biopsy path enhancement. Initial coronal post-contrast T1-weighted MRI (**a**) obtained soon after left transfrontal biopsy shows enhancement along the path of the biopsy needle (*arrow*). Follow-up coronal post-contrast T1-weighted MRI (**b**) obtained 3 months later shows that the enhancement has resolved, leaving behind a small area of low signal due to encephalomalacia (*arrow*)

5.2.2   Resection Cavities

5.2.2.1 Discussion

The space that remains after a tumor is surgically removed is known as the resection cavity. The resection cavity is often lined or packed with hemostatic agents (refer to Chap. 4) and contains variable amounts of cerebrospinal fluid and blood products, especially during the early postoperative period (Fig. 5.11). Oftentimes, resection cavities eventually shrink and collapse, becoming nearly imperceptible (Fig. 5.12), although some cavities stay the same size, particularly if they communicate with the ventricular system.

Variable amounts of tumor may remain adjacent to the cavity depending on whether gross total, near-total, or subtotal resection was performed. The extent of tumor resection depends

on several factors, including the location and type of tumor. Tumors that involve eloquent parts of the brain, that are in technically difficult areas to reach, or that involve critical structures, such as cranial nerves or major arteries, can limit the extent of tumor resection. Similarly, it is more difficult to achieve complete resection of infiltrative tumors than well-defined tumors. Ultimately, there is often a trade-off between removing as much tumor as possible versus preserving as much normal tissue and avoiding complications. Comparison with preoperative imaging should be performed when possible to help identify residual tumor.

Surgically induced parenchymal injury, postoperative hemorrhage, and enhancing conditions related to brain tumor surgery and adjunctive treatments are discussed in the following sections.

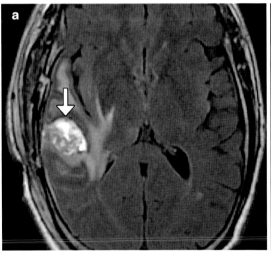 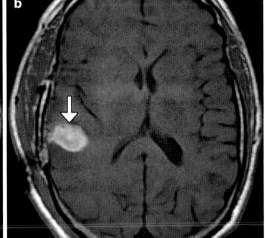

Fig. 5.11 Early surgical cavity with blood products. Axial FLAIR (**a**), T1-weighted (**b**), post-contrast T1-weighted (**c**), and GRE (**d**) MR images show subacute blood products within a right temporal resection cavity (*arrows*). There is no significant mass effect or enhancement

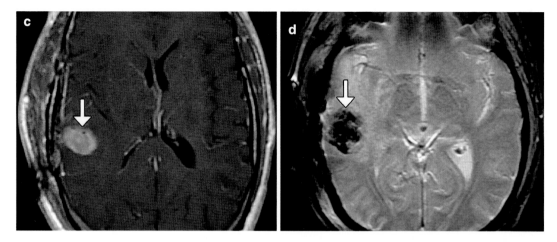

Fig. 5.11 (continued)

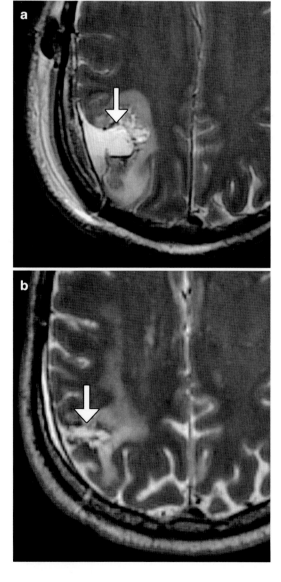

Fig. 5.12 Resection cavity evolution. Initial postoperative axial T2-weighted MRI (**a**) shows a fluid-filled resection cavity in the right parietal lobe *(arrow)*. Axial T2-weighted MRI obtained 7 months later (**b**) shows near-complete collapse of the resection cavity *(arrow)*

Surgically Induced Parenchymal Injury

Local areas of devitalized brain tissue surrounding the resection cavity are encountered on early postoperative MRI in up to 70% of cases of high-grade glioma resection as well as many other tumor resections. This phenomenon manifests as focal areas of restricted diffusion (Fig. 5.13). Enhancement of the devitalized tissue occurs in over 40% of cases between 1 week and several months. Furthermore, this phenomenon can lead to overestimation of residual non-enhancing tumor volume due to the presence of swelling and high signal on T2-weighted sequences during the early postoperative period. Visible encephalomalacia eventually forms around the surgical cavity in over 90% of cases of resection site infarcts. Larger, territorial infarcts are uncommon complications of tumor resection, but are predisposed by proximity to or encasement of major arterial branches and occasionally venous occlusion.

Vasogenic edema can result from forceful intraoperative retraction, which is sometimes performed in order to access large or deep tumors. The edema may be related to hyperemia of the brain surface after the release of retraction. On imaging obtained during the early postoperative period, retraction-induced vasogenic edema appears as swelling along the path of the retractors (Fig. 5.14). Unlike acute infarction, the vasogenic edema demonstrates elevated diffusivity rather than restricted diffusion.

A peculiar complication related to posterior fossa tumor resections is hypertrophic olivary degeneration, which results from disruption of the dentato-rubro-olivary pathway (Guillain-Mollaret triangle). This phenomenon can occur after surgical resection of cerebellar tumors. If the resection site involves the central tegmental tract, the ipsilateral olivary nucleus is affected, while if the superior cerebellar peduncle is involved, the contralateral olivary nucleus is affected. Thus, bilateral hypertrophic olivary degeneration results from disruption of the central tegmental tract and superior cerebellar peduncle. Tongue fasciculations are characteristic of hypertrophic olivary degeneration. On MRI, hypertrophic olivary degeneration manifests as T2 hyperintensity with or without enlargement of the anterolateral medulla (Fig. 5.15). The differential diagnosis includes ischemia, demyelination, tumor spread, and infection. The lack of enhancement with hypertrophic olivary degeneration may help differentiate this entity from the other possibilities, such as some neoplasms. In addition, most cases demonstrate associated atrophy of the contralateral dentate nucleus or cerebellar cortex. Signal changes on MRI develop approximately 1 month after surgery and can persist for many years. Hypertrophy of the olivary nucleus tends to develop after several months and can resolve after 2–3 years.

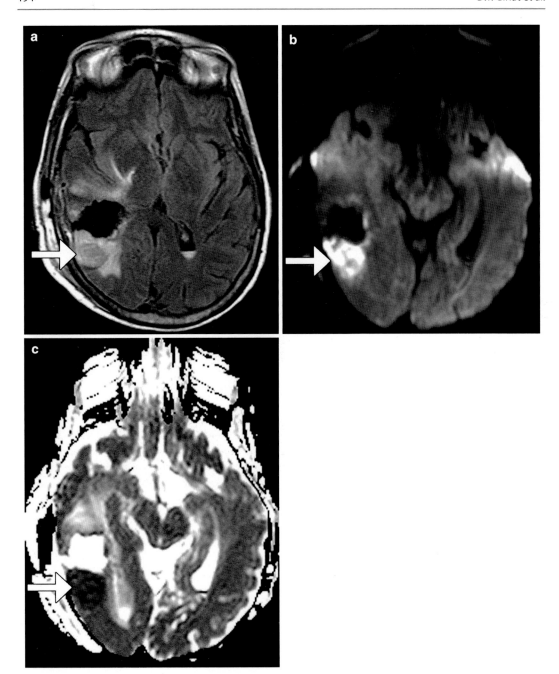

Fig. 5.13 Peri-resection infarction. The patient underwent recent resection of a right posterior temporal lobe glioblastoma. Axial FLAIR (**a**), DWI (**b**), and ADC (**c**) maps show an area of restricted diffusion posterior to the resection cavity (*arrows*)

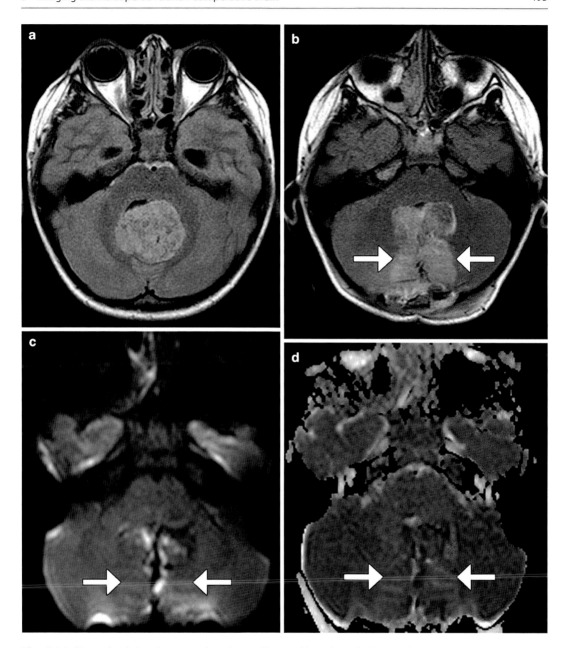

Fig. 5.14 Retraction-induced vasogenic edema. The patient has a history of fourth ventricular medulloblastoma. Preoperative axial FLAIR image (**a**) shows a large fourth ventricular mass, but no surrounding vasogenic edema. Postoperative FLAIR image (**b**) shows new areas of hyperintensity in the bilateral medial cerebellar hemispheres. The diffusion-weighted image (**c**) and ADC map (**d**) show corresponding mildly elevated diffusivity (*arrows*). Small areas of ischemia are also present medially

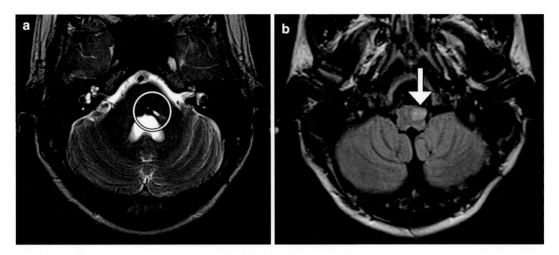

Fig. 5.15 Hypertrophic olivary degeneration. The patient presented with tongue fasciculations after resection of a right pontine cavernous malformation. Axial T2 MRI (**a**) shows the resection site *(encircled)*. Axial FLAIR MRI (**b**) shows high signal within an enlarged left olivary nucleus *(arrow)*

Postoperative Hemorrhagic Lesions

Hemorrhage is a relatively common occurrence with tumor resection and usually occurs at the craniotomy site. CT or MRI can readily depict these hemorrhages. The lack of contrast enhancement and susceptibility effects help distinguish hematomas from residual tumor (Fig. 5.16). Hemorrhage that results from incomplete tumor resection is sometimes termed "wounded tumor syndrome" and is more commonly encountered with vascular tumors, such as melanoma, renal cell carcinoma, and glioblastoma (Fig. 5.17). Other risk factors for postoperative hemorrhage include inadequate hemostasis, underlying coagulopathies, and hypertension.

Chronic hemorrhage after surgery can result in superficial siderosis and mainly occurs when there is a cystic cavity that contains friable vessels or residual/recurrent tumor (Fig. 5.18). Hemosiderin deposits can coat remote leptomeningeal surfaces, particularly the cerebellum and brainstem. On CT, superficial siderosis can appear as a mildly hyperattenuating coating of these structures, which may also become atrophic as a result. MRI is more sensitive for depicting hemosiderin deposits, which appear as very low signal intensity on all sequences. Blooming artifact on T2* GRE or SWI sequences accentuates the lesions. The significance of superficial siderosis is that it may cause symptoms such as ataxia and deafness.

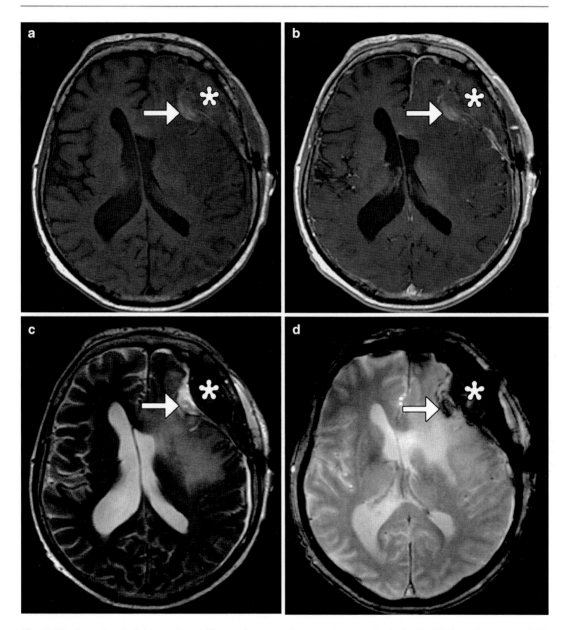

Fig. 5.16 Operative bed hemorrhage. The study was obtained to evaluate for residual tumor following recent meningioma resection. Copious oozing of blood was noted during surgery. Axial T1-weighted (**a**) and post-contrast T1-weighted (**b**), T2-weighted (**c**), and GRE (**d**) images show an intrinsically T1 hyperintense and T2 hypointense extradural collection (*) with blooming and mass effect upon the underlying brain. There is also a small amount of hemorrhage within the surgical cavity associated with hemostatic material (*arrows*)

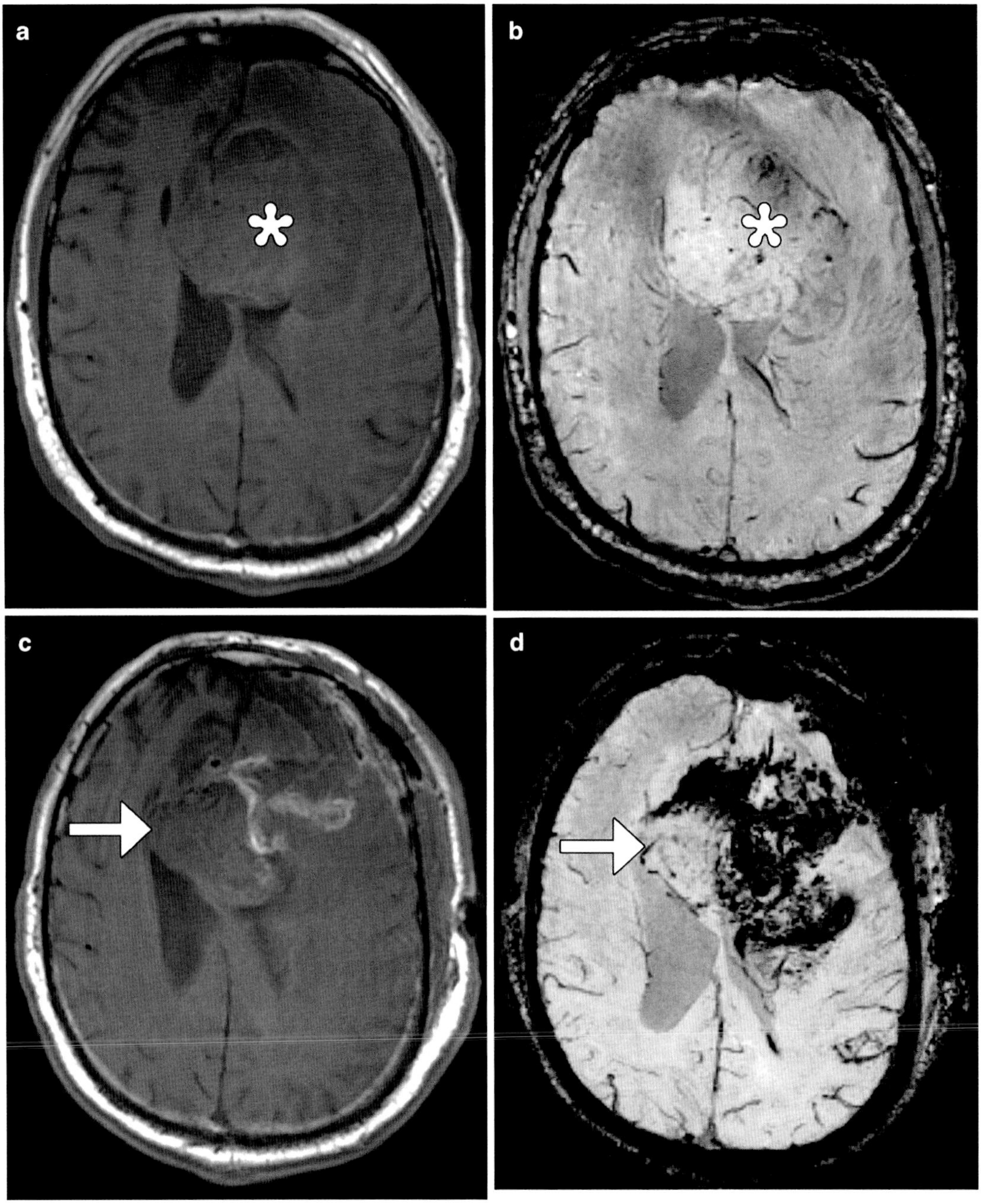

Fig. 5.17 Wounded tumor. The patient underwent subtotal resection of glioblastoma. Preoperative axial T1-weighted (**a**) and susceptibility-weighted imaging (**b**) show a large mass (*) in the left frontal lobe with only a few foci of microhemorrhage. Postoperative axial T1-weighted (**c**) and susceptibility-weighted imaging (**d**) show interval appearance of high T1 signal hemorrhage and extensive susceptibility effect within and adjacent to the residual tumor (*arrows*)

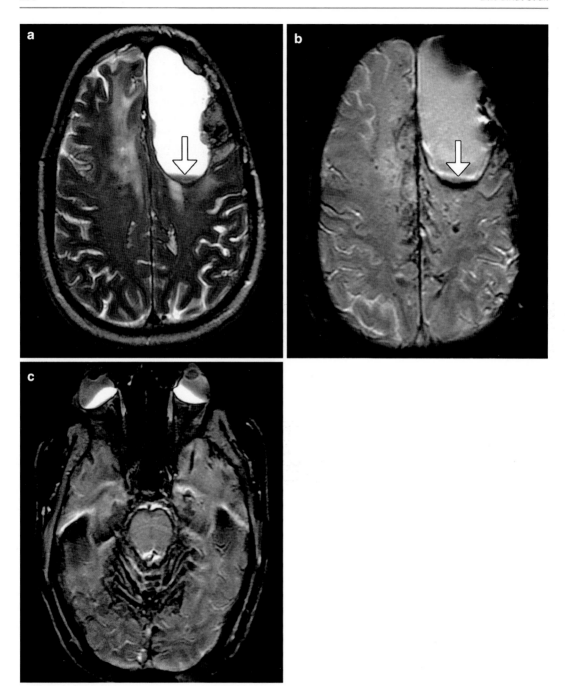

Fig. 5.18 Superficial siderosis. Axial T2-weighted MRI (**a**) and corresponding SWI (**b**) show a cystic left frontal lobe resection cavity with layering of blood products (*arrows*). In addition, there is blooming effect along the margins of the cavity and along the cerebral sulci. SWI at a more inferior level (**c**) shows extensive susceptibility effect in a leptomeningeal distribution in the brainstem and cerebellum

Enhancing Lesions in the Surgical Bed Region and Beyond

Many types of enhancing lesions can be encountered on imaging after surgery, as listed in Table 5.1 and depicted in Figs. 5.19, 5.20, 5.21, 5.22, and 5.23. Indeed, several of these conditions can coexist and make interpretation of the imaging a challenge. Differentiation of these conditions from recurrent enhancing tumor is based on morphology as well as timing. Advanced imaging techniques, such as perfusion MRI and MR spectroscopy, are often helpful for problem solving. Nevertheless, in some cases, biopsy or serial imaging can help elucidate ambiguous cases. It is also important to systematically evaluate the areas beyond the surgical bed on imaging exams, particularly with aggressive neoplasms, such as glioblastoma, which can undergo spread to remote parts of the brain, seed the scalp and face soft tissues, and undergo cerebrospinal fluid dissemination.

Table 5.1 Differential diagnosis of enhancing lesions on MRI after treatment for malignant glioma (Courtesy John W. Henson, MD and Jennifer Wulff, ARNP)

Condition	Onset	Other features
Granulation tissue	First postoperative week (usually after 2 or 3 days), intensifies over the ensuing weeks, and resolves over 3–5 months	The enhancement is typically linear and smooth, but can become more nodular by 1 week following surgery. Since residual enhancing tumor can be obscured or confounded by granulation tissue, baseline imaging is recommended within 48 h of surgery, before granulation tissue forms. Serial imaging can also help to differentiate granulation tissue from residual tumor in that tumor increases in size over time, while granulation tissue should remain stable and eventually resolves
Perioperative ischemia	2 weeks after surgery	Two-thirds of patients have focal infarcts around the resection cavity, and this can account for new post-op neurological deficits. Look for this on immediate post-op DWI. Can enhance after 10–14 days. Enhancement slowly resolves, leaving an area of encephalomalacia
Postoperative infection	1–3 weeks after surgery	Clinical deterioration and new enhancement 1–3 weeks after surgery should raise a question of infection. Wound breakdown and drainage, markedly tender wound, fever, and elevated ESR can occur. Focal infection may show restricted diffusion
Pseudoprogression	Within 3 months following completion of concomitant RT and TMZ	Inflammatory response to treatment. Often symptomatic. Occurs within the RT port. Cannot be distinguished from true progression by either routine MRI or advanced* MRI or FDG-PET. More likely in glioblastoma with methylated MGMT promoter. Wanes with time (scans are performed every month until change determines likely diagnosis). Good prognostic factor
True progression	Any time following surgery	Worsens with time. Routine MRI cannot distinguish from pseudoprogression and radiation necrosis, but tumor tends to have elevated blood volume on perfusion MRI. More likely in tumors without methylation of the MGMT promoter. Poor prognostic factor
Radiation necrosis	Usually >1 year after radiation therapy	Routine MRI cannot distinguish from progression; advanced MRI and FDG-PET can be very useful in distinguishing from progression. Can progress or wane over time. SMART (stroke-like migraines after radiation therapy) syndrome is an unusual, late complication of localized radiation therapy for brain tumors, in which patients present with headache and neurological deficits between about 2 and 10 years after treatment, usually greater than 50 Gy of radiation. Treated with observation, steroids, bevacizumab, or surgery

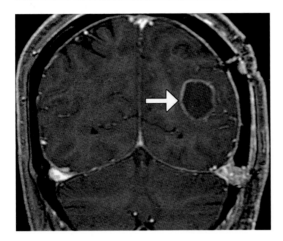

Fig. 5.19 Granulation tissue. The patient is status post meningioma resection 5 days prior to imaging. Coronal post-contrast T1-weighted MRI shows a thin circumferential rim of enhancement along the resection margin (*arrow*)

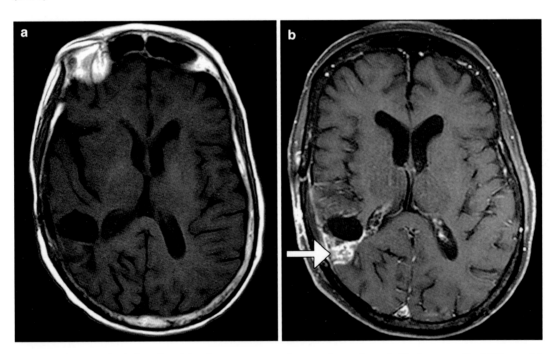

Fig. 5.20 Perioperative infarct. Pre- (**a**) and post-contrast (**b**) T1-weighted MR images obtained 1 month after surgery in the same case as in Fig. 5.13 show that the infarcted tissues enhance (*arrow*). Furthermore, the CBV map (**c**) shows corresponding hypoperfusion in the area (*arrow*)

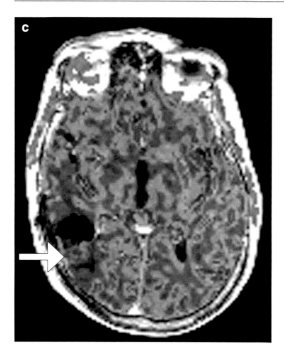

Fig. 5.20 (continued)

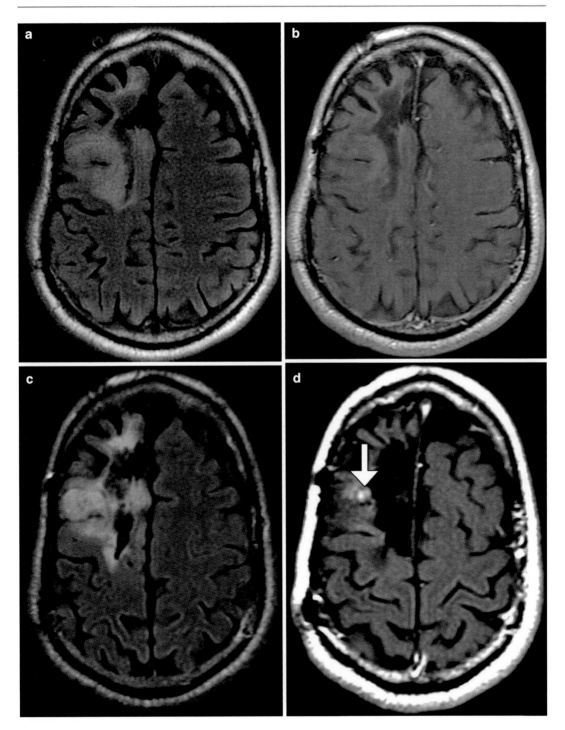

Fig. 5.21 Tumor progression. The patient underwent gross total resection of an oligoastrocytoma (WHO grade II/IV) in the right frontal lobe. Axial FLAIR (**a**) and post-contrast T1-weighted (**b**) MR images obtained approximately 10 years after resection show a right frontal resection cavity surrounded by non-enhancing FLAIR signal abnormality. Axial FLAIR (**c**) and post-contrast T1-weighted (**d**) MR images obtained approximately 1 year later show a new focus of enhancement adjacent to the resection cavity (*arrow*), but no obvious change in the FLAIR signal abnormality. Axial FLAIR (**e**), post-contrast T1-weighted (**f**), subtraction image (**g**), and CBV map (**h**) obtained approximately 6 months later demonstrate marked interval increase in volume of the FLAIR signal abnormality and enhancing adjacent to the resection cavity and associated elevated CBC (*arrows*)

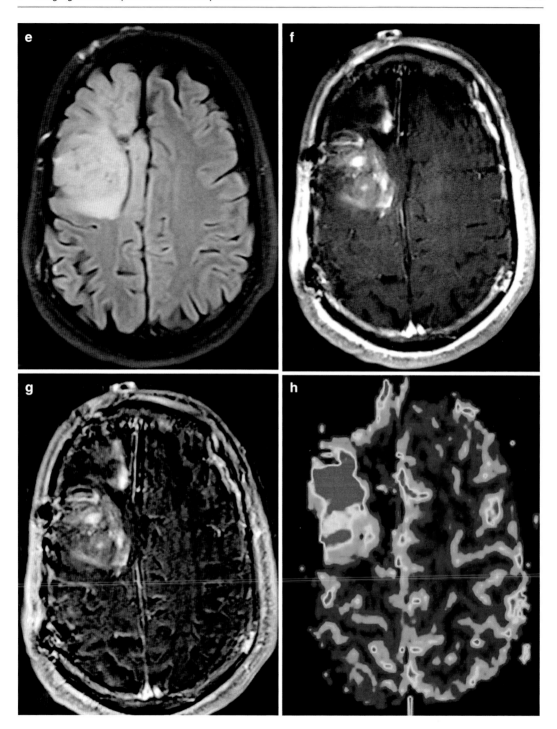

Fig. 5.21 (continued)

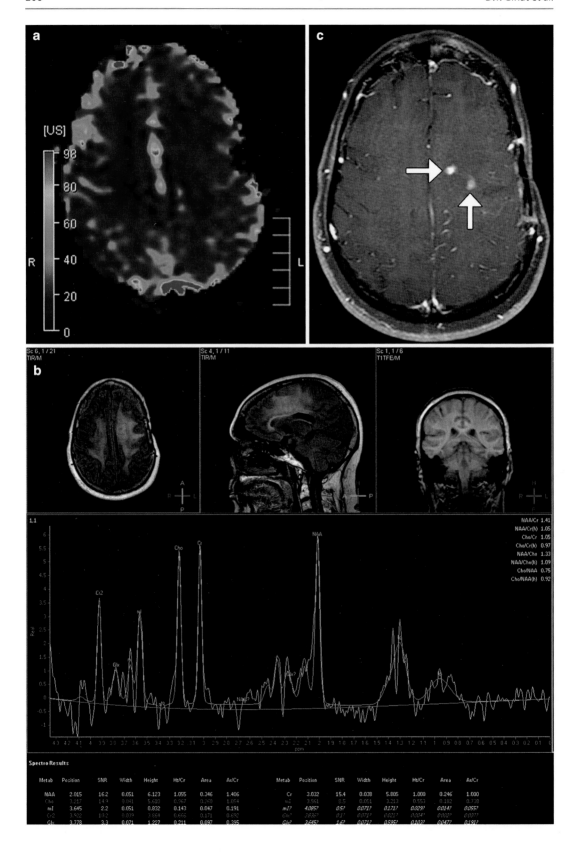

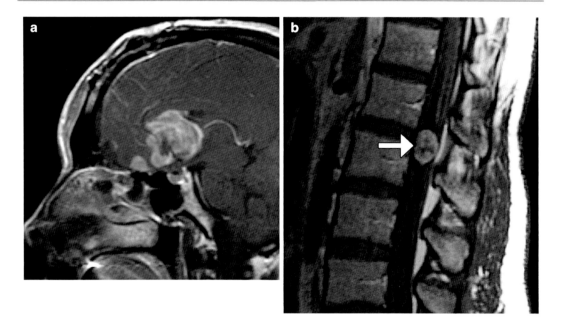

Fig. 5.23 Metastatic glioblastoma in the spinal canal. The patient presented with back and low extremity pain after gross total resection of a left frontal glioblastoma resection with recurrence. Sagittal post-contrast T1-weighted MRI (**a**) shows irregular enhancement involving the bilateral frontal lobes, extending to the meningeal surface. Sagittal post-contrast T1-weighted MRI (**b**) shows an intradural, extramedullary mass with irregular enhancement in the upper lumbar spinal canal (*arrow*)

Fig. 5.22 Radiation necrosis. The patient has a history of left frontal lobe glioblastoma that was resected and radiated approximately 1 year before. Axial (**a**) post-contrast T1-weighted MRI shows small areas of enhancement in the treatment bed region (*arrows*). There is no corresponding hypermetabolism on the blood volume map (**b**). MRI spectroscopy (**c**) over the abnormality shows a lactate peak, mildly reduced NAA peak, and a Cho peak that is not particularly elevated with respect to Cr

5.2.3 Ommaya Reservoirs

5.2.3.1 Discussion

Intrathecal chemotherapy can lengthen survival and alleviate symptoms in patients with widespread leptomeningeal metastases. The two primary means of delivering intrathecal chemotherapy are Ommaya reservoirs and repeat lumbar puncture. Ommaya reservoirs are implanted in the subcutaneous tissues of the scalp and contain a pump mechanism for drug delivery agents into the ventricular system through an intraventricular catheter (Fig. 5.24). Ommaya reservoirs offer many advantages over repeat lumbar punctures, including greater patient comfort, diminished risk for patients with thrombocytopenia, more consistent drug levels, and possibly greater clinical efficacy. Tumor cyst devices are similar to Ommaya shunts, but are used to inject chemotherapeutic agents directly into tumors.

Infection is a major complication of Ommaya catheter placement. The incidence of Ommaya-associated infection is 15% within the first year of placement (range 2–23%). *Staphylococcus aureus* and *Staphylococcus epidermidis* are the most common causative organisms. Manifestations of catheter-associated infection range from meningitis to abscess, for which imaging is useful for identifying fluid collections surrounding the catheter (Fig. 5.25). Debris in the fluid and enhancement helps differentiate infection from hygromas

(simple fluid collections), which can also occur with Ommaya catheter placement. Management consists of antibiotic therapy and possible hardware removal and debridement depending on the extent of the infection.

Focal brain necrosis due to chemotherapy extravasation secondary to Ommaya reservoir catheter obstruction is rare, with an incidence of 0.6% of patients. This condition is caused by displacement of the catheter tip into the brain parenchyma. Imaging demonstrates circumferential areas of necrosis surrounding the retracted Ommaya catheter, manifesting as patchy enhancement, high T2 signal, and restricted diffusion, representing cytotoxic edema (Fig. 5.26). A unique and serious complication of methotrexate extravasation is progressive leukoencephalopathy. This entity involves the white matter diffusely and can be either hemorrhagic or nonhemorrhagic.

Cerebrospinal fluid cysts can sometimes form around Ommaya catheters and may be caused by distal shunt obstruction, although this complication can also occur when the catheter is appropriately positioned, with or without hydrocephalus. The pericatheter cysts do not have perceptible walls or rim enhancement, but may have surrounding edema. Although the cysts may be asymptomatic, it is important to evaluate for predisposing factors that could be addressed, such as malpositioning of the Ommaya catheter (Fig. 5.27).

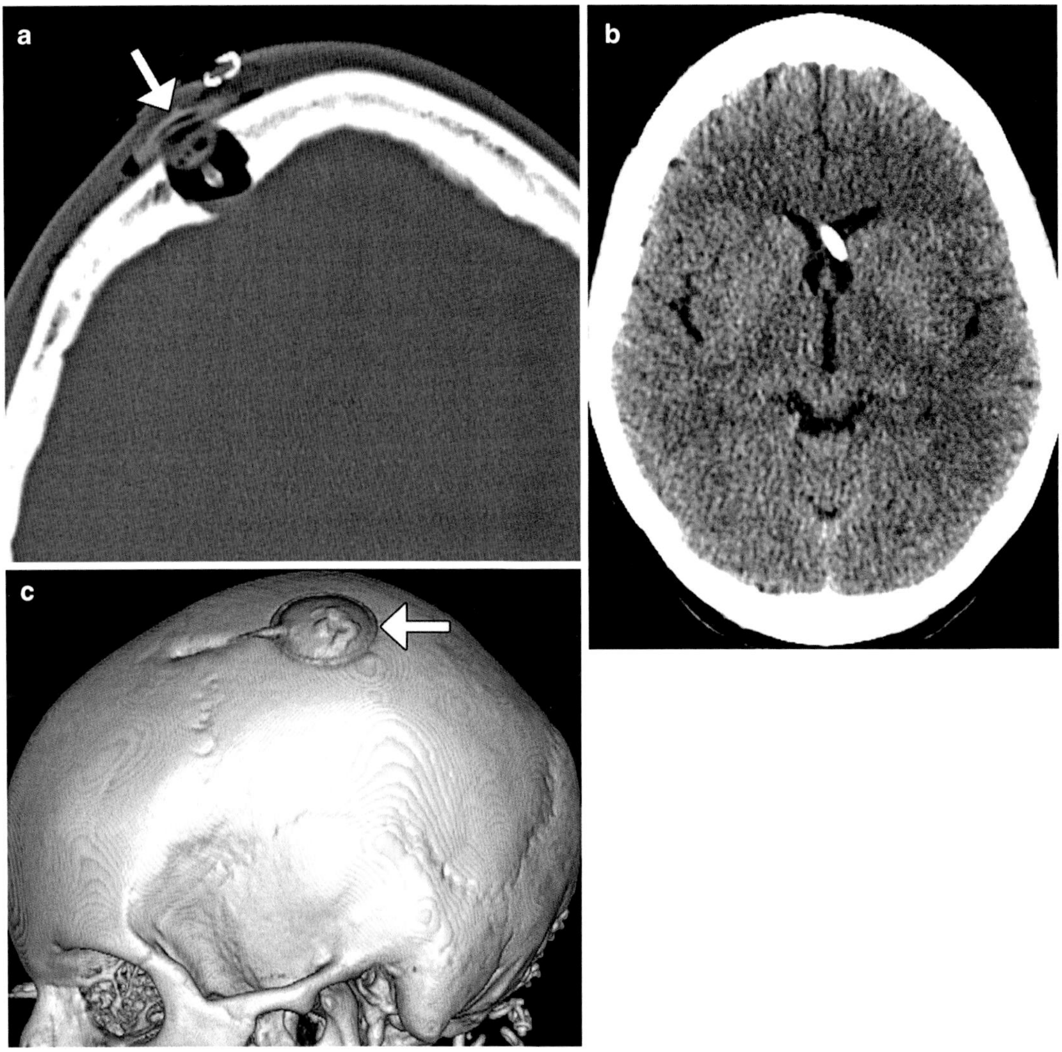

Fig. 5.24 Ommaya reservoir components. The patient has a history of leptomeningeal spread of breast cancer. Axial CT images show the Ommaya reservoir (*arrow*) positioned in the right frontal subcutaneous tissues (**a**). The drug delivery catheter enters the intracranial compart- ment via a burr hole. The tip of the catheter lies within the anterior horn of the left lateral ventricle (**b**). 3D CT image (**c**) shows the reservoir (*arrows*) and catheter entering the skull through a burr hole

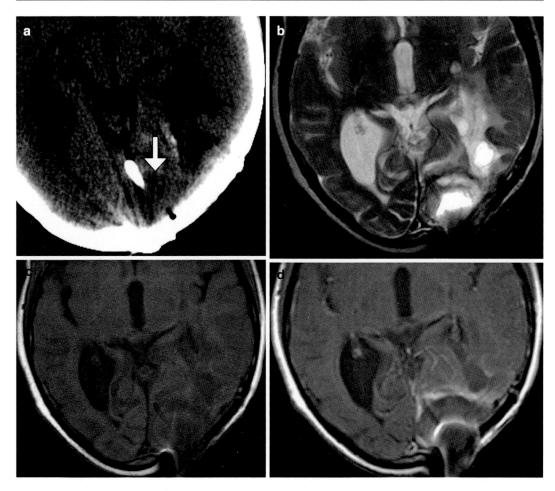

Fig. 5.25 Ommaya catheter infection. The patient presented with exposed Ommaya reservoir hardware and cellulitis. Axial CT image (**a**) shows a left parietal Ommaya catheter surrounded by a fluid collection (*arrow*), which is difficult to discern amidst streak artifact. Axial T2-weighted (**b**), T1-weighted (**c**), and post-contrast T1-weighted (**d**) MR images show a complex fluid collection with rim enhancement surrounding the Ommaya catheter, compatible with a pericatheter abscess

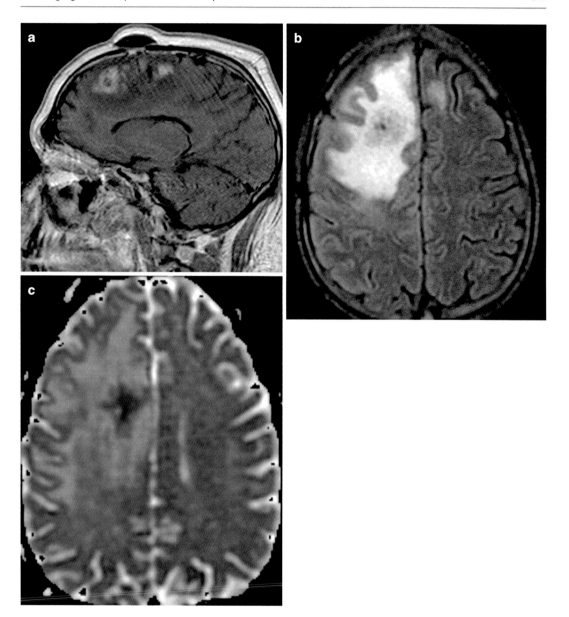

Fig. 5.26 Extravasation of methotrexate through blocked Ommaya reservoir with focal brain necrosis. Post-contrast sagittal T1-weighted MRI (**a**) shows edema and patchy enhancement surrounding the catheter. Axial FLAIR (**c**) better delineates the extent edema surrounding the Ommaya catheter, and the corresponding ADC map (**c**) shows restricted diffusion surrounding the path of the Ommaya catheter, consistent with cytotoxic edema

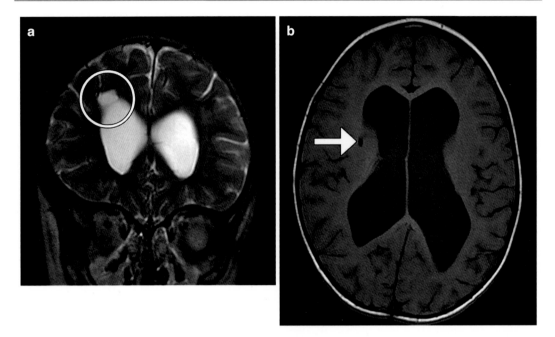

Fig. 5.27 Ommaya catheter-associated cyst and catheter malpositioning (**a**) shows a right frontal lobe periventricular cerebrospinal fluid cyst (*encircled*). Axial T1-weighted MRI (**b**) shows the catheter (*arrow*) has penetrated the right basal ganglia instead of the lateral ventricle. There is also hydrocephalus

5.2.4 Chemotherapy Wafers

5.2.4.1 Discussion

Chemotherapy wafers, such as carmustine implants (Gliadel), are sometimes implanted in the surgical bed after malignant brain neoplasm resection. The wafers are biodegradable sheets of polymers that are impregnated with the chemotherapy agent. Initially, the wafers appear as hypointense linear structures on T1- and T2-weighted MRI sequences, but they can change in signal intensity characteristics over time (Fig. 5.28).

The presence of wafers does not alter the pattern of tumor recurrence. Perfusion MRI is particularly useful to monitor the treatment effects and differentiate these from recurrent neoplasm. The presence of foci with elevated CBV suggests tumor recurrence. MR spectroscopy can also be useful for monitoring tumor response to chemotherapy wafers. For example, it has been noted that increased peritumoral NAA/Cr and decreased peritumoral Cho/NAA compared with normal brain tissue by 3–5 weeks suggest treatment response.

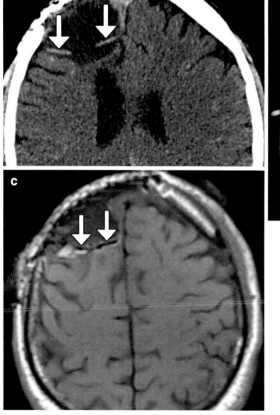
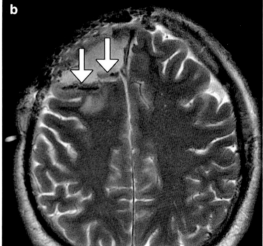

Fig. 5.28 Chemotherapy wafers. The patient has a history of glioblastoma status post resection and implantation of Gliadel wafers. Axial CT (**a**) shows hyperattenuating linear structures along the edges of the right frontal resection cavity (*arrows*). T2-weighted (**b**) and axial T1-weighted (**c**) MR images obtained 1 day after surgery demonstrate the low signal linear Gliadel wafers (*arrows*) lining the resection cavity

5.2.5   Brachytherapy Seeds

5.2.5.1 Discussion

Local radiation therapy can be administered for treatment of brain tumors via brachytherapy (interstitial) seed implantation. The seeds contain radioactive isotopes, such as I-125, and can be implanted temporarily (for approximately 1 week) or permanently. Temporary seeds are typically introduced and removed using plastic catheters passed through burr holes, while permanent seeds are implanted in the tumor/surgical bed. The seeds appear as tiny metallic cylinders on CT or signal voids on MRI (Fig. 5.29).

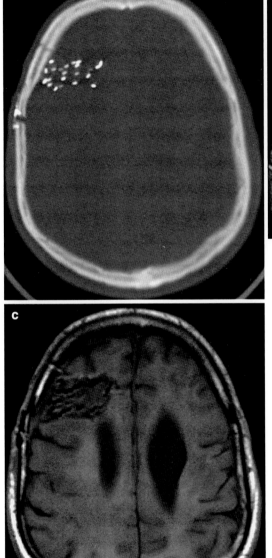
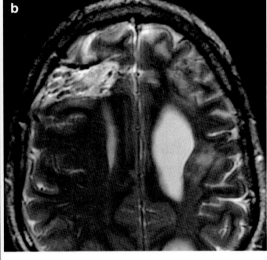

Fig. 5.29 Brachytherapy seeds. The patient has a history of metastatic sarcoma to the right frontal lobe and is status post right frontal craniotomy, gross total tumor resection, and placement of I-125 interstitial radiation seeds. Axial CT image (**a**) demonstrates numerous metallic interstitial seeds each measuring a few millimeters in length within the surgical cavity. On both T2-weighted (**b**) and T1-weighted (**c**) MRI, the seeds are of low signal intensity

5.2.6 GliaSite Radiation Therapy System

5.2.6.1 Discussion

The GliaSite radiation therapy system is used to administer intracranial brachytherapy for brain tumor treatment. The system is a catheter-based device that consists of an infusion port on one end and a double balloon on the other. Positioning markers are also included along the length of the catheter. The balloon, which contains the radioactive isotope solution, is positioned within the surgical cavity. The filled balloon is hyperattenuating on CT and displays fluid signal on MRI (Fig. 5.30). Normally, there can be enhancement in the tissues surrounding the balloon. The catheter and its position markers are also visible on both modalities. However, the balloon and surrounding tissues are better assessed on MRI, particularly when there is tumor recurrence. Perfusion MRI is especially helpful for evaluating enhancing lesions in the tumor bed, whereby elevated rCBV suggests recurrence of high-grade tumor.

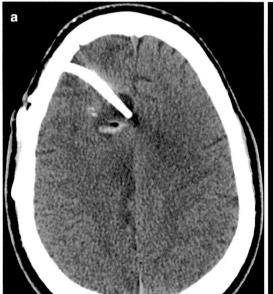 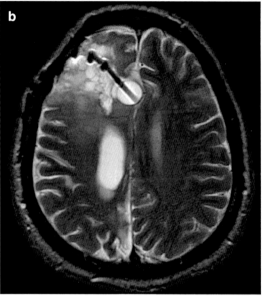

Fig. 5.30 GliaSite system. The patient has a history of right frontal glioblastoma, status post resection. Axial CT (**a**) and axial T2-weighted (**b**) and T1-weighted (**c**) MR images that show the fluid-filled GliaSite radiation therapy system balloon at the end of the low signal intensity catheter with positioning markers. Pre- (**d**) and post-contrast (**e**) T1-weighted images and CBV map (**f**) obtained 1 year later show an enhancing nodule with corresponding increased perfusion adjacent to the catheter in the surgical bed, consistent with recurrent tumor (*arrows*). Illustration of the GliaSite Radiation Therapy system (**g**)

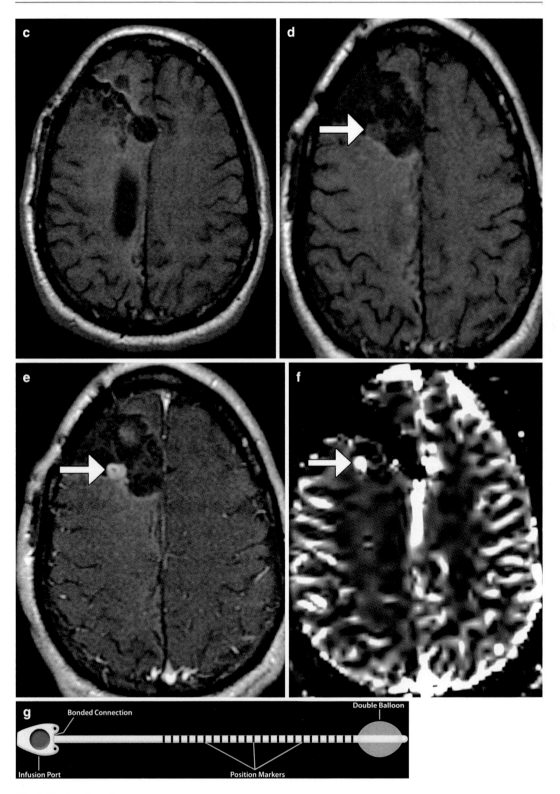

Fig. 5.30 (continued)

5.3 Neurodegenerative, Neuropsychiatric, and Epilepsy Surgery

5.3.1 Prefrontal Lobotomy

5.3.1.1 Discussion

Prefrontal lobotomy (leucotomy) is a now obsolete procedure that was introduced in 1935 as a treatment option for psychiatric illnesses, such as schizophrenia. The procedure essentially consists of ablating the frontal lobe white matter tracts using a probe-like device known as the leukotome via a transorbital or transcranial approach. This produces the appearance of band-like cavitary lesions in the frontal lobe white matter (Fig. 5.31). On MRI, FLAIR sequences show a hyperintense rim of gliosis surrounding the cavitary defects. Focal atrophy of the frontal lobe and corpus callosum is common and often pronounced. High-attenuation foci on CT and susceptibility effects on MRI can be observed along the lobotomy margins, which correspond to residual Pantopaque used for visualization of the lobotomy plane during the operation.

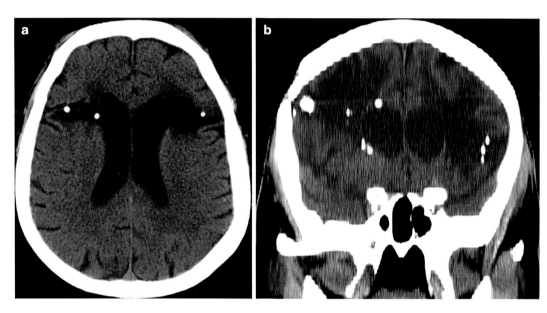

Fig. 5.31 Bilateral prefrontal lobotomy. The patient has a history of schizophrenia treated with bifrontal lobotomy many years before. Axial (**a**) and coronal (**b**) CT images show low-attenuation defects in the bilateral frontal lobe white matter. There are scattered punctate hyperattenuating foci in the surgical defects bilaterally, consistent with Pantopaque. There is also disproportionate enlargement of the bilateral frontal lobe sulci. Axial FLAIR (**c**), axial T1-weighted (**d**), and sagittal T1-weighted (**e**) MR images demonstrate linear cystic defects in the bilateral frontal lobes with surrounding white matter signal abnormality, consistent with gliosis. Axial GRE (**f**) shows small foci of susceptibility, which correspond to residual deposits of Pantopaque (*arrows*)

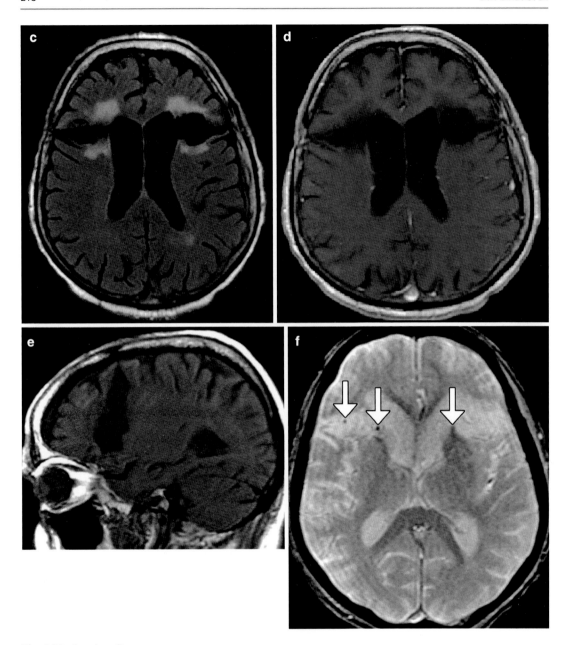

Fig. 5.31 (continued)

5.3.2 Pallidotomy

5.3.2.1 Discussion

Pallidotomy is a procedure that can be performed in Parkinson's disease patients who do not experience adequate symptom relief from medical therapy. The surgery consists of introducing probes via frontal burr holes for ablation of the posteroventral portion of the globus pallidus interna (Fig. 5.32). The goal of the procedure is to interrupt excessive inhibitory output from the basal ganglia. On CT, the pallidotomy lesions appear as hypoattenuating foci of encephalomalacia that become more pronounced over time. On MRI, acute pallidotomy lesions are usually hyperintense centrally on T1 and hypointense centrally on T2 due to hemorrhage surrounded by a rim of T2 hyperintensity and hypointensity on T1 and GRE, which represents edema. Restricted diffusion due to focal cytotoxic edema can also be encountered. Eventually, the lesion-edema complex evolves into a smaller focus of low T1 signal and high T2 signal. Lesion sizes can be variable depending upon technique implemented.

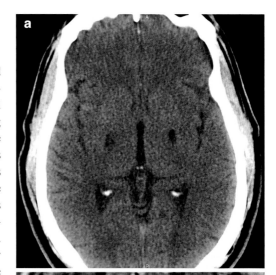
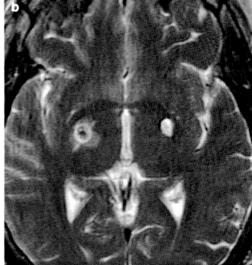
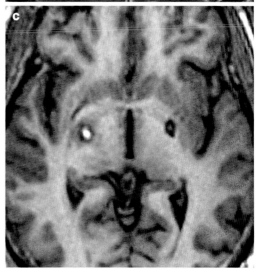

Fig. 5.32 Pallidotomy. The patient has a history of Parkinson's disease and underwent pallidotomy approximately 1 year prior to imaging on the left side and several days earlier on the right side. Axial CT image (**a**) shows hypoattenuating foci in the bilateral globus pallidi. The lesion on the right is more recent and slightly less hypoattenuating than the lesion on the left. Axial T2-weighted (**b**) and axial T1-weighted (**c**) images show subacute blood products within the right pallidotomy lesion surrounded by edema and fluid within the chronic left pallidotomy lesion

5.3.3 Cingulotomy

5.3.3.1 Discussion

Cingulotomy is a form of psychosurgery that is used to treat conditions, such as intractable obsessive-compulsive disorder. The procedure can be performed in a minimally invasive manner via thermal ablation. This process results in necrosis of the surrounding brain tissue, which appears as concentric rings of signal abnormality (Fig. 5.33). There can be T1 hyperintensity due to petechial hemorrhage, as well as T2 hyperintensity from edema and restricted diffusion due to ischemia during the early postoperative period, which then evolves over time. Diffusion tensor imaging is also useful for confirming interruption of the cingulum. In particular, the dorsolateral region of the cingulotomy lesion is associated with improved behavior.

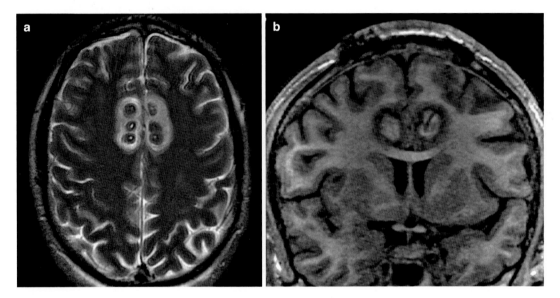

Fig. 5.33 Bilateral anterior cingulotomy. The patient has a history of medically intractable obsessive-compulsive disorder treated with bilateral stereotactic microelectrode-guided anterior dorsal cingulotomy. Axial T2-weighted (**a**) and coronal (**b**) and sagittal (**c**) T1-weighted MR images show concentric rings of signal changes at each microelectrode insertion site in the bilateral anterior cingulate gyri. The diffusion-weighted image (**d**) and ADC map (**e**) show circular zones of restricted diffusion consistent with ischemia. The color fractional anisotropy map (**f**) shows interruption of the bilateral anterior cingulate fiber tracts

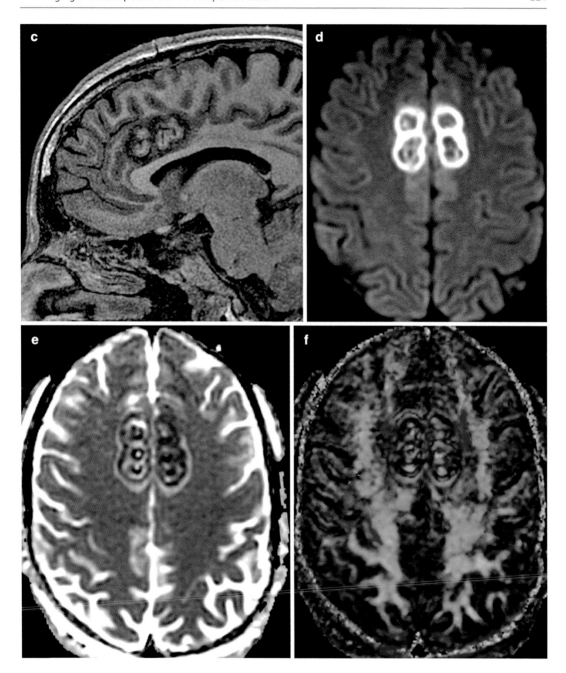

Fig. 5.33 (continued)

5.3.4   Subcaudate Tractotomy and Limbic Leucotomy

5.3.4.1 Discussion

Stereotactic subcaudate tractotomy is performed for treating severe cases of obsessive-compulsive disorder. The procedure consists of disrupting the fiber tracts between the orbitofrontal cortex and the thalamus, which are located approximately 5 mm anterior to the sella, 15 mm from the midline, and 10–11 mm above the planum sphenoidale (Fig. 5.34). Limbic leucotomy is a combination of cingulotomy and a ventral lesion similar to that of subcaudate tractotomy (Fig. 5.35). Following subcaudate tractotomy and limbic leucotomy, rostral atrophy can be identified on conventional imaging. In addition, diffusion tensor imaging can depict the absence of normal communicating white matter tracts between the inferior frontal lobes.

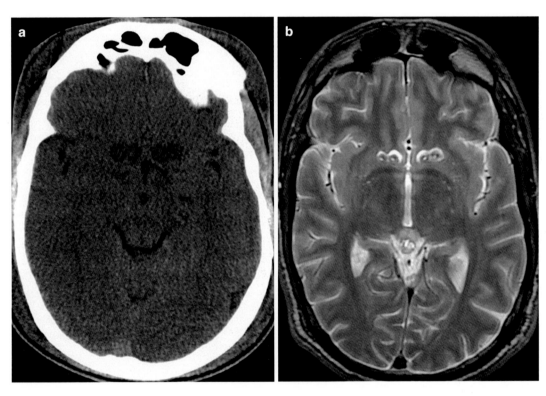

Fig. 5.34 Subcaudate tractotomy. The patient has a history of medically intractable obsessive-compulsive disorder. Axial (**a**) CT image shows paired hypoattenuating lesions in the bilateral subcaudate nucleus. T2-weighted images (**b**) demonstrate concentric T2 hyperintense zones surrounding the microelectrode insertion sites. Diffusion-weighted imaging (**c**) and corresponding ADC map (**d**) show that these zones have restricted diffusion, consistent with acute lesions

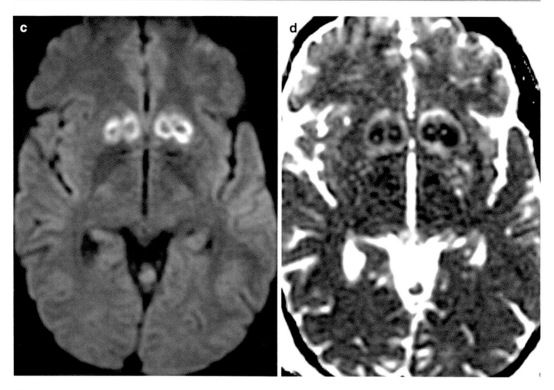

Fig. 5.34 (continued)

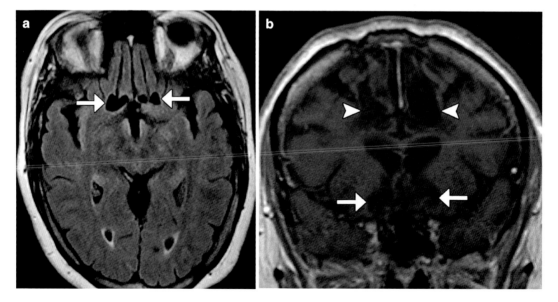

Fig. 5.35 Limbic leucotomy. Axial FLAIR (**a**), coronal T1-weighted (**b**), sagittal T1-weighted (**c**), and diffusion tensor directional color map (**d**) MR images show chronic lesions in the bilateral anterior cingulate gyri *(arrowheads)* and region of the anterior perforated substance *(arrows)*. There is also atrophy of the fornices

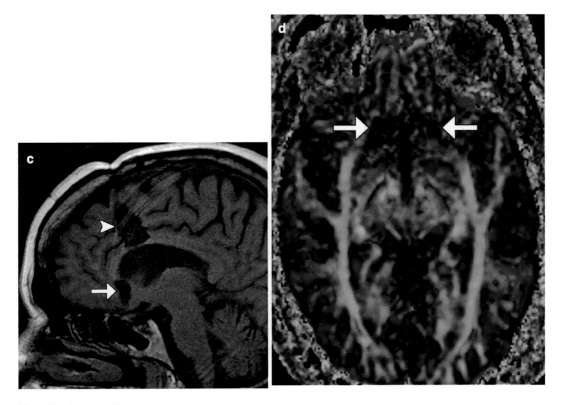

Fig. 5.35 (continued)

5.3.4.2 Thalamotomy

Essential tremor can be treated by lesioning of the ventralis intermedius nucleus of the thalamus. This can be accomplished via transcranial MR imaging-guided focused ultrasound lesion inducement, which is a noninvasive technique that generates heat at the site where numerous ultrasound beams intersect, utilizing MRI thermography guidance. Lesions are visible on T2-weighted images already apparent immediately after sonication and the lesions enhancement due to blood-brain barrier disruption. Over the course of a week after sonication, edema becomes more prominent, enhance, and become more distinct on T1-weighted images. Beyond 1 month after sonication, the lesions decrease in size (Fig. 5.36). Thalamotomy has effects on many other structures, which may be apparent on DTI. For example, there is decreased fractional anisotropy in the ipsilateral pre- and postcentral subcortical white matter in the hand knob area; the region of the corticospinal tract in the centrum semiovale, in the posterior limb of the internal capsule, and in the cerebral peduncle; the thalamus; the region of the red nucleus; the location of the central tegmental tract; and the region of the inferior olive. The magnitude of the DTI changes after thalamotomy correlates with the degree of clinical improvement in essential tremor. Skull characteristics, however, can affect the size of the lesions and should be evaluated prior to focused ultrasound.

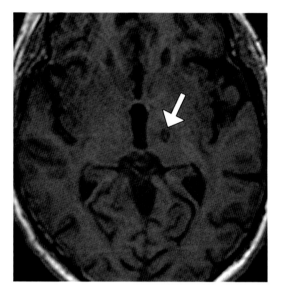

Fig. 5.36 Thalamotomy by focused ultrasound for essential tremor. Postoperative axial T1-weighted MRI shows a focal defect in the ViM nucleus of the left thalamus created by ultrasound (Courtesy of Daniel Cavalcante and Ryder Gwinn)

5.3.5 Deep Brain Stimulation (DBS)

5.3.5.1 Discussion

DBS is used to treat symptoms of Parkinson's disease, essential tremor, Tourette's, and intractable thalamic pain syndrome, among other conditions. Electrodes can be introduced via burr holes into the thalamus, globus pallidus, cerebellum, or subthalamic nucleus depending on the underlying condition (Figs. 5.37 and 5.38). Precise positioning of the electrodes can be achieved by the use of intraoperative stereotactic guidance and physiologic localization. The electrodes are comprised of insulated metallic wires that are connected to a pulse generator and battery pack that are buried in the subcutaneous tissues of the scalp, chest, or abdomen, depending on the model and number of pulse generators required. Although the electrodes are normally secured to the calvarium, displacement is a potential complication that can be readily assessed on CT (Fig. 5.39). Other complications include electrode fracture, "twiddler syndrome," and hemorrhage along the electrode tract, which is actually more common after removal (13%) than during insertion (2%), and ischemic infarction (0.4%) (Fig. 5.40).

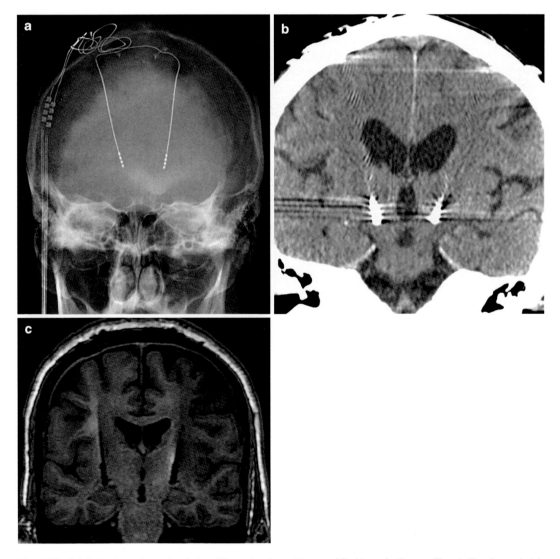

Fig. 5.37 Subthalamic nucleus stimulation. The patient has a history of Parkinson's disease. The skull radiograph (**a**), coronal CT (**b**), and coronal T1-weighted MRI (**c**) show bilateral DBS electrodes positioned in the subthalamic nuclei

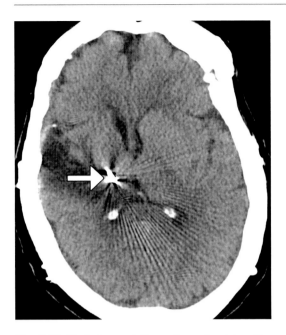

Fig. 5.38 Ventralis caudalis nucleus stimulator. The patient has had multiple aneurysms clipped and suffers from a thalamic pain syndrome secondary to hemorrhage and infarction. Axial CT image shows an electrode positioned in the right anterior thalamus (*arrow*). There is encephalomalacia across the right superior temporal gyrus, insula, and thalamus

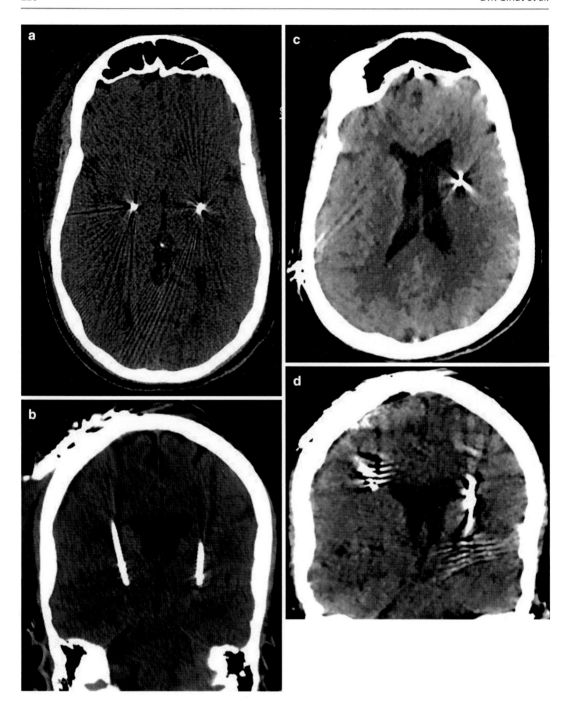

Fig. 5.39 Electrode migration. Initial postoperative axial (**a**) and coronal (**b**) CT images show satisfactory positioning of bilateral globus pallidus internus electrodes in a patient with dystonia. Subsequent axial (**c**) and coronal (**d**) CT images show marked interval retraction of the right electrode

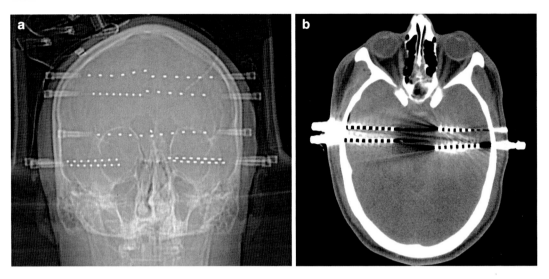

Fig. 5.46 Depth electrodes. Scout (**a**) and axial CT (**b**) images demonstrate numerous bilateral depth electrodes

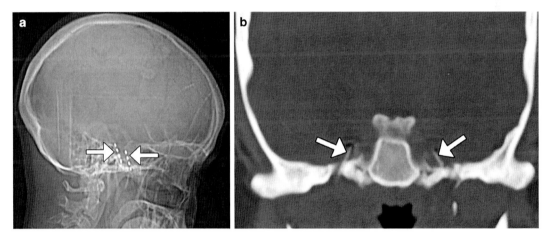

Fig. 5.47 Foramen ovale electrodes. Scout (**a**) and coronal CT (**b**) images show bilateral electrode wires (*arrows*) coursing through the foramen ovale

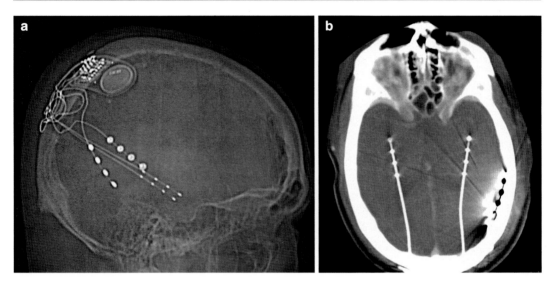

Fig. 5.48 NeuroPace. Scout (**a**) and axial (**b**) **CT** images demonstrate both subdural and depth electrodes in position. The pulse generator is implanted in the subgaleal space

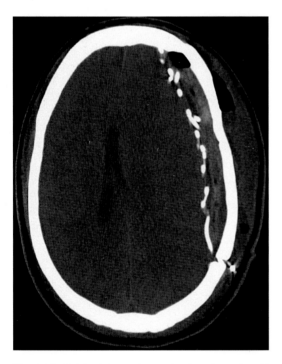

Fig. 5.49 Subdural hemorrhage related to electrode grid implantation. Axial CT image obtained after recent surgery shows a heterogeneous subdural fluid collection overlying the left hemisphere electrode grids and midline shift to the right

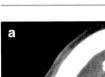

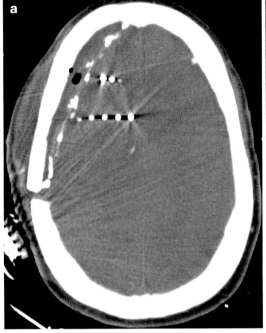

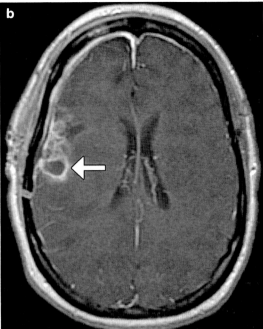

Fig. 5.50 Electrode-associated infection. The patient presented with fever and drainage from site of the subdural electrode insertion. Axial CT image (**a**) shows a gas-containing subdural collection overlying the deep brain electrodes. The subdural electrodes were then removed. The axial post-contrast T1-weighted MRI (**b**) shows a ring-enhancing collection in the right frontal lobe (*arrow*), as well as regional leptomeningeal and pachymeningeal enhancement

5.3.10 Corticectomy

5.3.10.1 Discussion

Corticectomy is performed to eliminate seizure foci and consists of resecting the neocortex in the region of an epileptogenic focus with sparring of the underlying white matter. The result can be appreciated on imaging, in which the bare white matter is surrounded by cerebrospinal fluid (Fig. 5.51).

Incomplete excision is the main predictor of poor surgical outcome, and reoperation may be appropriate for selected patients with intractable partial epilepsy who fail to respond to initial surgery. Comparison with the preoperative imaging is helpful, since the residual foci of cortical dysplasia can be subtle. Functional MRI and high-resolution sequences are particularly useful in planning additional surgery, since the eloquent areas can be delineated (Fig. 5.52).

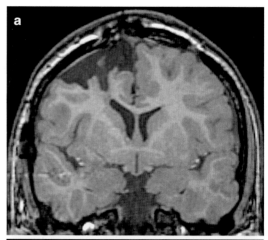

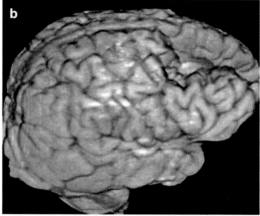

Fig. 5.51 Corticectomy. The patient has a history of tuberous sclerosis and intractable seizures. The patient underwent surgery in which a portion of the right frontal cortex was removed and carefully separated from the underlying white matter. Coronal (**a**) and 3D (**b**) T1-weighted MR images show decorticated white matter in the right frontal lobe

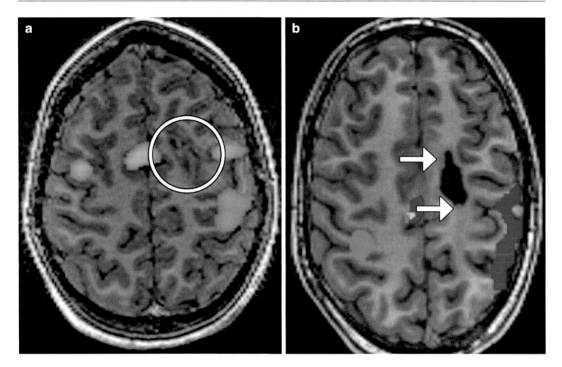

Fig. 5.52 Residual lesions after corticectomy. The patient is a right-handed white male with a long-standing history of intractable epilepsy secondary to a cortical dysplasia in the superior frontal region. Preoperative fMRI (**a**) shows a left frontal lobe cortical dysplasia (*arrow*). Postoperative fMRI (**b**) obtained after lesionectomy for excision of the epileptogenic focus shows small foci of residual cortical dysplasia (*arrows*) adjacent to the surgical cavity. However, the eloquent zones (*colored areas*) have been preserved

5.3.11 Selective Epilepsy Disconnection Surgery and Quadrantectomy

5.3.11.1 Discussion

The propagation of seizures associated with a diffusely abnormal quadrant of the brain can be impeded by selective disconnection of the underlying white matter tracts, as opposed to resection of entire regions of brain. Depending on the nature of the seizure focus, this can be accomplished via minimally invasive thermal ablation procedures for disrupting very focal white matter tracts (Fig. 5.53) or quadrantectomy for transecting wider areas of tissue, such as temporoparietooccipital disconnection for motor-sparing epilepsy surgery (Fig. 5.54). The disconnection foci or tracts can be readily depicted on postoperative MRI, if needed.

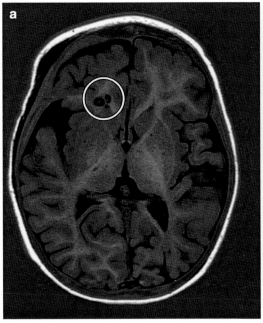
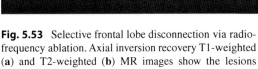
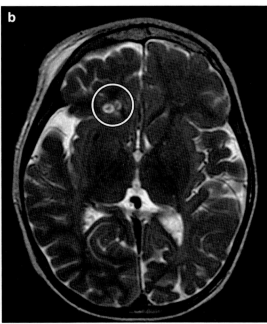

Fig. 5.53 Selective frontal lobe disconnection via radiofrequency ablation. Axial inversion recovery T1-weighted (**a**) and T2-weighted (**b**) MR images show the lesions (*encircled*) created in the right forceps minor in a patient with intractable epilepsy related to Sturge-Weber syndrome with a diffusely atrophic anterior right frontal lobe

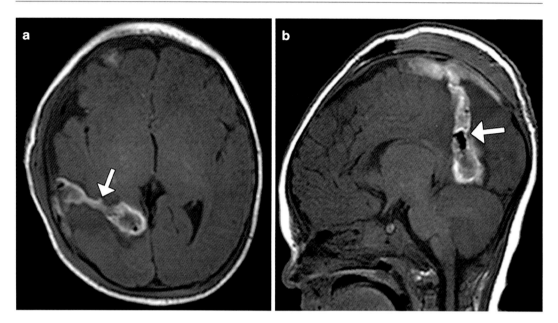

Fig. 5.54 Quadrantectomy. Axial (**a**) and sagittal (**b**) T1-weighted MR images show partial temporoparietooccipital disconnection, with blood products along the surgical margins (*arrows*)

5.3.12 Hypothalamic Hamartoma Thermal Ablation

5.3.12.1 Discussion

Hypothalamic hamartomas can be difficult to reach and remove via open surgical and endoscopic techniques. Thermal ablation offers a minimally invasive option in cases of associated epilepsy. Notably, it is not necessary to ablate the entire lesion, but it may be sufficient to interrupt the fiber tracks exiting the hamartoma. Therefore, one should not be surprised to find that the ablation zone occupies just a portion of the lesion on postoperative imaging (Fig. 5.55).

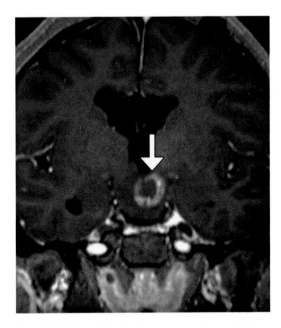

Fig. 5.55 Hypothalamic hamartoma laser ablation. Coronal post-contrast T1-weighted MRI shows the peripherally enhancing ablation zone at the neck of the large hypothalamic hamartoma. The patient's seizures improved after a transient increase in activity shortly after the procedure

5.3.13 Callosotomy

5.3.13.1 Discussion

Callosotomy, or surgical division of the corpus callosum, has been used successfully to treat intractable seizures, particularly drop attacks. Division of the corpus callosum can be partial (Fig. 5.56) or total and can be performed via thermal ablation (Fig. 5.57). MRI is the most suitable modality for depicting the extent of the surgical lesioning. The most common postoperative findings include surrounding T2 hyperintensity related to edema in over 20% of cases within 1 week and corpus callosum hematoma in 15% of cases. Other changes following callosotomy include atrophy and signal abnormalities in the cerebral white matter, perhaps related to Wallerian degeneration. The microstructural changes in the transected fibers can persist for many years after surgery and can be detected on diffusion tensor imaging, including fractional anisotropy and apparent diffusion coefficient maps. Therefore, diffusion tensor imaging is useful for depicting which fibers of the corpus callosum remain intact.

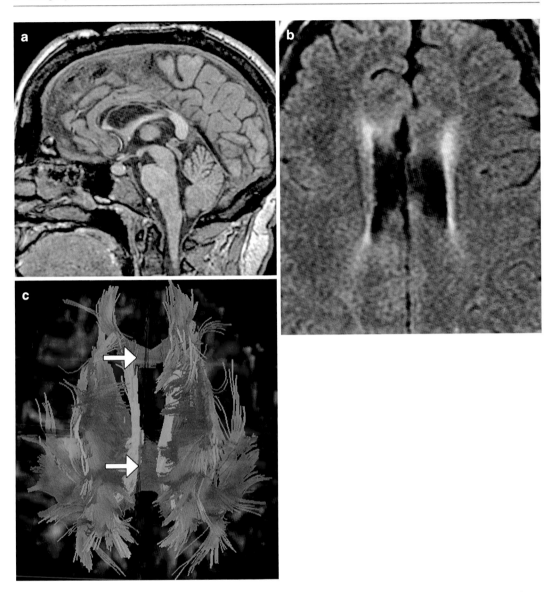

Fig. 5.56 Partial callosotomy. Sagittal T1-weighted (**a**) and axial FLAIR (**b**) images show a defect in the body of the body of the corpus callosum (*arrow*). Diffusion tensor imaging tractography map (**c**) shows interruption of corpus callosum body white matter tracts between the genu and splenium of the corpus callosum (*arrows*)

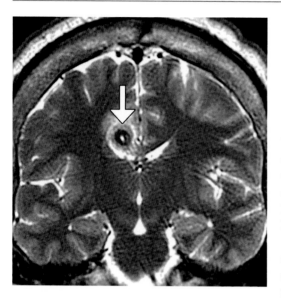

Fig. 5.57 Callosotomy via laser ablation. Coronal T2-weighted MRI shows the ablation zone with concentric areas of different signal characteristics in the right aspect of the corpus callosum body (*arrow*). Several other lesions were created along the corpus callosum

5.3.14 Anterior Temporal Lobectomy

5.3.14.1 Discussion

Anterior temporal lobectomy is performed for intractable seizures, particularly those caused by mesial temporal sclerosis. Varying degrees of temporal lobe resection can be performed, and a balance between minimizing the risk of postoperative deficits versus maximizing the likelihood of seizure control is sought. In general, the length of the resection is up to 4 cm in the dominant hemisphere and up to 6 cm in the nondominant hemisphere (Figs. 5.58 and 5.59).

There are certain imaging findings that can be encountered following temporal lobectomy. For example, increased enhancement of the choroid plexus has been reported in over 80% of cases of temporal lobectomies performed for seizure treatment within the first week of surgery. The pattern of enhancement is sometimes nodular or mass-like and can be mistaken for more serious pathology (Fig. 5.60). Concomitant enlargement of the choroid plexus occurs in the majority of cases, likely secondary to reactive hyperemia. An enlarged choroid plexus can also herniate into the surgical defect in the floor of the lateral ventricle temporal horn or atrium. Over time, gliosis forms along the edges of the resection cavity, which appears as increased signal and parenchymal volume loss (Fig. 5.61). Gliosis is commonly encountered and does not appear to be a signifi-

cant mechanism of recurrent epilepsy in patients with a seizure-free period after surgery. In addition, decreased fractional anisotropy is frequently observed ipsilateral to the surgery (Fig. 5.62). The decrease is especially pronounced among patients with postoperative visual field deficits. Due to the course of the posterior cerebral artery adjacent to the medial margin of the anterior temporal lobectomy, the vessel is potentially at risk of injury and consequent infarction (Fig. 5.63).

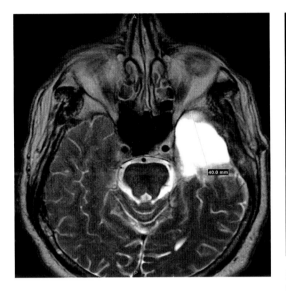

Fig. 5.58 Dominant hemisphere anterior temporal lobectomy. Axial T2-weighted MRI shows a left anterior temporal lobe surgical defect measures 4.0 cm in the anteroposterior dimension

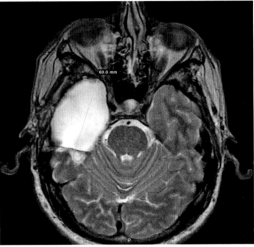

Fig. 5.59 Nondominant hemisphere anterior temporal lobectomy. Axial T2-weighted MRI shows a right anterior temporal lobe surgical defect that measures 6.0 cm in the anteroposterior dimension

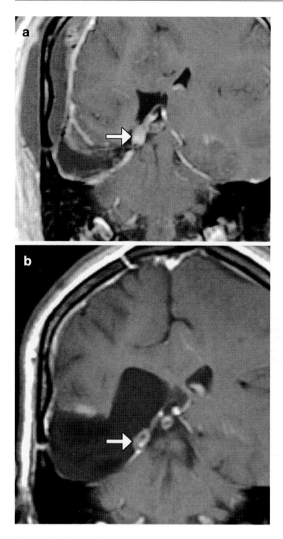

Fig. 5.60 Choroid plexus changes. Initial postoperative coronal contrast-enhanced T1-weighted MRI (**a**) shows right temporal lobectomy with herniation of the choroid plexus, which displays mass-like enhancement (*arrow*). Coronal contrast-enhanced T1-weighted MRI sequence obtained 3 months later (**b**) shows decreased swelling and enhancement of the choroid plexus changes (*arrow*)

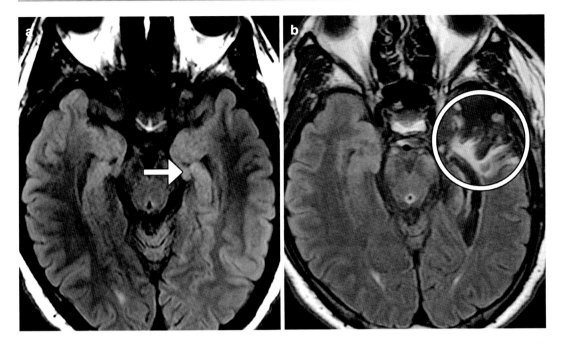

Fig. 5.61 Postoperative gliosis. The patient has a history of mesial temporal sclerosis. Preoperative axial FLAIR image (**a**) shows increased signal and decreased size of the left hippocampus (*arrow*). Postoperative axial FLAIR image (**b**) shows new high signal and volume loss along the left anterior temporal lobectomy margins (*encircled*)

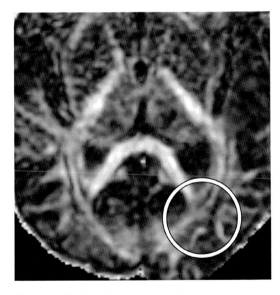

Fig. 5.62 Optic pathway changes after anterior temporal lobectomy. The patient has a history of left anterior temporal lobectomy. Fractional anisotropy map shows decreased anisotropy in the left optic pathway *(encircled)* ipsilateral to the temporal lobectomy

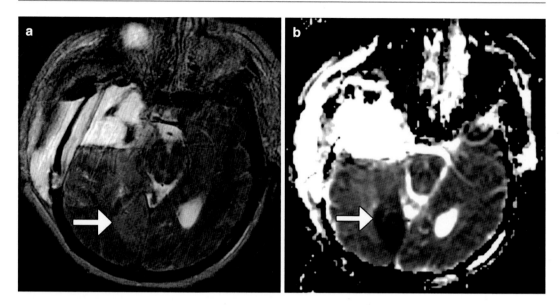

Fig. 5.63 Posterior cerebral artery territory infarction. Axial FLAIR image (**a**) shows evidence of recent right anterior temporal lobectomy and high signal in the right medial occipital lobe (*arrow*). ADC map (**b**) shows corresponding restricted diffusion (*arrow*)

5.3.15 Selective Amygdalohippocampectomy

5.3.15.1   Discussion

Selective amygdalohippocampectomy is a limited form of temporal lobectomy, which can be performed via transcortical, subtemporal, or transsylvian approaches or via laser ablation. Resection or laser ablation of at least some portions of the amygdala, anterior hippocampus, parahippocampal gyrus, and the subiculum is performed (Fig. 5.64). However, secondary encephalomalacia in the remaining portions of the temporal lobe is frequently observed due to Wallerian degeneration. Furthermore, injury to critical adjacent structures, such as the lateral geniculate nucleus with associated vision loss, can nevertheless occur with this selective procedure (Fig. 5.65).

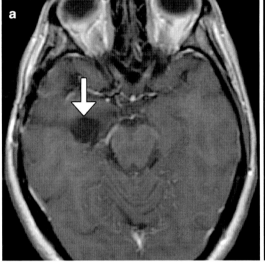
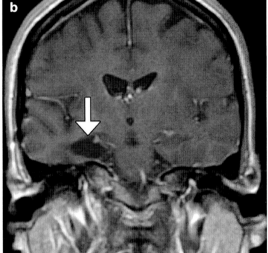

Fig. 5.64 Amygdalohippocampectomy. Axial (**a**) and coronal (**b**) T1-weighted MR images show a small resection cavity (*arrows*) in the left medial anterior temporal lobe structures, including the amygdala and hippocampus. The lateral portions of the temporal lobe are intact

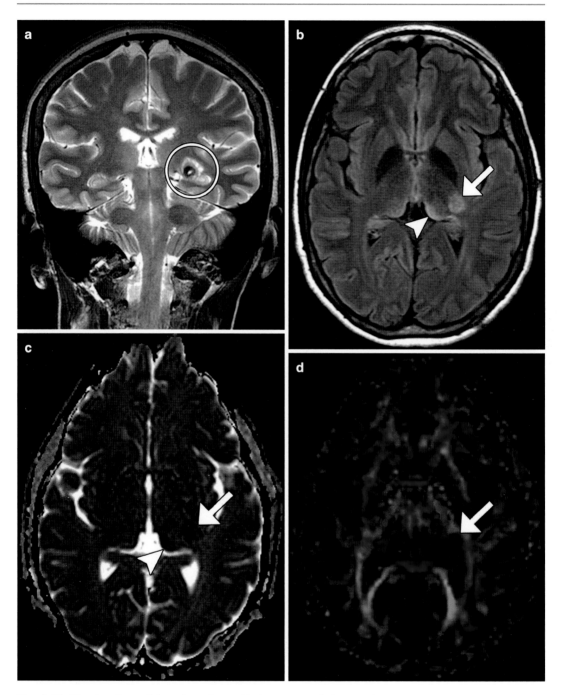

Fig. 5.65 Visual pathway injury from laser ablation amygdalohippocampectomy. The patient presented with new coronal T2-weighted MRI (**a**) shows the site of ablation involving the left hippocampus, as well as the adjacent temporal stem and lateral portion of the thalamus

(*encircled*). Indeed, there is high FLAIR signal (**b**) and restricted diffusion (**c**) and interruption (**d**) of a portion of the left optic radiations and lateral portions of the thalamus (*arrows*), as well as the pulvinar (*arrowheads*)

5.3.16 Hemispherectomy

5.3.16.1 Discussion

Hemispherectomy is mainly reserved for treating severe intractable seizure and rarely for gliomatosis cerebri. Several hemispherectomy techniques can be performed depending on the location and extent of seizure foci, and they can be total or partial. Techniques that use partial cortical removal and hemisphere disconnection are termed functional hemispherectomy or hemispherotomy (Fig. 5.66). On the other hand, techniques that result in complete cortical removal from the hemisphere are usually termed anatomical hemispherectomy, classical hemispherectomy, hemidecortication, or hemicorticectomy (Fig. 5.67).

On postoperative imaging, the hemispherectomy resection cavity fills with fluid during the first few days after surgery. With functional hemispherectomy, the remaining disconnected portions of the cerebral hemisphere eventually become atrophic. With complete anatomic hemispherectomy, duraplasty material is used to seal the interhemispheric fissure and prevent herniation of the remaining hemisphere.

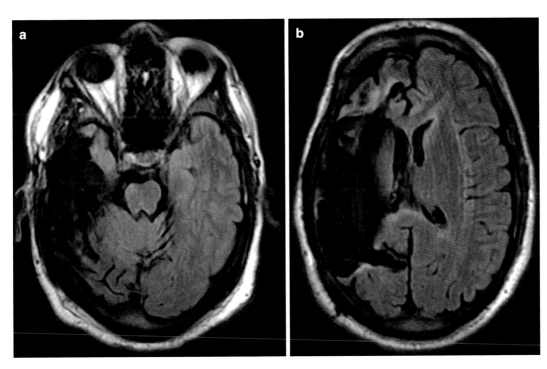

Fig. 5.66 Functional hemispherectomy. The patient has a history of Rasmussen's encephalitis recently treated with partial right hemispherectomy. Axial FLAIR images (**a** and **b**) show residual portions of the right frontal, temporal, and occipital lobes, which are partially detached from the remainder of the brain

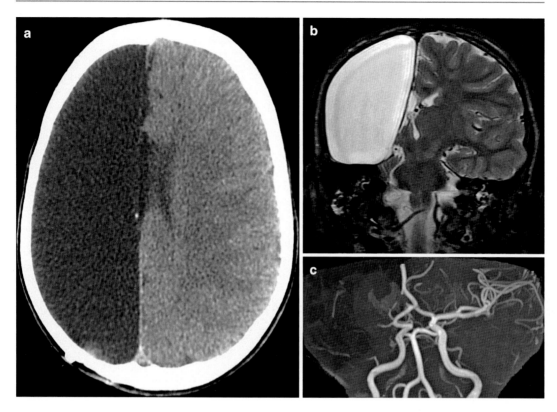

Fig. 5.67 Anatomical hemispherectomy. The patient has a history of intractable seizures related to Sturge-Weber syndrome treated via complete resection of the right cerebral hemisphere several years prior. Axial CT image (**a**) and coronal T2-weighted MRI (**b**) show complete absence of the right cerebral hemisphere. Duraplasty material (*arrow*) spans the interhemispheric fissure. 3D time-of-flight MRA (**c**) demonstrates the absence of the right MCA in the mid M1 segment status post ligation

Further Reading

Intraoperative MRI

Anzai Y, Lufkin R, DeSalles A, Hamilton DR, Farahani K, Black KL (1995) Preliminary experience with MR-guided thermal ablation of brain tumors. AJNR Am J Neuroradiol 16(1):39–48

Cabrera HN, Almeida AN, Silva CC, Fonoff ET, Martin Md, Leite Cda C, Teixeira MJ (2011) Use of intraoperative MRI for resection of gliomas. Arq Neuropsiquiatr 69(6):949–953

Ginat DT, Swearingen B, Curry W, Cahill D, Madsen J, Schaefer PW (2014) 3 tesla intraoperative MRI for brain tumor surgery. J Magn Reson Imaging 39(6) 1357–1365

Rahmathulla G, Recinos PF, Kamian K, Mohammadi AM, Ahluwalia MS, Barnett GH (2014) MRI-guided laser interstitial thermal therapy in neuro-oncology: a review of its current clinical applications. Oncology 87(2):67–82

Tovar-Spinoza Z, Carter D, Ferrone D, Eksioglu Y, Huckins S (2013) The use of MRI-guided laser-induced thermal ablation for epilepsy. Childs Nerv Syst 29(11):2089–2094.

Brain Tumor Surgery

Stereotactic Biopsy

Bernstein M, Parrent AG (1994) Complications of CT-guided stereotactic biopsy of intra-axial brain lesions. J Neurosurg 81(2):165–168

Field M, Witham TF, Flickinger JC, Kondziolka D, Lunsford LD (2001) Comprehensive assessment of hemorrhage risks and outcomes after stereotactic brain biopsy. J Neurosurg 94(4):545–551

McGirt MJ, Woodworth GF, Coon AL, Frazier JM, Amundson E, Garonzik I, Olivi A, Weingart JD (2005) Independent predictors of morbidity after image-guided stereotactic brain biopsy: a risk assessment of 270 cases. J Neurosurg 102(5):897–901

Resection Cavities

Dolinskas CA, Simeone FA (1998) Surgical site after resection of a meningioma. AJNR Am J Neuroradiol 19(3):419–426

Gibbs VC (2005) Patient safety practices in the operating room: correct-site surgery and nothing left behind. Surg Clin North Am 85(6):1307–19, xiii

Herman M, Pozzi-Mucelli RS, Skrap M (1996) CT and MRI findings after stereotactic resection of brain lesions. Eur J Radiol 23(3):228–234

Muzumdar D (2007) Safety in the operating room: neurosurgical perspective. Int J Surg 5(4):286–288

Surgically-Induced Parenchyma Injury

Akar S, Drappatz J, Hsu L, Blinder RA, Black PM, Kesari S (2008) Hypertrophic olivary degeneration after resection of a cerebellar tumor. J Neurooncol 87(3): 341–345

Catsman-Berrevoets CE, van Breemen M, van Veelen ML, Appel IM, Lequin MH (2005) Supratentorial arterial ischemic stroke following cerebellar tumor resection in two children. Pediatr Neurosurg 41(4): 206–211

Harada S, Nakamura T 1994 Retraction induced brain edema. Acta Neurochir Suppl (Wien) 60:449–451

Sherchan P, Kim CH, Zhang JH 2013 Surgical brain injury and edema prevention. Acta Neurochir Suppl 118:129–133

Tsui EY, Cheung YK, Mok CK, Yuen MK, Chan JH (1999) Hypertrophic olivary degeneration following surgical excision of brainstem cavernous hemangioma: a case report. Clin Imaging 23(4):215–217

Ulmer S, Braga TA, Barker FG 2nd, Lev MH, Gonzalez RG, Henson JW (2006) Clinical and radiographic features of peritumoral infarction following resection of glioblastoma. Neurology 67(9):1668–1670

Vaidhyanath R, Thomas A, Messios N (2010) Bilateral hypertrophic olivary degeneration following surgical resection of a posterior fossa epidermoid cyst. Br J Radiol 83(994):e211–e215

Postoperative Hemorrhagic Lesions

Fukamachi A, Koizumi H, Nukui H (1985) Postoperative intracerebral hemorrhages: a survey of computed tomographic findings after 1074 intracranial operations. Surg Neurol 23(6):575–580

Koebbe CJ, Sherman JD, Warnick RE (2001) Distant wounded glioma syndrome: report of two cases. Neurosurgery 48(4):940–943; discussion 943–944

Papanastassiou V, Kerr R, Adams C (1996) Contralateral cerebellar hemorrhagic infarction after pterional craniotomy: report of five cases and review of the literature. Neurosurgery 39(4):841–851; discussion 851–852

Enhancing Lesions in the Surgical Bed Region and Beyond

Ananthnarayan S, Bahng J, Roring J, Nghiemphu P, Lai A, Cloughesy T, Pope WB (2008) Time course of imaging changes of GBM during extended bevacizumab treatment. J Neurooncol 88(3):339–347

Belhawi SM, Hoefnagels FW, Baaijen JC, Aliaga ES, Reijneveld JC, Heimans JJ, Barkhof F, Vandertop WP, Hamer PC (2011) Early postoperative MRI overestimates residual tumor after resection of gliomas with no or minimal enhancement. Eur Radiol 21(7): 1526–1534

Birbilis TA, Matis GK, Eleftheriadis SG, Theodoropoulou EN, Sivridis E (2010) Spinal metastasis of glioblastoma multiforme: an uncommon suspect? Spine (Phila Pa 1976) 35(7):E264–E269

Brandsma D, van den Bent MJ (2009) Pseudoprogression and pseudoresponse in the treatment of gliomas. Curr Opin Neurol 22(6):633–638

Hygino da Cruz LC Jr, Rodriguez I, Domingues RC, Gasparetto EL, Sorensen AG (2011) Pseudoprogression and pseudoresponse: imaging challenges in the assessment of posttreatment glioma. AJNR Am J Neuroradiol 32(11): 1978–1985

Elster AD, DiPersio DA (1990) Cranial postoperative site: assessment with contrast-enhanced MR imaging. Radiology 174(1):93–98

Ginat DT, Kelly HR, Schaefer PW, Davidson CJ, Curry W (2012) Recurrent scalp metastasis from glioblastoma following resection. Clin Neurol Neurosurg 115(4):461–463.

Hein PA, Eskey CJ, Dunn JF, Hug EB (2004) Diffusion-weighted imaging in the follow-up of treated high-grade gliomas: tumor recurrence versus radiation injury. AJNR Am J Neuroradiol 25(2):201–209

Hustinx R, Pourdehnad M, Kaschten B, Alavi A (2005) PET imaging for differentiating recurrent brain tumor from radiation necrosis. Radiol Clin North Am 43(1):35–47

Iwamoto FM, Abrey LE, Beal K, Gutin PH, Rosenblum MK, Reuter VE, DeAngelis LM, Lassman AB (2009) Patterns of relapse and prognosis after bevacizumab failure in recurrent glioblastoma. Neurology 73(15):1200–1206

Jain R, Scarpace LM, Ellika S, Torcuator R, Schultz LR, Hearshen D, Mikkelsen T (2010) Imaging response criteria for recurrent gliomas treated with bevacizumab: role of diffusion weighted imaging as an imaging biomarker. J Neurooncol 96(3):423–431

Kerklaan JP, Lycklama á Nijeholt GJ, Wiggenraad RG, Berghuis B, Postma TJ, Taphoorn MJ (2011) SMART syndrome: a late reversible complication after radiation therapy for brain tumors. J Neurol 258(6): 1098–1104

Kong DS, Kim ST, Kim EH, Lim DH, Kim WS, Suh YL, Lee JI, Park K, Kim JH, Nam DH (2011) Diagnostic dilemma of pseudoprogression in the treatment of newly diagnosed glioblastomas: the role of assessing relative cerebral blood flow volume and oxygen-6-methylguanine-DNA methyltransferase promoter methylation status. AJNR Am J Neuroradiol 32(2):382–387

Maslehaty H, Cordovi S, Hefti M (2011) Symptomatic spinal metastases of intracranial glioblastoma: clinical characteristics and pathomechanism relating to GFAP expression. J Neurooncol 101(2):329–333

Mullins ME, Barest GD, Schaefer PW, Hochberg FH, Gonzalez RG, Lev MH (2005) Radiation necrosis versus glioma recurrence: conventional MR imaging clues to diagnosis. AJNR Am J Neuroradiol 26(8):1967–1972

Pope WB, Kim HJ, Huo J, Alger J, Brown MS, Gjertson D, Sai V, Young JR, Tekchandani L, Cloughesy T, Mischel PS, Lai A, Nghiemphu P, Rahmanuddin S, Goldin J (2009) Recurrent glioblastoma multiforme: ADC histogram analysis predicts response to bevacizumab treatment. Radiology 252(1):182–189

Smith EA, Carlos RC, Junck LR, Tsien CI, Elias A, Sundgren PC (2009) Developing a clinical decision model: MR spectroscopy to differentiate between recurrent tumor and radiation change in patients with new contrast-enhancing lesions. AJR Am J Roentgenol 192(2):W45–W52

Sugahara T, Korogi Y, Tomiguchi S, Shigematsu Y, Ikushima I, Kira T, Liang L, Ushio Y, Takahashi M (2000) Posttherapeutic intraaxial brain tumor: the value of perfusion-sensitive contrast-enhanced MR imaging for differentiating tumor recurrence from nonneoplastic contrast-enhancing tissue. AJNR Am J Neuroradiol 21(5):901–909

Young RJ, Gupta A, Shah AD, Graber JJ, Zhang Z, Shi W, Holodny AI, Omuro AM (2011) Potential utility of conventional MRI signs in diagnosing pseudoprogression in glioblastoma. Neurology 76(22):1918–1924

Ommaya Reservoirs

Bleyer WA, Pizzo PA, Spence AM et al. (1978) The Ommaya reservoir: newly recognized complications and recommendations for insertion and use. Cancer 41(6):2431–2437

Chowdhary S, Chalmers LM, Chamberlain PA (2006) Methotrexate-induced encephaloclastic cyst: a complication of intraventricular chemotherapy. Neurology 67(2):319

DeAngelis LM (1998) Current diagnosis and treatment of leptomeningeal metastasis. J Neurooncol 38(2–3): 245–252

Goeser CD, McLeary MS, Young LW (1998) Diagnostic imaging of ventriculoperitoneal shunt malfunctions and complications. Radiographics 18(3):635–651

Lishner M, Perrin RG, Feld R, Messner HA, Tuffnell PG, Elhakim T, Matlow A, Curtis JE (1990) Complications associated with Ommaya reservoirs in patients with cancer. The Princess Margaret Hospital experience and a review of the literature. Arch Intern Med 150(1): 173–176

Mechleb B, Khater F, Eid A, David G, Moorman JP (2003) Late onset Ommaya reservoir infection due to Staphylococcus aureus: case report and review of Ommaya Infections. J Infect 46(3):196–198

Ommaya AK (1984) Implantable devices for chronic access and drug delivery to the central nervous system. Cancer Drug Deliv 1(2):169–179

Sandberg DI, Bilsky MH, Souweidane MM, Bzdil J, Gutin PH (2000) Ommaya reservoirs for the treatment of leptomeningeal metastases. Neurosurgery 47(1):49–54; discussion 54–55

Stone JA, Castillo M, Mukherji SK (1999) Leukoencephalopathy complicating an Ommaya reservoir and chemotherapy. Neuroradiology 41(2):134–136

Ziereisen F, Dan B, Azzi N, Ferster A, Damry N, Christophe C (2006) Reversible acute methotrexate leukoencephalopathy: atypical brain MR imaging features. Pediatr Radiol 36(3):205–212

Chemotherapy Wafers

Attenello FJ, Mukherjee D, Datoo G, McGirt MJ, Bohan E, Weingart JD, Olivi A, Quinones-Hinojosa A, Brem H (2008) Use of Gliadel (BCNU) wafer in the surgical treatment of malignant glioma: a 10-year institutional experience. Ann Surg Oncol 15(10):2887–2893

Engelhard HH (2000) The role of interstitial BCNU chemotherapy in the treatment of malignant glioma. Surg Neurol 53(5):458–464

Giese A, Kucinski T, Knopp U, Goldbrunner R, Hamel W, Mehdorn HM, Tonn JC, Hilt D, Westphal M (2004) Pattern of recurrence following local chemotherapy with biodegradable carmustine (BCNU) implants in patients with glioblastoma. J Neurooncol 66(3):351–360

Brachytherapy Seeds

Darakchiev BJ, Albright RE, Breneman JC, Warnick RE (2008) Safety and efficacy of permanent iodine-125 seed implants and carmustine wafers in patients with recurrent glioblastoma multiforme. J Neurosurg 108(2):236–242

Patel S, Breneman JC, Warnick RE, Albright RE Jr, Tobler WD, van Loveren HR, Tew JM Jr (2000) Permanent iodine-125 interstitial implants for the treatment of recurrent glioblastoma multiforme. Neurosurgery 46(5):1123–1128; discussion 1128–1130

GliaSite Radiation Therapy System

Matheus MG, Castillo M, Ewend M, Smith JK, Knock L, Cush S, Morris DE (2004) CT and MR imaging after placement of the GliaSite radiation therapy system to treat brain tumor: initial experience. AJNR Am J Neuroradiol 25(7):1211–1217

Rogers LR, Rock JP, Sillis AK et al. (2006) Results of a phase ii trial of the GliaSite radiation therapy system for treatment of newly diagnosed brain metastases. J Neurosurgery 105(3):375–384

Tatter SB, Shaw EG, Rosenblum ML et al. (2003) An inflatable balloon catheter and liquid 125I radiation source (GilaSite radiation therapy system) for treatment of recurrent malignant glioma; multicenter safety and feasibility trial. J Neurosurg 99(2):297–303

Wernicke AG, Sherr DL, Schwartz TH et al. (2010) Feasibility and safety of GilaSite brachytherapy in treatment of CNS tumors following neurosurgical resection. J Cancer Res Ther 6(1):65–74

Neurodegenerative, Neuropsychiatric, and Epilepsy Surgery

Prefrontal Lobotomy

Dorsey JF, Centner PJ (1951) Pantopaque-gelfoam method for the roentgen visualization of the plane of lobotomy. Am J Roentgenol Radium Ther 65(2):277–278

Duncan AW, Schoene WC, Rumbaugh CL (1980) The computerized tomographic appearance of frontal lobotomy. Comput Tomogr 4(4):255–260

Kucharski A (1984) History of frontal lobotomy in the United States, 1935–1955. Neurosurgery 14(6):765–772

Manoj AL, Okubadejo A (2001) Bilateral frontal lobe lesions. QJM 94(8):449

Uchino A, Kato A, Yuzuriha T, Takashima Y, Kudo S (2001) Cranial MR imaging of sequelae of prefrontal lobotomy. AJNR Am J Neuroradiol 22(2):301–304

Pallidotomy

Cohn MC, Hudgins PA, Sheppard SK, Starr PA, Bakay RA (1998) Pre- and postoperative MR evaluation of stereotactic pallidotomy. AJNR Am J Neuroradiol 19(6):1075–1080

Krauss JK, Desaloms JM, Lai EC, King DE, Jankovic J, Grossman RG (1997) Microelectrode-guided posteroventral pallidotomy for treatment of Parkinson's disease: postoperative magnetic resonance imaging analysis. J Neurosurg 87(3):358–367

Cingulotomy

Harat M, Rudas M, Rybakowski J (2008) Psychosurgery: the past and present of ablation procedures. Neuro Endocrinol Lett 29(Suppl 1):105–122

Leiphart JW, Valone FH 3rd (2010) Stereotactic lesions for the treatment of psychiatric disorders. J Neurosurg 113(6):1204–1211

Mashour GA, Walker EE, Martuza RL (2005) Psychosurgery: past, present, and future. Brain Res Brain Res Rev 48(3):409–419

Sundararajan SH, Belani P, Danish S, Keller I. 2015 Early MRI Characteristics after MRI-Guided Laser-Assisted Cingulotomy for Intractable Pain Control. AJNR Am J Neuroradiol;36(7):1283–1287.

Yang JC, Ginat DT, Dougherty DD, Makris N, Eskandar EN. 2014 Lesion analysis for cingulotomy and limbic leucotomy: comparison and correlation with clinical outcomes, J Neurosurg;120(1):152–163.

Subcaudate Tractotomy and Limbic Leucotomy

Cauley KA, Waheed W, Salmela M, Filippi CG (2010) MR imaging of psychosurgery: rostral atrophy following stereotacic subcaudate tractotomy. Br J Radiol 83(995):e239–e242

Harat M, Rudas M, Rybakowski J (2008) Psychosurgery: the past and present of ablation procedures. Neuro Endocrinol Lett 29 Suppl 1:105–122

Thalamotomy

Jung HH, Chang WS, Rachmilevitch I, Tlusty T, Zadicario E, Chang JW. 2015 Different magnetic resonance imaging patterns after transcranial magnetic resonance-guided focused ultrasound of the ventral intermediate nucleus of the thalamus and anterior limb of the internal capsule in patients with essential tremor or obsessive-compulsive disorder. J Neurosurg;122(1):162–168

Lipsman N, Schwartz ML, Huang Y, Lee L, Sankar T, Chapman M, Hynynen K, Lozano AM: MR-guided focused ultrasound thalamotomy for essential tremor: a proof-of-concept study. Lancet Neurol 2013;12(5):462–468.

Wintermark M, Huss DS, Shah BB, Tustison N, Druzgal TJ, Kassell N, Elias WJ. Thalamic connectivity in patients with essential tremor treated with MR imaging-guided focused ultrasound: in vivo fiber tracking by using diffusion-tensor MR imaging. Radiology 2014;272(1):202–209.

Deep Brain Stimulation (DBS)

Ackermans L, Temel Y, Visser-Vandewalle V. Deep brain stimulation in Tourette's syndrome. Neurotherapeutics 2008;5:339–344.

Cleary DR, Ozpinar A, Raslan AM, Ko AL (2015) Deep brain stimulation for psychiatric disorders: where we are now. Neurosurg Focus 38(6):E2

Elias WJ, Lozano AM (2010) Deep brain stimulation: the spectrum of application. Neurosurg Focus 10;29(2): Introduction

Fenoy AJ, Simpson RK Jr (2014) Risks of common complications in deep brain stimulation surgery: management and avoidance. J Neurosurg 120(1):132–139

Kim JP, Chang WS, Park YS, Chang JW (2011) Impact of ventralis caudalis deep brain stimulation combined with stereotactic bilateral cingulotomy for treatment of post-stroke pain. Stereotact Funct Neurosurg 90(1):9–15

Liu JK, Soliman H, Machado A, Deogaonkar M, Rezai AR (2012) Intracranial hemorrhage after removal of deep brain stimulation electrodes. J Neurosurg 116(3): 525–528

Lyons MK (2011) Deep brain stimulation: current and future clinical applications. Mayo Clin Proc 86(7):662–672

Maciunas RJ, Maddux BN, Riley DE, et al (2007) Prospective randomized double-blind trial of bilateral thalamic deep brain stimulation in adults with Tourette syndrome. J Neurosurg 107:1004–1014

Maddux B, Riley D, Whitney CM, Maciunas RJ (2007) Double-blind trial of thalamic DBS for Tourette syndrome: one-year follow-up. Neurology 68(suppl 1):A155

Pahwa R, Lyons KE, Wilkinson SB, Simpson RK Jr, Ondo WG, Tarsy D, Norregaard T, Hubble JP, Smith DA, Hauser RA, Jankovic J (2006) Long-term evaluation of deep brain stimulation of the thalamus. J Neurosurg 104(4): 506–512

Porta M, Brambilla A, Cavanna AE, et al (2009) Thalamic deep brain stimulation for treatment-refractory Tourette syndrome: two-year outcome. Neurology 73:1375–1380

Saint-Cyr JA, Hoque T, Pereira LC et al. (2002) Localization of clinically effective stimulating electrodes in the human subthalamic nucleus on magnetic resonance imaging. J Neurosurg 97:1152–1166

Welter ML, Mallet L, Houeto JL, et al (2008) Internal pallidal and thalamic stimulation in patients with Tourette syndrome. Arch Neurol 65:952–957

Zhang K, Bhatia S, Oh MY, Cohen D, Angle C, Whiting D (2010) Long-term results of thalamic deep brain stimulation for essential tremor. J Neurosurg 112(6): 1271–1276

Epidural Motor Cortex Stimulator

Brown JA, Pilitsis JG (2005) Motor cortex stimulation for central and neuropathic facial pain: a prospective study of 10 patients and observations of enhanced sensory and motor function during stimulation. Neurosurgery 56(2):290–297; discussion 290–297

Lefaucheur JP, Drouot X, Cunin P, Bruckert R, Lepetit H, Creange A, Wolkenstein P, Maison P, Keravel Y, Nguyen JP (2009) Motor cortex stimulation for the treatment of refractory peripheral neuropathic pain. Brain 132(Pt 6):1463–1471

Neural Interface System (BrainGate)

Chadwick EK, Blana D, Simeral JD, Lambrecht J, Kim SP, Cornwell AS, Taylor DM, Hochberg LR, Donoghue JP, Kirsch RF (2011) Continuous neuronal ensemble control of simulated arm reaching by a human with tetraplegia. J Neural Eng 8(3):034003

Simeral JD, Kim SP, Black MJ, Donoghue JP, Hochberg LR (2011) Neural control of cursor trajectory and click by a human with tetraplegia 1000 days after implant of an intracortical microelectrode array. J Neural Eng 8(2):025027

Microcatheter Subthalamic Infusion of Glutamate Decarboxylase

During MJ, Kaplitt MG, Stern MB, Eidelberg D (2001) Subthalamic GAD gene transfer in Parkinson disease patients who are candidates for deep brain stimulation. Hum Gene Ther 12(12):1589–1591

LeWitt PA, Rezai AR, Leehey MA, Ojemann SG, Flaherty AW, Eskandar EN, Kostyk SK, Thomas K, Sarkar A, Siddiqui MS, Tatter SB, Schwalb JM, Poston KL, Henderson JM, Kurlan RM, Richard IH, Van Meter L, Sapan CV, During MJ, Kaplitt MG, Feigin A (2011) AAV2-GAD gene therapy for advanced Parkinson's disease: a double-blind, sham-surgery controlled, randomized trial. Lancet Neurol 10(4):309–319

Seizure Monitoring Electrodes and NeuroPace

Davies KG, Phillips BL, Hermann BP (1996) MRI confirmation of accuracy of freehand placement of mesial temporal lobe depth electrodes in the investigation of intractable epilepsy. Br J Neurosurg 10(2): 175–178

Kushen MC, Frim D (2007) Placement of subdural electrode grids for seizure focus localization in patients with a large arachnoid cyst. Technical note. Neurosurg Focus 22(2):E5

Lee WS, Lee JK, Lee SA, Kang JK, Ko TS (2000) Complications and results of subdural grid electrode implantation in epilepsy surgery. Surg Neurol 54(5): 346–351

Placantonakis DG, Shariff S, Lafaille F, Labar D, Harden C, Hosain S, Kandula P, Schaul N, Kolesnik D, Schwartz TH (2010) Bilateral intracranial electrodes for lateralizing intractable epilepsy: efficacy, risk, and outcome. Neurosurgery 66(2):274–283

Steven DA, Andrade-Souza YM, Burneo JG, McLachlan RS, Parrent AG (2007) Insertion of subdural strip electrodes for the investigation of temporal lobe epilepsy. Technical note. J Neurosurg 106(6):1102–1106

Velasco TR, Sakamoto AC, Alexandre V Jr, Walz R, Dalmagro CL, Bianchin MM, Araújo D, Santos AC, Leite JP, Assirati JA, Carlotti C Jr (2006) Foramen ovale electrodes can identify a focal seizure onset when surface EEG fails in mesial temporal lobe epilepsy. Epilepsia 47(8):1300–1307

Waziri A, Schevon CA, Cappell J, Emerson RG, McKhann GM 2nd, Goodman RR (2009) Initial surgical experience with a dense cortical microarray in epileptic

patients undergoing craniotomy for subdural electrode implantation. Neurosurgery 64(3):540–545

Wiggins GC, Elisevich K, Smith BJ (1999) Morbidity and infection in combined subdural grid and strip electrode investigation for intractable epilepsy. Epilepsy Res 37(1):73–80

Corticectomy

Bourgeois M, Di Rocco F, Sainte-Rose C (2006) Lesionectomy in the pediatric age. Childs Nerv Syst 22(8):931–935

Kloss S, Pieper T, Pannek H, Holthausen H, Tuxhorn I (2002) Epilepsy surgery in children with focal cortical dysplasia (FCD): results of long-term seizure outcome. Neuropediatrics 33(1):21–26

Krsek P, Maton B, Jayakar P, Dean P, Korman B, Rey G, Dunoyer C, Pacheco-Jacome E, Morrison G, Ragheb J, Vinters HV, Resnick T, Duchowny M (2009) Incomplete resection of focal cortical dysplasia is the main predictor of poor postsurgical outcome. Neurology 72(3):217–223

Montes JL, Rosenblatt B, Farmer JP, O'Gorman AM, Andermann F, Watters GV, Meagher-Villemure K (1995) Lesionectomy of MRI detected lesions in children with epilepsy. Pediatr Neurosurg 22(4): 167–173

Siegel AM, Cascino GD, Meyer FB, McClelland RL, So EL, Marsh WR, Scheithauer BW, Sharbrough FW (2004) Resective reoperation for failed epilepsy surgery: seizure outcome in 64 patients. Neurology 63(12):2298–2302

Selective Disconnection

Dorfer C, Czech T, Mühlebner-Fahrngruber A, Mert A, Gröppel G, Novak K, Dressler A, Reiter-Fink E, Traub-Weidinger T, Feucht M (2013) Disconnective surgery in posterior quadrantic epilepsy: experience in a consecutive series of 10 patients. Neurosurg Focus 34(6):E10.

Mohamed AR, Freeman JL, Maixner W, Bailey CA, Wrennall JA, Harvey AS (2011) Temporoparietooccipital disconnection in children with intractable epilepsy. J Neurosurg Pediatr 7(6):660–670.

Hypothalamic Hamartoma Thermal Ablation

Kameyama S, Murakami H, Masuda H, Sugiyama I (2009) Minimally invasive magnetic resonance imaging-guided stereotactic radiofrequency thermocoagulation for epileptogenic hypothalamic hamartomas. Neurosurgery 65(3):438–49; discussion 449

Rolston JD, Chang EF. Stereotactic laser ablation for hypothalamic hamartoma. Neurosurg Clin N Am 2016;27(1):59–67.

Callosotomy

Asadi-Pooya AA, Sharan A, Nei M, Sperling MR (2008) Corpus callosotomy. Epilepsy Behav 13(2):271–278

Harris RD, Roberts DW, Cromwell LD (1989) MR imaging of corpus callosotomy. AJNR Am J Neuroradiol 10(4):677–680

Khurana DS, Strawsburg RH, Robertson RL, Madsen JR, Helmers SL (1999) MRI signal changes in the white matter after corpus callosotomy. Pediatr Neurol 21(4):691–695

Pizzini FB, Polonara G, Mascioli G, Beltramello A, Foroni R, Paggi A, Salvolini U, Tassinari G, Fabri M (2010) Diffusion tensor tracking of callosal fibers several years after callosotomy. Brain Res 1312:10–17

Anterior Temporal Lobectomy

Alsaadi TM, Ulmer JL, Mitchell MJ, Morris GL, Swanson SJ, Mueller WM (2001) Magnetic resonance analysis of postsurgical temporal lobectomy. J Neuroimaging 11(3):243–247

Hennessy MJ, Elwes RD, Binnie CD, Polkey CE (2000) Failed surgery for epilepsy. A study of persistence and recurrence of seizures following temporal resection. Brain 123(Pt 12):2445–2466

Saluja S, Sato N, Kawamura Y, Coughlin W, Putman CM, Spencer DD, Sze G, Bronen RA (2000) Choroid plexus changes after temporal lobectomy. AJNR Am J Neuroradiol 21(9):1650–1653

Taoka T, Sakamoto M, Nakagawa H, Nakase H, Iwasaki S, Takayama K, Taoka K, Hoshida T, Sakaki T,

Kichikawa K (2008) Diffusion tensor tractography of the Meyer loop in cases of temporal lobe resection for temporal lobe epilepsy: correlation between postsurgical visual field defect and anterior limit of Meyer loop on tractography. AJNR Am J Neuroradiol 29(7):1329–1334

Selective Amygdalohippocampectomy

Adada B (2008) Selective amygdalohippocampectomy via the transsylvian approach. Neurosurg Focus 25(3):E5

Renowden SA, Matkovic Z, Adams CB, Carpenter K, Oxbury S, Molyneux AJ, Anslow P, Oxbury J (1995) Selective amygdalohippocampectomy for hippocampal sclerosis: postoperative MR appearance. AJNR Am J Neuroradiol 16(9):1855–1861

Hemispherectomy

Bien CG, Schramm J (2009) Treatment of Rasmussen encephalitis half a century after its initial description: promising prospects and a dilemma. Epilepsy Res 86(2–3):101–112

De Almeida AN, Marino R Jr, Aguiar PH, Jacobsen Teixeira M (2006) Hemispherectomy: a schematic review of the current techniques. Neurosurg Rev 29(2):97–102; discussion 102

Kossoff EH, Vining EP, Pillas DJ, Pyzik PL, Avellino AM, Carson BS, Freeman JM (2003) Hemispherectomy for intractable unihemispheric epilepsy etiology vs outcome. Neurology 61(7):887–890

Rasmussen T, Villemure JG (1989) Cerebral hemispherectomy for seizures with hemiplegia. Cleve Clin J Med 56(Suppl Pt 1):S62–S68; discussion S79–S83

Imaging of Cerebrospinal Fluid Shunts, Drains, and Diversion Techniques

6

Daniel Thomas Ginat, Per-Lennart A. Westesson, and David Frim

6.1 Types of Procedures

6.1.1 External Ventricular Drainage

6.1.1.1 Discussion

External ventricular drains (EVD) are used for a variety of purposes, including temporary decompression of an enlarged ventricular system and acute hydrocephalus from tumor obstruction in order to better define the resection or following subarachnoid hemorrhage. An EVD catheter is inserted into the ventricular space via a transcranial approach after creating a burr hole along the coronal suture at the mid-pupillary line or secondarily along the parieto-occipital junction one-third of the way from the ear to the vertex. Imaging may be performed to assess the status of the ventricular system, as well as to evaluate for complications, which include infection, hemorrhage, excess drainage, catheter obstruction, cerebrospinal fluid leak, and malpositioning, which may require repositioning.

D.T. Ginat, M.D., M.S. (✉)
Department of Radiology, University of Chicago
Pritzker School of Medicine, Chicago, IL, USA
e-mail: dtg1@uchicago.edu

P.-L.A. Westesson, M.D., Ph.D., DDS
Division of Neuroradiology, University of Rochester
Medical Center, Rochester, NY, USA

D. Frim, M.D., Ph.D.
Section of Neurosurgery, University of Chicago
Pritzker School of Medicine, Chicago, IL, USA

© Springer International Publishing Switzerland 2017
D.T. Ginat, P.-L.A. Westesson (eds.), *Atlas of Postsurgical Neuroradiology*,
DOI 10.1007/978-3-319-52341-5_6

6.1.2 Ventriculoperitoneal (VP) Shunts

6.1.2.1 Discussion

VP shunting consists of diverting cerebrospinal fluid from an intracranial compartment to the peritoneum via a catheter and is commonly performed to treat hydrocephalus. VP shunt devices consist of a ventricular catheter, valve, and a distal catheter (Figs. 6.1 and 6.2). The catheter portion of a VP shunt is composed of extruded Silastic tubing impregnated with a radiopaque material, such as barium, in order to confer conspicuity on radiographic studies. Integrated reservoirs can also be added to the proximal shunt catheter, which enables percutaneous access and testing of the shunt system. The built-in reservoirs are usually positioned within the subgaleal space (Fig. 6.3).

Programmable valves contain radiopaque chiral markers that enable the valve opening pressure setting or performance level to be determined radiographically (Figs. 6.4, 6.5, 6.6, and 6.7). Some models have devices that allow these settings to be determined without radiographs. Antisiphon devices are also incorporated into some models in order to prevent cerebrospinal fluid overdrainage, when the patient is upright. While programmable shunts are generally MRI compatible up to 3T, there is a potential risk for inadvertent change of settings during MRI scanning. Thus, it is imperative to verify the settings following MRI. The pressure settings can be adjusted noninvasively using a magnetic tool. Furthermore, recent innovations have made available programmable valves that are resistant to environmental magnetic influences.

Gliosis often forms around the ventricular shunt catheter tract, but generally does not have clinical significance. The gliosis typically appears as circumferential low attenuation on CT and high signal on T2-weighted MRI measuring up to several millimeters in thickness (Fig. 6.8).

Up to one-third of VP shunts fail within 1 year of placement, and shunt revision is necessary in up to 70–80% of patients during their lifetime. Overall, programmable VP shunts have a similar failure rate as standard shunts. However, the pressure adjustment capability of programmable VP shunts leads to patient improvement in over 50% of cases. Complications include the following, for which examples are depicted later in this chapter:

- Infection (most common: 5–47%)
- Obstruction (usually proximal: emergency condition due to resulting increased ICP)
- Subcutaneous cerebrospinal fluid collections
- Catheter disconnection/migration/retraction (anywhere from mouth to anus!)
- Incisional hernia
- Bowel obstruction/volvulus
- Viscus perforation
- Cerebrospinal fluid pseudocysts
- Conduit for metastatic spread

Imaging plays an important role in evaluating patients with VP shunts. Radiographic shunt series are commonly performed as an initial screening for suspected shunt failure. However, these studies are less sensitive than cross-sectional imaging modalities. Nuclear medicine shunt studies are uncommonly performed but can be used to assess for shunt patency. Radiotracer, usually Tc-99m DTPA or In-111 DTPA, is injected into to the reservoir (Fig. 6.9). Normally, the radiotracer material spills freely throughout the peritoneal cavity. A focal collection of radiotracer suggests the presence of a pseudocyst. Reflux may normally occur into the ventricles and the reservoir emptying half-time of less than 10 min, although this may vary depending on the type of shunt. A similar concept for evaluating shunt patency is the "shuntogram," which involves injection of contrast material into the shunt valve, and tracking the flow of the contrast via serial radiographs of the cranial, chest, and abdominal components of the shunt system is obtained over the course of approximately 15 min.

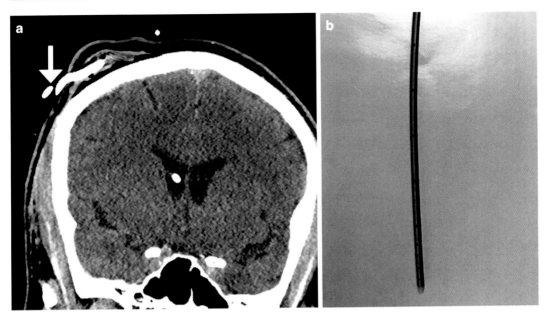

Fig. 6.1 External ventricular drain. Coronal CT image (**a**) shows the catheter within the right lateral ventricle and the external portion (*arrow*). Photograph of an external ventricular drain (**b**) (Courtesy of Marc Moisi)

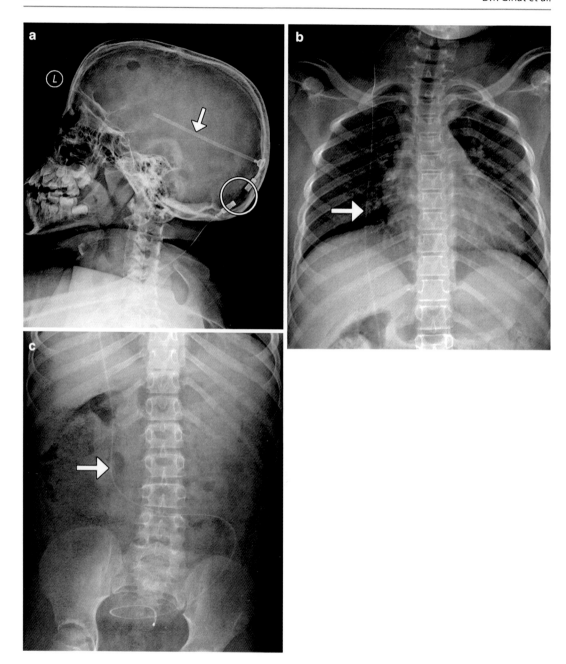

Fig. 6.2 Shunt series. Selected radiographs (**a–c**) show the proximal portion of the shunt catheter overlies the lateral ventricle (*arrow*); exits through a burr hole; tunnels into the subcutaneous tissues of the head, neck, chest, and abdomen (*arrow*); and terminates within the peritoneal cavity (*arrow*). Radiolucent portions (*encircled*) of the shunt should not be mistaken for discontinuities

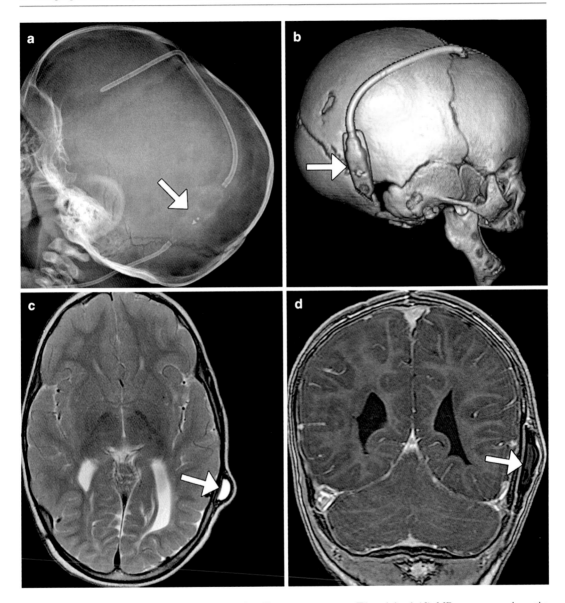

Fig. 6.3 Delta 1.5 valve VP shunt. Lateral skull radiograph (**a**) and 3D CT (**b**) images demonstrate the reservoir component (*arrows*) of the VP shunt containing performance level markers. Axial T2-weighted (**c**) and coronal post-contrast T1-weighted (**d**) MR sequences show the cerebrospinal fluid-filled reservoir (*arrows*) positioned in the subgaleal space

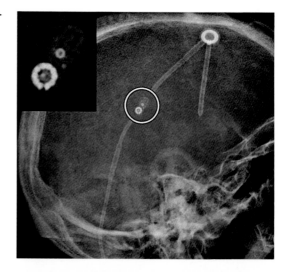

Fig. 6.4 Codman Hakim programmable shunt valve. Lateral radiograph with magnified view (*inset*) shows the components of the device (*encircled*) with pressure setting markers

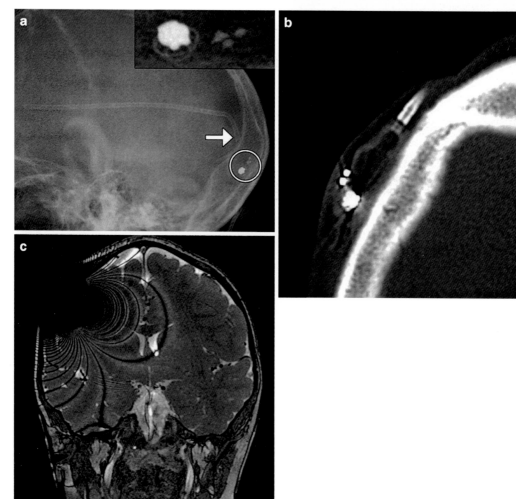

Fig. 6.5 Strata valve programmable shunt. Lateral radiograph (**a**) with magnified view (*inset*) of the VP shunt valve (*encircled*). The pressure setting can be read on the radiograph, but not on the axial CT image (**b**). The magnetic components of the programmable shunt produce extensive susceptibility artifacts on MRI (**c**)

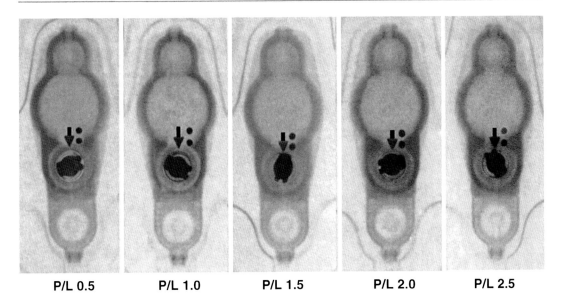

| P/L 0.5 | P/L 1.0 | P/L 1.5 | P/L 2.0 | P/L 2.5 |

Fig. 6.6 Valve performance level setting chart (Courtesy of Medtronic)

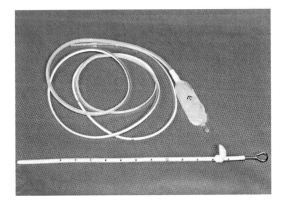

Fig. 6.7 Photograph of ventriculoperitoneal shunt components (Courtesy of Patricia Smith and Sarah Paengatelli)

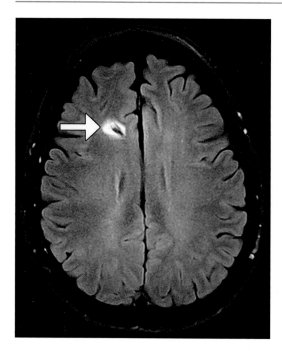

Fig. 6.8 Catheter-associated gliosis. Axial FLAIR MRI shows circumferential high signal surrounding the shunt catheter tract (*arrow*)

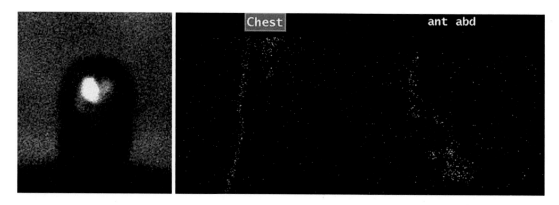

Fig. 6.9 Patent shunt catheter depicted on a nuclear medicine shunt study. Sequential ^{99m}Tc DTPA shunt images obtained over a 30-min period after injection of radiotracer into the ventricles via a shunt catheter show unimpeded passage of radiotracer from the ventricular system into the peritoneal cavity

6.1.3   Atypical Ventricular Shunts

6.1.3.1 Discussion

Other parts of the body can be used as terminals for the distal portions of ventricular shunt catheters. Ventriculoatrial, ventriculopleural, ventriculovesical, and ventriculo-gallbladder shunts are plausible alternatives for diverting cerebrospinal fluid away from the ventricles in patients with hydrocephalus, particularly when ventriculoperitoneal shunts fail.

* Ventriculoatrial Shunts (Fig. 6.10): The distal tip of a ventriculoatrial shunt should terminate in the right atrium or even in the superior vena cava.   Complications   particular   to ventriculoatrial shunts include pulmonary embolism and endocarditis.
* Ventriculopleural Shunts (Fig. 6.11): The terminus is within the pleural space. Variable amounts of cerebrospinal fluid may accumulate in the pleural space, in which up to 20% are symptomatic. This complication is more

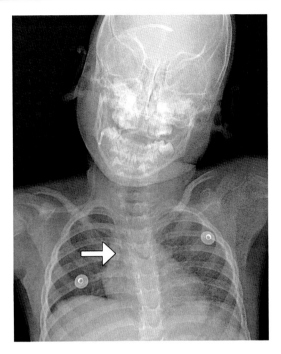

Fig. 6.10 Ventriculoatrial shunt. Frontal radiograph shows a ventricular shunt tip (*arrow*) at the level of the atriocaval junction (*arrow*)

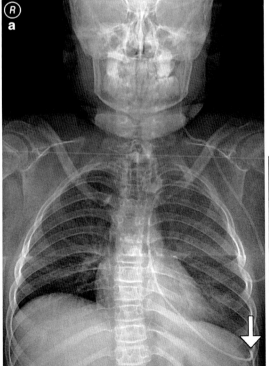

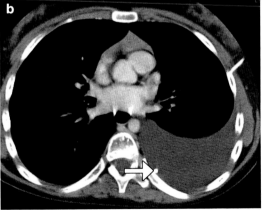

Fig. 6.11 Ventriculopleural shunt. Frontal radiograph (**a**) and axial CT (**b**) show a shunt catheter with distal end (*arrows*) located within the left pleural space, where there is cerebrospinal fluid

prevalent in infants due to the smaller surface area for fluid resorption.

- Ventriculoureteral Shunts: The terminus of the shunt is located in the ureter through a Roux-en-Y anastomosis. Diversion of cerebrospinal fluid can result in electrolyte abnormalities and cystitis.

- Ventriculocholecystic Shunts: Shunt tip terminations in the gallbladder have a satisfactory long-term success rate of over 60%. The most common complications include obstruction and cholecystitis, with an incidence of about 10% each.

6.1.4 Ventriculosubgaleal Shunts

6.1.4.1 Discussion

Ventriculosubgaleal shunting is diversion of intraventricular cerebrospinal fluid into the subgaleal space for temporary absorption by the subcutaneous tissues of the scalp. These shunts are a relatively straightforward, effective, and safe option for temporary treatment of hydrocephalus. Ventriculosubgaleal shunting can avoid the need for external drainage or frequent cerebrospinal fluid aspiration in unstable neonates until the cerebrospinal fluid characteristics and abdomen are suitable for ventriculoperitoneal shunting. On CT and MRI, the ventriculosubgaleal shunt catheter can be traced from the ventricular system to the subgaleal space, where there is often a variable amount of cerebrospinal fluid accumulation (Fig. 6.12).

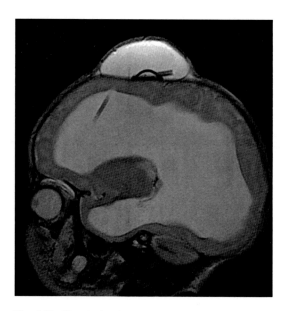

Fig. 6.12 Ventriculosubgaleal shunt. Sagittal T2-weighted MRI in a neonate show a pocket of subgaleal cerebrospinal fluid surrounding the ventriculosubgaleal shunt reservoir (Courtesy of Tina Young Poussaint MD)

6.1.5   Ventriculo-cisternal (Torkildsen) Shunts

6.1.5.1 Discussion

The Torkildsen shunt was initially conceived to bypass aqueductal stenosis and allow cerebrospinal fluid to drain directly through an extracranial pathway from the lateral ventricle to the cervical subarachnoid space. While this technique has been replaced by endoscopic third ventriculocisternostomy, the Torkildsen shunt approach is occasionally necessary in cases of complex hydrocephalus. The Torkildsen shunt typically courses from a lateral ventricle to the cisterna magna at the level of the foramen magnum (Fig. 6.13). These shunts are introduced into the lateral ventricle via a parieto-occipital burr hole and then exit to the extracranial space via that burr hole to course into the foramen magnum where the shunting tube is introduced into the cervical subarachnoid space. Occasionally, a C1 laminectomy is required for this procedure. The proximity of the distal end of the shunt to the cervicomedullary junction can predispose to upper spinal cord compression, rarely resulting in cervical myelopathy. Imaging can be used to evaluate such symptoms.

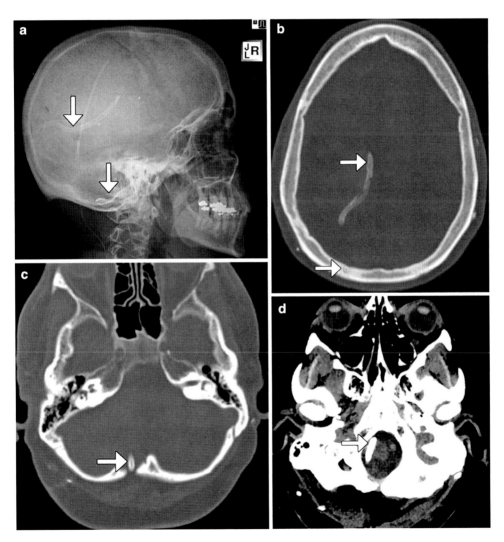

Fig. 6.13 Ventriculo-cisternal shunt. The patient has a history of chronic headaches and multiple shunts, including a Torkildsen shunt that was placed many years before. Lateral radiograph (**a**) and axial CT images (**b–d**) demonstrate the course of the internal shunt catheter (*arrows*) from the right lateral ventricle, inferiorly behind the cerebral hemisphere and cerebellum, and terminating at the level of the foramen magnum. There is a right occipital burr hole, through which the catheter was introduced

6.1.6 Percutaneously Accessed Cerebrospinal Fluid Reservoirs

6.1.6.1 Discussion

The subcutaneous cerebrospinal fluid devices consist of reservoirs positioned over the calvarium in the subgaleal space and catheters inserted into the intracranial compartment. The catheters can be inserted into the ventricular system or tumor cyst for decompression and connected to the reservoirs (Fig. 6.14). The reservoir can be accessed percutaneously using a needle. Ventricular reservoirs can also be converted into ventriculosubgaleal shunts or ventriculoperitoneal shunts, as many of these also have side ports. Complications of ventricular reservoirs include skin erosion and intracranial migration, which may require endoscopic retrieval, as well as generic complications encountered with all shunting systems.

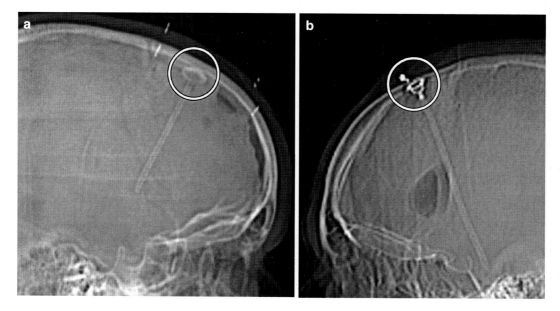

Fig. 6.14 Percutaneous cerebrospinal fluid reservoir with catheter in ventricular system. Scout images in two different patients (**a**, **b**) show the reservoirs (*encircled*) in the scalp connected to ventricular catheters

6.1.7   Subdural-Peritoneal Shunts

6.1.7.1 Discussion

Subdural-peritoneal shunting devices can be used to treat chronic subdural hematomas that are sufficiently degraded to a fluid state, such that the collection can flow into the peritoneal space (Fig. 6.15). Compared with burr hole decompression and drainage alone, subdural-peritoneal shunts result in a lower recurrence rate. Complications include acute subdural hematoma, subdural empyema, and cerebral edema.

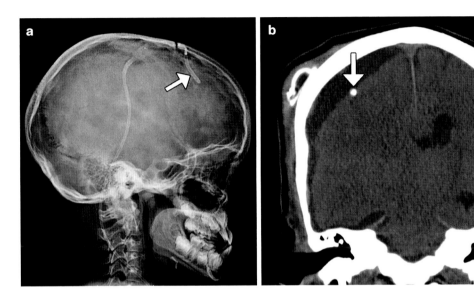

Fig. 6.15 Subdural-peritoneal shunt for chronic hematoma. Lateral radiograph (**a**) shows that the catheter tip lies just beneath the calvarium, in the subdural space (*arrow*). The rest of the catheter is tunneled in the subcutaneous tissues and runs toward the abdomen. The corresponding coronal CT image (**b**) shows the catheter tip (*arrow*) located within the right frontal convexity fluid collection

6.1.8 Cystoperitoneal and Cystoventriculostomy Shunts

6.1.8.1 Discussion

In rare instances, arachnoid cysts can cause symptoms and require surgical intervention. In some reports, cystoperitoneal (subarachnoid-peritoneal) shunting has proven effective for decompression of arachnoid cysts into the peritoneal cavity (Fig. 6.16). Meningoceles and cystic schwannomas are also sometimes amenable to cystoperitoneal shunting. Internal drainage of arachnoid cysts into regional ventricles or cisterns via stereotactic cystoventriculostomy is another feasible treatment approach, in which a drain is inserted in the cyst lumen and directed into an adjacent ventricle or cistern (Fig. 6.17).

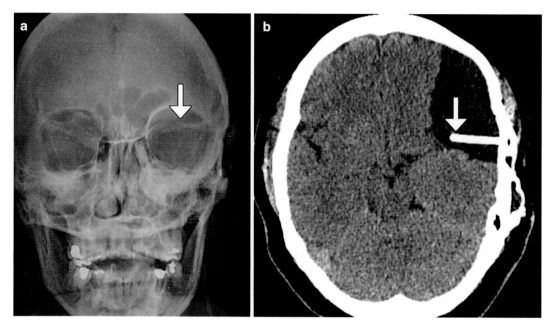

Fig. 6.16 Cystoperitoneal shunting. The patient has a history of ventriculoperitoneal shunt placement for arachnoid cyst and presents with headache. Frontal radiograph (**a**) shows that the tip of the shunt catheter (*arrow*) projects over the left hemisphere, not in the expected location of the ventricular system. Axial CT image (**b**) shows a cystoperitoneal shunt catheter (*arrow*) within a large left frontotemporal convexity arachnoid cyst

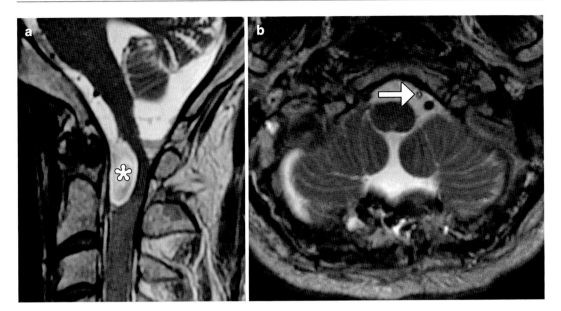

Fig. 6.17 Cystocisternal shunt. The patient has a history of arachnoid cyst secondary to Candida meningitis with obstruction of cerebrospinal fluid at the level of craniocervical junction, resulting in cord compression. Preoperative sagittal T2-weighted image (**a**) shows a cerebrospinal fluid intensity collection at the craniocervical junction, which exerts mass effect upon the spinal cord and medulla (*). Postoperative axial (**b**) T2-weighted MRI demonstrates a drainage catheter (*arrow*) within the subarachnoid space anterior to the cervicomedullary junction

6.1.9 Syringosubarachnoid and Syringopleural Shunts

6.1.9.1 Discussion

Direct intervention for syringohydromyelia is generally considered a rescue procedure and can be accomplished via syringosubarachnoid or syringopleural shunting. Syringosubarachnoid shunting can be used to treat syringohydromyelia related to a variety of causes, such as tumor, trauma, and Chiari malformations. This procedure serves to free the obstructed cerebrospinal fluid pathways via myelotomy and insertion of a Silastic T-shaped tube. The tube extends from the syringohydromyelia cavity to the subarachnoid space, into which the excess cerebrospinal fluid drains (Fig. 6.18). The T-shaped configuration of the tube allows cerebrospinal fluid to drain from both superior and inferior directions in the syrinx.

Syringopleural shunts can also be used to treat syringomyelia by extending a catheter from the syrinx to the pleural cavity as a negative pressure terminus (Fig. 6.19).

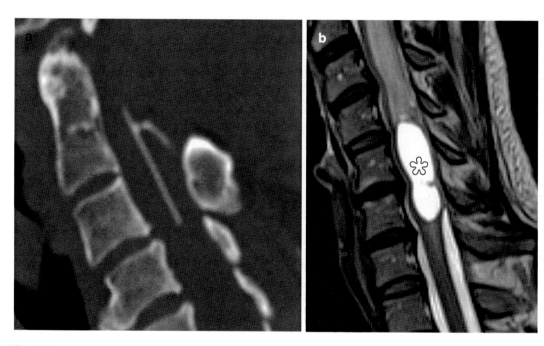

Fig. 6.18 Syringosubarachnoid shunt. Two patients' status post T-tube insertion for cervical spine syringomyelia decompression. Sagittal (**a**) CT image in one patient shows the hyperattenuating portions of the T-tube. Sagittal preoperative T2-weighted MRI (**b**) in another patient shows a large syrinx (*) in the cervical spinal cord, which was successfully decompressed following T-tube insertion (*arrow*), as shown on the postoperative T2-weighted MRI (**c**). There is also new kyphotic deformity after multilevel laminectomy

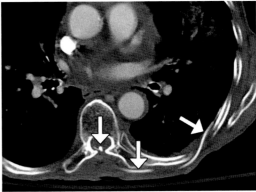

Fig. 6.19 Syringopleural shunt. Axial CT image shows a shunt catheter that extends from the spinal canal along the left back subcutaneous tissues into the pleural cavity (*arrows*)

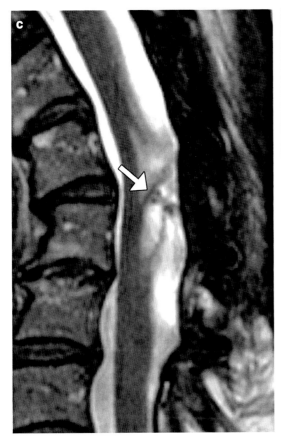

Fig. 6.18   (continued)

6.1.10 Lumboperitoneal Shunts

6.1.10.1 Discussion

Lumboperitoneal shunting is an alternative method for treating pseudotumor cerebri and communicating hydrocephalus separate from ventriculoperitoneal shunting. The procedure consists of introducing an intrathecal catheter and tunneling a distal catheter through the abdominal subcutaneous tissues and into the peritoneal cavity (Fig. 6.20). Lumboperitoneal shunt catheters can incorporate percutaneous programmable or gravity-actuated antisiphon components, in order to regulate pressure and reduce the risk of overdrainage (Figs. 6.21 and 6.22). Reported complications include malfunction, malposition, hemorrhage, and infection.

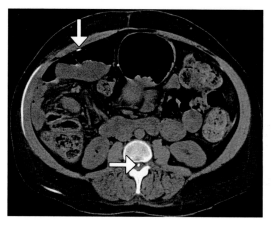

Fig. 6.20 Lumboperitoneal shunt. The patient has a history of pseudotumor cerebri and cerebrospinal fluid rhinorrhea. Axial CT image shows the shunt catheter (*arrows*) extending from the spinal canal, through the subcutaneous tunnel, and into the peritoneum

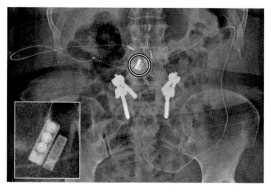

Fig. 6.22 Lumboperitoneal shunt catheter with gravity-actuated horizontal-vertical (*HV*) valve system. Frontal radiograph shows the lumboperitoneal shunt catheter in position with gravity-actuated valve component (*encircled*), which is magnified in the *inset*

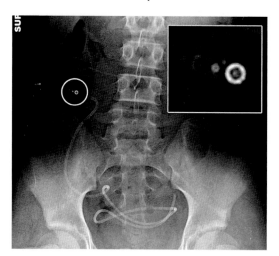

Fig. 6.21 Lumboperitoneal shunt catheter with percutaneously programmable valve. Frontal radiograph shows the lumboperitoneal shunt catheter in position with a programmable valve component (*encircled*), which is magnified in the *inset*

6.1.11 Third Ventriculocisternostomy

6.1.11.1 Discussion

Endoscopic fenestration of the anterior floor of the third ventricle (Liliequist's membrane) creates an alternative route for cerebrospinal fluid into the subarachnoid space via the prepontine cistern. This procedure bypasses obstruction at the level of the Sylvian aqueduct and restores cerebrospinal fluid flow out of the ventricular system. Third ventriculocisternostomy is a minimally invasive alternative to shunt implantation and is indicated for patients with aqueductal stenosis, obstructive tumors, and obstructive cysts.

The hemodynamic changes induced by third ventriculocisternostomy can be detected on MRI (Fig. 6.23). In particular, the sagittal phase-contrast cine sequence is the gold standard for evaluating cerebrospinal fluid flow dynamics. Following successful third ventriculostomy, a flame-shaped jet of high signal (flow) intensity across the floor of the third ventricle is characteristic. A jet of cerebrospinal fluid can also manifest on T2-weighted sequences. With high-resolution heavily T2-weighted cisternogram-type sequences, the normal Liliequist's membrane can be identified. Following third ventriculostomy, the membrane will appear disrupted.

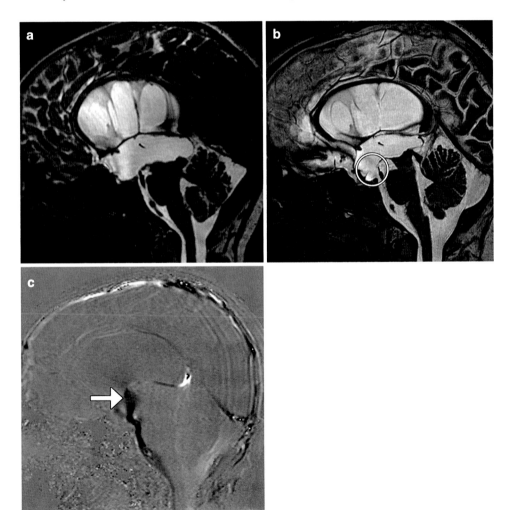

Fig. 6.23 Third ventriculocisternostomy. Preoperative sagittal FIESTA (**a**) shows enlargement of the third and lateral ventricles. Postoperative sagittal FIESTA (**b**) shows a defect in Liliequist's membrane (*encircled*) and decrease in size of the third and lateral ventricles. The postoperative sagittal phase-contrast MRI (**c**) shows the a strong jet of cerebrospinal fluid (*arrow*) across the third ventriculostomy

6.1.12 Endoscopic Septum Pellucidum and Intraventricular Cyst Fenestration

6.1.12.1 Discussion

Endoscopic fenestration can be performed to treat symptomatic septum pellucidum cysts. The procedure consists of creating a burr hole, introducing a cannula and endoscope into the lateral ventricles, and coagulating the septum pellucidum to allow communication between the right and left lateral ventricles. Postoperative MRI can show the disrupted membranes of the septum pellucidum and decrease in size of the cyst after successful fenestration (Fig. 6.24). Arachnoid and porencephalic cysts can be successfully fenestrated to create a communication with the ventricular system or cisterns, averting the need for a shunt catheter. Rarely, tumor cysts are decompressed into the ventricular system as a last resort (Fig. 6.25). This approach is generally avoided due to the risk of subsequent hydrocephalus secondary to malabsorption from the cyst contents.

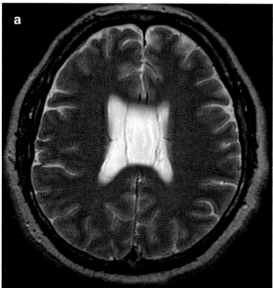 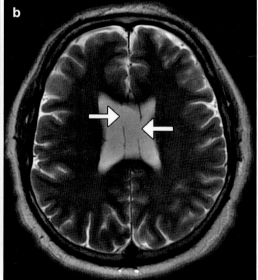

Fig. 6.24 Endoscopic septum pellucidum cyst fenestration. Preoperative T2-weighted MRI (**a**) shows a dilated cavum septum pellucidum cyst. Postoperative T2-weighted MRI (**b**) shows bilateral defects in the septum pellucidum (*arrows*) resulting in decompression of the cyst

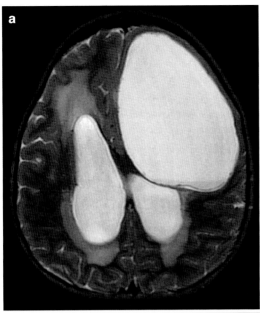

6.1.13 Aqueductoplasty

6.1.13.1 Discussion

Aqueductoplasty with or without stenting is a treatment option for isolated fourth ventricle resulting from membranous aqueductal stenosis. Balloon dilatation can be performed to expand the obstructed aqueduct of Sylvius (Fig. 6.26). Alternatively, a small-caliber flexible endoscope can be used to create a perforation in the offending membrane and to introduce a stent. Following aqueductoplasty, the third and lateral ventricles usually decrease in size. If inserted, the aqueductal stent is visible as a radioattenuating tubular structure on CT that extends from the fourth ventricle to the floor of the third ventricle and should not be misconstrued as a migrated shunt fragment in the appropriate setting.

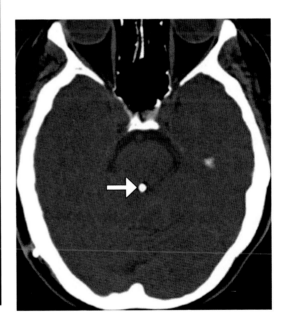

Fig. 6.25 Endoscopic cyst fenestration into the ventricular system. Preoperative axial T2-weighted MRI (**a**) shows a large cystic lesion that compresses the left frontal lobe and abuts the left lateral ventricle. Postoperative axial T2-weighted MRI (**b**) shows interval decrease in size of the cystic lesion, which now communicates with the left lateral ventricle through a surgical defect

Fig. 6.26 Aqueductoplasty and stenting. Axial CT image shows a stent within the aqueduct of Sylvius (*arrow*)

6.1.14 Endoscopic Choroid Plexus Cauterization

6.1.14.1 Discussion

Choroid plexus surgery is an option for treating hydrocephalus in patients with suspected cerebrospinal fluid overproduction and patients lacking a septum pellucidum. Choroid plexus cauterization can be performed endoscopically and consists of coagulating a portion of the choroid plexus. On imaging, truncation of the treated choroid plexus can be appreciated (Fig. 6.27). Interestingly, following choroid plexus cauterization alone, ventricular size does not necessarily decrease significantly, although sulci become more prominent indicating decreased cerebrospinal fluid pressure. Nevertheless, choroid plexus cauterization is often performed in conjunction with ventriculocisternostomy.

Choroid plexus papillomas can cause hydrocephalus due to overproduction of cerebrospinal fluid with rates of over 1.0 mL/min as well as subarachnoid obstruction. Total surgical resection of the tumor and vascular pedicle is the treatment of choice. Coagulation of the tumor can facilitate resection. After resection, the hydrocephalus usually resolves (Fig. 6.28). Additional treatment for hydrocephalus after resection may be required due to intraventricular hemorrhage, inflammation from surgery, and mechanical distortion of the ventricular system.

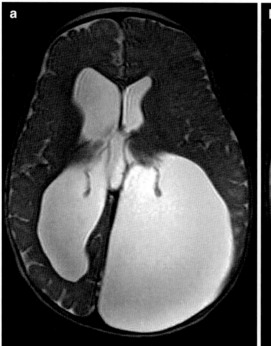
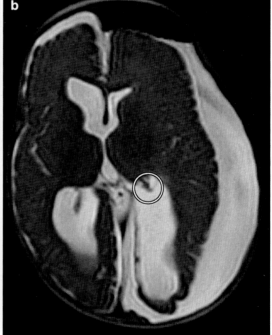

Fig. 6.27 Choroid plexus cauterization. Preoperative axial T2-weighted MRI (**a**) shows dilatation of the lateral ventricles, particularly the atrium of the left lateral ventricle, resulting in cranial vault deformity. Postoperative axial T2-weighted MRI (**b**) shows interval truncation of the left lateral ventricle choroid plexus secondary to fulguration (*encircled*). Sequelae of left ventricular fenestration are also demonstrated, with resultant decompression of the ventricular system and development of extra-axial cerebrospinal fluid

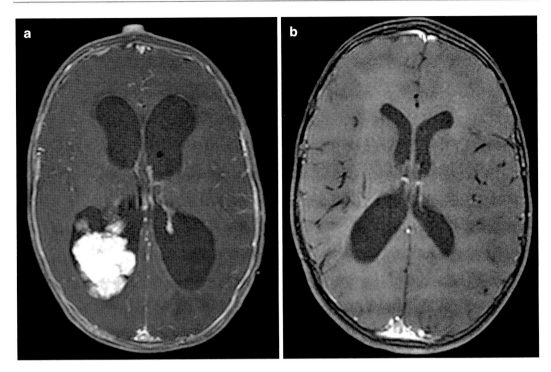

Fig. 6.28 Choroid plexus tumor resection. Preoperative axial post-contrast T1-weighted MRI (**a**) shows a lobulated mass within the right lateral ventricle and marked enlargement of the ventricular system. Postoperative post-contrast T1-weighted MRI (**b**) shows interval resection of the tumor and markedly decreased ventricular size

6.2   Complications Related to Cerebrospinal Fluid Diversion Surgeries

6.2.1   Corpus Callosum Changes Secondary to Shunt Catheterization

6.2.1.1   Discussion

Due to its proximity to lateral ventricle shunt trajectories, the corpus callosum is prone to injury during catheter insertion. This can result in linear areas of high T2 signal in the corpus callosum adjacent to the catheter. Corpus callosal swelling can also occur after ventricular shunting for long-standing obstructive hydrocephalus. This appears as enlargement and hypoattenuation on CT images corresponding to increased T2 and decreased T1 signal on MRI that are often oriented transversely with a striated pattern, mainly within the body of the corpus callosum (Fig. 6.29). The etiology for the signal changes is likely attributable to compression of the corpus callosum against the rigid falx cerebri from hydrocephalus prior to shunting. These changes are typically not associated with symptoms and should not be misinterpreted as neoplasm, white matter disease, or leukoencephalopathy in particular, the corpus callosum can acquire a scalloping deformity, which is best appreciated on sagittal images. Furthermore, the changes often resolve over time.

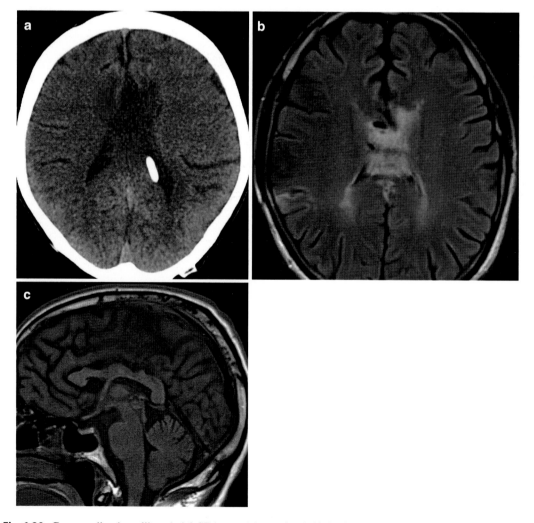

Fig. 6.29 Corpus callosal swelling. Axial CT image (**a**) shows low attenuation and enlargement of the body of the corpus callosum. Axial T2-weighted MRI (**b**) shows striated high signal in the corpus callosum. Sagittal T1-weighted MRI (**c**) shows scalloping deformity of the corpus callosum

6.2.2   Shunt-Associated Intracranial Hemorrhage

6.2.2.1 Discussion

Intraparenchymal, subdural, and intraventricular hemorrhage associated with placement of VP shunts is an uncommon complication, with an estimated incidence of 0.3–4% (Fig. 6.30). Intracranial hemorrhage may present soon after ventricular catheterization or it can be delayed. Predisposing factors include underlying parenchymal friability, venous occlusion, coagulopathy, multiple catheter passes, choroid plexus injury, and malpositioning near a vascular structure. Intraparenchymal hemorrhage associated with VP shunting typically runs parallel to the length of the tubing and can be circumferential. Frequently, choroid plexus hemorrhage can lead to disseminated intraventricular hemorrhage and can contribute to shunt malfunction.

The development of chronic calcified subdural hematomas is a potential long-term complication of ventriculoperitoneal shunting. The calcifications tend to occur at the margins of the fluid collection (Fig. 6.31), but may sometimes be more confluent. When bilateral, these have been termed "armored brain." Although the calcified subdural hematomas can produce symptoms, they generally do not require further intervention.

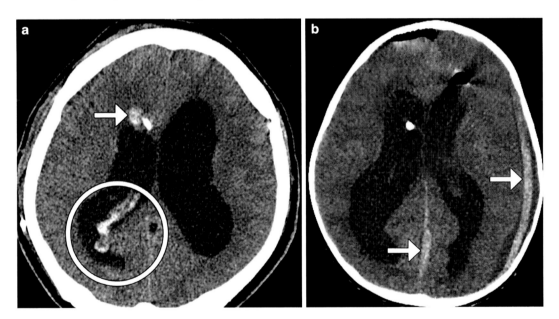

Fig. 6.30 Shunt-associated hemorrhage. Axial CT image (**a**) obtained 2 days following VP shunt placement shows a focus of right frontal lobe hemorrhage adjacent to the catheter (*arrow*). There is also hemorrhage within the choroid plexus and the posterior horn of the right lateral ventricle (*encircled*). Axial CT image in a different patient (**b**) shows subdural hematomas (*arrows*) that formed shortly after shunt catheter insertion.

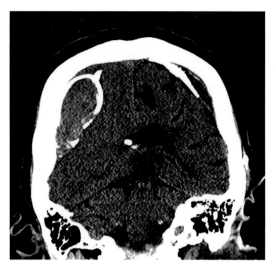

Fig. 6.31 Chronic calcified subdural hematoma. Coronal CT image shows peripherally calcified bilateral cerebral convexity subdural collections in a patient with long-standing ventricular shunting

6.2.3   Intraventricular Fat Migration

6.2.3.1 Discussion

Fragments of subcutaneous adipose tissue can uncommonly migrate into the intracranial cisterns and ventricular system either during placement of a cerebrospinal fluid shunt catheter, since the catheter is tunneled through subcutaneous fat. This complication is apparent on MRI and CT as nodules with fat characteristics within the ventricles or cisterns (Fig. 6.32) can be adherent to the ventricular walls. Nevertheless, patients are often not symptomatic from this.

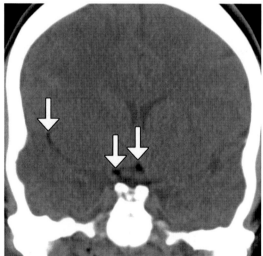

Fig. 6.32 Intraventricular fat. The patient underwent recent lumboperitoneal shunt insertion. Coronal CT image shows fat-attenuation material within the suprasellar cistern and right Sylvian fissure (*arrows*)

6.2.4   MRI-Induced Programmable Valve Setting Alteration

6.2.4.1 Discussion

Recurrent hydrocephalus in patients with indwelling ventricular shunts is a sign of shunt failure. Of note, high-field-strength MRI can alter the pressure setting of most percutaneous programmable cerebrospinal fluid shunts and may also result in acute hydrocephalus, mimicking shunt malfunction, if the setting is not checked and reset after the scan (Fig. 6.33). The accumulation of cerebrospinal fluid can lead to ventricular enlargement, unless there is extensive preexisting ventricular scarring that limits ventricular expansion. Enlargement of the temporal horns is among the earliest findings of this complication. Other signs include effacement of the sulci and transependymal flow of cerebrospinal fluid. Hydrocephalus can result in sutural diastasis and enlargement of cranial diameter in children.

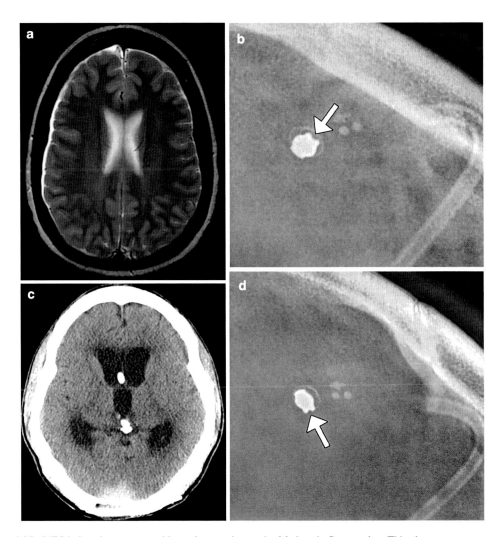

Fig. 6.33 MRI-induced programmable valve setting alteration. The patient with a percutaneously programmable cerebrospinal fluid shunt, presented acutely obtunded after undergoing MRI at 1.5T the previous day. The pressure settings were not checked following MRI. The following day, the patient was minimally responsive and was noted that the pressure setting changed from 0.5 to 2.5 on the Medtronic Strata valve. This change was presumably secondary to the magnetic field. Axial T2-weighted MRI (**a**) shows no ventricular dilatation. Shunt survey (**b**) obtained before the MRI shows a pressure setting of 0.5. Axial CT image (**c**) obtained the day after the MRI shows acute massive hydrocephalus and the subsequent shunt survey (**d**) shows a pressure setting of 2.5

6.2.5 Ventricular Loculations and Isolated Ventricles

6.2.5.1 Discussion

The formation of loculations of cerebrospinal fluid within the ventricular system can lead to shunt failure. The compartmentalized collection of cerebrospinal fluid can lead to symptoms of hydrocephalus and may be caused by adhesions from prior hemorrhage or infection, for example. CT ventriculography performed by injecting contrast into the shunt catheter can be used to delineate the presence of loculations by the lack of communication of the contrast material with the rest of the ventricular system (Fig. 6.34). Similarly, an isolated or trapped ventricle is an uncommon phenomenon that can occur in the setting of ventricular shunting with adhesion formation and represents a form of focal hydrocephalus. The significance of this complication is that it can exert mass effect upon surrounding structures. On imaging, disparate sizes of the ventricles are apparent, and contrast does not enter the trapped ventricle on CT ventriculography if the contrast is injected into the other portions of the ventricular system (Fig. 6.35). The level of obstruction is often at the foramen of Monro, but can occur anywhere in the ventricular system. Treatment may consist of ventricular catheter repositioning, septostomy, foramen of Monro reconstruction, or implantation of a catheter into the affected ventricle. Isolated ventricles that are not enlarging can be difficult to differentiate from asymmetric ventricles, which may also be encountered after shunting and do not require treatment. Midline shift and progressive increase in size of the ventricle suggest trapping over simple asymmetry of the ventricles. If there is any doubt, short interval imaging follow-up can be performed.

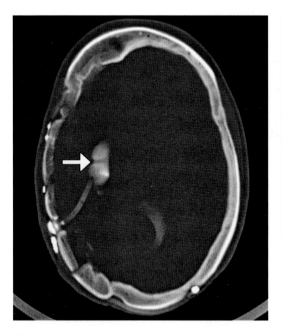

Fig. 6.34 Ventricular loculation. Axial CT ventriculogram shows the injected contrast confined to a cystic compartment (*arrow*)

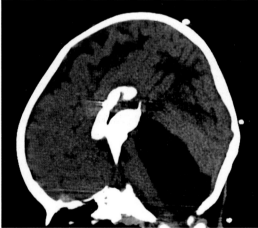

Fig. 6.35 Isolated fourth ventricle. Sagittal CT ventriculogram shows the injected contrast confined to the third and lateral ventricles and a markedly expanded fourth ventricle

6.2.6   Slit Ventricle Syndrome

6.2.6.1 Discussion

Slit ventricle syndrome can be defined as a hydro-cephalus patient that presents with headache and narrow ventricles on imaging, with a functioning cerebrospinal fluid shunting device, but an elevated cerebrospinal fluid pressure when tested by lumbar puncture. This relatively rare condition may result from reduced brain compliance, often due to the use of a siphoning-valve shunting device at an early age. On imaging, the ventricles appear to be very small and do not increase in proportion to the increased intraventricular pressure (Fig. 6.36). The condition can be very serious and should not be misinterpreted as small ventricles simply due to overshunting.

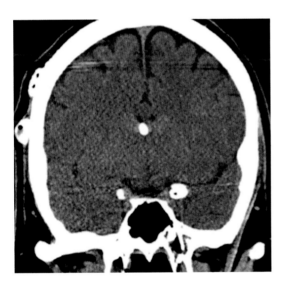

Fig. 6.36 Slit ventricle syndrome. The patient had clinical evidence of intracranial hypertension. Coronal CT image shows small size of the ventricular system with right transparietal shunt catheter in position

6.2.7   Chronic Overshunting and Associated Findings

6.2.7.1 Discussion

Chronically shunted patients occasionally can develop intracranial hypotension secondary to long-term overdraining of cerebrospinal fluid that manifests as diffuse meningeal thickening and enhancement (Fig. 6.37). This process may extend into the cervical spine and rarely results in cervical myelopathy. Otherwise, headache is a common symptom. However, elderly patients are usually asymptomatic due to brain atrophy.

Chronic low-pressure ventricular shunting in children may also lead to hyperostosis cranii ex vacuo. This process is usually diffuse and involves predominantly the inner table of both the skull base and calvarium (Fig. 6.38). On CT, the new bone formation can display a layered appearance. In infants, there may be associated premature closure of the sutures (Fig.6.39), which in turn can result in a cranial stenosis syndrome of elevated intracranial pressure.

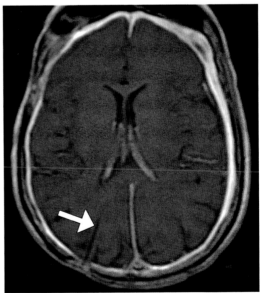

Fig. 6.37 Intracranial hypotension. There is diffuse thickening and avid enhancement of the meninges. A right parietal ventriculostomy catheter (*arrow*) is present

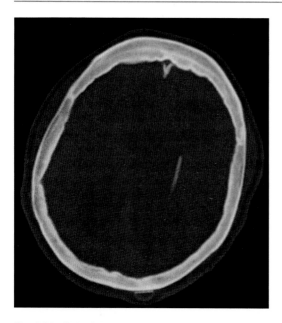

Fig. 6.38 Calvarial hyperostosis. Axial CT image shows diffuse calvarial thickening in a patient with long-standing ventricular shunting

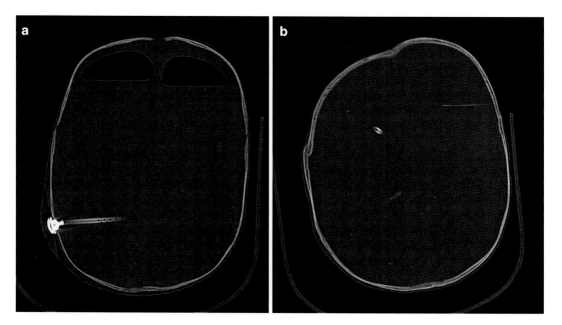

Fig. 6.39 Post-shunt craniosynostosis. Axial CT image (**a**) after recent ventriculoperitoneal shunt insertion shows patent cranial sutures. Follow-up axial CT image (**b**) obtained several months later shows interval closure of the cranial sutures

6.2.8   Shunt-Associated Infections

6.2.8.1 Discussion

Shunt-associated infections may be classified as proximal or distal, and it is important to image both ends of the shunt system in suspected cases of infection. Proximal ventricular shunt-associated infections mainly include ventriculitis (ependymitis) and meningitis. Cerebritis and abscess are less common complications. Overall, the incidence of VP shunt-associated infection ranges from 2% to 40% per shunting procedure. Distal shunt-associated infections include cellulitis and subcutaneous and intra-abdominal abscesses, which can be readily demonstrated on CT (Figs. 6.40 and 6.41). Intra-abdominal and subcutaneous abscess related to the ventricular catheter appear as rim-enhancing fluid collections with surrounding fat stranding on CT. The most common causative organisms are *Staphylococcus aureus* and *epidermidis*. On imaging, ventriculitis can manifest as periventricular enhancement and restricted diffusion associated with intraventricular layering debris (Fig. 6.42). Treatment generally consists of removal of the entire shunt device, an interim period of external ventricular drainage and antibiotic therapy, and eventual replacement of the shunting device at a different site.

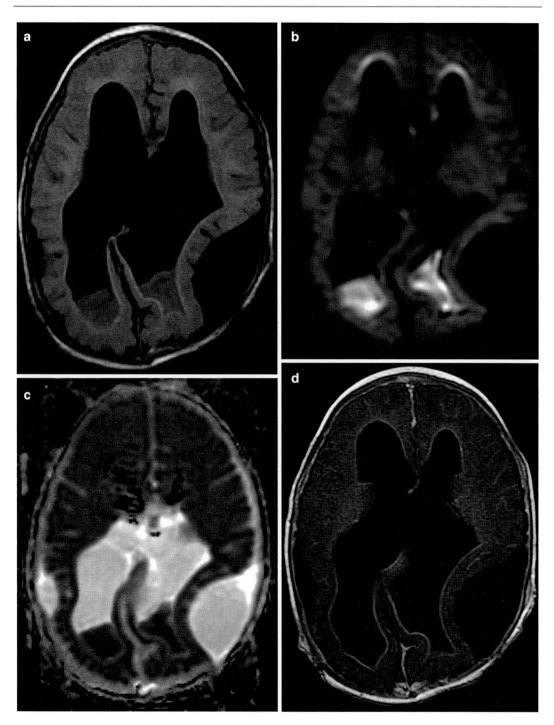

Fig. 6.40 Ventriculitis. Axial FLAIR (**a**), DWI (**b**), and ADC map (**c**) show layering debris with restricted diffusion in the occipital horns of the bilateral lateral ventricles. Axial T1-weighted post-contrast axial MRI (**d**) show diffuse enhancement along the walls of the bilateral lateral ventricles. There are also bilateral cererbral convexity subdural fluid collections, left larger than right

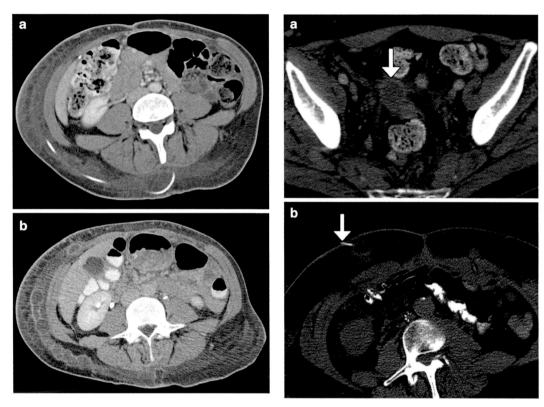

Fig. 6.41 Cellulitis and subcutaneous abscesses. Axial CT image (**a**) shows extensive skin thickening and subcutaneous stranding along the path of the lumboperitoneal shunt. Subsequent axial CT image obtained after removal of the device (**b**) shows development of multiple rim-enhancing fluid collections along the prior shunt tract. *Staphylococcus aureus* was cultured from the wounds

Fig. 6.42 Intraperitoneal abscess. Axial contrast-enhanced CT image of the pelvis (**a**) shows an abscess in the midpelvis (*arrow*). Axial CT of the abdomen (**b**) shows externalization of the distal end of the ventriculoperitoneal shunt. The tip of the catheter exits the skin of the right lower quadrant (*arrow*)

6.2.9 Shunt Malposition and Migration

6.2.9.1 Discussion

Proper positioning of shunt catheters within the ventricles can be challenging particularly in patients with small ventricles. It has been reported that suboptimal ventriculoperitoneal shunt positioning occurs in about 25% of cases and that in about 8% of cases, the catheter tip is located entirely outside the ventricular system, either too far proximal or distal. Catheter malposition can compromise cerebrospinal fluid drainage and lead to injury of brain parenchyma and associated symptomatology (Fig. 6.43).

Distal shunt catheter migration has been reported to occur in many different locations, including into the scrotum, vagina, heart, lungs/pleura, rectum, and abdominal wall, among others. Retraction into the abdominal wall can lead to the formation of a pseudocyst within the subcutaneous tissues (Fig. 6.44). Migration of the distal shunt into the rectum must be preceded by bowel perforation. Bowel and liver perforation by VP shunt catheters are rare occurrences (Fig. 6.45). Imaging is useful to localize the migrated shunt device components and associated complications. Management may include laparotomy with catheter removal and replacement into another absorptive site.

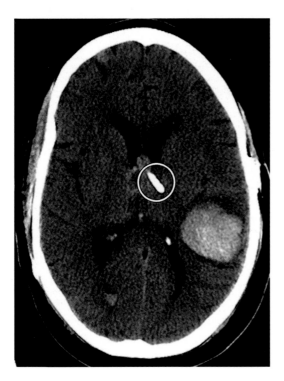

Fig. 6.43 Shunt catheter malposition. Axial CT image shows the tip of the shunt catheter in the left thalamus (*encircled*). There is a hematoma in the left temporal lobe

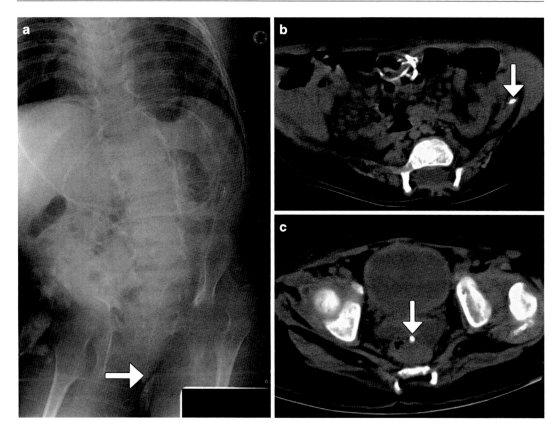

Fig. 6.44 Bowel perforation. Frontal radiograph (**a**) shows coiling of a VP shunt catheter in the midabdomen. The catheter then courses in the pelvis and projects in the rectum/anus region (*arrow*). Axial CT images (**b, c**) show the catheter within the left colon and rectum (*arrows*) (Courtesy of Nina Klionsky, MD)

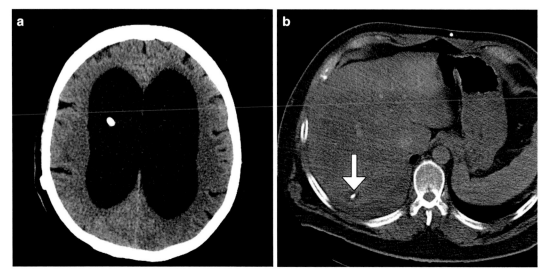

Fig. 6.45 Catheter liver puncture. The patient presented with worsening neurological status after attempted ventriculoperitoneal shunting at another institution. Axial CT image of the head (**a**) shows marked verntriculomegaly despite recent ventricular shunt insertion. Axial CT image of the abdomen (**b**) shows the distal portion of the catheter within the liver parenchyma, surrounded by a small amount of cerebrospinal fluid (*arrow*)

6.2.10 Shunt Catheter Mechanical Failure

6.2.10.1 Discussion

Mechanical failure of cerebrospinal fluid shunt catheters can be due to kinking or disconnection or breakage. While kinking is typically an early complication, disconnection and breakage of the tubing tend to be late complications that are usually related to aging/degradation of the catheter material and less often mechanical trauma. Radiographs as part of shunt series are usually adequate for depicting these complications (Figs. 6.46 and 6.47). Disconnected or fractured shunts have abnormal lucent gaps. Comparison with prior shunt series can be helpful for discerning subtle defects. It should be noted that some VP shunts contain radiolucent components that should not be misinterpreted as discontinuities.

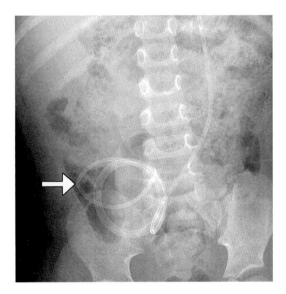

Fig. 6.46 Catheter kink. Frontal radiograph shows a sharp bend (*arrow*) in a distal ventriculoperitoneal shunt catheter

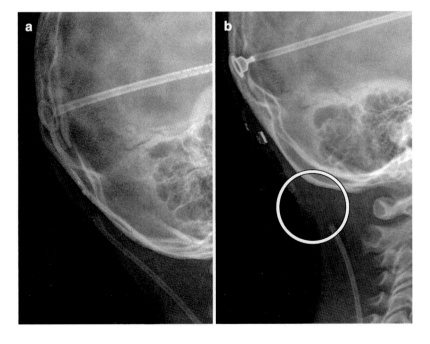

Fig. 6.47 Shunt fracture. Initial lateral radiograph (**a**) shows intact shunt hardware. Follow up lateral radiograph (**b**) when the patient presented with new neurological symptoms shows interval fracture and retraction of the catheter tubing in the neck (*encircled*)

6.2.11 Intraparenchymal Pericatheter Cysts and Interstitial Cerebrospinal Fluid

6.2.11.1 Discussion

Intraparenchymal pericatheter cysts are rare complications of shunt surgery. These typically result from increased resistance to outflow or obstruction and are often preceded by cerebrospinal fluid edema around the catheter. On imaging, these cysts appear as ovoid collections with characteristics of cerebrospinal fluid around the shunt catheter (Fig. 6.48). Low attenuation on CT and high T2 signal on MRI in the surrounding brain parenchyma can also be present. The pericatheter cysts are reversible with shunt revision or may resolve spontaneously with conservative management.

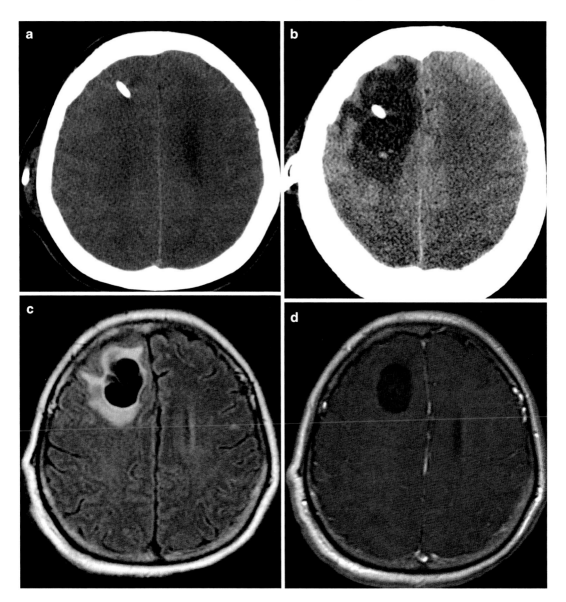

Fig. 6.48 Pericatheter cyst and interstitial cerebrospinal fluid. Initial axial CT (**a**) image shows an unremarkable course of the right transfrontal VP shunt catheter. Axial CT (**b**) obtained 3 weeks later shows interval development of a low-attenuation collection surrounding the shunt catheter. The corresponding axial T2 FLAIR (**c**) and post-contrast T1-weighted (**d**) MR images show that the collection follows cerebrospinal fluid signal. Although there is high T2 signal in the surrounding white matter, there is no associated enhancement to suggest abscess

6.2.12 Peritoneal Pseudocysts

6.2.12.1 Discussion

Intraperitoneal pseudocysts associated with shunt catheters are localized, walled-off collections of cerebrospinal fluid within the peritoneal cavity, which is often readily depicted on CT or ultrasound (Fig. 6.49). Nuclear medicine or other shunt studies confirm a communication between the catheter and pseudocyst.

Pseudocysts are variable in size and appearance. Small, loculated collections tend to be infected, while large cysts may be sterile cerebrospinal fluid collections, although infection with a pseudocyst should be considered regardless of size. Large intraperitoneal pseudocysts may cause bowel obstruction, ventriculomegaly, and increased intracranial pressure, independent of infectious complications.

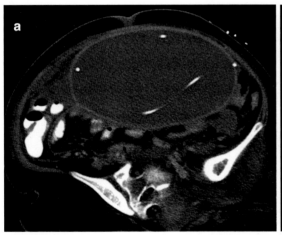 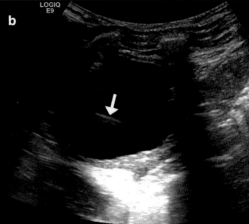

Fig. 6.49 Peritoneal pseudocyst. Axial CT image (**a**) shows a large, well-defined fluid collection that contains the distal portion of the shunt catheter. Ultrasound image in a different patient (**b**) shows an intra-abdominal fluid collection surrounding the shunt catheter (*arrow*)

6.2.13 Cerebrospinal Fluid Leak Syndrome

6.2.13.1 Discussion

Cerebrospinal fluid leakage is an uncommon complication of cerebrospinal fluid shunting procedures. Patients characteristically present with signs of postural cerebrospinal fluid hypotension. On imaging, fluid collections with cerebrospinal fluid characteristics can be found in the soft tissues adjacent to the catheter, essentially anywhere along the course of the catheter (Fig. 6.50). There can be associated catheter disconnection or dislodgement.

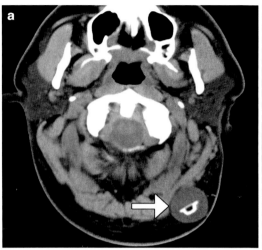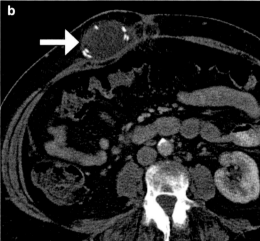

Fig. 6.50 Shunt device associated cerebrospinal fluid leakage. Axial CT image (**a**) shows a cerebrospinal fluid attenuation collection (*arrow*) surrounding the reservoir in the left upper neck. Axial CT image in a different patient (**b**) shows the distal end of the VP shunt has migrated and coiled within the right anterior abdominal wall subcutaneous tissues, resulting in accumulation of cerebrospinal fluid (*arrow*)

6.2.14 Tumor Seeding

6.2.14.1 Discussion

Ventriculoperitoneal shunts can rarely serve as a conduit for tumor dissemination. Various intracranial tumors can metastasize to the abdomen via the shunts, including glioblastoma, PNET, and germinoma, among others. Conversely, intracranial spread of intra-abdominal tumors into the intracranial compartment via the shunts has been reported. Cross-sectional imaging can be used to localize and characterize the metastatic deposits (Fig. 6.51).

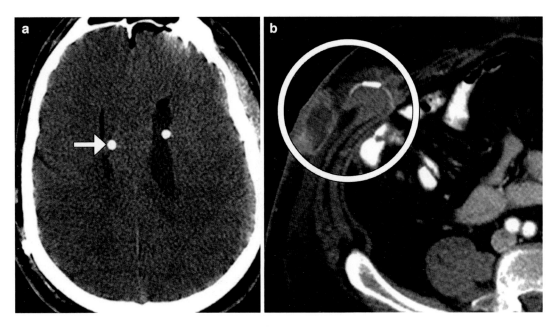

Fig. 6.51 Tumor seeding. Axial CT image of the brain (**a**) shows the shunt catheter tip (*arrow*) penetrating a corpus callosum glioblastoma. Axial post-contrast CT image of the abdomen (**b**) shows irregular masses within the right abdomen subcutaneous tissues along the course of the shunt (*encircled*), consistent with metastatic deposits

6.2.15 Shunt Catheter Calcification

6.2.15.1   Discussion

Dystrophic calcifications can form around the silicone tubing of shunt catheters within the subcutaneous tissues, particularly those impregnated with barium (Fig. 6.52). This phenomenon is likely attributable to a fibrotic reaction to the tube. Calcifications are most commonly encountered in the region of the clavicles. The presence of calcification surrounding shunt catheters may be associated with malfunction, pain, and fever. Removal of the affecting tubing can relieve symptoms although the catheter can be difficult to remove due to associated fibrosis. The condition is readily depicted on radiographs or CT in which the calcifications are usually coarse, irregular, and scattered along the length of the shunt tubing.

6.2.16 Pulmonary Embolism from Ventriculoatrial Shunting

6.2.16.1   Discussion

In rare cases, the presence of a catheter in the deep venous system and right atrium can predispose to thrombus formation along the intracardiac portion of the catheter and lead to pulmonary embolism. Patients may present with chest pain and shortness of breath. Pulmonary embolism protocol CT is the modality of choice for evaluating pulmonary artery filling defects (Fig. 6.53).

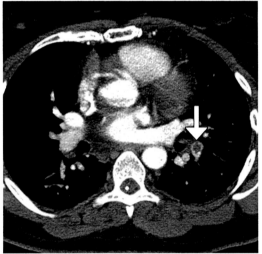

Fig. 6.53 Pulmonary embolism associated with ventriculoatrial shunting. The patient presented with shortness of breath after shunt placement. Axial post-contrast CT image shows a filling defect in a left pulmonary artery branch (*arrow*)

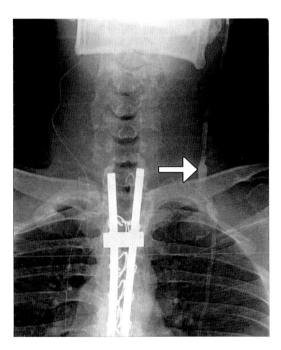

Fig. 6.52 Pericatheter dystrophic calcifications. Frontal radiograph of the neck shows diffuse dystrophic calcifications along the left VP shunt tube (*arrow*). A normal-appearing right shunt catheter is present on the contralateral side

6.2.17 Chiari Decompression Surgery and Associated Complications

6.2.17.1 Discussion

The goal of neurosurgical intervention in patients with Chiari type 1 malformation is to reduce symptomatic cerebrospinal fluid pressure gradients across the craniocervical junction. Decompression typically involves suboccipital craniectomy and C1 laminectomy, with or without duraplasty. Regardless of the particular technique implemented, decompression should result in a widened neo-foramen magnum, with improved cerebrospinal fluid flow, which can be assessed qualitatively or quantitatively via phase-contrast imaging, as well as diminished syringomyelia (Fig. 6.54).

There are several adjunct procedures that can be implemented in conjunction with Chiari decompression, particularly as a second resort, including craniocervical decompression without or with duraplasty, fourth ventricular stenting, endoscopic third ventriculostomy, tonsillar reduction, and syringohydromyelia decompression. In particular, fourth ventricular stenting can be performed when there is obstruction of the fourth ventricular outflow in patients with refractory syringohydromyelia. Silastic tubes that are typically used for this purpose are visible on conventional MRI sequences as low-signal-intensity structures on T1- and T2-weighted sequences (Fig. 6.55).

Tonsillar cauterization or reduction leads to a characteristic finding on early postoperative imaging, which is essentially related to ischemia at the margins of the resected tissues, along with microhemorrhages (Fig. 6.56). Enhancement along the margins of the cauterized tissue can also be observed in the perioperative period. Over time, the ischemia evolves to encephalomalacia with further shrinkage of the inferior cerebellum and greater flow across the neo-foramen magnum.

Complications of Chiari decompression include hemorrhage, infection, stroke, cerebrospinal fluid leak with pseudomeningocele formation, hydrocephalus, craniocervical instability, arachnoid adhesion formation, inflammatory or granulomatous reaction to implanted materials, and cerebellar ptosis or cerebellar slump syndrome. Some of these complications may warrant revision surgery, and some are discussed in more detail in the following pages.

Infarction is a rare complication of Chiari I malformation decompression, but is more likely to occur during complex revision surgeries. The posterior inferior cerebellar artery territory is most often involved, and the extent is typically beyond the areas affected by ischemia induced by cauterization performed for tonsillar reduction. DWI and FLAIR MRI sequences are useful for evaluating perioperative infarcts (Fig. 6.57).

Pseudomeningoceles consist of cerebrospinal fluid collections that extend into the upper neck and scalp soft tissues from the site of decompression. This phenomenon occurs even if duraplasty is performed, since a completely watertight closure is not always possible to achieve. The pseudomeningoceles can occasionally produce enough mass effect to aggravate the syringohydromyelia. Furthermore, the pseudomeningoceles can also fluctuate in size over time, particularly with changes related to intracranial shunting (Fig. 6.58).

Arachnoid adhesions can tether the cerebellum to overlying dura and impede cerebrospinal fluid flow. The adhesions are best depicted on high-resolution cisternogram type sequences, such as FIESTA, CISS, or DRIVE, and appear as low-signal-intensity bands that distort the parenchyma. These are often located posterior to the cerebellum or at the craniocervical junction and attach to the overlying dura or dural graft (Fig. 6.59).

Cerebellar slump syndrome can manifest with aggravated symptoms after decompression surgery for Chiari I malformation due to further inferior descent of the cerebellum, which can compress the upper spinal cord and distort the brainstem, as demonstrated on MRI (Fig. 6.60). This complication can be predisposed by a neo-foramen magnum that is too large.

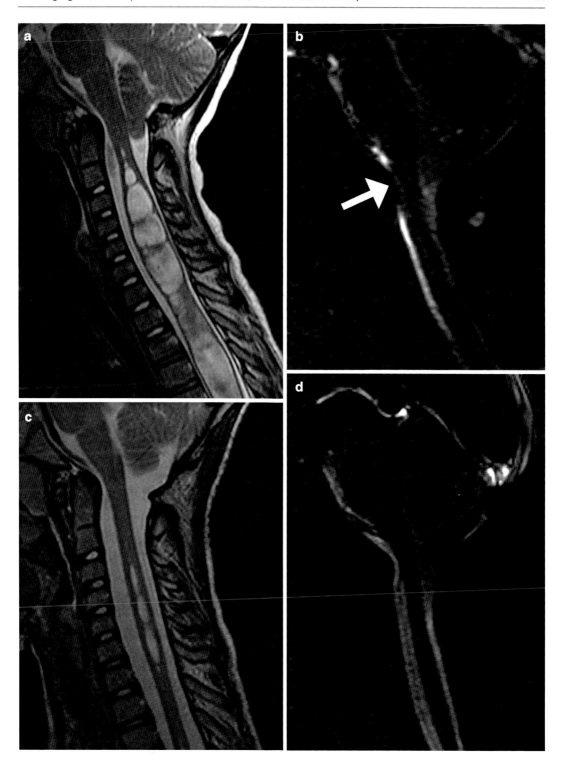

Fig. 6.54 Expected findings following Chiari decompression surgery. Preoperative sagittal T2-weighted MRI (**a**) and phase-contrast flow image (**b**) show low-lying cerebellar tonsils with impeded cerebrospinal fluid flow across the foramen magnum and extensive syringohydromyelia.

Postoperative, preoperative sagittal T2-weighted MRI (**c**) and phase-contrast flow image (**d**) show a widened neo-foramen magnum with improved cerebrospinal fluid flow and decrease in the degree of syringohydromyelia

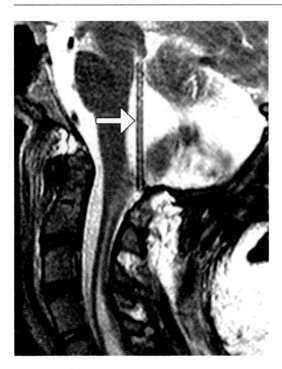

Fig. 6.55 Fourth ventricular stent. Sagittal T2-weighted MRI shows a stent (*arrows*) traversing the fourth ventricle. Chiari decompression surgery was also performed

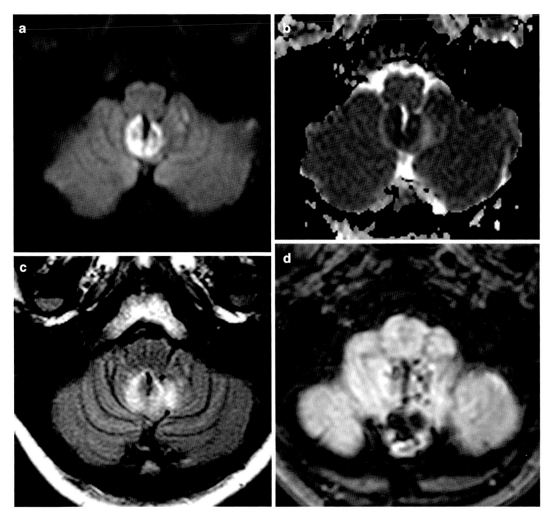

Fig. 6.56 Tonsillar reduction. Axial DWI (**a**), ADC map (**b**), FLAIR (**c**), and SWI (**d**) show areas of ischemia at the margins of the bilateral cerebellar tonsils with a few associated microhemorrhages

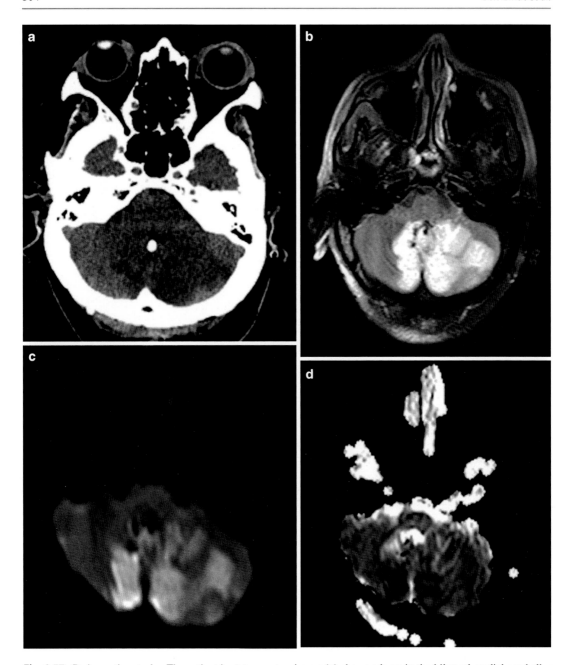

Fig. 6.57 Perioperative stroke. The patient is status post re-exploration of Chiari decompression, direct midline myelotomy for syrinx drainage, exploration/reestablishment of fourth ventricular outflow by stenting from fourth ventricle to the cervical subarachnoid space. Axial CT image (**a**) shows edema in the bilateral medial cerebellar hemispheres. Axial FLAIR (**b**), DWI (**c**), and ADC map (**d**) show corresponding acute infarction in the bilateral cerebellar hemispheres

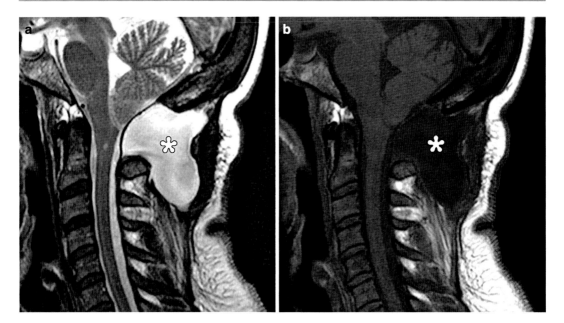

Fig. 6.58 Pseudomeningocele. Sagittal T2-weighted (**a**) and T1-weighted (**b**) MR images show a cerebrospinal fluid collection extending from the suboccipital craniectomy into the subcutaneous tissues of the posterior neck (*)

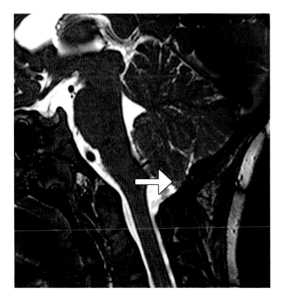

Fig. 6.59 Adhesions. Sagittal FIESTA image shows distortion of the inferior cerebellum associated with a hypointense band that extends to the overlying dura (*arrow*)

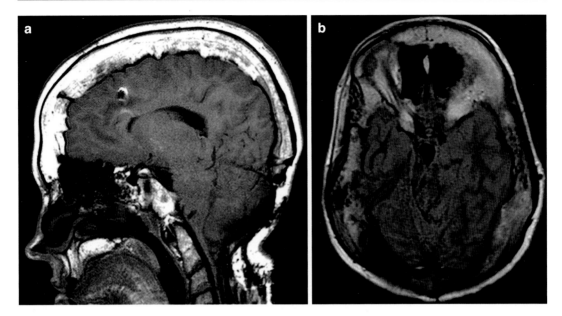

Fig. 6.60 Cerebellar slump syndrome. Sagittal T1-weighted (**a**) and axial FLAIR (**b**) MR images show distortion of the brainstem and inferior positioning and crowding of the posterior fossa contents. The calvarium is markedly thickened, presumably due to chronic shunting effects and decreased intracranial pressure

Further Reading

Types of Procedures

External Ventricular Drainage
Dasic D, Hanna SJ, Bojanic S, Kerr RS (2006) External ventricular drain infection: the effect of a strict protocol on infection rates and a review of the literature. Br J Neurosurg 20(5):296–300

Gigante P, Hwang BY, Appelboom G, Kellner CP, Kellner MA, Connolly ES (2010) External ventricular drainage following aneurysmal subarachnoid haemorrhage. Br J Neurosurg 24(6):625–632

Rappaport ZH, Shalit MN (1989) Perioperative external ventricular drainage in obstructive hydrocephalus secondary to infratentorial brain tumours. Acta Neurochir 96(3–4): 118–121

Ventriculoperitoneal Shunts
Ahn ES, Bookland M, Carson BS, Weingart JD, Jallo GI (2007) The Strata programmable valve for shunt-dependent hydrocephalus: the pediatric experience at a single institution. Childs Nerv Syst 23(3): 297–303

Bartynski WS, Valliappan S, Uselman JH, Spearman MP (2000) The adult radiographic shuntogram. AJNR Am J Neuroradiol 21(4):721–726

Desai KR, Babb JS, Amodio JB (2007) The utility of the plain radiograph "shunt series" in the evaluation of suspected ventriculoperitoneal shunt failure in pediatric patients. Pediatr Radiol 37(5):452–456

Goeser CD, McLeary MS, Young LW (1998) Diagnostic imaging of ventriculoperitoneal shunt malfunctions and complications. Radiographics 18(3):635–651

Lollis SS, Mamourian AC, Vaccaro TJ, Duhaime AC (2010) Programmable CSF shunt valves: radiographic identification and interpretation. AJNR Am J Neuroradiol 31(7):1343–1346

Maller VV, Agarwal A, Kanekar S (2016) Imaging of ventricular shunts. Semin Ultrasound CT MR 37(2): 159–173

Mangano FT, Menendez JA, Habrock T, Narayan P, Leonard JR, Park TS, Smyth MD (2005) Early programmable valve malfunctions in pediatric hydrocephalus. J Neurosurg 103(6 Suppl):501–507

Turner MS (1995) The treatment of hydrocephalus: a brief guide to shunt selection. Surg Neurol 43(4):314–319; discussion 319–323

Wallace AN, McConathy J, Menias CO, Bhalla S, Wippold FJ 2nd (2014) Imaging evaluation of CSF shunts. AJR Am J Roentgenol 202(1):38–53.

Atypical Ventricular Shunts
Girotti ME, Singh RR, Rodgers BM (2009) The ventriculo-gallbladder shunt in the treatment of refractory hydrocephalus: a review of the current literature. Am Surg 75(8):734–737

Hoffman HJ, Hendrick EB, Humphreys RP (1983) Experience with ventriculo-pleural shunts. Childs Brain 10(6):404–413

Küpeli E, Yilmaz C, Akçay S (2010) Pleural effusion following ventriculopleural shunt: case reports and review of the literature. Ann Thorac Med 5(3):166–170

Zhang J, Qu C, Wang Z, Wang C, Ding X, Pan S, Ji Y (2009) Improved ventriculoatrial shunt for cerebrospinal fluid diversion after multiple ventriculoperitoneal shunt failures. Surg Neurol 72(Suppl 1):S29–S33; discussion S33–S34

Ventriculosubgaleal Shunts

Fulmer BB, Grabb PA, Oakes WJ, Mapstone TB (2000) Neonatal ventriculosubgaleal shunts. Neurosurgery 47(1):80–83; discussion 83–84

Rizvi SA, Wood M (2010) Ventriculosubgaleal shunting for post-haemorrhagic hydrocephalus in premature neonates. Pediatr Neurosurg 46(5):335–339

Savitz MH, Malis LI (2000) Subgaleal shunting: a 20-year experience. Neurosurg Focus 9(6):ecp1

Ventriculo-Cisternal (Torkildsen) Shunts

Morota N, Ihara S, Araki T (2010) Torkildsen shunt: re-evaluation of the historical procedure. Childs Nerv Syst 26(12):1705–1710

Schulder M, Maniker AH, Lee HJ (1999) Cervical myelopathy due to migration of Torkildsen's shunt: case report. Surg Neurol 51(1):27–30

Percutaneously Accessed Cerebrospinal Fluid Reservoirs

Gnanalingham KK, Lafuente J, Harkness W (2003) Intraventricular migration of a Rickham reservoir: endoscopic retrieval. Childs Nerv Syst 19(12):831–833

Köksal V, Oktem S (2010) Ventriculosubgaleal shunt procedure and its long-term outcomes in premature infants with post-hemorrhagic hydrocephalus. Childs Nerv Syst 26(11):1505–1515

Perria C (1988) Modified Holter Rickham reservoir: a device percutaneous photodynamic treatment of cystic malignant brain tumors. J Neurosurg Sci 32(3):99–101

Subdural-Peritoneal Shunts

Santarius T, Qureshi HU, Sivakumaran R, Kirkpatrick PJ, Kirollos RW, Hutchinson PJ (2010) The role of external drains and peritoneal conduits in the treatment of recurrent chronic subdural hematoma. World Neurosurg 73(6):747–750

Sauter KL (2000) Percutaneous subdural tapping and subdural peritoneal drainage for the treatment of subdural hematoma. Neurosurg Clin N Am 11(3):519–524

Cystoperitoneal and Cystoventriculostomy Shunts

Barrett C, Prasad KS, Hill J, Johnson I, Heaton JM, Crossman JE, Mendelow AD (2010) Image-guided drainage of cystic vestibular schwannomata. Acta Neurochir 152(1):177–180

Guzel A, Trippel M, Ostertage CB (2007) Suprasellar arachnoid cyst: a 20-year follow-up after stereotactic internal drainage: case report and review of the literature. Turk Neurosurg 17(3):211–218

Helland CA, Wester K (2007) A population based study of intracranial arachnoid cysts: clinical and neuroimaging outcomes following surgical cyst decompression in adults. J Neurol Neurosurg Psychiatry 78:1129–1135

Zhang J, Zhao SY, Yuan XH (2006) Stereotactic cyst/ventricular-peritoneal shunting for the treatment of prepontine arachnoid cyst: case report. Surg Neurol 66(6):616–618; discussion 618

Syringosubarachnoid and Syringopleural Shunts

Cacciola F, Capozza M, Perrini P, Benedetto N, Di Lorenzo N (2009) Syringopleural shunt as a rescue procedure in patients with syringomyelia refractory to restoration of cerebrospinal fluid flow. Neurosurgery 65(3):471–476; discussion 476

Ergün R, Akdemir G, Gezici AR, Tezel K, Beskonakli E, Ergungor F, Taskin Y (2000) Surgical management of syringomyelia-Chiari complex. Eur Spine J 9(6):553–557

Hida K, Iwasaki Y (2001) Syringosubarachnoid shunt for syringomyelia associated with Chiari I malformation. Neurosurg Focus 11(1):E7

Lumboperitoneal Shunt

Eggenberger ER, Miller NR, Vitale S (1996) Lumboperitoneal shunt for the treatment of pseudotumor cerebri. Neurology 46(6):1524–1530

Gallmann W, Gonzalez-Toledo E, Riel-Romero R (2010) Intraventricular fat from retrograde flow through a lumboperitoneal shunt. J Neuroimaging 21(3):287–289

Uretsky S (2009) Surgical interventions for idiopathic intracranial hypertension. Curr Opin Ophthalmol 20(6):451–455

Wang VY, Barbaro NM, Lawton MT, Pitts L, Kunwar S, Parsa AT, Gupta N, McDermott MW (2007) Complications of lumboperitoneal shunts. Neurosurgery 60(6):1045–1048; discussion 1049

Third Ventriculostomy

Farin A, Aryan HE, Ozgur BM, Parsa AT, Levy ML (2006) Endoscopic third ventriculostomy. J Clin Neurosci 13(7):763–770

Foroutan M, Mafee MF, Dujovny M (1998) Third ventriculostomy, phase-contrast cine MRI and endoscopic techniques. Neurol Res 20(5):443–448

Fushimi Y, Miki Y, Takahashi JA, Kikuta K, Hashimoto N, Hanakawa T, Fukuyama H, Togashi K (2006) MR imaging of Liliequist's membrane. Radiat Med 24(2): 85–90

Jallo GI, Kothbauer KF, Abbott IR (2005) Endoscopic third ventriculostomy. Neurosurg Focus 19(6):E11

Stivaros SM, Sinclair D, Bromiley PA, Kim J, Thorne J, Jackson A (2009) Endoscopic third ventriculostomy: predicting outcome with phase-contrast MR imaging. Radiology 252(3):825–832

Endoscopic Septum Pellucidum and Cyst Fenestration

Koch CA, Moore JL, Krähling KH, Palm DG (1998) Fenestration of porencephalic cysts to the lateral ventricle: experience with a new technique for treatment of seizures. Surg Neurol 49(5):524–532; discussion 532–533

Lancon JA, Haines DE, Lewis AI, Parent AD (1999) Endoscopic treatment of symptomatic septum pellucidum cysts: with some preliminary observations on the ultrastructure of the cyst wall: two technical case reports. Neurosurgery 45(5):1251–1257

Weyerbrock A, Mainprize T, Rutka JT (2006) Endoscopic fenestration of a symptomatic cavum septum pellucidum: technical case report. Neurosurgery 59(4 Suppl 2):ONSE491; discussion ONSE491

Aqueductoplasty

Fritsch MJ, Schroeder HW (2012) Endoscopic aqueductoplasty and stenting. World Neurosurg 2013;79(2 Suppl):S20.e15–8.

Schulz M, Goelz L, Spors B, Haberl H, Thomale UW (2012) Endoscopic treatment of isolated fourth ventricle: clinical and radiological outcome. Neurosurgery (4):847–858; discussion 858–859

Sansone JM, Iskandar BJ (2005) Endoscopic cerebral aqueductoplasty: a trans-fourth ventricle approach. J Neurosurg 103(5 Suppl):388–392.

Endoscopic Choroid Plexus Cauterization

Morota N, Fujiyama Y (2004) Endoscopic coagulation of choroid plexus as treatment for hydrocephalus: indication and surgical technique. Childs Nerv Syst 20(11–12):816–820

Pople IK, Ettles D (1995) The role of endoscopic choroid plexus coagulation in the management of hydrocephalus. Neurosurgery 36(4):698–701; discussion 701–702

Fourth Ventricular Stenting

Mohanty A, Satish S, Manwaring KH (2012) 167 Isolated fourth ventricle: to shunt or stent? Neurosurgery 71(2):E566

Sacco D, Scott RM (2003) Reoperation for Chiari malformations. Pediatr Neurosurg 39(4):171–178

Complications

Corpus Callosum Changes Secondary to Shunt Catheterization

Lane JI, Luetmer PH, Atkinson JL (2001) Corpus callosal signal changes in patients with obstructive hydrocephalus after ventriculoperitoneal shunting. AJNR Am J Neuroradiol 22(1):158–162

Numaguchi Y, Kristt DA, Joy C, Robinson WL (1993) Scalloping deformity of the corpus callosum following ventricular shunting. AJNR Am J Neuroradiol 14(2):355–362

Shunt-Associated Intracranial Hemorrhage and Gliosis

Fukuhara T, Vorster SJ, Luciano MG (2000) Critical shunt-induced subdural hematoma treated with combined pressure-programmable valve implantation and endoscopic third ventriculostomy. Pediatr Neurosurg 33(1):37–42

Misaki K, Uchiyama N, Hayashi Y, Hamada J (2010) Intracerebral hemorrhage secondary to ventriculoperitoneal shunt insertion - four case reports. Neurol Med Chir (Tokyo) 50(1):76–79

Savitz MH, Bobroff LM (1999) Low incidence of delayed intracerebral hemorrhage secondary to ventriculoperitoneal shunt insertion. J Neurosurg 91(1):32–34

Sharma RR, Mahapatra A, Pawar SJ, Sousa J, Athale SD. Symptomatic calcified subdural hematomas. Pediatr Neurosurg 1999;31(3):150–154.

Petraglia AL, Moravan MJ, Jahromi BS. Armored brain: a case report and review of the literature. Surg Neurol Int 2011;2:120.

Intraventricular Fat Migration

Goeser CD, McLeary MS, Young LW (1998) Diagnostic imaging of ventriculoperitoneal shunt malfunctions and complications. Radiographics 18(3):635–651

MRI-Induced Programmable Valve Setting Alteration

Lavinio A, Harding S, Van Der Boogaard F, Czosnyka M, Smielewski P, Richards HK, Pickard JD, Czosnyka ZH (2008) Magnetic field interactions in adjustable hydrocephalus shunts. J Neurosurg Pediatr 2(3): 222–228

Lefranc M, Ko JY, Peltier J, Fichten A, Desenclos C, Macron JM, Toussaint P, Le Gars D, Petitjean M (2010) Effect of transcranial magnetic stimulation on four types of pressure-programmable valves. Acta Neurochir 152(4):689–697

Murtagh FR, Quencer RM, Poole CA (1979) Cerebrospinal fluid shunt function and hydrocephalus in the pediatric age group: a radiographic/clinical correlation. Radiology 132(2):385–388

Ventricular Loculations and Isolated Ventricles

Hubbard JL, Houser OW, Laws ER Jr (1987) Trapped fourth ventricle in an adult: radiographic findings and surgical treatment. Surg Neurol 28(4):301–306

Maurice-Williams RS, Choksey M (1986) Entrapment of the temporal horn: a form of focal obstructive hydrocephalus. J Neurol Neurosurg Psychiatry 49(3): 238–242

Oi S, Abbott R (2004) Loculated ventricles and isolated compartments in hydrocephalus: their pathophysiology and the efficacy of neuroendoscopic surgery. Neurosurg Clin N Am 15(1):77–87

Slit Ventricle Syndrome

Goeser CD, McLeary MS, Young LW (1998) Diagnostic imaging of ventriculoperitoneal shunt malfunctions and complications. Radiographics 8(3):635–651

Rekate HL (2008) Shunt-related headaches: the slit ventricle syndromes. Childs Nerv Syst 24(4):423–430

Chronic Overshunting and Associated Findings

Di Preta JA, Powers JM, Hicks DG (1994) Hyperostosis cranii ex vacuo: a rare complication of shunting for hydrocephalus. Hum Pathol 25(5):545–547

Hochman MS, Naidich TP (1999) Diffuse meningeal enhancement in patients with overdraining, longstanding ventricular shunts. Neurology 52(2): 406–409

Lucey BP, March GP Jr, Hutchins GM (2003) Marked calvarial thickening and dural changes following chronic ventricular shunting for shaken baby syndrome. Arch Pathol Lab Med 127(1):94–97

Seyithanoglu H, Guzey FK, Emel E, Ozkan N, Aycan A (2010) Chronic ossified epidural hematoma after ventriculoperitoneal shunt insertion: a case report. Turk Neurosurg 20(4):519–523

Vinchon M, Dhellemmes P, Laureau E, Soto-Ares G (2007) Progressive myelopathy due to meningeal thickening in shunted patients: description of a novel entity and the role of surgery. Childs Nerv Syst 23(8):839–845

Weinzweig J, Bartlett SP, Chen JC, Losee J, Sutton L, Duhaime AC, Whitaker LA. Cranial vault expansion in the management of postshunt craniosynostosis and slit ventricle syndrome. Plast Reconstr Surg 2008;122(4):1171–1180.

Shunt-Associated Infections

Goeser CD, McLeary MS, Young LW (1998) Diagnostic imaging of ventriculoperitoneal shunt malfunctions and complications. Radiographics 18(3):635–651

Puca A, Anile C, Maira G, Rossi G (1991) Cerebrospinal fluid shunting for hydrocephalus in the adult: factors related to shunt revision. Neurosurgery 29(6):822–826

Shunt Malposition and Migration

Alakandy LM, Iyer RV, Golash A (2008) Hemichorea, an unusual complication of ventriculoperitoneal shunt. J Clin Neurosci 15(5):599–601

Ghritlaharey RK, Budhwani KS, Shrivastava DK, Gupta G, Kushwaha AS, Chanchlani R, Nanda M (2007) Trans-anal protrusion of ventriculo-peritoneal shunt catheter with silent bowel perforation: report of ten cases in children. Pediatr Surg Int 23(6):575–580

Sathyanarayana S, Wylen EL, Baskaya MK, Nanda A (2000) Spontaneous bowel perforation after ventriculoperitoneal shunt surgery: case report and a review of 45 cases. Surg Neurol 54(5):388–396

Wan KR, Toy JA, Wolfe R, Danks A (2011) Factors affecting the accuracy of ventricular catheter placement. J Clin Neurosci 18(4):485–488

Shunt Catheter Disconnection and Retained Fragments

Boch AL, Hermelin E, Sainte-Rose C, Sgouros S (1998) Mechanical dysfunction of ventriculoperitoneal shunts caused by calcification of the silicone rubber catheter. J Neurosurg 88(6):975–982

Goeser CD, McLeary MS, Young LW (1998) Diagnostic imaging of ventriculoperitoneal shunt malfunctions and complications. Radiographics 18(3):635–651

Intraparenchymal Pericatheter Cysts and Interstitial Cerebrospinal Fluid

Iqbal J, Hassounah M, Sheikh B (2000) Intraparenchymal pericatheter cyst. A rare complication of ventriculoperitoneal shunt for hydrocephalus. Br J Neurosurg 14(3):255–258

Sinha AK, Lall R, Benson R, O'Brien DF, Buxton N (2008) Intraparenchymal pericatheter cyst following ventriculoperitoneal shunt insertion: does it always merit shunt revision? Zentralbl Neurochir 69(3): 152–154; discussion 154

Pseudocysts

Chung JJ, Yu JS, Kim JH, Nam SJ, Kim MJ (2009) Intraabdominal complications secondary to ventriculoperitoneal shunts: CT findings and review of the literature. AJR Am J Roentgenol 193(5):1311–1317

Goeser CD, McLeary MS, Young LW (1998) Diagnostic imaging of ventriculoperitoneal shunt malfunctions and complications. Radiographics 18(3):635–651

Kariyattil R, Steinbok P, Singhal A, Cochrane DD (2007) Ascites and abdominal pseudocysts following ventriculoperitoneal shunt surgery: variations of the same theme. J Neurosurg 106(5 Suppl):350–353

Mobley LW 3rd, Doran SE, Hellbusch LC (2005) Abdominal pseudocyst: predisposing factors and treatment algorithm. Pediatr Neurosurg 41(2):77–83

Cerebrospinal Fluid Leak Syndrome

Liao YJ, Dillon WP, Chin CT, McDermott MW, Horton JC (2007) Intracranial hypotension caused by leakage of cerebrospinal fluid from the thecal sac after lumboperitoneal shunt placement. Case report. J Neurosurg 107(1): 173–177

Tumor Seeding

Murray MJ, Metayer LE, Mallucci CL, Hale JP, Nicholson JC, Kirollos RW, Burke GA (2011) Intra-abdominal metastasis of an intracranial germinoma via ventriculoperitoneal shunt in a 13-year-old female. Br J Neurosurg 25(6):747–749

Nawashiro H, Otani N, Katoh H, Ohnuki A, Ogata S, Shima K (2002) Subcutaneous seeding of pancreatic carcinoma along a VP shunt catheter. Lancet Oncol 3(11):683

Newton HB, Rosenblum MK, Walker RW (1992) Extraneural metastases of infratentorial glioblastoma multiforme to the peritoneal cavity. Cancer 69(8): 2149–2153

Shunt Catheter Calcifications

Shimotake K, Kondo A, Aoyama I, Nin K, Tashiro Y, Nishioka T (1988) Calcification of a ventriculoperitoneal shunt tube. Case report. Surg Neurol 30(2):156–158

Pulmonary Embolism from Ventriculoatrial Shunting

Soppi E, Järventie G, Siitonen L. Multiple pulmonary embolism in patients with ventriculoatrial shunts: a report on two cases. J Intern Med 1989;225(6): 423–425.

Yavuzgil O, Ozerkan F, Ertürk U, Işlekel S, Atay Y, Buket S. A rare cause of right atrial mass: thrombus formation and infection complicating a ventriculoatrial shunt for hydrocephalus. Surg Neurol 1999;52(1):54–60; discussion 60–61.

Chiari Decompression Surgery and Associated Complications

Kumar R, Kalra SK, Vaid VK, Mahapatra AK (2008) Chiari I malformation: surgical experience over a decade of management. Br J Neurosurg 22(3): 409–414

Mazzola CA, Fried AH (2003) Revision surgery for Chiari malformation decompression. Neurosurg Focus 15(3):E3

McGirt MJ, Nimjee SM, Fuchs HE, George TM (2006) Relationship of cine phase-contrast magnetic resonance imaging with outcome after decompression for Chiari I malformations. Neurosurgery 59(1):140–146; discussion 140–146

Munshi I, Frim D, Stine-Reyes R, Weir BK, Hekmatpanah J, Brown F (2000) Effects of posterior fossa decompression with and without duraplasty on Chiari malformation-associated hydromyelia. Neurosurgery 46(6):1384–1389; discussion 1389–1389

Paré LS, Batzdorf U (1998) Syringomyelia persistence after Chiari decompression as a result of pseudomeningocele formation: implications for syrinx pathogenesis: report of three cases. Neurosurgery 43(4): 945–948

Parker SR, Harris P, Cummings TJ, George T, Fuchs H, Grant G (2011) Complications following decompression of Chiari malformation Type I in children: dural graft or sealant? J Neurosurg Pediatr 8(2):177–183

Rozenfeld M, Frim DM, Katzman GL, Ginat DT (2015) MRI findings after surgery for Chiari malformation type I. AJR Am J Roentgenol 205(5):1086–1093.

Wicklund MR, Mokri B, Drubach DA, Boeve BF, Parisi JE, Josephs KA (2011) Frontotemporal brain sagging syndrome: an SIH-like presentation mimicking FTD. Neurology 76(16): 1377–1382

Imaging of the Postoperative Skull Base and Cerebellopontine Angle

7

Daniel Thomas Ginat, Peleg M. Horowitz, Gul Moonis, and Suresh K. Mukherji

7.1 Anterior Craniofacial Resection

7.1.1 Discussion

Anterior cranial (craniofacial) resection is the treatment of choice for aggressive tumors, such as sinonasal undifferentiated carcinoma (SNUC) and esthesioneuroblastoma, that are adjacent to or extend into the anterior cranial fossa. This approach is also sometimes used for resection of suprasellar tumors. The procedure consists of extensive removal of the anterior skull base and nasal cavity and paranasal sinus structures along with tumor resection. This may require both transnasal and anterior skull base (i.e., transbasal, cranio-orbital) approaches. The dura is repaired using dural patch grafts, which may consist of pericranial or fascial autograft, acellular cadaveric dermal allograft, xenograft (bovine pericardium), or synthetic collagen-based matrix. The defect in the floor of the anterior cranial fossa can be closed with vascularized pericranial or nasoseptal rotational flaps, titanium mesh, bone graft, synthetic implant, or a combination of these (Figs. 7.1, 7.2, 7.3, and 7.4). In cases of large defects, free flap reconstruction may be used. Vascularized pericranial flaps, which are created by stripping away the periosteum from the outer table of the calvarium, typically demonstrate enhancement on MRI.

During anterior cranial resection, the frontal lobes may be retracted to some degree, which predisposes to local ischemia at the site of retractor placement. Aggressive retraction, which might be implemented for removal of large tumors, can avulse the lenticulostriate vessels, leading to basal ganglia infarcts (Fig. 7.5).

Infection acquired after anterior cranial resection is predisposed by concurrent partial anterior frontal lobectomy, prior craniotomy, persistent cerebrospinal fluid fistula, and high doses of radiation therapy. Alloplastic materials used for reconstruction and devitalized tissues are also risk factors for postoperative infection, potentially serving as niduses for microorganisms. Wound infections tend to occur along the lateral forehead where the skin incisions are made (Fig. 7.6), while intracranial infections are often

D.T. Ginat, M.D., M.S. (✉)
Department of Radiology,
University of Chicago, Chicago, IL, USA
e-mail: dtg1@uchicago.eduG

P.M. Horowitz, M.D., Ph.D.
Department of Surgery,
University of Chicago, Chicago, IL, USA

G. Moonis, M.D.
Department of Radiology, Columbia Presbyterian,
New York, NY, USA

S.K. Mukherji, M.D., M.B.A., F.A.C.R.
Department of Radiology, Michigan State University,
East Lansing, MI, USA

© Springer International Publishing Switzerland 2017
D.T. Ginat, P.-L.A. Westesson (eds.), *Atlas of Postsurgical Neuroradiology*,
DOI 10.1007/978-3-319-52341-5_7

in the midline, due to the proximity to the sinonasal passages and potential fistula formation (Fig. 7.7).

Follow-up imaging is important for monitoring tumor recurrence. MRI is the study of choice for postoperative surveillance (Fig. 7.8). Following craniofacial resection, MRI often demonstrates enhancing soft tissue related to granulation tissue formation at the resection site in the superior nasal cavity that is difficult to differentiate from residual or recurrent tumors, such as esthesioneuroblastoma. FDG-PET/CT can also be useful for evaluating for the presence of posttreatment tumor, although infection and inflammation of the resection bed can be hypermetabolic, similar to recurrent tumor.

Radiation therapy is often administered for malignant tumors treated via anterior craniofacial resection. This can result in radiation necrosis, which has a characteristic pattern of white matter signal abnormality and ring-enhancing lesions in the distribution of radiation field and mainly occurs 6 months to 1 year after treatment (Fig. 7.9).

Another important complication of anterior cranial fossa resection is encephalocele, particularly if only a pericranial flap was used to repair the skull base defect. On CT, a postoperative encephalocele appears as nonspecific soft tissue attenuation with variable amounts of surrounding cerebrospinal fluid attenuation. Thus, MRI is useful for making the diagnosis since the continuity of the lesion with the intracranial brain parenchyma can be readily established and differentiated from tumor recurrence or sinus mucosal disease (Fig. 7.11).

Since anterior cranial fossa resection typically involves access through the paranasal sinuses in addition to craniotomies, there is the risk of transgressing the lamina papyracea and orbital entry. This may injure the rectus muscles and other orbital contents (Fig. 7.11). Other complications associated with FESS can also occur with anterior cranial fossa resection. As the normal air flow through the nasal sinuses is frequently disrupted, mucocele formation and chronic inflammatory changes in the paranasal sinuses are common.

Fig. 7.1 Illustration of the anterior cranial fossa approach with skull base reconstruction using pericranial flap and dural patch, titanium mesh, and bone graft

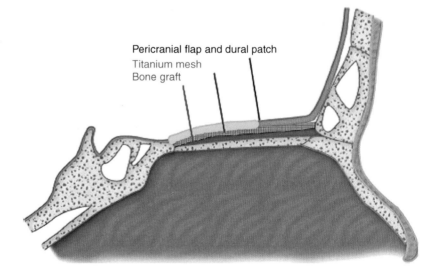

Pericranial flap and dural patch
Titanium mesh
Bone graft

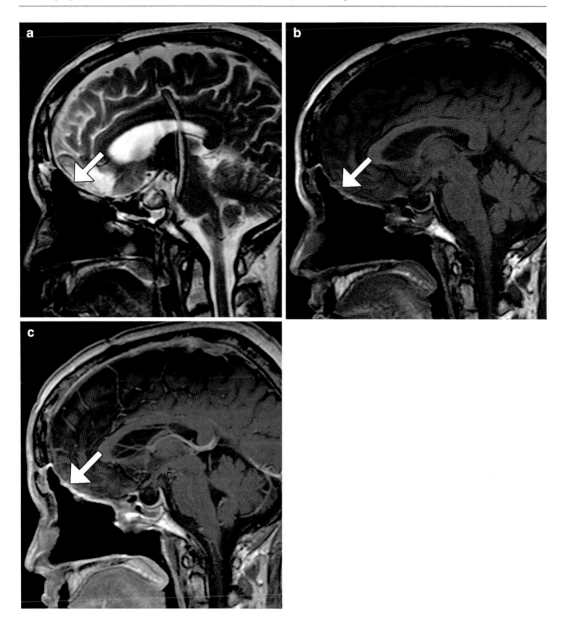

Fig. 7.2 Anterior cranial resection with vascularized pericranial flap. Sagittal T2-weighted (**a**), T1-weighted (**b**), and post-contrast T1-weighted (**c**) MR images show pericranial flap reconstruction of the anterior cranial fossa (*arrows*). The flap appears as a thin sheet that enhances

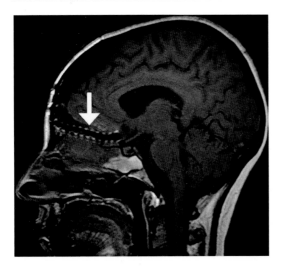

Fig. 7.3 Anterior cranial resection with mesh reconstruction. Sagittal (**b**) T1-weighted MRI shows the low-signal-intensity mesh positioned along the floor of the anterior cranial fossa (*arrow*)

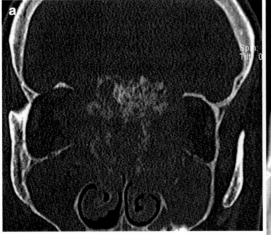

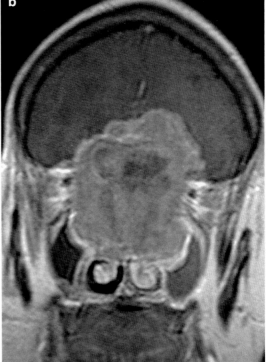

Fig. 7.4 Anterior cranial resection with bone graft reconstruction. The patient has a history of a large sinonasal undifferentiated carcinoma (SNUC) involving the anterior skull base treated via anterior craniofacial resection. Preoperative coronal CT image (**a**) and coronal post-contrast T1-weighted (**b**) MRI show the heterogeneously enhancing paranasal sinus mass extending through the cribriform plate and into the anterior skull base. Postoperative coronal (**c**) CT image shows extensive para-nasal sinus and skull base resections. There are no residual ethmoid cells. A split calvarial bone graft harvested from the frontal bone was used to close the skull base defect. Postoperative coronal post-contrast T1-weighted (**d**) MRI also shows the extensive anterior craniofacial resection. The low-signal-intensity anterior skull base bone graft lies superior to the pericranial flap. There is mucosal thickening, but no evidence of residual or recurrent tumor

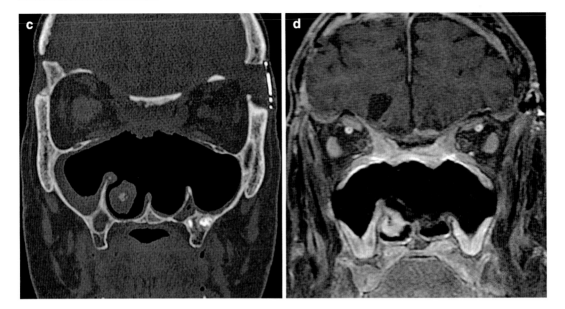

Fig. 7.4 (continued)

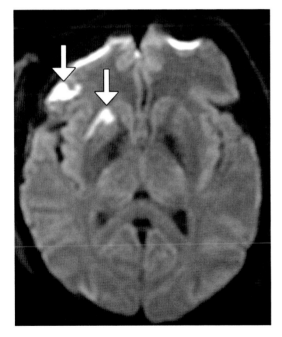

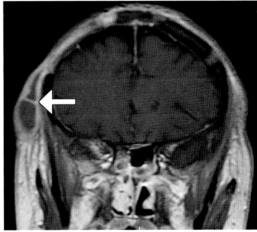

Fig. 7.6 Scalp abscess. Coronal post-contrast T1-weighted MRI shows a loculated, rim-enhancing collection in the right scalp adjacent to an osteotomy site (*arrow*)

Fig. 7.5 Cerebral infarction. Axial diffusion-weighted image obtained after recent anterior cranial resection shows restricted diffusion in the right putamen and opercular region of the right frontal lobe, likely secondary to retraction (*arrows*)

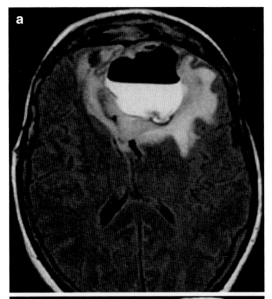

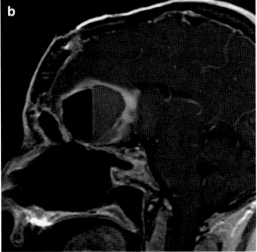

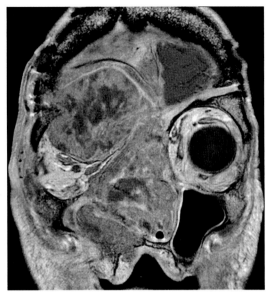

Fig. 7.8 Squamous cell carcinoma recurrence after anterior cranial fossa resection. Coronal post-contrast T1-weighted MRI shows a large heterogeneously enhancing craniofacial mass that extends across the craniotomy into the intracranial compartment and right orbit

Fig. 7.7 Intraparenchymal abscess with fistula. The patient presented with fever after esthesioneuroblastoma resection. Axial T2 FLAIR (**a**) and sagittal (**b**) post-contrast T1-weighted MR images show a large left anterior frontal lobe rim-enhancing cavity containing an air-fluid level. There is extensive signal abnormality surrounding the abscess, which represents cerebritis

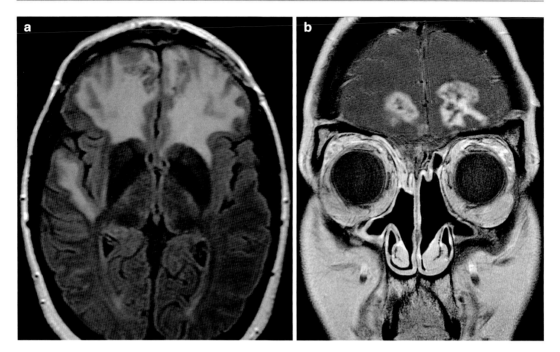

Fig. 7.9 Radiation necrosis. Axial T2 FLAIR (**a**) and coronal (**b**) contrast-enhanced T1-weighted MR images show extensive bifrontal edema and heterogeneous peripherally enhancing lesions, which are in the distribution of the radiation field after anterior cranial resection

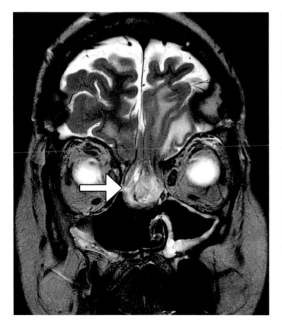

Fig. 7.10 Encephalocele after anterior cranial resection. Coronal T2-weighted MRI demonstrates a large encephalocele (*arrow*) through the anterior cranial fossa defect

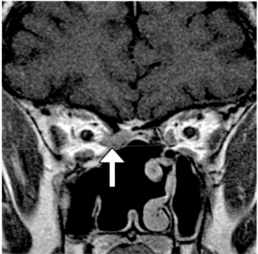

Fig. 7.11 Rectus muscle injury. The patient presented with right restrictive esotropia following anterior cranial resection and radiation treatment of a squamous cell carcinoma. Coronal post-contrast T1-weighted MR image shows enhancing, amorphous soft tissue material in the right posterior ethmoid air cells that represents scar, which retracts the medial rectus muscle (*arrow*) through a defect in the lamina papyracea

7.2   Decompression of Cystic Craniopharyngiomas

7.2.1   Discussion

Resection of craniopharyngiomas often poses a surgical dilemma since gross total resection is difficult to achieve with large tumors without injury to surrounding structures. Consequently, residual tumor often remains despite additional radiation and chemotherapy. Nevertheless, the main gain of surgery is to the associated reduce mass effect. Subtotal decompression can be accomplished via transsphenoidal or transcranial cyst fenestration, with or without permanent catheter implantation (Figs. 7.12 and 7.13), and can be a suitable alternative to resection for providing patients with symptomatic relief, such as visual recovery. While CT is adequate for confirming the positioning of catheters, multiplanar and multisequence MRI is better suited for delineating the cystic versus solid components, which can evolve considerably following treatment and have complex features on follow-up exams. Ultimately, the goal of follow-up imaging is to determine if growth has occurred with associated complications, such as hydrocephalus, and if there is a dominant cystic component that could be targeted in a minimally invasive manner (Fig. 7.14). Postoperative abscess can potentially mimic cyst progression on MRI, but the clinical presentation and presence of new restricted diffusion may help suggest infection (Fig. 7.15).

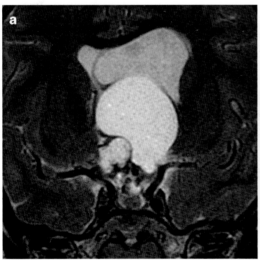
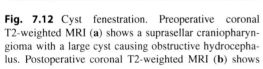
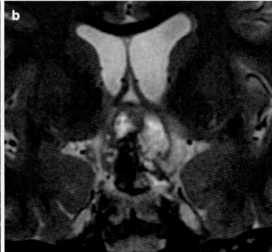

Fig. 7.12 Cyst fenestration. Preoperative coronal T2-weighted MRI (**a**) shows a suprasellar craniopharyngioma with a large cyst causing obstructive hydrocephalus. Postoperative coronal T2-weighted MRI (**b**) shows marked interval decompression of the cystic component. Although residual tumor is apparent, there is decreased mass effect

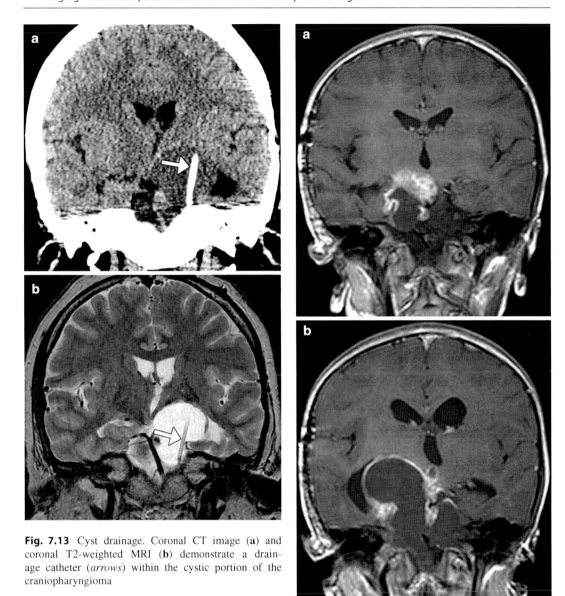

Fig. 7.13 Cyst drainage. Coronal CT image (**a**) and coronal T2-weighted MRI (**b**) demonstrate a drainage catheter (*arrows*) within the cystic portion of the craniopharyngioma

Fig. 7.14 Postoperative cyst growth. The patient underwent prior transcranial craniopharyngioma debulking, with residual enhancing and cystic suprasellar components (**a**). While the solid component decreased in size after radiation therapy, the cystic component increased in size and caused obstructive hydrocephalus (**b**), as shown on the coronal post-contrast T1-weighted MR images

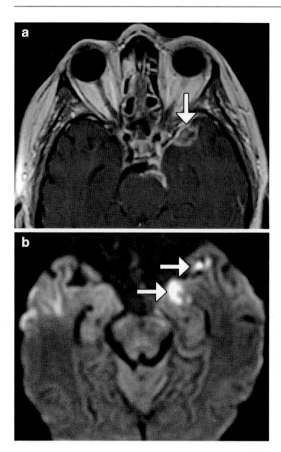

Fig. 7.15 Postoperative infection. Initial coronal
contrast-enhanced T1-weighted MRI (**a**) obtained after
anterior craniopharyngioma cyst fenestration shows a
residual solid enhancing nodular component of the craniopharyngioma (*arrow*). Axial post-contrast T1-weighted
MRI (**a**) and DWI (**b**) obtained after craniopharyngioma
cyst decompression show leptomeningeal enhancement
and a rim-enhancing fluid collection with restricted diffusion from abscess formation (*arrows*)

7.3 Transsphenoidal Tumor Resection

7.3.1 Discussion

The transsphenoidal approach is widely used for resecting pituitary tumors (hypophysectomy) and other sellar and parasellar lesions. Transsphenoidal surgery consists of accessing the sella via the nasal cavity and paranasal sinuses and typically involves some degree of resecting the posterior bony septum back to the sphenoid face and performing sphenoidotomy (Fig. 7.16). The process of drilling through bone during the transsphenoidal approach can leave behind metallic debris that has detached from the surgical instruments. These metal particles can be deposited anywhere along the path of the access route, such as in the nasal cavity and sphenoid sinus. Although it is usually too minute to be apparent on radiographs, the metal debris can cause noticeable artifact on MRI (Fig. 7.17).

Giant adenomas or other large lesions of the pituitary region are sometimes not amenable to resection via transsphenoidal approach alone. Such tumors require craniotomy and/or a combined approach that includes transsphenoidal and transcranial routes (Fig. 7.18). Less invasive endoscopic transsphenoidal-transventricular combined approaches can also be performed in selected cases.

Fat graft is commonly used to pack skull base defects after transsphenoidal resection of pituitary region tumors. The packing serves to prevent cerebrospinal fluid leakage, hemorrhage, and prolapse of intracranial contents into larger defects. Fat grafts are hyperintense on both T1- and T2-weighted sequences and decrease in size over time, such that in most cases, the fat grafts resorb completely after 1 year following surgery (Fig. 7.19).

Other materials used to seal and fill the sella include gelatin sponge (Fig. 7.20), muco-

sal pedicle flaps (Fig. 7.21), and titanium mesh (Fig. 7.22), each of which has particular imaging features. Then move it right after the sentence: Fat grafts are hyperintense on both T1- and T2-weighted sequences and decrease in size over time, such that in most cases, the fat grafts resorb completely after 1 year following surgery (Fig. 7.19). Bone remodeling is a chronic process that sometimes occurs after transsphenoidal resection. This phenomenon manifests as thickening, ossification, and high T1 signal intensity, most commonly along the planum sphenoidale (Figs 7.16 and 7.19).

Nasal stents and sinonasal fluid related to bloody mucus drainage can be encountered on early postoperative imaging (Fig. 7.23).

The early postoperative imaging appearance of the pituitary after transsphenoidal resection is variable, ranging from no enhancement to nodular enhancement to peripheral rim enhancement. There can also be postoeprative reexpansion of the normal pituitary gland, thickening of the pituitary stalk, and swelling of the optic apparatus. In addition, there may be a postoperative mass caused by residual tumor, edema, hemorrhage, implant material, granulation tissue, or a combination of these. In particular, granulation tissue can be difficult to differentiate from residual tumor on imaging initially. However, on follow-up, granulation tissue typically involutes, while residual tumor is expected to persist or grow (Fig. 7.24). In particular, early postoperative dynamic MRI after transsphenoidal pituitary adenoma resection can be useful for differentiating residual tumor from postoperative surgical changes. Residual tumor from subtotal resection of pituitary macroadenomas is usually distributed lateral to the sella, where it is difficult to attain and left behind in order to minimize complications (Fig. 7.25). Indeed, the primary goal of the surgery is not necessarily to remove the entire tumor, but to alleviate the mass effect upon the optic chiasm.

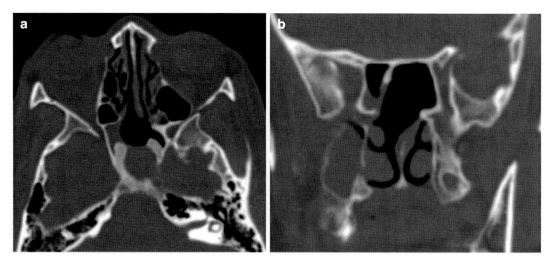

Fig. 7.16 Transsphenoidal approach. Axial (**a**) and coronal (**b**) CT images show posterior nasal septostomy and sphenoidotomy. There is also a surgical defect in the anterior wall of the expanded sella, which otherwise has thickened walls

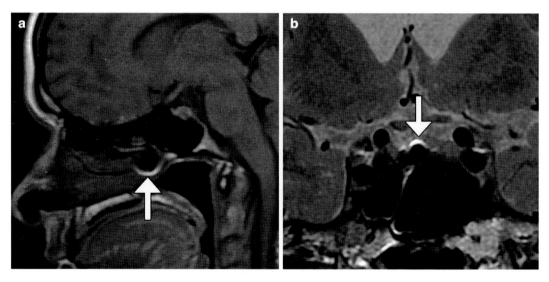

Fig. 7.17 Residual metal debris after transsphenoidal surgery. Sagittal T1-weighted MRI (**a**) shows metallic artifact in the posterior nasal cavity (*arrow*). Coronal T2-weighted MRI in a different patient (**b**) shows metal susceptibility artifact along the floor of the sella (*arrow*)

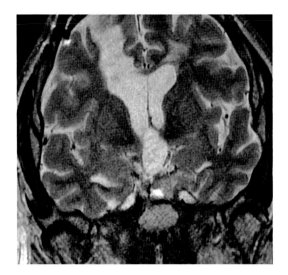

Fig. 7.18 Combined transventricular-transsphenoidal resection. Coronal T2-weighted MRI shows a linear passage through the right frontal lobe toward the sellar region, where there is residual tumor

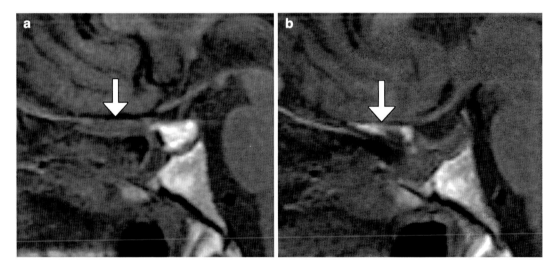

Fig. 7.19 Fat graft shrinkage and bone remodeling. Initial postoperative sagittal T1-weighted MRI (**a**) shows the T1 hyperintense fat graft within the sella and normal intermediate signal intensity of the planum sphenoidale (*arrow*). Postoperative sagittal T1-weighted MRI (**b**) obtained 2 years after surgery shows interval fat graft shrinkage and development of high signal intensity in the planum sphenoidale (*arrow*)

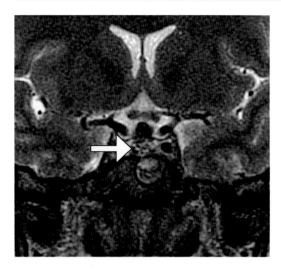

Fig. 7.20 Merocel packing. Coronal T2-weighted MRI shows the packing in the sella and sphenoid sinus, which appears as a heterogeneous blob (*arrow*)

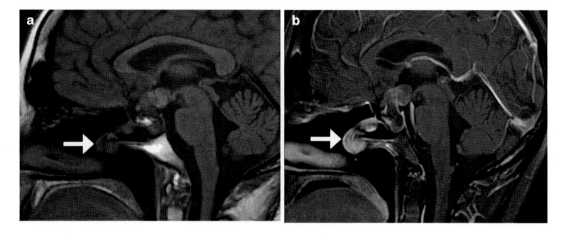

Fig. 7.21 Pedicled mucosal flap. Sagittal pre-contrast T1-weighted (**a**) and post-contrast sagittal T1-weighted (**b**) MR images show an enhancing pedicled mucosal flap (*arrows*) transposed into the sphenoid sinus

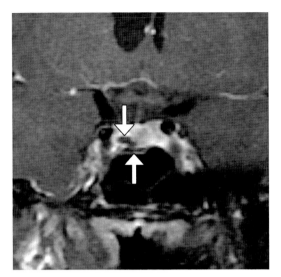

Fig. 7.22 Titanium mesh sellar reconstruction. Coronal T1-weighted MRI shows sheets of titanium mesh (*arrows*) along the floor of the sella

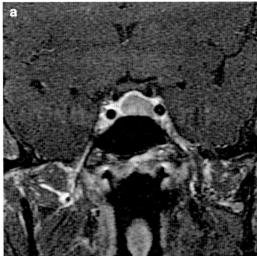

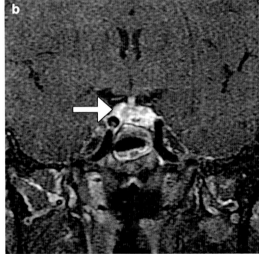

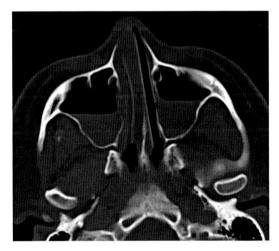

Fig. 7.23 Expected early posteroperative sinonasal findings after transsphenoidal surgery. Axial CT image shows fluid in the bilateral maxillary sinus and bialteral nasal stens

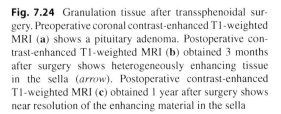

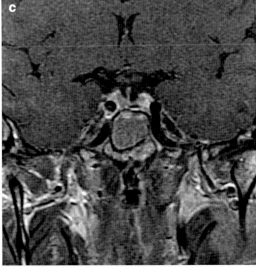

Fig. 7.24 Granulation tissue after transsphenoidal surgery. Preoperative coronal contrast-enhanced T1-weighted MRI (**a**) shows a pituitary adenoma. Postoperative contrast-enhanced T1-weighted MRI (**b**) obtained 3 months after surgery shows heterogeneously enhancing tissue in the sella (*arrow*). Postoperative contrast-enhanced T1-weighted MRI (**c**) obtained 1 year after surgery shows near resolution of the enhancing material in the sella

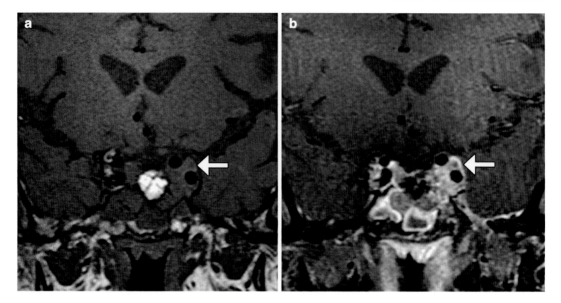

Fig. 7.25 Subtotal pituitary macroadenoma resection. Coronal T1-weighted (**a**) and post-contrast fat-suppressed T1-weighted (**b**) MR images show enhancing residual tumor extending into the left cavernous sinus (*arrow*), without mass effect upon the optic apparatus. There is fat packing in the sella, which drops in signal with fat suppression in contradistinction to the residual tumor, which enhances

7.4 Transsphenoidal Resection Complications

7.4.1 Discussion

Sellar hematomas are not uncommon after transsphenoidal resection. When large, these can cause mass effect upon surrounding structures and produce symptoms. Subacute hematomas in the sella can display high signal on T1- and T2-weighted MRI sequences and should not be mistaken for fat graft or residual tumor (Fig. 7.26). Gradient echo (GRE) or susceptibility-weighted imaging (SWI) techniques can sometimes be useful for identifying blood products on MRI, although susceptibility effects from air in the adjacent sphenoid sinus can limit assessment.

Arterial injury during transsphenoidal resection is uncommon, but can manifest as pseudoaneurysm and/or subarachnoid hemorrhage, which can lead to vasospasm. Most arterial complications related to transsphenoidal surgery involve the internal carotid artery, but the ophthalmic, posterior communicating, and anterior cerebral arteries may also be affected. Arterial injury may occur during dural opening, tumor resection, or reconstruction of the sinuses and may be predisposed by anatomic variants of the sinuses and internal carotid arteries and large tumors that involve the cavernous sinus. Therefore, meticulous preoperative planning with imaging is important for minimizing arterial injury.

Once arterial injury is suspected during transsphenoidal resection, angiography is essential for identifying the presence of pseudoaneurysms. The speculum and packing material may be kept within the sphenoid sinus in order to prevent exsanguination, and excess packing may result in arterial stenosis or occlusion. Endovascular control of bleeding may be achieved by either balloon occlusion or coil embolization of the affected internal carotid artery, coil embolization of the pseudoaneurysm, or stenting alone of the affected segment of the internal carotid artery (Fig. 7.27). Peritumoral hemorrhage can lead to delayed cerebral vasospasm and associated progressive worsening neurological deficits.

Malposition or migration of packing material for transsphenoidal resection is uncommon. The displaced packing material can exert mass effect upon the optic chiasm, resulting in visual symptoms that may differ from the preoperative deficits (Fig. 7.28). Alternatively, the packing material can extend posteriorly and compress the brainstem (Fig. 7.29). Such complications can be readily demonstrated on multiplanar CT or MRI. However, in some cases, displacement of packing material can potentially mimic tumor invasion.

Mucosal inflammation is fairly common after transsphenoidal resection and most commonly involves the sphenoid sinuses (Fig. 7.30). On the other hand, mucocele formation after transsphenoidal resection is a rare or perhaps under-reported complication. Scar tissue can obstruct the egress of mucous secretions, resulting in their accumulation. On MRI, mucoceles are often homogeneously iso- to hyperintense on T1- and T2-weighted sequences and display peripheral enhancement. These may sometimes be multilocular. The main differential consideration is a postoperative hematoma, although these can be distinguished by their time course. Hematomas tend to resorb over time, while mucoceles persist or even expand. Susceptibility-weighted imaging can also be helpful, whereby hematomas are hypointense, while mucoceles do not. Postoperative mucoceles can cause symptoms, such as headache and diplopia, but they can be successfully treated via incision and drainage.

Although prophylactic antibiotics are routinely given before transsphenoidal surgery, the incidence of postoperative meningitis is in the range of 0.4–9%. This complication can manifest as leptomeningeal enhancement in the basilar cistern region on MRI (Fig. 7.31). The presence of postoperative cerebrospinal fluid leakage is an important risk factor for meningitis after transsphenoidal surgery.

Cerebrospinal fluid leak is a known complication of transsphenoidal resections. This is a serious complication that can predispose to meningitis and intracranial hypotension. The beta-2-transferrin assay is an accurate test for confirming the presence of cerebrospinal fluid leaks. Imaging also plays an important role in the workup of cerebrospinal fluid leak: it is used to confirm the diagnosis, localize the site of cerebrospinal fluid leak, identify a potential cause, and help plan surgical repair. Several imaging modalities are available to evaluate cerebrospinal fluid leak, including high-resolution CT, CT cisternography, MRI, and radionuclide cisternography (Fig. 7.32). However, high-resolution CT is the first-line imaging modality and can correctly predict the site of cerebrospinal fluid leak in over 90% of cases. When beta-2 transferrin is positive and high-resolution CT demonstrates a single bony defect without any sign of encephalocele, no other imaging is necessary. CT cisternography is reserved for patients with a negative high-resolution CT or multiple bony defects and active cerebrospinal fluid leakage. The sensitivity of CT cisternography is only about 50% in patients with intermittent cerebrospinal fluid leak. MR cisternography should be performed if high-resolution CT shows a bony defect with an associated soft tissue opacity in order to exclude the possibility of meningocele or encephalocele. Contrast-enhanced sequences are useful for detecting dural enhancement at the site of the leak. Nuclear cisternography using In-111 is sometimes performed for complex cases and to help determine whether there is indeed a cerebrospinal fluid leak.

A variety of endocrinological disturbances can occur after transsphenoidal resection. In the acute postoperative setting, a minority of patients experience diabetes insipidus. This is associated with absence of the posterior pituitary bright spot on imaging. On the other hand, hyponatremia related to transsphenoidal surgery tends to have a delayed onset. Panhypopituitarism can result from transection of the hypophysis. This can best be evaluated using high-resolution MRI sequences, such as CISS and thin-section

T1-weighted images (Fig. 7.33). In addition, an ectopic posterior pituitary bright spot can be observed in this condition.

Ptosis of the optic chiasm is not an uncommon finding following pituitary tumor resection. This phenomenon tends to occur when a large portion of the pituitary sella contents have been evacuated resulting in a nearly or completely empty sella (Fig. 7.34). Ptosis is recognized by a convex-down configuration of the optic chiasm on a coronal or sagittal plane. When severe, this condition has the potential to cause visual deficits. The problematic empty sella with optic chiasm ptosis can be treated via chiasmopexy. This procedure consists of supporting the optic chiasm in near-anatomic position via transsphenoidal Silastic struts and coils, among other materials (Fig. 7.35). Acute visual loss related to transsphenoidal surgery can result from infarction of the optic apparatus if the blood supply is disrupted during tumor resection. This can be assessed on coronal T2-weighted MRI, which may show new signal abnormality in the optic apparatus (Fig. 7.36).

Fibrosis following transsphenoidal pituitary surgery is not an uncommon finding on postoperative MRI. Fibrosis can manifest as linear or amorphous areas within the sella. The imaging appearance is often indistinguishable from implant materials or residual tumor. Occasionally, adhesion bands form that extend across the sella or diaphragm to the brain or residual tumor. Adhesions appear as linear structures with low to intermediate signal intensity on T1-weighted and T2-weighted MRI sequences and enhance less and/or slower than the pituitary stalk (Fig. 7.37). These adhesions can hamper subsequent surgical resection of residual tumor. Fibrosis may also prevent normal pituitary gland re-expansion and cause stalk deviation.

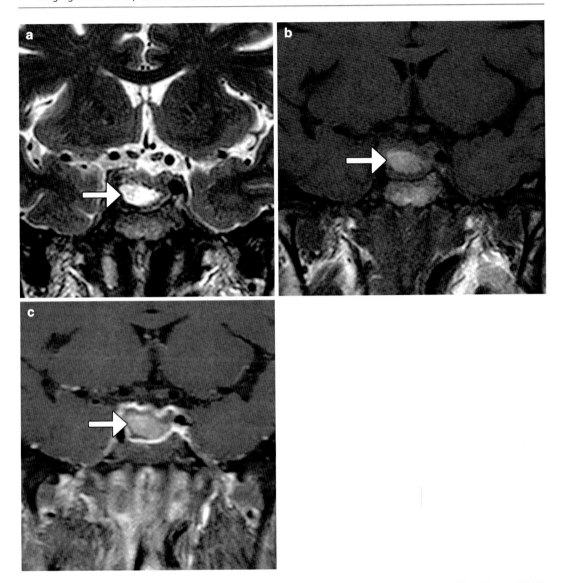

Fig. 7.26   Postoperative hematoma. Coronal T2-weighted (**a**), T1-weighted (**b**), and post-contrast T1-weighted (**c**) MR images show the intrinsically hyperintense fluid collection in the sella (*arrows*) after recent transsphenoidal surgery

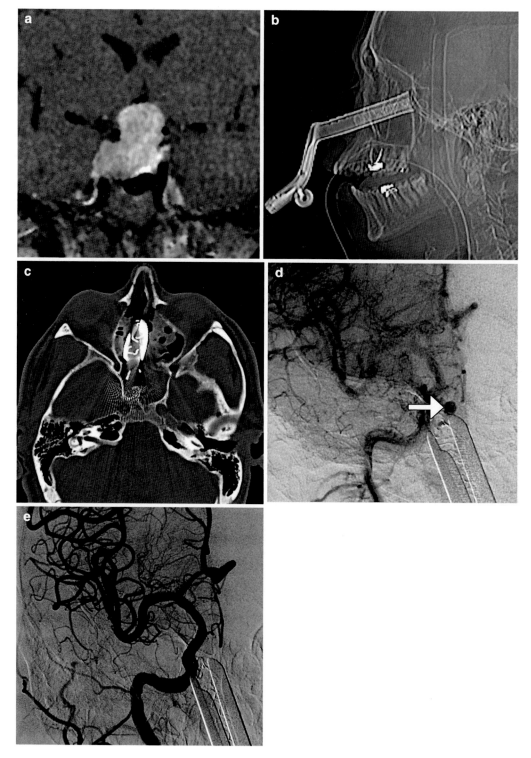

Fig. 7.27 Carotid artery injury. Preoperative coronal post-contrast T1-weighted MRI (**a**) shows a large pituitary adenoma that extends into the cavernous sinuses. Postoperative scout (**b**) and axial CT image (**c**) show transsphenoidal speculum. Digital subtraction carotid angiograms show a right cavernous carotid pseudoaneurysm (*arrow*) adjacent to the speculum (**d**). The pseudoaneurysm was successfully treated via endovascular coiling (**e**)

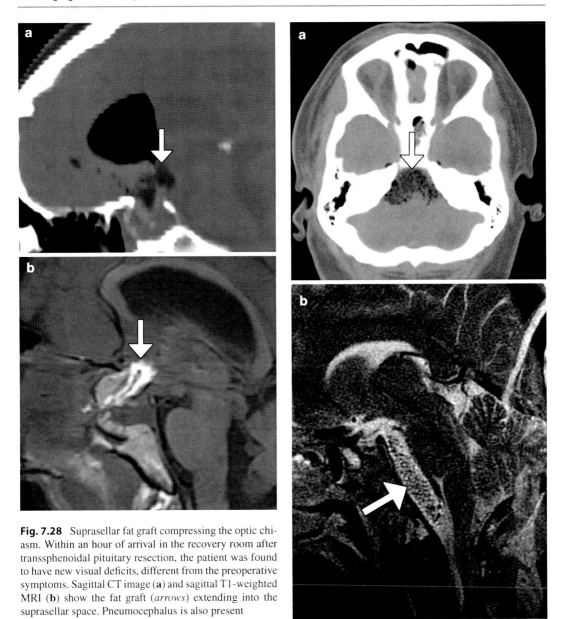

Fig. 7.28 Suprasellar fat graft compressing the optic chiasm. Within an hour of arrival in the recovery room after transsphenoidal pituitary resection, the patient was found to have new visual deficits, different from the preoperative symptoms. Sagittal CT image (**a**) and sagittal T1-weighted MRI (**b**) show the fat graft (*arrows*) extending into the suprasellar space. Pneumocephalus is also present

Fig. 7.29 Merocel migration and brainstem compression. Axial CT image (**a**) shows low-intensity sponge-like material posterior to the sella that compresses the brainstem (*arrow*). Similarly, the sagittal T2-weighted MRI (**b**) shows the spongy hypointense packing material extending posteriorly, exerting mild mass effect upon the brainstem (*arrow*)

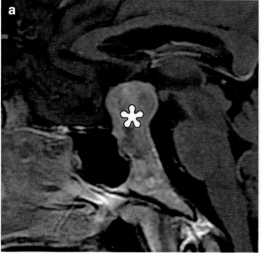 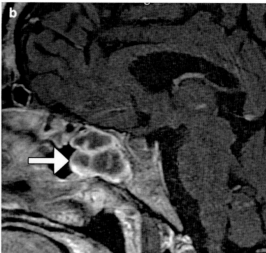

Fig. 7.30 Sinus inflammation. The patient presented with symptoms of congestion following transsphenoidal pituitary adenoma resection. Preoperative sagittal contrast-enhanced T1-weighted MRI (**a**) shows a pituitary macroadenoma (*) but a clear sphenoid sinus. Postoperative sagittal post-contrast coronal T1-weighted MRI (**b**) demonstrates complete extensive mucosal thickening of the sphenoid sinus (*arrow*)

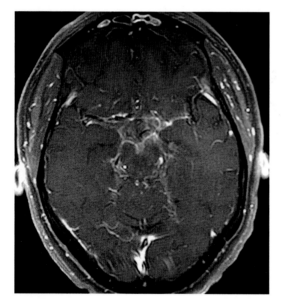

Fig. 7.31 Postoperative infection. Axial post-contrast fat-suppressed T1-weighted MRI shows diffuse leptomeningeal enhancement centered about the basal cisterns due to meningitis

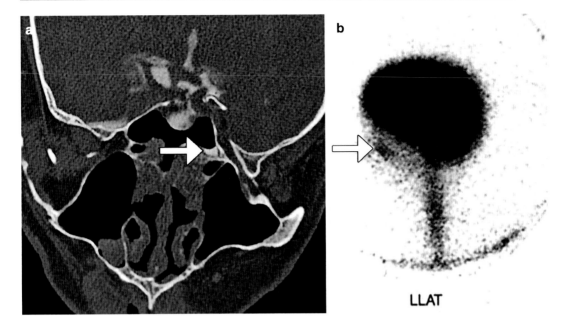

Fig. 7.32 Cerebrospinal fluid leak. The patient underwent transsphenoidal resection of a pituitary adenoma. Approximately 1 week after surgery, the patient presented with a cerebrospinal fluid leak. Oblique coronal CT (**a**) cisternogram image with the patient scanned in a prone position shows pooling of contrast around the fat graft that has partially herniated inferiorly into the sphenoid sinus through a bony defect in the floor of the sella with a meningocele and spillage of contrast into the sphenoid sinus (*arrow*). The patient was scanned in a prone position in order to direct a maximum amount of contrast to the site of suspected cerebrospinal fluid leakage. Nuclear medicine cisternogram (**b**) also shows radiotracer activity localizing to the paranasal sinuses (*arrow*). Cerebrospinal fluid was also seen percolating around the fat graft during the subsequent surgery

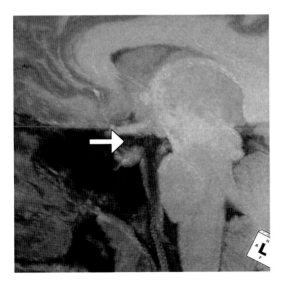

Fig. 7.33 Pituitary stalk transection. The patient is status post-transsphenoidal decompression of sellar/suprasellar Rathke's cleft cyst complicated by transection of the pituitary stalk and secondary panhypopituitarism. The thick-slab sagittal MIP T1-weighted MRI shows interruption of the infundibulum (*arrow*)

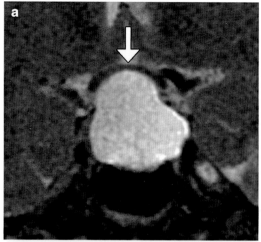

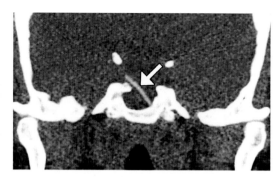

Fig. 7.35 Chiasmopexy. Coronal CT image shows a strip of Silastic (*arrow*) in the sella, which was used to support a sagging optic chiasm

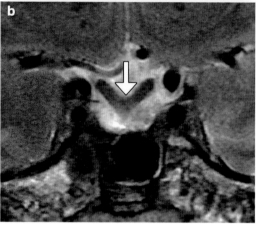

Fig. 7.34 Optic chiasm ptosis. Preoperative coronal T2-weighted MRI (**a**) shows a large macrocystic pituitary adenoma that uplifts the optic chiasm (*arrow*). Postoperative coronal T2-weighted MRI (**b**) demonstrates ptosis of the optic chiasm (*arrow*) into an otherwise empty sella

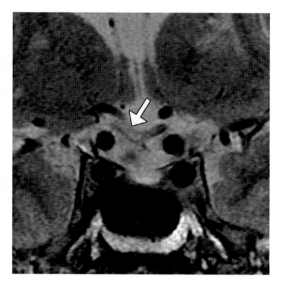

Fig. 7.36 Optic nerve ischemia. The patient presented with new visual deficits after transsphenoidal surgery. Coronal T2-weighted MRI shows hyperintensity and swelling of the right optic chiasm (*arrow*)

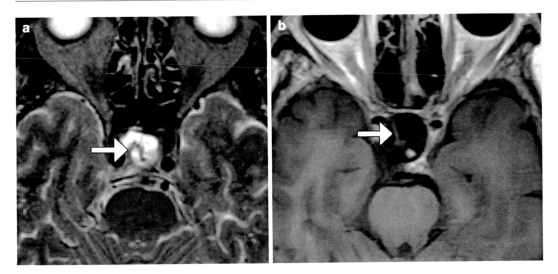

Fig. 7.37 Postoperative fibrosis. Axial T2-weighted (**a**) and post-contrast T1-weighted (**b**) MR images show an intermediate intensity band (*arrows*) traversing the sella anterior to the pituitary stalk

7.5 Middle Cranial Fossa Reconstruction

7.5.1 Discussion

Reconstruction of the middle cranial fossa can be performed using titanium mesh, bone grafts, hydroxyapatite cement, free flaps (most commonly fat or myocutaneous), temporalis muscle or fascia grafts, and pericranial flaps, often in combination (Figs. 7.38, 7.39, and 7.40). Titanium mesh reconstruction is particularly useful for reproducing the natural contours of the middle cranial fossa thereby providing good cosmetic results. The incidence of complications secondary to these reconstruction techniques is generally low, but includes instability of the repair, encephalomalacia, cerebrospinal fluid leaks, infection, and lesion recurrence.

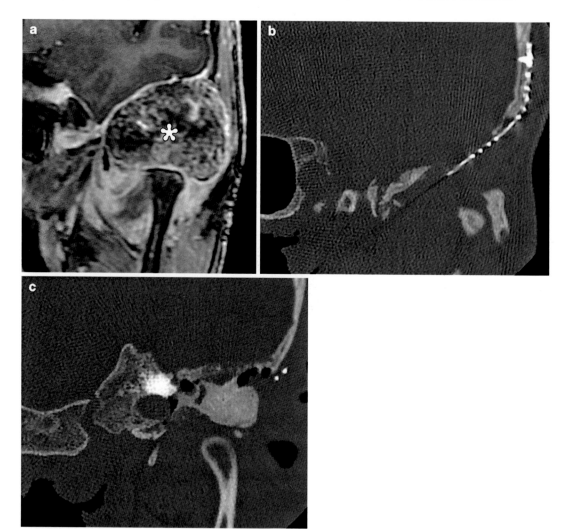

Fig. 7.38 Middle cranial fossa reconstruction with titanium mesh and bone graft. The patient underwent middle cranial fossa reconstruction with mesh and bone graft for resection of TMJ pseudogout. Preoperative coronal postcontrast T1-weighted MRI (**a**) shows a large mass (*) in the left temporomandibular joint that erodes into the middle cranial fossa. Postoperative coronal (**b**, **c**) CT images demonstrate interval resection of the tophus. There is reconstruction of the middle fossa floor with a titanium plate and bone graft

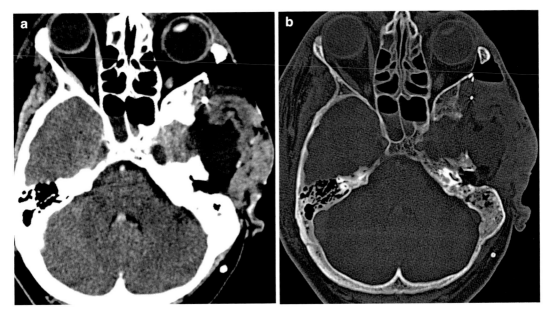

Fig. 7.39 Middle cranial fossa reconstruction with myo-cutaneous flap. The patient has a history of recurrent glioblastoma involving the left middle cranial fossa. Reconstruction was performed using a rectus abdominis myocutaneous flap. Axial CT images in the soft tissue (**a**) and bone (**b**) windows demonstrate resection of a portion of the left middle cranial fossa skull base and application of a myocutaneous flap

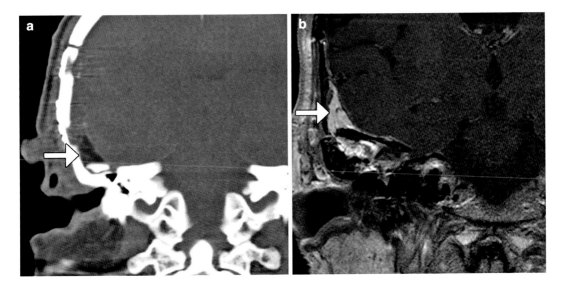

Fig. 7.40 Middle cranial fossa reconstruction with fat and bone grafts. Coronal CT (**a**) image and coronal T1-weighted MRI (**b**) show fat graft (*arrows*) as well as bone graft positioned in right the middle cranial fossa for treatment of a postoperative cerebrospinal fluid leak

7.6 Surgical Approaches for Vestibular Schwannoma Resection

7.6.1 Discussion

Several surgical approaches can be used to resect vestibular schwannomas, including the middle cranial fossa approach, the translabyrinthine approach, and the retrosigmoid approach.

The middle cranial fossa approach for cerebellopontine angle and perimesencephalic tumors consists of temporal craniotomy, extradural temporal lobe retraction, dissection of the petrous ridge dura, and drilling of the roof of the internal auditory canal, which is covered with a fascia or fat graft after the tumor is resected. The main advantages of this approach include a higher likelihood of hearing preservation and access to the fundus of the internal auditory canal for small intracanalicular tumors. Overall, this approach carries a higher risk for facial nerve injury, and retraction injury resulting in temporal lobe gliosis is found in most patients on follow-up imaging (Fig. 7.41). This approach also has limited applicability for the resection of large tumors but can be combined with the retrosigmoid approach in selected cases.

The translabyrinthine approach provides maximal exposure to the cerebellopontine angle, although it sacrifices hearing capacity. This approach is used to resect intralabyrinthine, intracochlear, and larger cerebellopontine angle tumors, as well as vestibular schwannomas in cases where hearing is poor or has been lost. The translabyrinthine approach entails complete mastoidectomy and labyrinthectomy with fat graft packing. In addition, the sigmoid sinus, tegmen tympani, and portions of the internal auditory canal can be skeletonized. The ossicles are sometimes removed, and packing material is left in the middle ear cavity in order to minimize cerebrospinal fluid leakage. Fat grafts are typically used to fill the mastoidectomy bowl, middle ear, and sometimes the internal auditory canal (Fig. 7.42). On post-contrast MRI sequences, enhancement along the periphery of the fat graft is typical and likely attributable to the presence of granulation

tissue. This enhancement usually lasts up to 1–2 years and tends to be linear and diffuse, but it can also have a "whorled" appearance. Often, the fat graft shrinks over time, losing its triangular configuration and allowing air or fluid to enter the mastoid bowl.

The retrosigmoid approach for cerebellopontine angle tumors consists of creating a bone flap and performing a dural incision over the ipsilateral cerebellar hemisphere, posterior to the sigmoid sinus and inferior to the transverse sinus. The mastoid air cells are commonly entered, and bone wax is applied along the edges in order to prevent leakage of cerebrospinal fluid. The cerebellar hemisphere is retracted medially, and the medial portion of the posterior internal auditory canal wall is resected, once the intracranial portion of the tumor is resected. However, an internal labyrinthectomy is often necessary in order to access the fundus of the internal auditory canal. Fat graft is also sometimes inserted into the cerebellopontine angle region if air cells are encountered in the wall of the resected medial internal auditory canal. Occasionally, prominence of the cerebrospinal fluid lateral to a flattened cerebellar hemisphere results from retraction and often gradually dissipates over time (Fig. 7.43).

Although there is no consensus for when to obtain baseline postoperative imaging, it is generally recommended that this is performed between 6 months and 1 year. Patients with known subtotal resection, nodular or mass-like enhancement in the internal acoustic canal, or a history of neurofibromatosis type II undergo serial imaging thereafter. Residual tumor is deliberatively left in some cases, particularly in the lateral internal auditory canal, which is difficult to access via a retrosigmoid approach, in order to minimize the risk of facial nerve and vascular injury. Fat-suppressed post-contrast T1-weighted MRI sequences are particularly useful for the evaluation of tumor (Fig. 7.44).

Various surgical complications can be encountered on postoperative imaging. For example, fat grafts can undergo necrosis, which may appear as cystic change within and adjacent to the residual fat graft (Fig. 7.45). Rarely, aseptic lipoid meningitis can result from fragmentation and dispersal of the fat graft in the subarachnoid space (Fig. 7.46). Other complications may include leakage of cerebrospinal fluid into the mastoid air cells and middle ear (Fig. 7.47), particularly in patients with overpneumatized air cells that are transgressed by the surgical approach, pseudomeningocele from leakage of cerebrospinal fluid into the overlying scalp (Fig. 7.48), her-

niation of the cerebellum into the surgical cavity (Fig. 7.49), endolymphatic sac fenestration with loss of T2 signal (Fig. 7.50), infectious of inflammatory labyrinthitis (Fig. 7.51), labyrinthitis ossificans (Fig. 7.52), wound infection (Fig. 7.53), territorial infarction (Fig. 7.54), and venous sinus thrombosis (Fig. 7.55).

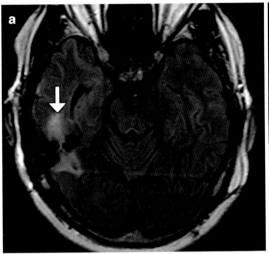 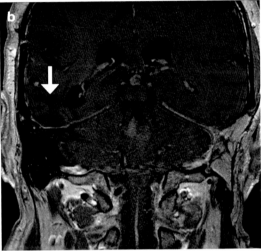

Fig. 7.41 Middle cranial fossa approach. Axial FLAIR (**a**) and coronal post-contrast T1-weighted (**b**) MR images demonstrate encephalomalacia and volume loss in the right inferior temporal lobe (*arrows*) ipsilateral to the middle cranial fossa approach for cerebellopontine angle schwannoma resection. Sequelae of translabyrinthine resection are also noted on the left side without associated brain parenchymal injury

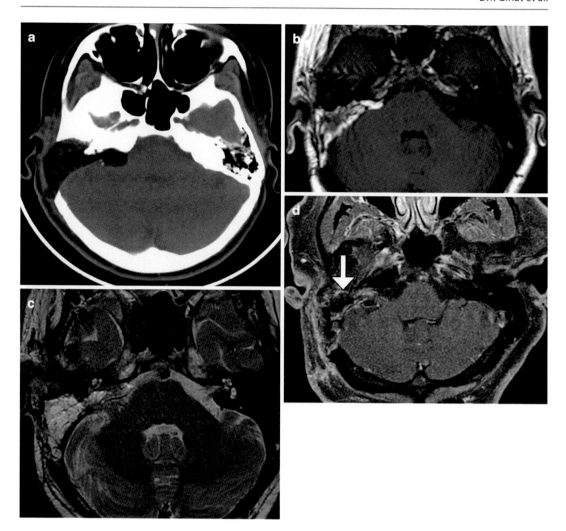

Fig. 7.42 Translabyrinthine approach with fat graft reconstruction. Axial CT (**a**) and T1-weighted MRI (**b**) show obliteration of the internal auditory canal and mastoid bowl with fat graft. The axial T2-weighted MRI (**c**) shows absence of the right vestibule and semicircular canals, but the right cochlea remains intact. Granulation tissue enhancement. Axial contrast-enhanced fat-saturated T1-weighted MRI (**d**) shows linear enhancement along the periphery of the fat graft (*arrow*) and along the overlying incision plane, which likely represents granulation tissue

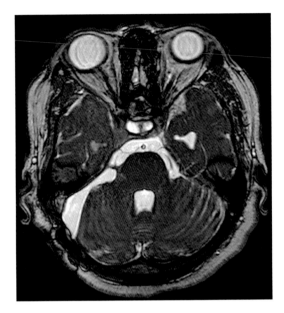

Fig. 7.43 Retrosigmoid approach. Axial T2-weighted MRI shows prominent extra-axial cerebrospinal fluid adjacent to the flattened edge of the right cerebellar hemisphere, which is attributable to intraoperative retraction of the cerebellum

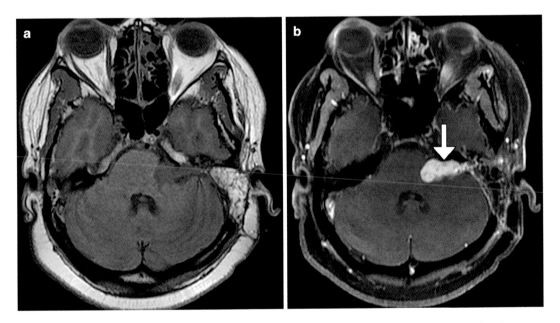

Fig. 7.44 Residual schwannoma. Axial pre- (**a**) and post-contrast (**b**) T1-weighted MR images show enhancing tumor in the left cerebellopontine angle cistern (*arrow*) and fat graft along the surgical approach

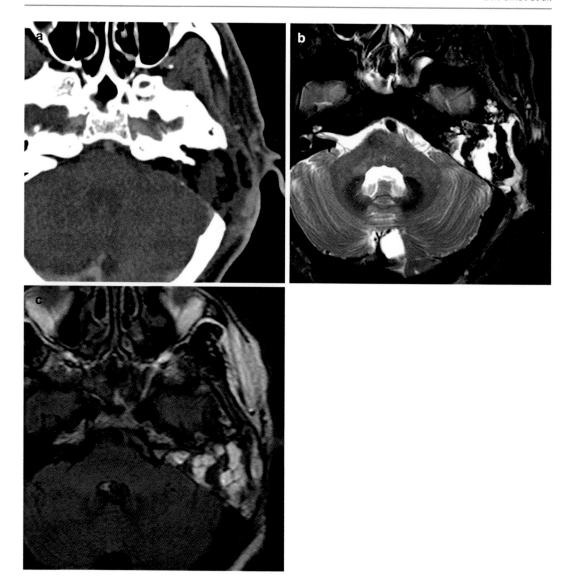

Fig. 7.45 Fat graft necrosis. Axial CT image (**a**), axial T2-weighted (**b**), and T1-weighted (**c**) MR images show bands of fluid within the left translabyrinthine fat graft

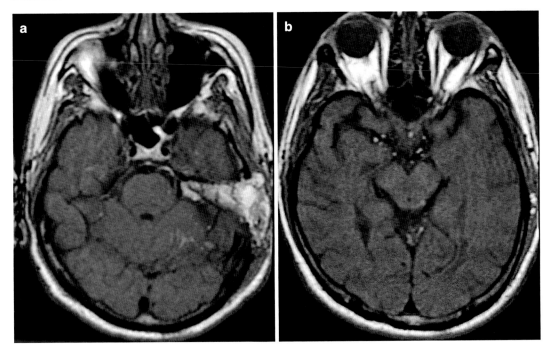

Fig. 7.46 Fat graft aseptic lipoid meningitis. Axial (**a, b**) T1-weighted MR images demonstrate numerous high T1 signal foci scattered in the subarachnoid spaces including the suprasellar cistern, which represent fragments of the fat graft used during translabyrinthine resection

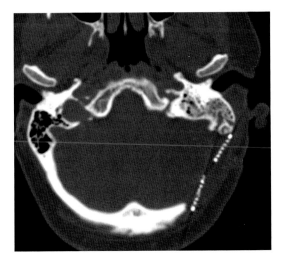

Fig. 7.47 Mastoid entry and cerebrospinal fluid leak. The patient presented with cerebrospinal fluid otorrhea after right acoustic schwannoma resection. Axial CT image shows left retrosigmoid craniotomy traverses the left mastoid air cells. There is opacification of the remaining left mastoid air cells and middle ear, which was not present prior to surgery

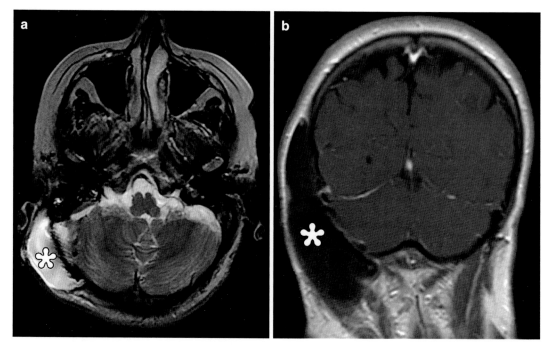

Fig. 7.48 Pseudomeningocele. Axial T2-weighted (**a**) and coronal (**b**) T1-weighted MR images show the large subgaleal fluid collection (*) that has cerebrospinal fluid signal characteristics and extends far superiorly within the subgaleal space

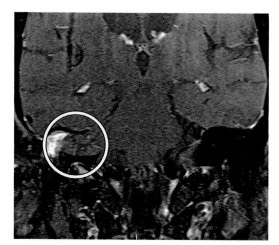

Fig. 7.49 Encephalocele is a rare complication of the translabyrinthine approach. Coronal post-contrast T1-weighted MRI shows a dural defect through which the right cerebellar hemisphere (*encircled*) herniates into the translabyrinthine resection site, facilitated by shrinkage of the fat graft

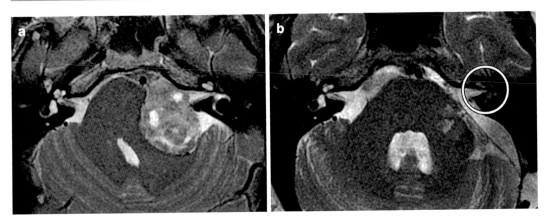

Fig. 7.50 Postoperative endolymphatic sac fluid signal loss. Preoperative axial T2-weighted MRI (**a**) shows a large left vestibular schwannoma with mass effect on the pons and middle cerebellar peduncle, which are otherwise intact. There is normal signal within the bilateral inner ear structures. Postoperative axial T2-weighted MRI (**b**) shows interval resection of the mass. There is diminished signal within the left cochlea, labyrinth, and semicircular canals (*encircled*)

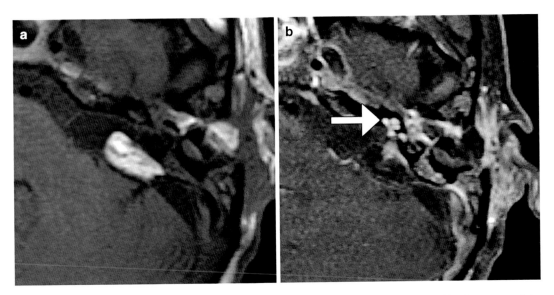

Fig. 7.51 Labyrinthitis. Axial pre- (**a**) and post-contrast (**b**) T1-weighted MR images show avid enhancement of the labyrinthine structures (*arrow*)

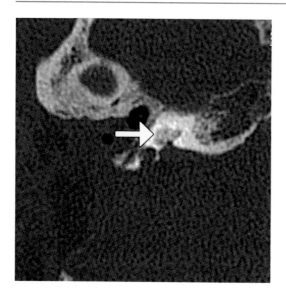

Fig. 7.52 Labyrinthitis ossificans. Axial CT image demonstrates sclerosis of the right cochlea (*arrow*) following translabyrinthine surgery

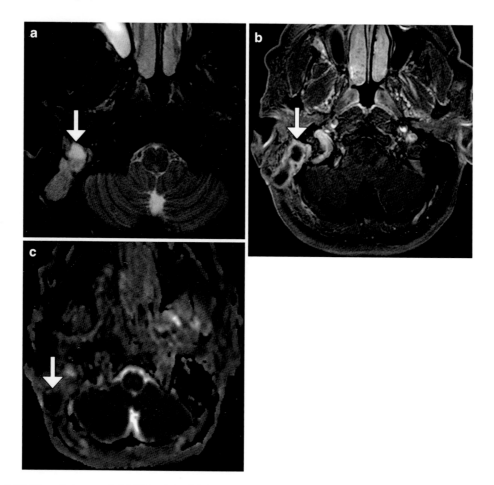

Fig. 7.53 Wound abscess. Axial T2-weighted (**a**), axial (**b**) and coronal (**c**) post-contrast T1-weighted, and ADC map (**d**) show a rim-enhancing fluid collection with debris and an area of restricted diffusion in the right translabyrinthine resection site (*arrows*)

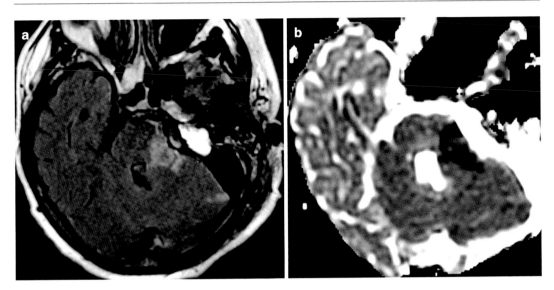

Fig. 7.54 Infarction. Axial T2 FLAIR MRI (**a**) shows high signal in the left lateral pons, middle cerebral peduncle, and portions of the lateral cerebellar hemisphere. The corresponding ADC map (**b**) shows restricted diffusion

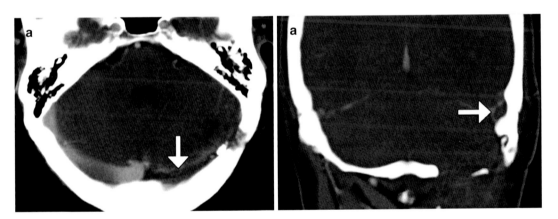

Fig. 7.55 Venous sinus thrombosis. Axial (**a**) and coronal (**b**) CT venogram images show a filling defect in the left transverse sinus adjacent to the retrosigmoid craniotomy (*arrows*)

7.7 Radiosurgery for Vestibular Schwannomas

7.7.1 Discussion

Radiosurgery can be administered as a noninvasive, image-guided treatment for selected cases of vestibular schwannomas. The technique consists of applying high-dose photon radiation to the lesion from different angles. The treated tumors may continue to increase in size for up to 2 years, followed by regression (Fig. 7.60).

Development of high T2 signal intensity in the adjacent brain parenchyma occurs in about 30% of cases. Transient loss of enhancement and central necrosis are also common. The presence of tumor necrosis and alterations in enhancement properties do not necessarily correlate with clinical outcome. Although the changes in contrast enhancement are not predictive of clinical outcome, imaging follow-up is recommended in order to differentiate true ongoing tumor progression from transient treatment-related swelling.

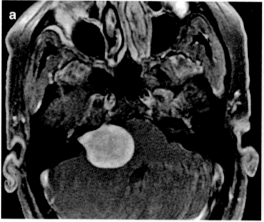
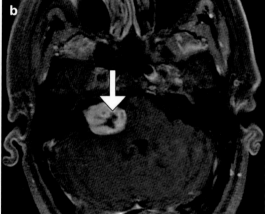
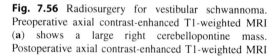

Fig. 7.56 Radiosurgery for vestibular schwannoma. Preoperative axial contrast-enhanced T1-weighted MRI (**a**) shows a large right cerebellopontine mass. Postoperative axial contrast-enhanced T1-weighted MRI (**b**) shows interval central non-enhancement within the mass (*arrow*). There is also decrease in size and mass effect on the right middle cerebellar peduncle and brainstem

Further Reading

Anterior Craniofacial Resection

Cantù G, Solero CL, Mariani L, Salvatori P, Mattavelli F, Pizzi N, Riggio E (1999) Anterior craniofacial resection for malignant ethmoid tumors–a series of 91 patients. Head Neck 21(3):185–191

Cantù G, Riccio S, Bimbi G, Squadrelli M, Colombo S, Compan A, Rossi M, Pompilio M, Solero CL (2006) Craniofacial resection for malignant tumours involving the anterior skull base. Eur Arch Otorhinolaryngol 263(7):647–652

Langstein HN, Chang DW, Robb GL (2001) Coverage of skull base defects. Clin Plast Surg 28(2):375–387, x

Moyer JS, Chepeha DB, Teknos TN (2004) Contemporary skull base reconstruction. Curr Opin Otolaryngol Head Neck Surg 12(4):294–299

Pitman KT, Costantino PD, Lassen LF (1995) Sinonasal undifferentiated carcinoma: current trends in treatment. Skull Base Surg 5(4):269–272

Scher RL, Cantrell RW (1992) Anterior skull base reconstruction with the pericranial flap after craniofacial resection. Ear Nose Throat J 71(5):210–212, 215–217

Schuster JJ, Phillips CD, Levine PA. MR of esthesioneuroblastoma (olfactory neuroblastoma) and appearance after craniofacial resection. AJNR Am J Neuroradiol 1994;15(6):1169–1177.

Decompression of Cystic Sellar/ Suprasellar Lesions

al-Wahhabi B, Choudhury AR, al-Moutaery KR, Aabed M, Faqeeh A (1993) Giant craniopharyngioma with blindness reversed by surgery. Childs Nerv Syst 9(5):292–294

Ohmori K, Collins J, Fukushima T (2007) Craniopharyngiomas in children. Pediatr Neurosurg 43(4):265–278

Transsphenoidal Resection

Bonneville F, Cattin F, Marsot-Dupuch K, Dormont D, Bonneville JF, Chiras J (2006) T1 signal hyperintensity in the sellar region: spectrum of findings. Radiographics 26(1):93–113

Kremer P, Forsting M, Ranaei G, Wüster C, Hamer J, Sartor K, Kunze S (2002) Magnetic resonance imaging after transsphenoidal surgery of clinically nonfunctional pituitary macroadenomas and its impact on detecting residual adenoma. Acta Neurochir 144(5):433–443

Rajaraman V, Schulder M (1999) Postoperative MRI appearance after transsphenoidal pituitary tumor resection. Surg Neurol 52(6):592–598; discussion 598–599

Romano A, Chibbaro S, Marsella M, Oretti G, Spiriev T, Iaccarino C, Servadei F (2010) Combined endoscopic transsphenoidal-transventricular approach for resection of a giant pituitary macroadenoma. World Neurosurg 74(1):161–164

Steiner E, Knosp E, Herold CJ, Kramer J, Stiglbauer R, Staniszewski K, Imhof H (1992) Pituitary adenomas: findings of postoperative MR imaging. Radiology 185(2):521–527

Yoon PH, Kim DI, Jeon P, Lee SI, Lee SK, Kim SH (2001) Pituitary adenomas: early postoperative MR imaging after transsphenoidal resection. AJNR Am J Neuroradiol 22(6): 1097–1104

Transsphenoidal Resection Complications

Ahmad FU, Pandey P, Mahapatra AK (2005) Post operative 'pituitary apoplexy' in giant pituitary adenomas: a series of cases. Neurol India 53(3):326–328

Bonneville F, Cattin F, Marsot-Dupuch K, Dormont D, Bonneville JF, Chiras J (2006) T1 signal hyperintensity in the sellar region: spectrum of findings. Radiographics 26(1):93–113

Buchinsky FJ, Gennarelli TA, Strome SE, Deschler DG, Hayden RE (2001) Sphenoid sinus mucocele: a rare complication of transsphenoidal hypophysectomy. Ear Nose Throat J 80:886–888

Cappabianca P, Cavallo LM, Colao A, de Divitiis E. Surgical complications associated with the endoscopic endonasal transsphenoidal approach for pituitary adenomas. J Neurosurg. 2002;97(2):293–298.

Connor SE (2010) Imaging of skull-base cephalocoeles and cerebrospinal fluid leaks. Clin Radiol 65(10): 832–841

Crowley RW, Dumont AS, Jane JA Jr (2009) Bilateral intracavernous carotid artery pseudoaneurysms as a result of sellar reconstruction during the transsphenoidal resection of a pituitary macroadenoma: case report. Minim Invasive Neurosurg 52(1):44–48

Goel A, Deogaonkar M, Desai K (1995) Fatal postoperative 'pituitary apoplexy': its cause and management. Br J Neurosurg 9(1):37–40

Hald JK, Nakstad PH, Kollevold T, Bakke SJ, Skalpe IO (1992) MR imaging of pituitary macroadenomas before and after transsphenoidal surgery. Acta Radiol 33(5):396–399

Kadyrov NA, Friedman JA, Nichols DA, Cohen-Gadol AA, Link MJ, Piepgras DG (2002) Endovascular treatment of an internal carotid artery pseudoaneurysm following transsphenoidal surgery. Case report. J Neurosurg 96(3):624–627

Kessler L, Legaludec V, Dietemann JL, Maitrot D, Pinget M (1999) Sphenoidal sinus mucocele after transsphenoidal surgery for acromegaly. Neurosurg Rev 22(4): 222–225

La Fata V, McLean N, Wise SK, DelGaudio JM, Hudgins PA (2008) CSF leaks: correlation of high-resolution CT and multiplanar reformations with intraoperative endoscopic findings. AJNR Am J Neuroradiol 29(3): 536–541

Lloyd KM, DelGaudio JM, Hudgins PA (2008) Imaging of skull base cerebrospinal fluid leaks in adults. Radiology 248(3):725–736

Puri AS, Zada G, Zarzour H, Laws E, Frerichs K (2012) Cerebral vasospasm after transsphenoidal resection of pituitary adenomas: report of 3 cases and review of the literature. Neurosurgery 71:173–180

Raymond J, Hardy J, Czepko R, Roy D (1997) Arterial injuries in transsphenoidal surgery for pituitary adenoma; the role of angiography and endovascular treatment. AJNR Am J Neuroradiol 18(4):655–665

Saeki N, Hoshi S, Sunada S, Sunami K, Murai H, Kubota M, Tatsuno I, Iuchi T, Yamaura A (2002) Correlation of high signal intensity of the pituitary stalk in macroadenoma and postoperative diabetes insipidus. AJNR Am J Neuroradiol 23(5):822–827

Steiner E, Knosp E, Herold CJ, Kramer J, Stiglbauer R, Staniszewski K, Imhof H (1992) Pituitary adenomas: findings of postoperative MR imaging. Radiology 185(2):521–527

Steiner E, Math G, Knosp E, Mostbeck G, Kramer J, Herold CJ (1994) MR-appearance of the pituitary gland before and after resection of pituitary macroadenomas. Clin Radiol 49(8):524–530

Taylor SL, Tyrrell JB, Wilson CB (1995) Delayed onset of hyponatremia after transsphenoidal surgery for pituitary adenomas. Neurosurgery 37(4):649–653; discussion 653–654

van Aken MO, de Marie S, van der Lely AJ, Singh R, van den Berge JH, Poublon RM, Fokkens WJ, Lamberts SW, de Herder WW. Risk factors for meningitis after transsphenoidal surgery. Clin Infect Dis 1997 Oct;25(4):852–856.

Yoon PH, Kim DI, Jeon P, Lee SI, Lee SK, Kim SH (2001) Pituitary adenomas: early postoperative MR imaging after transsphenoidal resection. AJNR Am J Neuroradiol 22(6):1097–1104

Zada G, Du R, Laws ER Jr (2011) Defining the "edge of the envelope": patient selection in treating complex sellar-based neoplasms via transsphenoidal versus open craniotomy. J Neurosurg 114(2):286–300

Zona G, Testa V, Sbaffi PF, Spaziante R (2002) Transsphenoidal treatment of empty sella by means of a silastic coil: technical note. Neurosurgery 51(5): 1299–1303; discussion 1303

Middle Cranial Fossa Reconstruction

Chang DW, Langstein HN, Gupta A, De Monte F, Do KA, Wang X, Robb G (2001) Reconstructive management of cranial base defects after tumor ablation. Plast Reconstr Surg 107(6):1346–1355; discussion 1356–1357

Jacobsen N, Mills R (2006) Management of stenosis and acquired atresia of the external auditory meatus. J Laryngol Otol 120(4):266–271

Lipira A, Limbrick D, Haughey B, Custer P, Chicoine MR (2009) Titanium mesh reconstruction to maintain scalp contour after temporalis musculofascial flap reconstruction of the floor of the middle cranial fossa: a technical note and report of two cases. Skull Base 19(4):303–309

Surgical Approaches for Vestibular Schwannoma Resection

Friedman RA, Goddard JC, Wilkinson EP, Schwartz MS, Slattery WH 3rd, Fayad JN, Brackmann DE (2011) Hearing preservation with the middle cranial fossa approach for neuro fibromatosis type 2. Otol Neurotol 32:1530–1537

Silk PS, Lane JI, Driscoll CL (2009) Surgical approaches to vestibular schwannomas: what the radiologist needs to know. Radiographics 29(7):1955–1970

Bennett ML, Jackson CG, Kaufmann R, Warren F (2008) Postoperative imaging of vestibular schwannomas. Otolaryngol Head Neck Surg 138(5):667–671

Hwang PH, Jackler RK (1996) Lipoid meningitis due to aseptic necrosis of a free fat graft placed during neurotologic surgery. Laryngoscope 106(12 Pt 1):1482–1486

Schmerber S, Palombi O, Boubagra K, Charachon R, Chirossel JP, Gay E (2005) Long-term control of vestibular schwannoma after a translabyrinthine complete removal. Neurosurgery 57(4):693–698

Weissman JL, Hirsch BE, Fukui MB, Rudy TE (1997) The evolving MR appearance of structures in the internal auditory canal after removal of an acoustic neuroma. AJNR Am J Neuroradiol 18(2):313–323

Miller RS, Pensak ML (2006) An anatomic and radiologic evaluation of access to the lateral internal auditory canal via the retrosigmoid approach and description of an internal labyrinthectomy. Otol Neurotol 27(5):697–704

Silk PS, Lane JI, Driscoll CL (2009) Surgical approaches to vestibular schwannomas: what the radiologist needs to know. Radiographics 29(7):1955–1970

Radiosurgery for Vestibular Schwannomas

Meijer OW, Weijmans EJ, Knol DL, Slotman BJ, Barkhof F, Vandertop WP, Castelijns JA (2008) Tumor-volume changes after radiosurgery for vestibular schwannoma: implications for follow-up MR imaging protocol. AJNR Am J Neuroradiol 29(5):906–910

Nakamura H, Jokura H, Takahashi K, Boku N, Akabane A, Yoshimoto T (2000) Serial follow-up MR imaging after gamma knife radiosurgery for vestibular schwannoma. AJNR Am J Neuroradiol 21(8):1540–1546

Imaging of the Postoperative Ear and Temporal Bone

8

Daniel Thomas Ginat, Gul Moonis,
Suresh K. Mukherji, and Michael B. Gluth

8.1 Osseointegrated Bone Conduction Hearing Implants

8.1.1 Discussion

Osseointegrated bone conduction hearing implants (BAHA, Cochlear Corporation, Australia and Ponto, Oticon Corporation, Sweden) are implantable hearing devices used in patients with conductive, mixed, or unilateral sensorineural hearing loss who cannot wear traditional air-conducting hearing aids. These devices function in conductive hearing loss by direct transmission of sound via bone conduction to the ipsilateral inner ear, bypassing the external auditory canal and middle ear. In unilateral profound sensorineural hearing loss, they work by

D.T. Ginat, M.D., M.S. (✉)
Department of Radiology, University of Chicago,
Chicago, IL, USA
e-mail: dtg1@uchicago.edu

G. Moonis, M.D.
Department of Radiology, Columbia Presbyterian,
New York, NY, USA

S.K. Mukherji, M.D., M.B.A., F.A.C.R.
Department of Radiology, Michigan State University,
East Lansing, MI, USA

M.B. Gluth, M.D.
Department of Surgery, Division of Otolaryngology,
University of Chicago, Chicago, IL, USA

transcranial bone conduction of sound to the contralateral normal functioning cochlea.

The traditional forms of these devices consist of a titanium screw-like implants anchored into the squamous portion of the temporal bone, as well as percutaneous external flange fixture abutments to which removable sound processors/vibrators will attach. However, in newer versions, these devices may lack a percutaneous component and instead feature a magnetic disk that is attached to the osseointegrated screw completely contained just under the scalp (BAHA Attract, Cochlear Corporation, Australia), working via transcutaneous passage of sound vibration. All of these osseointegrated hearing implants can be identified on imaging with a typical implant depth of 3–4 mm into the cortex of the skull (Fig. 8.1). However, the magnetic component of newer non-percutaneous versions will generate a lot of imaging artifact. All osseointegrated hearing implants that have been approved for use in the USA are MRI compatible when the external sound processor is removed. The most common complication of these devices is adjacent soft tissue and skin reactions resulting in cellulitis or infection. Other complications include loss of osseointegration due to adjacent bone necrosis which can result in screw loosening and extrusion. Intracranial abscess has also been reported, but this is a rare complication of BAHA implantation.

© Springer International Publishing Switzerland 2017
D.T. Ginat, P.-L.A. Westesson (eds.), *Atlas of Postsurgical Neuroradiology*,
DOI 10.1007/978-3-319-52341-5_8

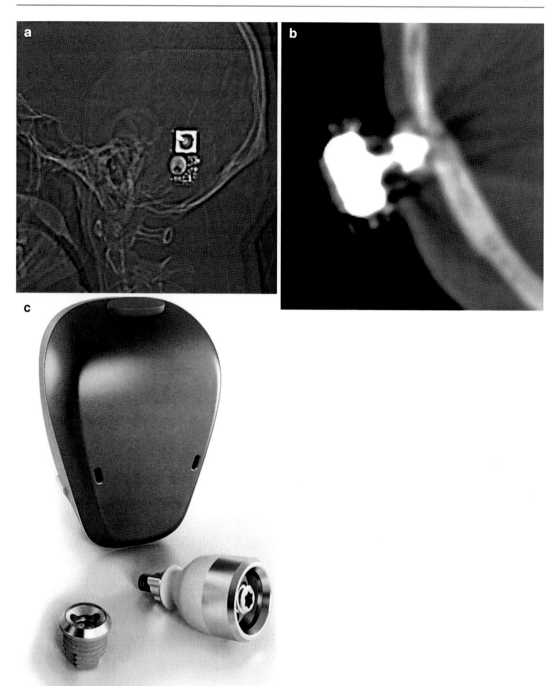

Fig. 8.1 The patient has a history of conductive hearing loss due to aural atresia. Lateral scout image (**a**) shows the BAHA device in position (*arrow*). Axial CT image (**b**) shows the screw embedded in the temporal bone (*arrow*) and the overlying abutment (*arrowhead*). Photograph of BAHA device components (**c**) (Courtesy of Cochlear Corp)

8.2   Auriculectomy

8.2.1   Discussion

Auriculectomy consists of resection of all or part of the pinna. This procedure is usually performed for resection of external ear cutaneous malignancies, such as basal cell carcinoma or squamous cell carcinoma. Parotidectomy and neck dissection may be performed in conjunction with auriculectomy if there is extension of tumor along the fascial planes or if regional lymph node metastasis is suspected. In addition, lateral temporal bone resection is often per-formed if there is extension of tumor from the outer pinna into the external auditory canal. Depending upon the extent of resection, the resulting surgical defect can be closed primarily (Fig. 8.2) or via a variety of reconstruction tech-niques using skin grafts or soft tissue flaps (Fig. 8.3), for example. Furthermore, auricular prostheses can also be applied for cosmetic pur-poses, and these may be held in place with osseointegrated magnetic implants (Vistafix, Cochlear Corporation, Australia). Ultimately, postoperative imaging, particularly CT or MRI, is typically obtained to evaluate for tumor recur-rence in this group of patients.

Fig. 8.2 Auriculectomy. Axial CT image (**a**) shows a right auricular squamous cell carcinoma (*arrow*). Postoperative axial CT image (**b**) shows complete absence of the right auricle

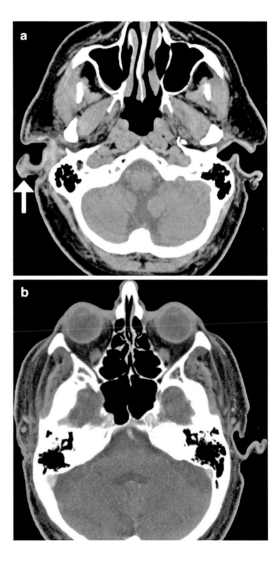

Fig. 8.3 Auricular reconstruction with rib graft. Axial (**a**) and 3D (**b**) CT images show cartilage and bone fragments within the remodeled right auricle

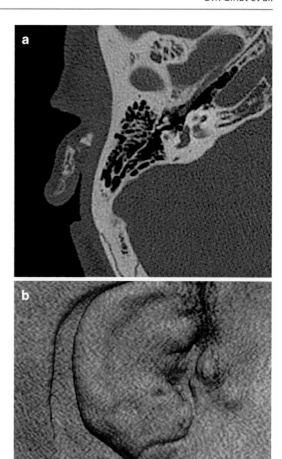

8.3 Auricular Reconstruction

8.3.1 Discussion

Ear reconstruction is performed to reproduce the normal appearance of the auricle for conditions such as microtia. Autogenous rib cartilage reconstruction has been one of the more traditional methods. The cartilage grafts often appear calcified (Fig. 8.3). High-density porous polyethylene (Medpor) is a more recent option. Medpor is a stable alloplastic implant material that can integrate with host tissues and is relatively resistant to infection. For auricular reconstruction, the prosthesis is enveloped in a temporoparietal fascial flap with full-thickness skin graft coverage in order to provide good cosmetic results and minimize the risk of implant extrusion. On CT, Medpor ear prostheses demonstrate attenuation values between fat and soft tissue and are shaped to resemble the natural morphology of the auricle (Fig. 8.4).

Fig. 8.4 Auricular reconstruction with porous polyethylene. Coronal (**a**) and sagittal (**b**) CT images show a low-attenuation left auricular implant that has near-anatomic configuration

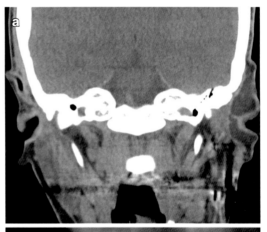
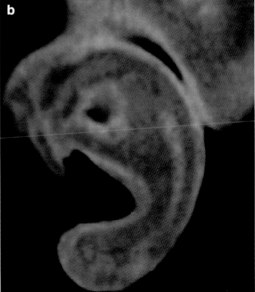

8.4   Canaloplasty and Meatoplasty

8.4.1   Discussion

Canaloplasty and meatoplasty consist of surgically widening the bony external auditory canal and soft tissue/cartilaginous meatus, respectively. This can be performed for treating congenital or acquired canal stenosis and other lesions such as exostoses. Canaloplasty is also often performed as part of a transcanal approach in order to augment surgical exposure during middle ear surgery. Meatoplasty is often performed in conjunction with canal wall down mastoidectomy to provide postoperative access to the resultant mastoid cavity for evacuation of debris in the office. The resulting appearance on CT is an external auditory canal with a relatively capacious lumen (Fig. 8.5). In particular, thinning, irregularity, and/or flattening of the bone, soft tissue thickening, and bony wall defects are common findings on postoperative imaging and should not be mistaken for pathology. Complications of canaloplasty include canal restenosis, temporomandibular joint violation, osteonecrosis, and facial nerve palsy—especially if the distal aspect of the mastoid portion of the facial nerve courses lateral to the tympanic annulus thereby being at risk of drill trauma in the posterior-inferior aspect of the external auditory canal. If persistent pain, trismus, or delayed healing is encountered after canaloplasty, radiologic assessment of the integrity of the anterior canal wall is made to determine if the temporomandibular joint has been violated and assessment of whether this has resulted in a prolapse of joint capsule into the canal lumen. Chronic otitis externa and failed epithelialization after canaloplasty may suggest the possibility of iatrogenic osteonecrosis from excessive burning of the bone by a drill bur that was applied with insufficient irrigation, which will appear as a lytic defect on CT.

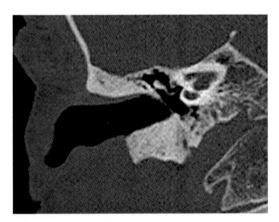

Fig. 8.5 Canaloplasty and meatoplasty. Coronal CT image shows a capacious meatus and external auditory canal with straightening of the floor and loss of the inferior tympanic sulcus

8.5   Atresiaplasty

8.5.1   Discussion

Atresiaplasty consists of creating an external auditory canal and tympanic membrane in order to restore hearing in selected patients with congenital external aural atresia. An opening is drilled through the atresia plate, a new tympanic membrane is usually created using temporalis fascia, and the external auditory canal is often lined with split-thickness skin grafts (Fig. 8.6). Complications of the procedure include external auditory canal restenosis, lateralization and perforation of the tympanic membrane, ossicular chain refixation, sensorineural hearing loss, facial nerve injury, and cholesteatoma, usually in the created external auditory canal, which appears as globular soft tissue on CT, sometimes with associated bone erosions (Fig. 8.7).

Fig. 8.6 Atresiaplasty. Preoperative axial (**a**) and coronal (**b**) CT images show bony atresia of the left external auditory canal with intact ossicles. Postoperative axial (**c**) and coronal (**d**) CT images show interval resection of the atretic plate and partial mastoidectomy, resulting in a passage that communicates with the exterior and neotympanic membrane

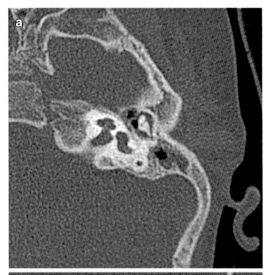

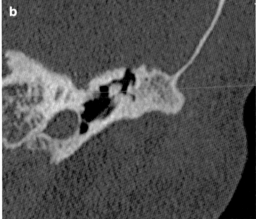

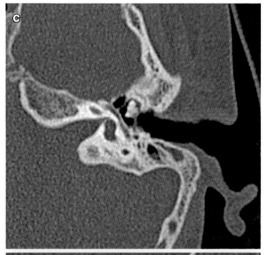

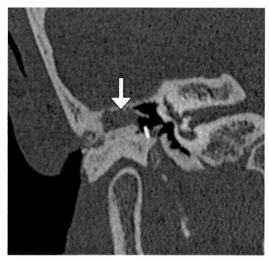

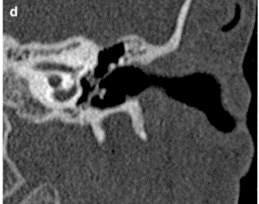

Fig. 8.7 Cholesteatoma after atresiaplasty. Coronal CT image shows soft tissue material (*arrow*) within the surgically created external auditory canal, which proved to be a cholesteatoma. There is also scar tissue that tethers the ossicular prosthesis in an abnormal position

Fig. 8.6 (continued)

8.6 Myringotomy and Tympanostomy Tubes

8.6.1 Discussion

Tympanostomy tubes (pressure equalization tubes) are commonly used to treat the manifestations of Eustachian tube dysfunction including recurrent acute otitis media or chronic otitis media with effusion by providing an alternative outlet for middle drainage and intratympanic pressure equalization via the external auditory canal. Tube placement follows myringotomy, in which an opening is made in the tympanic membrane. Tympanostomy tubes are available in a variety of shapes, sizes, and materials, including plastics and metals, which are readily apparent on CT (Figs. 8.8, 8.9, and 8.10). However, the presence of fluid or malpositioning may make identification of these tubes difficult. The tubes may be found incidentally on CT. Thus, recognizing tympanostomy tubes on imaging is important as to not confuse these with unintended foreign bodies or ossicular dislocation. CT may also be performed to confirm the presence of tympanostomy tubes that are not readily visible on physical exam and to evaluate for suspected complications, such as persistent effusions within the middle ear or mastoid, cholesteatoma, or diffuse tympanosclerosis (Fig. 8.11). Occasionally a tube may be detected in the middle ear space due to a rare incidence of medial migration, but more often a result of accidental loss of a tube within the middle ear during placement. Tympanostomy tubes are normally expelled spontaneously from the tympanic membrane after 3–24 months (Fig. 8.12) depending on the design and shape of the particular tube utilized. The main complications of tympanostomy tubes include formation of a foreign body granuloma on the tympanic membrane immediately adjacent to the tube or chronic otorrhea due to unresolved underlying chronic otitis media or mastoiditis.

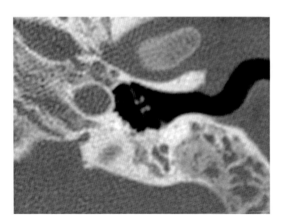

Fig. 8.8 Plastic grommet. Axial CT image shows a Teflon grommet appropriately situated across the tympanic membrane

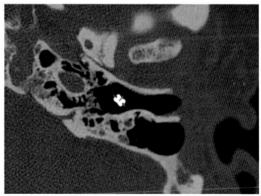

Fig. 8.9 Metal grommet. Axial CT image shows a metal grommet in the tympanic membrane

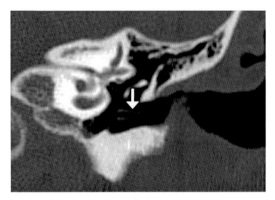

Fig. 8.10 Plastic shaft tympanostomy tube. Coronal CT image shows a long shaft Teflon tube (*arrow*)

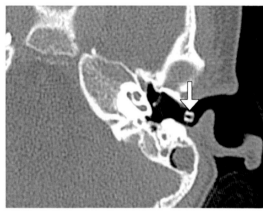

Fig. 8.12 Extrusion of tympanostomy tube. Axial CT image shows a tympanostomy tube in the external auditory canal (*arrow*)

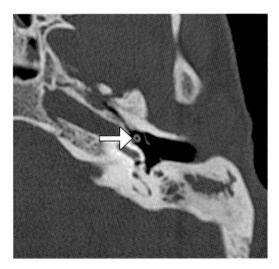

Fig. 8.11 Medial dislocation of tympanostomy tube. Axial CT image shows a tympanostomy tube in the hypotympanum (*arrow*). Note the myringotomy, which appears as a gap in the tympanic membrane

8.7   Myringoplasty and Tympanoplasty

8.7.1   Discussion

Myringoplasty is a simple procedure that is limited to tympanic membrane repair without exploration or manipulation of the middle ear space. Myringoplasty is most often applied to very small tympanic membrane defects caused by extruded tympanostomy tubes. In contrast, tympanoplasty involves reconstruction of the tympanic membrane with concurrent middle ear exploration and possible ossicular chain reconstruction. Several types of tympanoplasty procedures can be performed, which are depicted in Figs. 8.13, 8.14, 8.15, 8.16, 8.17, 8.18, 8.19, and 8.20 and described in Table 8.1. Among these, Type 1 and Type 3 tympanoplasties are overwhelmingly the most commonly performed. Some forms of mastoidectomy may be performed concurrent with tympanoplasty if chronic suppurative otitis media and/or cholesteatoma is present.

The most common materials used for tympanoplasty include autologous temporalis fascia and auricular cartilage grafts—with the later gaining progressive popularity among ear surgeons when dealing with chronic middle ear disease due to their resistance to the effects of negative middle ear pressure. Tympanoplasty grafts appear slightly thicker than the normal native tympanic membranes, especially if cartilage is utilized. However, excessive thickness may signify scarring within the middle ear or postoperative myringitis. Silastic sheeting is sometimes implanted during tympanoplasty in order to prevent the formation of adhesions as part of a staged surgical process wherein removal is performed months later during a second-stage middle ear exploration and ossicular chain reconstruction procedure.

High-resolution CT is the main imaging modality used for studying the architectural changes from tympanoplasty and evaluating suspected causes of graft failure and persistent conductive hearing loss, such as recurrent perforation, middle ear effusion, tympanosclerosis affecting the ossicular chain, tympanic membrane lateralization, and tympanic membrane blunting. The latter two of these are more likely to be encountered if canaloplasty was performed at that same time as tympanic membrane repair or if the malleus has been completely removed.

Fig. 8.13 Type I tympanoplasty with temporalis fascia. The patient has a history of long-standing right-sided tympanic membrane perforation. Since the patient was a possible candidate for cochlear implantation, repair of the tympanic membrane perforation was necessary. Preoperative axial CT image (**a**) demonstrates a perforation of the right tympanic membrane. Axial CT image obtained after tympanoplasty (**b**) shows a tympanic membrane graft composed of temporalis fascia, which is slightly thicker than native tympanic membrane

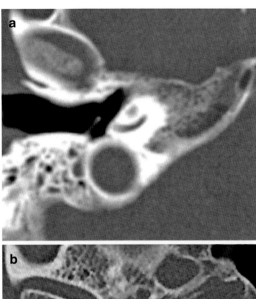

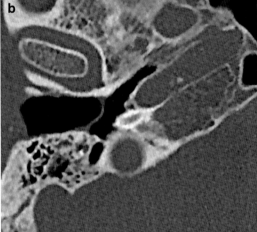

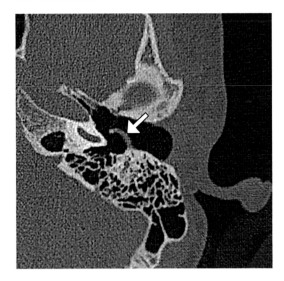

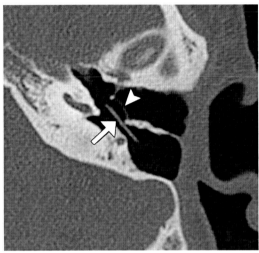

Fig. 8.14 Type I tympanoplasty with cartilage graft. Axial CT image shows the reconstructed posterior portion of the left tympanic membrane as a thick sheet (*arrow*). Note the relative thickness of the normal anterior portion of the tympanic membrane

Fig. 8.15 Type I tympanoplasty with silastic implant for preventing adhesions. Axial CT image shows the implant (*arrow*) inserted into the middle ear cavity, medial to the reconstructed tympanic membrane (*arrowhead*)

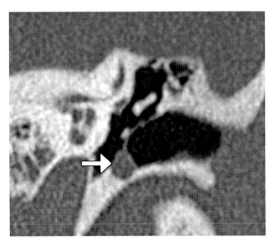

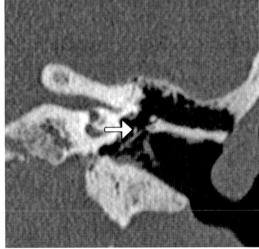

Fig. 8.16 Iatrogenic intratympanic cholesteatoma following tympanoplasty. Coronal CT image shows expansile soft tissue (*arrow*) along the inferior tympanic annulus, splaying the tympanic membrane graft

Fig. 8.17 Type II tympanoplasty. Coronal CT image shows the long process of the incus (*arrow*) in contact with the tympanic membrane graft

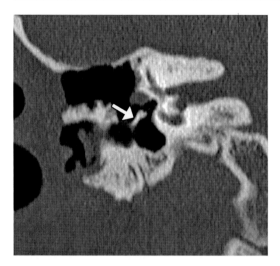

Fig. 8.18 Type III tympanoplasty minor columella with bone strut. Coronal CT image shows a bone graft (*arrow*) interposed between the tympanic membrane and stapes head

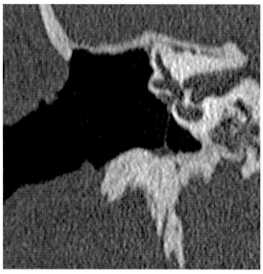

Fig. 8.20 Type IV tympanoplasty. Coronal CT image shows the tympanic membrane graft applied to the stapes footplate such that the footplate is exteriorized into the mastoid cavity and external auditory canal. Note the small middle ear space (cavum minor) created during Type IV tympanoplasty

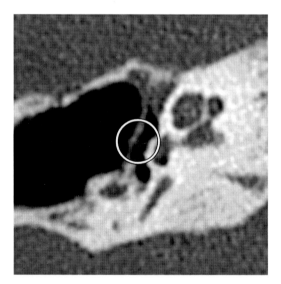

Fig. 8.19 Type III tympanoplasty stapes columella. Axial CT image demonstrates a reconstructed tympanic membrane with cartilage graft applied directly to the head of the stapes (*encircled*)

Table 8.1 Wullstein classification of types of tympanoplasty

Type	Description	Diagram
I	Repair of the tympanic membrane without altering the ossicles. Most common type performed	
II	Repair of the tympanic membrane with drumhead reconstructed onto intact incus (malleus usually absent). This procedure is only rarely performed	
III	Repair of the tympanic membrane and ossicular chain in a manner that couples the stapes to the drumhead. Variations include *minor columella* (usually a PORP prosthesis or sculpted incus interposition autograft) where drumhead is connected to intact stapes superstructure *major columella*, usually a TORP prosthesis, where the drumhead is connected to stapes footplate without intact superstructure, or *stapes columella* where drumhead is placed directly upon the intact stapes superstructure	

(continued)

Table 8.1 (continued)

Type	Description	Diagram
IV	Tympanic membrane repair graft is applied directly to the stapes footplate such that it is exteriorized into the ear canal while shielding of the round window niche using a thick graft, resulting in small middle ear space termed cavum minor. Usually performed along with canal wall down mastoidectomy	
V	Same as type IV tympanoplasty except stapes footplate is removed and oval window is sealed with soft tissue graft. Performed when the stapes footplate is ankylosed	

8.8   Ossicular Interposition

8.8.1   Discussion

Ossicular interposition grafting is a form of ossicular reconstruction (Type 3 tympanoplasty mechanism) that consists of resecting the malleus head or incus and then reinserting it between the stapes and either the malleus manubrium or tympanic membrane after it has been sculpted with a drill bur. The most common form of this technique is incus interposition grafting, in which the long process is amputated and a notch is cut into the short process such that it can be wedged between the manubrium of the malleus and the stapes superstructure (Fig. 8.21). If the stapes superstructure is absent, the long process of the incus is positioned in contact with the stapes footplate, and the notched short process is positioned below the manubrium (notched incus with long process); however, results of incus interposition are much poorer if the stapes superstructure is absent and the technique is only rarely utilized. The malleus head can also be used as an interposition graft by drilling a small groove at the point where the head was amputated from the malleus neck, thereby allowing the graft to be set securely between the stapes superstructure and the undersurface of the tympanic membrane. Complications related to ossicular interposition include encasement by granuloma, iatrogenic cholesteatoma, graft necrosis (Fig. 8.22), and graft dislocation (Fig. 8.23).

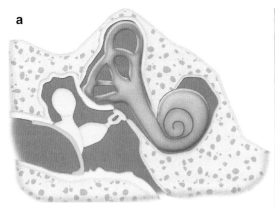
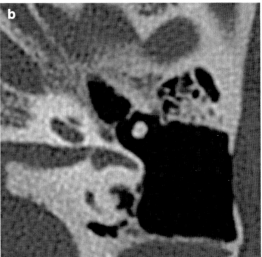

Fig. 8.21 Incus interposition. Illustration of incus interposition (**a**). Axial (**b**) CT image shows that only the malleus is present in the epitympanic space due to disarticulation of the malleoincudal joint. Axial (**c**) and coronal (**d**) CT images show that the sculpted incus (*arrows*) articulates with the head of the stapes

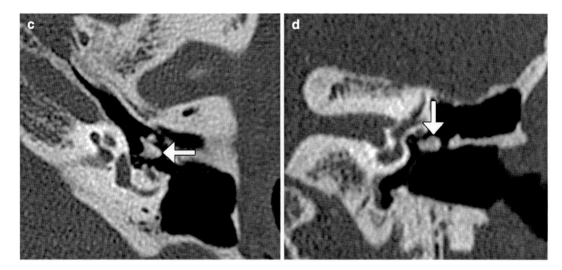

Fig. 8.21 (continued)

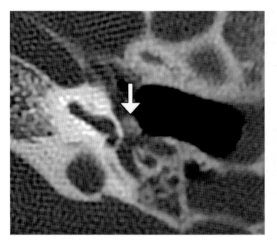

Fig. 8.22 Osteonecrosis of incus interposition graft. Axial CT image shows a demineralized incus interposition graft (*arrow*)

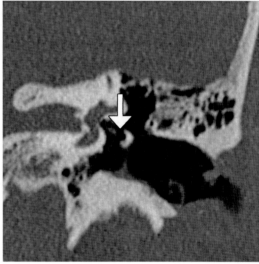

Fig. 8.23 Incus interposition dislocation. Coronal CT image shows an air gap between the head of the stapes and the remodeled incus (*arrow*)

8.9   Ossicular Reconstruction with a Synthetic Prosthesis: Partial Ossicular Reconstruction Prosthesis (PORP), Total Ossicular Reconstruction Prosthesis (TORP), Incudostapedial Joint Reconstruction Prosthesis, and Vibrating Ossicular Reconstruction Prosthesis

8.9.1   Discussion

PORPs and *TORPs* are synthetic implants used for ossicular chain reconstruction typically composed of a head to engage the tympanic membrane and a shaft to engage the stapes. Most modern prostheses are composed of dense hydroxyapatite, titanium, or some combination of the two. Hydroxyapatite has the advantage of being compatible with direct contact to the tympanic membrane, whereas titanium has a tendency to erode through the drumhead if directly in contact; therefore, an overlying protective cartilage cap is mandatory if a titanium head is utilized and optional with hydroxylapatite. On CT, cartilage appears as a thickened segment of tympanic membrane overlying the prosthesis. Plastipore, Teflon, polyethylene, stainless steel, gold, platinum, nitinol, and cortical bone have also been used. Some PORPs and TORPs feature a notched head that is intended to stabilize the implant by engaging the malleus manubrium, while others are placed in direct contact with the posterior/superior quadrant of the tympanic membrane. PORPs extend to the head of the intact stapes and are set upon the superstructure with an open cradle located at the end of the shaft. TORPs extend from the tympanic membrane to the stapes footplate where a cylindrical distal end of the shaft is set (Fig. 8.24). Occasionally a separate "footplate shoe" prosthesis is used in combination with a TORP to prevent it from slipping off of the footplate, since TORPs are often considered less secure than PORPs. A final class of incudostapedial joint reconstruction prosthesis exists to deal with the common scenario of isolated incus erosion involving the long process—including its articulation with the stapes superstructure. These prostheses can be observed spanning from the residual incus long process to the stapes capitulum. However, synthetic hydroxylapatite bone cement products are also commonly utilized for this purpose. Selected examples of various prostheses are shown in Figs. 8.25, 8.26, 8.27, 8.28, and 8.29 and listed in Table 8.2.

Vibrating ossicular reconstruction prostheses (VORPs) are part of an electronic implantable hearing device (Vibrant Soundbridge, Med-El, Austria) that may be used to treat conductive hearing loss in cases where the prognosis for a favorable hearing outcome with a PORP or a TORP is extremely poor, such as severe congenital middle ear anomalies or end-stage middle ear disease. A VORP can also be used in cases of mixed hearing loss where the amplification needs are beyond the capability of a conventional hearing aid. VORPs consist of an external sound processor that is held magnetically over an implanted receiver-stimulator located under the postauricular scalp. The receiver-stimulator is connected by a wire to a magnetic vibrating floating mass transducer that is either connected to the ossicular chain or placed directly onto the round window membrane (Fig. 8.30).

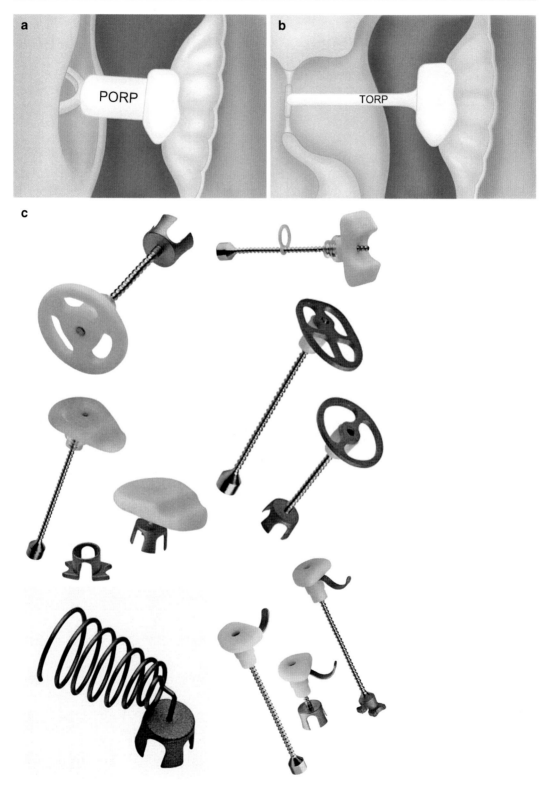

Fig. 8.24 Schematics of *PORP* (**a**) and *TORP* (**b**). The PORP inserts between the tympanic membrane or cartilage graft complex and the head of the stapes. In contrast, the TORP inserts between the tympanic membrane or car-tilage graft complex and the stapes footplate at the oval window. Photographs of various ossicular prostheses (**c**) (Courtesy of Grace Medical)

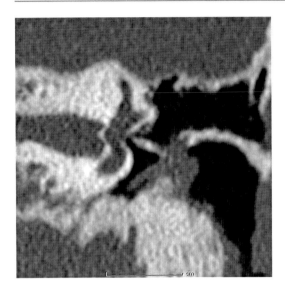

Fig. 8.25 Cortical bone sculpted TORP. Coronal CT image shows a linear bone fragment that extends between the tympanic membrane cartilage graft and stapes footplate

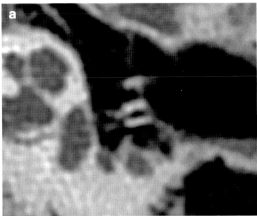

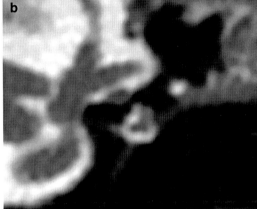

Fig. 8.27 Applebaum PORP. Axial (**a**) and coronal (**b**) CT images show the characteristic hollow L-shaped hydroxyapatite prosthesis, which articulates with the stapes medially and incus laterally

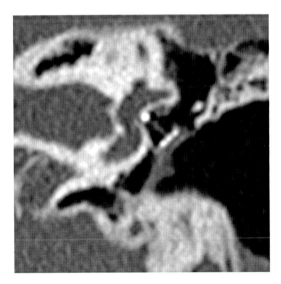

Fig. 8.26 Goldenberg TORP. Coronal CT image shows the flathead prosthesis attached to the tympanic membrane with cartilage graft reconstruction and shaft well seated upon the stapes footplate

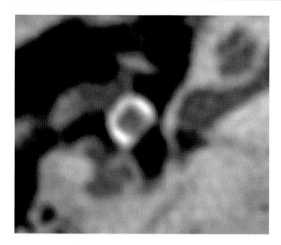

Fig. 8.28 Black oval-top PORP. Axial CT image shows the tympanic membrane and tragal cartilage graft draped over the C-shaped hydroxyapatite head of the prosthesis. The piston of the prosthesis, which articulates with the head of the stapes, is not conspicuous

Table 8.2 Examples of ossicular prostheses

Prosthesis	Description
Applebaum	Hydroxylapatite incudostapedial joint reconstruction prosthesis spanning from the incus long process to stapes head. Features a characteristic L-shaped configuration
Black oval top	Available as PORP or TORP. Features a bulky head with a "horseshoe" or C shape
Dornhoffer	Available as PORP or TORP with notched hydroxylapatite head and a titanium shaft
Goldenberg	Available as PORP or TORP. Triangular notched hydroxylapatite head with off-centered Plastipore shaft

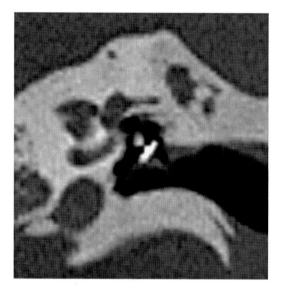

Fig. 8.29 Dornhoffer PORP. Stenver reformatted CT image shows the hydroxyapatite head in contact with the reconstructed tympanic membrane and the titanium cradle in contact with the stapes superstructure

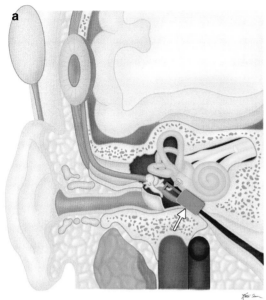
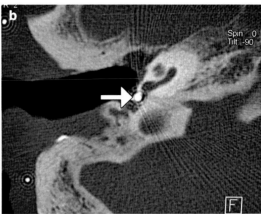

Fig. 8.30 VORP. The illustration (**a**) shows the components of the VORP including the floating mass transducer (*arrow*) in the round window niche attached to the incus. Axial CT image (**b**) shows the floating mass transducer in the round window niche (*arrow*) (Courtesy of Christine Toh, MD)

8.10   Stapedectomy, Stapedotomy, and Stapes Prosthesis

8.10.1 Discussion

Stapes reconstruction is performed for treatment of conductive hearing loss in patients with otosclerosis, stapes fracture, adhesions, or tympanosclerosis. Stapedectomy usually consists of resecting the entire stapes, while stapedotomy involves removing the superstructure and creating a small hole into the stapes footplate. Stapedotomy often involves minimally traumatic surgical techniques, such as hands-free laser application.

Stapes prostheses typically extend from the incus to the stapedotomy defect in the footplate and ideally do not extend medially into the vestibule more than 0.25 mm. Several types of sta-

pes prostheses are available, but most fall into the categories of being either a bucket or piston (Fig. 8.31). Bucket prostheses are set just under the lenticular process of the incus with a small wire that secures it, while pistons usually consist of a smaller barrel and a wire that is crimped around the long process (Figs. 8.32, 8.33 and 8.34). Alternatively, stapes prostheses can be attached to the malleus if the incus is not available for reconstruction (Fig. 8.35). Stapes prostheses can be made from a variety of materials including titanium, Teflon, fluoroplastic, and nitinol. Virtually all stapes prostheses are MRI compatible, except for the McGee stainless steel prostheses dating from 1987. Nevertheless, the metal components of the prosthesis can produce susceptibility artifact that obscures detail of surrounding structures and can resemble labyrinthitis ossificans (Fig. 8.36).

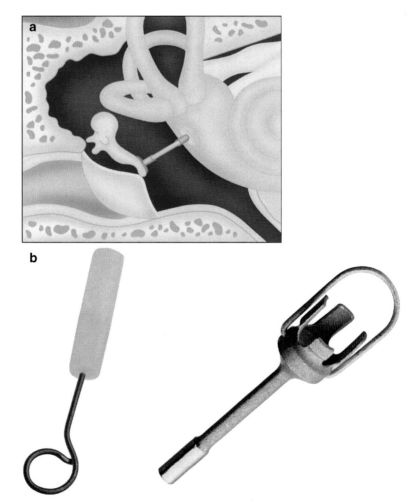

Fig. 8.31 Schematic of a stapes piston prosthesis (**a**). Photographs of piston and bucket handle stapes prostheses (**b**) (Courtesy of Grace Medical)

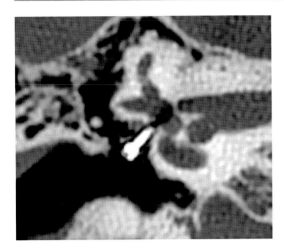

Fig. 8.32 Robinson bucket handle prosthesis. Coronal CT image shows a metallic prosthesis that extends from the long process of the incus to the oval window, where there is beam-hardening artifact

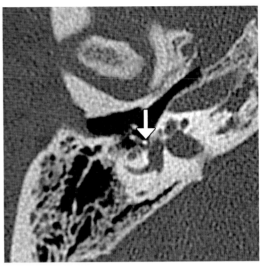

Fig. 8.34 Smart nitinol wire piston prosthesis. Axial CT image shows the prosthesis in position (*arrow*) in contact with the stapes footplate

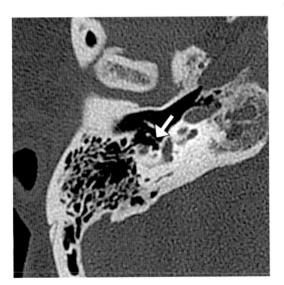

Fig. 8.33 Schuknecht Teflon wire stapes piston prosthesis. Axial CT image shows the filamentous prosthesis in position (*arrow*)

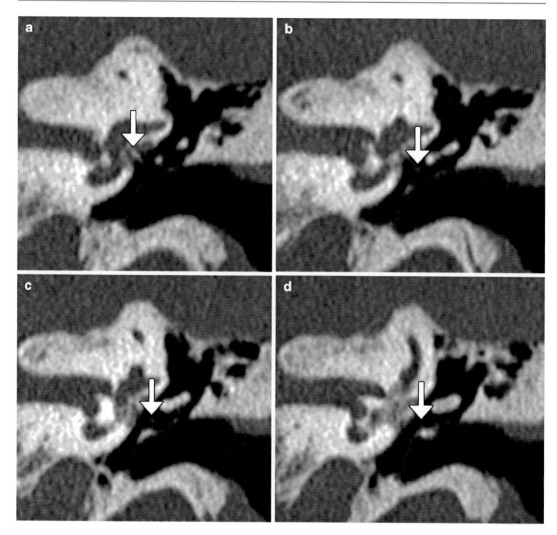

Fig. 8.35 Stapedectomy with malleus grip prosthesis. Serial coronal CT images (**a–d**) demonstrate a wire prosthesis (*arrows*) extending from the stapes footplate to the malleus

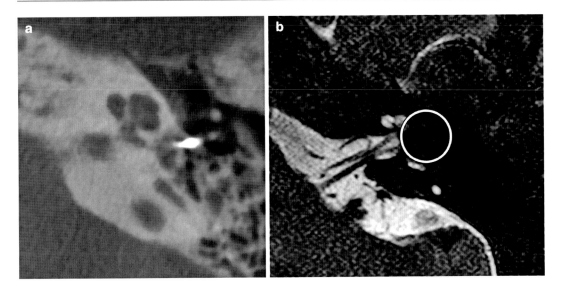

Fig. 8.36 Susceptibility artifact from stapes prosthesis mimicking labyrinthitis ossificans. Axial CT image (**a**) shows a large metallic Robinson prosthesis. The corresponding axial CISS image (**b**) shows obscuration of a portion of the cochlea due to the artifact (*encircled*)

8.11 Ossicular Prosthesis Complications

8.11.1 Discussion

CT imaging may be obtained after ossicular chain reconstruction if a poorer-than-expected hearing outcome results in order to determine if the prosthesis has slipped or if there is another potential cause of hearing loss such as middle ear effusion, fixation of prosthesis or ossicular remnant by scar tympanosclerosis (especially involving the malleus or incus head in the epitympanum), or recurrent cholesteatoma. Encasement of a prosthesis by granulation tissue or cholesteatoma can cause conductive hearing loss whether or not the ossicular prosthesis is displaced.

Complications of ossicular prostheses depend on the particular type of prosthesis, but generally include migration into the vestibule (TORP or stapes prosthesis) (Fig. 8.37), perilymphatic fistula (Fig. 8.38), subluxation, dislocation, extrusion or other form of malposition (Figs. 8.39, 8.40, 8.41, 8.42, 8.43, 8.44, 8.45, and 8.46), encasement/displacement by granulation tissue or recurrent cholesteatoma (Figs. 8.47 and 8.48), tympanic membrane dehiscence (Fig. 8.49), and bending or fracture of the prostheses (Fig. 8.50). Prosthesis subluxation or dislocation is the most common complication responsible for up to 60% of postoperative hearing loss and occurs most commonly in the first 6–8 weeks before fibrosis occurs. Stapes prostheses most commonly displace posterior and inferior to the oval window. Alternatively, these prostheses can migrate into the vestibule, which can cause vertigo and possibly a concurrent perilymphatic fistula. Vestibular penetration is a serious complication that represents 10% of stapes prosthesis complications. Signs of perilymphatic fistula include the presence of air in the labyrinth (pneumolabyrinth) and rarely middle ear effusion. The portion of the prosthesis at the stapes footplate can reliably penetrate the vestibule without causing symptoms is 0.25 mm, but slightly deeper penetration may be asymptomatic in some cases. Prosthesis extrusion through the tympanic membrane occurs in 2.6–7% of cases depending on the type of prosthesis and method of tympanoplasty. The main risk factor for prosthesis extrusion is ongoing Eustachian tube dysfunction. CT is the modality of choice for evaluating most of these complications, especially in the late postoperative period. However, MRI is generally better for characterizing granulation tissue and cholesteatoma.

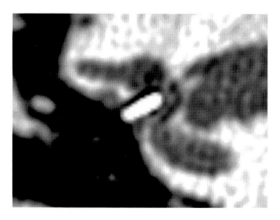

Fig. 8.37 Vestibular perforation. Coronal CT image shows medial displacement of the stapes prosthesis into the vestibule through the oval window

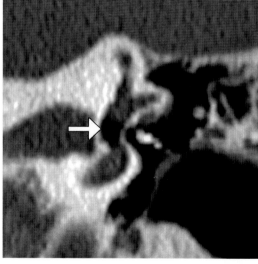

Fig. 8.38 Perilymphatic fistula. The patient presented with acute vertigo after stapedectomy. Coronal CT image shows air within the vestibule (*arrow*) and a laterally displaced stapes prosthesis

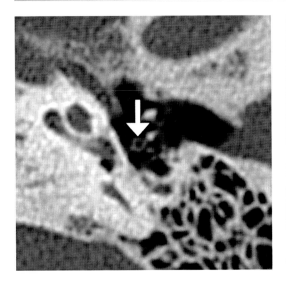

Fig. 8.39 Stapes prosthesis separation from the incus. Axial CT image shows an empty prosthesis wire loop (*arrow*) adjacent to the incus (Courtesy of Mary Elizabeth Cunnane, M.D.)

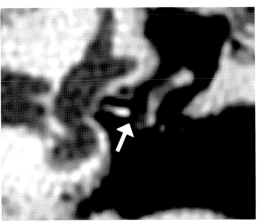

Fig. 8.41 Stapes prosthesis detachment from the incus. Coronal CT image shows an air gap (*arrow*) between the lenticular process of the incus and McGee stapes prosthesis

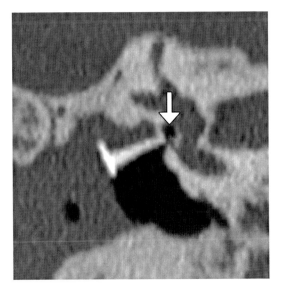

Fig. 8.40 Lateralized TORP. Coronal CT image shows an air gap (*arrow*) between the shaft of the hydroxyapatite prosthesis and the oval window. There is also extensive nonspecific opacification of the widened external auditory canal

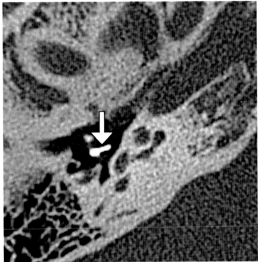

Fig. 8.42 Stapes bucket prosthesis dislocation. Axial CT image shows the distal end of the prosthesis (*arrow*) projecting far anterior to the region of the oval widow

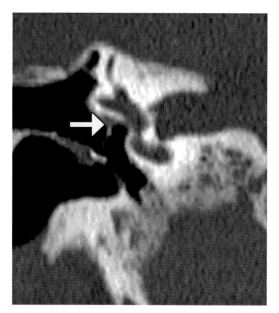

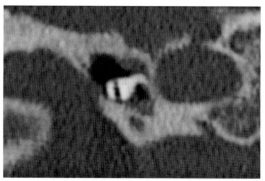

Fig. 8.44 Dislocated PORP. Coronal CT image shows the Wehr's short single-notch incus prosthesis in the hypotympanum, adjacent to the Eustachian tube orifice

Fig. 8.43 TORP facial nerve impingement. Coronal CT image shows the medial ends of the prosthesis contacting the tympanic segment of the facial nerve canal (*arrow*)

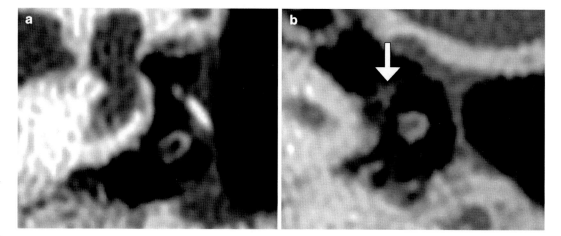

Fig. 8.45 PORP detachment from stapes. Coronal (**a**) and axial (**b**) CT images show the shaft of the prosthesis separated and angled away from the oval window, far removed from the stapes (*arrow*)

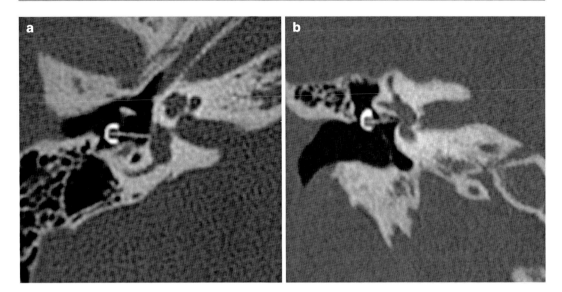

Fig. 8.46 Extruded TORP. Axial (**a**) and coronal (**b**) CT images show the black oval-top prosthesis head that extends lateral to the tympanic membrane, while the shaft still contacts the footplate

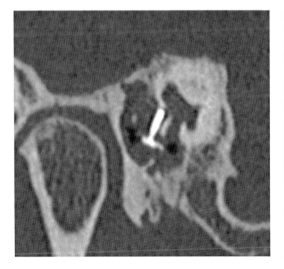

Fig. 8.47 Dislocated TORP encased in soft tissue. Poschl plane CT image shows a hydroxyapatite TORP orientated upside down and encased by nonspecific soft tissue

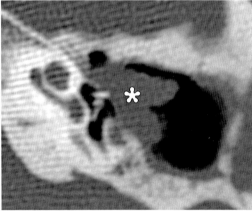

Fig. 8.48 Recurrent cholesteatoma with TORP displacement. Axial CT image shows a cholesteatoma (*) that displaces the ossicular prosthesis

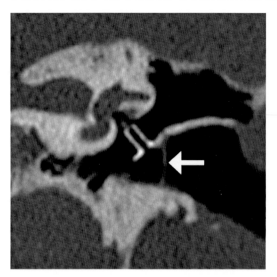

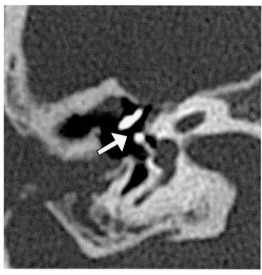

Fig. 8.49 Ossicular prosthesis tympanic membrane detachment. Coronal CT image shows separation of the tympanic membrane graft (*arrow*) from the head of the prosthesis

Fig. 8.50 Prosthesis fracture. Axial CT image shows an air gap (*arrow*) between the head and shaft of the prosthesis

8.12 Atticotomy

8.12.1 Discussion

Atticotomy, also known as epitympanectomy, consists of removing the bone of the lateral attic wall (scutum) in order to provide visualization of the attic contents and aditus ad antrum (Fig. 8.51). This procedure is most often used to treat attic cholesteatoma or fixation of the ossicular heads. Often, but not always, the body of the incus and head of the malleus are resected during atticotomy if they are involved with disease or if wider surgical exposure is needed. Atticotomy may be applied as a stand-alone procedure through the external auditory canal, or it may be part of a more extensive combined approach that additionally involves canal wall-up mastoidectomy. Canal wall defects that result from atticotomy can easily be reconstructed with auricular cartilage or soft tissue grafts, but rarely these defects are intentionally left open if the surgeon intends to exteriorize part or all of the attic into the external auditory canal. Following atticotomy, CT or MRI may be performed to evaluate for the presence of recurrent cholesteatoma. Atticotomy is sometimes difficult to distinguish from autoatticotomy where long-standing negative middle ear pressure or cholesteatoma has generated an atticotomy defect.

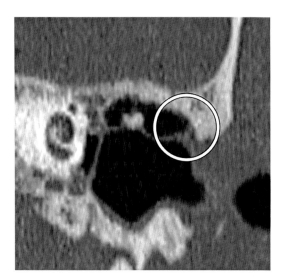

Fig. 8.51 Atticotomy. Coronal CT image shows partial absence of the left ossicles and surgical resection of the scutum (*encircled*). The epitympanum is clear, but the reconstructed tympanic membrane is atelectatic

8.13   Eustachian Tube Occlusion Procedures

8.13.1   Discussion

A patulous Eustachian tube can cause autophony and a sense of ear fullness. Intolerable symptoms can be treated via fat, Teflon, or hydroxyapatite injection into the Eustachian tube and surrounding soft tissues in order to create mass effect upon an incompetent tubal valve. Alternatively, the Eustachian tube can be occluded using Silastic tubes (Fig. 8.52). Injected hydroxyapatite appears as streaky or focal hyperattenuation on CT (Fig. 8.53). The material can resorb over time. Injected Teflon appears mildly hyperattenuating on CT and sometimes incites a foreign body reaction, which results in an encapsulated granuloma after 3–6 months following injection (Fig. 8.54). Such lesions can also appear intensely hypermetabolic on PET. Other complications include inadequate occlusion of the Eustachian tube and breakage or migration of the catheters and plugs, which can lead to recurrent symptoms and impingement upon the ossicles (Figs. 8.55 and 8.56).

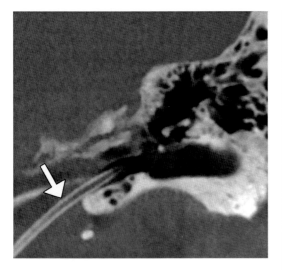

Fig. 8.52 Eustachian tube catheter. Stenver plane CT image shows the catheter (*arrow*) coursing through the Eustachian tube

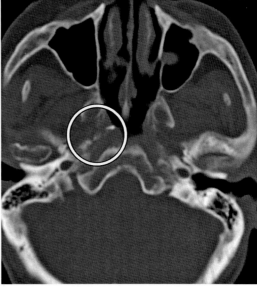

Fig. 8.53 Hydroxyapatite injection. Axial CT image shows the high-attenuation focus of hydroxyapatite in the left parapharyngeal soft tissues along the expected course of the Eustachian tube (*encircled*)

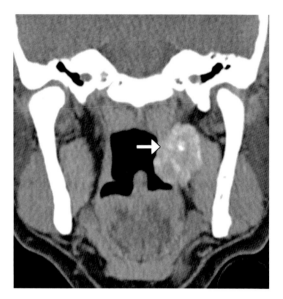

Fig. 8.54 Teflon injection with granuloma formation. Coronal CT image shows a hyperattenuating mass in the left nasopharyngeal region. Biopsy confirmed the presence of foreign body reaction. (Courtesy of Juan Small MD)

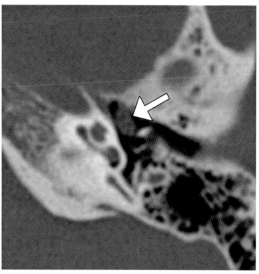

Fig. 8.56 Displaced transtympanic Eustachian tube plug. Axial CT image shows the soft attenuation plug (*arrow*) within the mesotympanum, abutting the ossicular chain, rather than within the Eustachian tube orifice

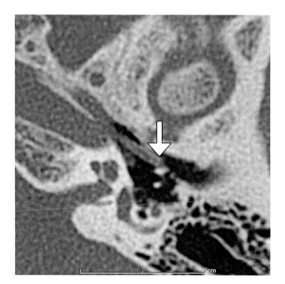

Fig. 8.55 Eustachian tube catheter migration. Axial CT image shows the catheter (*arrow*) impinging upon the ossicles and tympanic membrane

8.14 Mastoidectomy and Mastoid Obliteration

8.14.1 Discussion

There are two main types of mastoidectomy: canal wall-up mastoidectomy (also called intact canal wall mastoidectomy) in which the native bony external auditory canal is preserved (except for perhaps a partial atticotomy defect) or canal wall-down mastoidectomy in which the superior and posterior segments of the bony canal wall are resected such that the mastoidectomy cavity and portions of the middle ear are thereby rendered exteriorized into the external auditory canal. Canal wall-down mastoidectomy can be further divided into radical and modified radical mastoidectomy based on whether or not the entire middle ear space is exteriorized with the ossicles removed (radical) or the middle ear space is par-

tially maintained via tympanic membrane reconstruction (modified radical) (Figs. 8.57, 8.58, 8.59, 8.60, and 8.61). Sometimes, the surgeon chooses to obliterate all or part of the mastoid cavity or exteriorized attic with fascia, bone chips, cartilage, or soft tissue rotational flaps in order to reduce the postoperative risk of having a high-maintenance chronically unstable canal wall-down mastoid cavity (Figs. 8.62 and 8.63). Thin-section CT and MRI are the most useful modalities for evaluating patients with potential complications following mastoidectomy. In particular, T2-weighted turbo spin echo and gradient echo sequences with multiplanar reformats are best suited for evaluating the middle ear structures, while high resolution T2-weighted steady state sequences are optimal for imaging the inner ear. The use of T1-weighted sequences without and with contrast is recommended for an overall assessment.

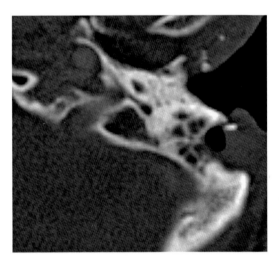

Fig. 8.57 Partial canal wall-up mastoidectomy. Axial CT image shows that the lateral cortex of the mastoid has been resected. The mastoid air cells are otherwise nearly intact. Sometimes a limited mastoidectomy such as this is performed to drain a mastoid abscess

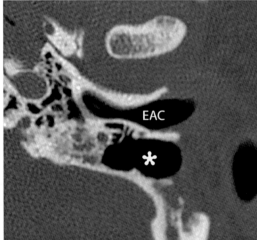

Fig. 8.58 Canal wall-up mastoidectomy. Axial CT image shows an intact posterior wall of the external auditory canal (EAC) and an air-filled mastoid bowl (*). Sometimes the mastoid cavity can lack aeration after canal wall-up mastoidectomy if the lateral soft tissues scar inward to fill the cavity

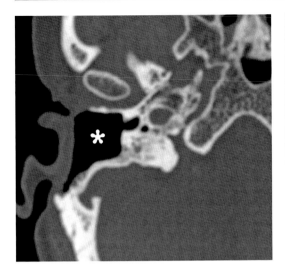

Fig. 8.59 Canal wall-down mastoidectomy. Axial CT image shows resection of the posterior wall of the external auditory canal, such that the mastoid bowl (*) communicates with the external auditory canal

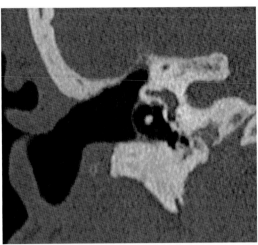

Fig 8.61 Modified radical mastoidectomy. Coronal CT image shows the repositioned right tympanic membrane margin overlying the horizontal semicircular canal and resection of the mastoid air cells

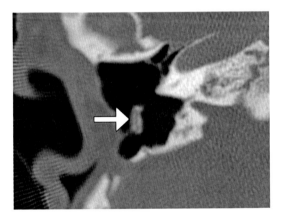

Fig. 8.60 Radical mastoidectomy. Axial CT image shows the absence of the ossicles, but preservation of the facial nerve, which has been skeletonized (*arrow*) as it courses through the mastoid bowl

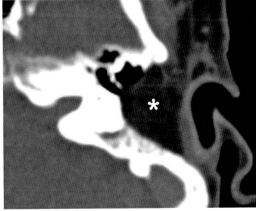

Fig. 8.62 Mastoid obliteration with fat graft. Axial CT image shows fat graft present within the mastoidectomy bowl (*). Sometimes fat is used to obliterate a mastoid cavity even if it is a canal wall-up procedure if a cerebrospinal fluid leak is present

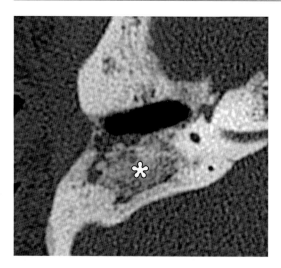

Fig. 8.63 Mastoid obliteration with bone dust. Axial CT image shows the bone dust (*) packing the mastoidectomy bowl. The bone dust was harvested from the surface of the mastoid cortex

8.15 Mastoidectomy Complications

8.15.1 Discussion

Imaging after mastoidectomy may be performed to evaluate for a variety of complications, including abscess formation surrounding the mastoidectomy bowl, including intracranially (Fig. 8.64), chronic infection of a canal wall-down mastoidectomy cavity, which may be associated with an unstable cavity and high facial ridge (Fig. 8.65), excess granulation tissue (Fig. 8.66), recurrent cholesteatoma, (Figs. 8.67 and 8.68), and facial nerve injury (Fig. 8.69), which can lead to formation of reparative neuromas (Fig. 8.70), cerebrospinal fluid leakage (Fig. 8.71), and encephaloceles (Fig. 8.72). Profound sensorineural hearing loss and vestibular weakness can also occur if the surgeon violates the labyrinth with the drill.

It is common for exteriorized mastoid cavities to become infected on a chronic or recurrent basis, and this may lead to the need for frequent office visits to clean debris, to treat granulation tissue, and to apply antimicrobial medications. The stability of a canal wall-down mastoidectomy cavity is highly dependent on surgical technique, and there are several factors notable on CT imaging that may be implicated in cavity instability including a large open mastoid tip filled with debris, a small or absent meatoplasty, a high residual ridge of the bone overlying the mastoid segment of the facial nerve (defined as 2 mm or greater proximal to the chorda tympani facial nerve junction), numerous residual diseased air cells, the absent or perforated tympanic membrane, or residual cholesteatoma.

Historically, recurrent cholesteatoma was encountered in one-third to one-half of patients treated with canal wall-up mastoidectomy and roughly 10% of those treated with canal wall-down mastoidectomy. Due to the high failure rate of canal wall-up surgery, a planned second-look procedure or planned radiologic imaging is usually part of the treatment scheme. Imaging usually consists of CT or MRI with non-EPI diffusion-weighted imaging usually obtained 9–12 months after surgery. Recurrent cholesteatomas tend to show restricted diffusion, while granulation tissue does not. CT has a high negative predictive value when it shows a clear middle ear and mastoid cavity. However, CT is nonspecific, while MRI is well suited for elucidating the differential when there is soft tissue in the postoperative cavity. Although both recurrent cholesteatomas and granulation tissue are typically hyperintense on T2-weighted and hypo-/isointense on T1-weighted MRI sequences, recurrent cholesteatomas tend to show rim enhancement, while postoperative granulation tissue fills in with contrast. It is also important to distinguish recurrent cholesteatomas from encephaloceles and cholesterol granulomas. Residual cholesteatoma after surgical removal is most often found in the sinus tympani, the oval window niche, the anterior epitympanum, and the supratubal recess/protympanum, but can even be extratemporal. Residual cholesteatoma found within the mastoid itself, although possible, is surprisingly uncommon except in extensive cases or in cases that involve complex canal wall-down mastoidectomy cavities. The main differential diagnosis of recurrent cholesteatoma is postsurgical granulation tissue and encephalocele.

Facial nerve injury is an uncommon complication of tympanomastoidectomy. The tympanic and proximal mastoid segments of the facial nerve are most likely to be involved. This may result in a reparative granuloma. Nerve cable grafts are sometimes used to repair the transected nerves. On CT, reparative neuromas appear as bulbous enlargement of the nerve, and on MRI, enhancement of the lesion can be appreciated. Thus, the location and presence of enhancement help differentiate post-mastoidectomy reparative neuroma from recurrent cholesteatoma.

If postoperative cerebrospinal fluid leak is suspected, as discussed earlier, thin-section CT with multiplanar reformatted imaging is the first-line imaging modality for evaluation. CT cisternography is helpful when there are multiple defects. However, thin-section coronal double inversion recovery MRI is particularly useful for evaluating suspected encephalocele after mastoidectomy, which usually results from tegmen dehiscence. This information is important for guiding subsequent surgical repair. Tegmen defects can be repaired using a variety of techniques, including fibrin glue, fascia grafts, muscle graft, fat graft, bone graft, hydroxyapatite (Fig. 8.73), or a combination of these. Some of these materials can resorb over time, predisposing to recurrent cerebrospinal fluid leak and/or encephalocele.

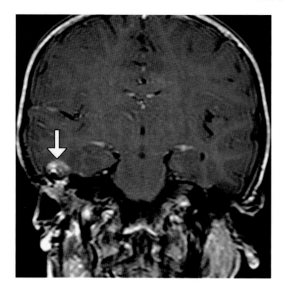

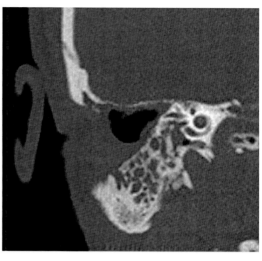

Fig. 8.65 Unstable mastoid cavity. Coronal CT image shows opacification of the residual mastoid air cells and debris along the margins of the mastoidectomy bowl

Fig. 8.64 Coronal post-contrast T1-weighted MR image shows a peripherally enhancing lesion in the right temporal lobe (*arrow*) overlying the right canal mastoidectomy bowl in a patient with a history of mastoiditis

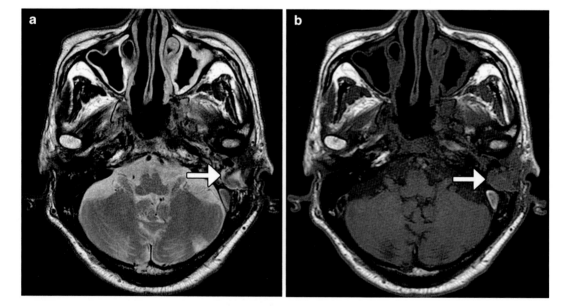

Fig. 8.66 Granulation tissue. Axial T2-weighted (**a**), T1-weighted (**b**), and post-contrast fat-suppressed T1-weighted (**c**) MR images show enhancing soft tissue in the left mastoidectomy bowl (*arrows*)

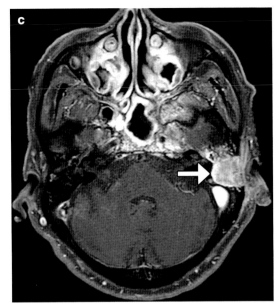

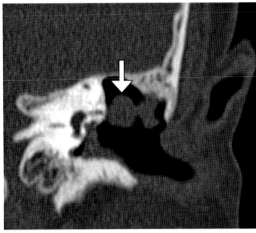

Fig. 8.67 Recurrent cholesteatoma. Axial CT image (**a**) shows globular opacification of the mastoidectomy bowl (*arrow*)

Fig. 8.66 (continued)

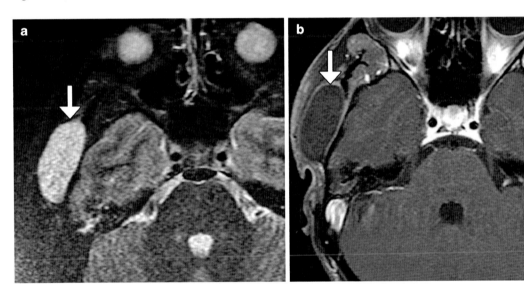

Fig. 8.68 Extratemporal cholesteatoma recurrence. The patient has a history of right mastoidectomy for cholesteatoma. Axial T2-weighted MRI (**a**), post-contrast fat-suppressed T1-weighted MRI (**b**), and ADC map (**c**) show a cystic lesion in the right preauricular subcutaneous tissues with restricted diffusion (*arrows*)

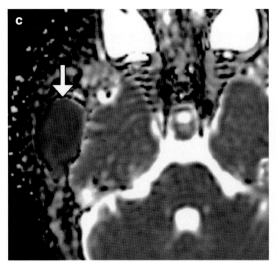

Fig. 8.68 (continued)

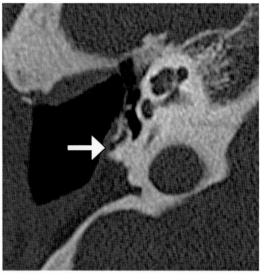

Fig. 8.69 Facial nerve dehiscence. The patient presented with right facial nerve palsy after canal wall-down mastoidectomy. Axial CT image shows a defect in the bone overlying the pyramidal turn of the facial nerve (*arrow*), which is covered by skin graft

Fig. 8.70 Facial nerve injury with reparative neuroma. Axial CT image shows enlargement of the tympanic segment of the facial nerve (*arrow*), which is dehiscent following mastoidectomy and tympanoplasty. Axial post-contrast T1-weighted MRI (**b**) shows enhancement of the lesion (*arrow*)

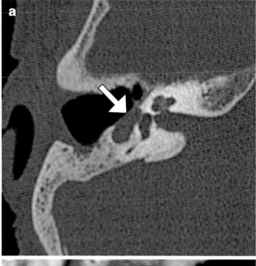

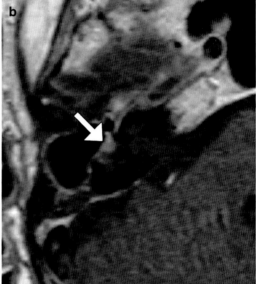

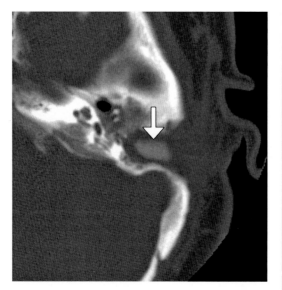

Fig. 8.71 Cerebrospinal fluid leak after mastoidectomy. The patient presented with otorrhea after transmastoid biopsy. Axial image from a CT cisternogram with intrathecal injection of contrast demonstrates a small dehiscence in the tegmen tympani and contrast in the mastoid defect (*arrow*)

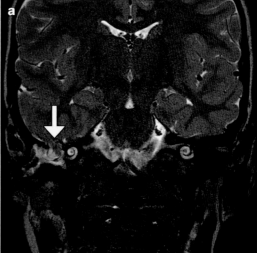

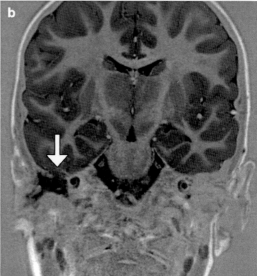

Fig. 8.72 Encephalocele after mastoidectomy. Coronal T2-weighted (**a**) and double inversion recovery (DIR) T1-weighted (**b**) MR images show a defect in the tegmen with extension of the brain and cerebrospinal fluid in the mastoid bowl (*arrows*)

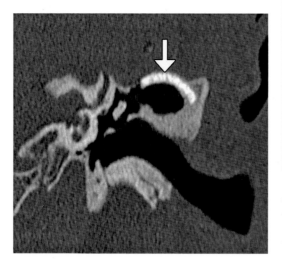

Fig. 8.73 Repair of tegmen defect with hydroxyapatite. Coronal CT image shows a large defect in the tegmen following canal wall-up mastoidectomy, which has been repaired using hydroxyapatite (*arrow*) as well as temporal fascia

8.16   Temporal Bone Resection

8.16.1 Discussion

Treatment of external auditory canal malignancies will often include temporal bone resection. Usually these cases involve squamous cell carcinoma of the external ear, but sometimes parotid malignancies that secondarily extend into the ear and temporal bone. Temporal bone resection is typically classified as lateral, subtotal, or total (radical), some of which are depicted in Figs. 8.74 and 8.75 and listed in Table 8.3. Lateral temporal bone resection involves en bloc removal of the tympanic membrane and entire external auditory canal and is appropriate for tumors limited to the external auditory canal that have not penetrated the middle ear or mastoid. As a consequence of lateral temporal bone resection, the temporomandibular joint is rendered continuous with the tympanomastoid space, while mastoidectomy and auriculectomy

defects are also present. Subtotal temporal bone resection involves extension of lateral temporal bone resection margins to include the middle ear and mastoid structures, the facial nerve, and the labyrinth. Total temporal bone resection involves further extension of subtotal temporal bone resection margins to include the sigmoid sinus/jugular bulb and the intrapetrous carotid artery, but this radical procedure is almost never performed in the modern era. All types of temporal bone resection may be extended to also include additional resection of adjacent involved structures, such as the mandibular condyle or dura. Parotidectomy and neck dissection are usually performed alongside temporal bone resection, and reconstruction may involve primary closure with or without a skin graft if the defect is small, but most often require a myocutaneous flap. Imaging plays an important role in the postoperative follow-up for tumor recurrence (Fig. 8.76). This may involve a combination of CT, MRI, and PET.

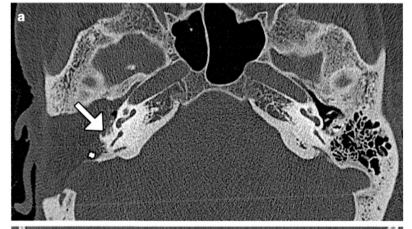
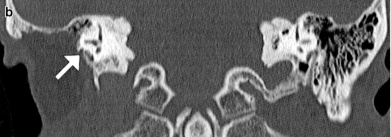

Fig. 8.74 Lateral temporal bone resection. Postoperative axial (**a**) and coronal (**b**) CT images demonstrate essentially complete resection of the tympanic bone and ossicles. The temporomandibular joint is continuous with tympanomastoid defect. The facial nerve is preserved, but skeletonized (*arrows*). The inner ear structures are also preserved. A radial forearm free flap has been packed into the surgical cavity

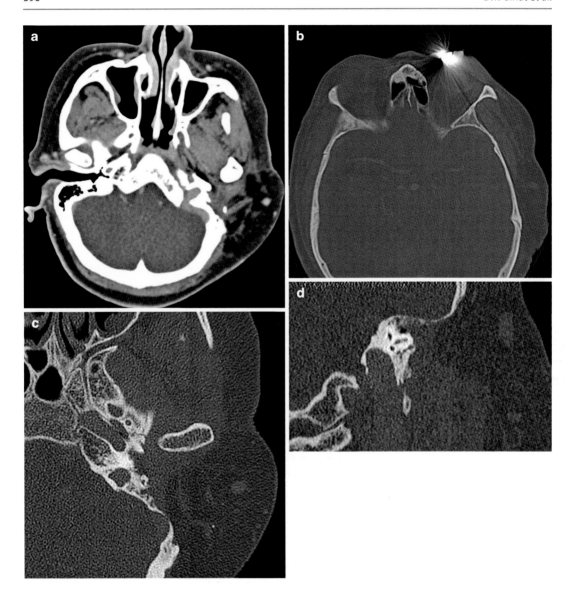

Fig. 8.75 Subtotal temporal bone resection. Axial CT head images (**a**, **b**) show left subtotal temporal bone resection with myocutaneous flap reconstruction. Labyrinth is absent. Since the facial nerve was sacrificed, an eyelid weight was implanted. Axial (**c**) and coronal (**d**) temporal bone CT images show extensive resection of the temporal bone structures, including the expected course of the facial nerve

Table 8.3 Types of temporal bone resection

Temporal bone resection type	Description
Lateral	Removal of the entire external auditory canal and tympanic membrane including attached malleus. Intratemporal facial nerve and inner ear are preserved
Subtotal	Same as lateral temporal bone resection with additional resection of the facial nerve, all middle ear structures, and inner ear. Great vessels are preserved
Total	Same as subtotal temporal bone resection with additional resection of the great vessels (sigmoid sinus/jugular bulb and intrapetrous internal carotid artery)

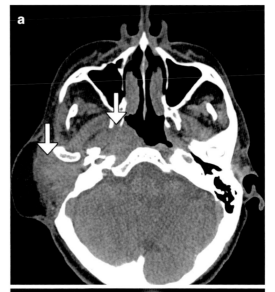

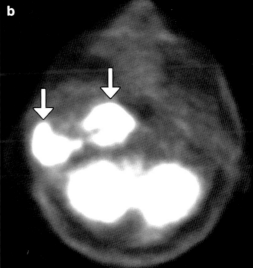

Fig. 8.76 Tumor recurrence after lateral temporal bone resection. The patient has a history of squamous cell carcinoma. Axial CT image (**a**) shows subtle soft tissue attenuation in the resection cavity that extends into the parapharyngeal space (*arrows*) and displaces the flap laterally. The corresponding PET image (**b**) shows considerable hypermetabolic activity within the lesion (*arrows*), which is now very conspicuous. There is normal activity within the cerebellum

8.17 Cochlear Implants

8.17.1 Discussion

Cochlear implants are electronic devices that can provide the sense of sound to patients with severe sensorineural hearing loss by direct stimulation of the cochlear nerve. Cochlear implants consist of an external microphone, external speech processor, external transducer coil, internal receiver-stimulator, and electrode array within the cochlea. The components, particularly the position of the electrodes, are well seen on the modified Stenver or Arcelin view (Fig. 8.77). The removable external component of a cochlear implant houses a microphone, a speech microprocessor, and a radio-emitting coil that not only sends a signal to the implanted receiver-stimulator but also powers the device transcutaneously. The external coil is held in place magnetically. The implanted receiver-stimulator contains a magnet, a computer chip, and an electrode array, which is surgically threaded into the cochlea. The electrodes of this array contain anywhere from 8 to 24 metallic leads that vary depending on the actual device in place. These electrodes are visible on CT as a string of metallic beads.

Typical surgery for cochlear implantation consists of performing a canal-wall-up mastoidectomy and posterior tympanotomy drilled through the facial recess, which is defined as the space between the facial nerve and the chorda tympani. This allows visualization of the round window niche where the electrode is introduced into the scala tympani of the basal turn of the cochlea either via the round window membrane itself or a small cochleostomy drilled immediately adjacent to the round window (Fig. 8.78). The degree of electrode extension into the cochlea will vary depending on the surgeon's wishes based on the length of the particular electrode array chosen and the portion of the cochlea that one wishes to stimulate. For routine cases, it is typical for the electrode to complete at least a 270 degree turn within the cochlea, such that all the electrodes are seated within the cochlea. In patients with labyrinthitis ossificans, a cochleostomy with drill out of the ossified basal turn may be required (Fig. 8.79). A recess is sometimes drilled into the bone posterior to the mastoid cavity where the body of the receiver-stimulator is to be set within a periosteal pocket in order to allow the device to sit flush along the surface of the skull.

Several imaging techniques have been used to depict cochlear implants, including conventional radiography, phase-contrast radiography, cone beam CT, fusion of conventional radiographs and CT images, and spiral CT. Most cochlear implants are only compatible with MRI if the internal magnet is removed through a minor procedure, but at some centers 1.5 T MRI images have been safely obtained by tightly wrapping the head overlying the implant and closely observing the patient during the scan. Alternatively, the electrodes can be left in position, while the rest of the cochlear implant device is removed for the MRI. The electrodes produce negligible artifacts on MRI at 1.5 T (Fig. 8.80). It is undesirable to remove the electrodes for prolonged periods of time because it can be difficult to reinsert the device. Newer cochlear implants may be MRI compatible without removing the internal magnet, even up to 3 T; however, there can be artifact from the indwelling magnet that can limit the usefulness of the MRI if obtained to view structures of the head and neck. The specific model MRI guidelines should nevertheless be verified prior to scanning with MRI.

Fig. 8.77 Cochlear implant components. Modified Stenver (Arcelin) view (**a**) shows the implanted antenna and magnet (*arrowhead*) and electronic components of the receiver-stimulator (*), as well as the electrode array coiled within the cochlea (*arrow*). Photograph of a cochlear implant with an enlarged view of the scalar electrodes in the inset (**b**) (Courtesy of Advanced Bionics)

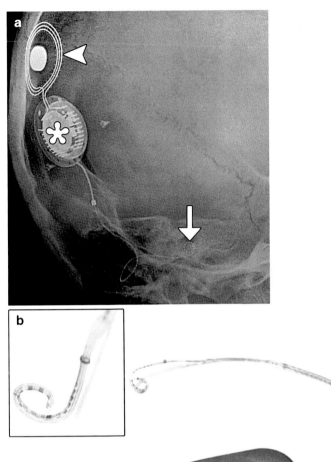
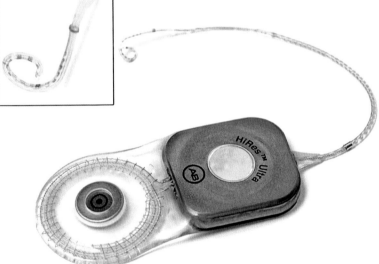

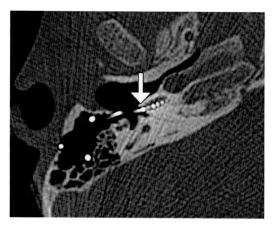

Fig. 8.78 Cochlear implant insertion through the round window. Axial CT image shows that the electrode courses through the mastoid bowl, across the facial recess, and into the cochlea via a widened round window (*arrow*)

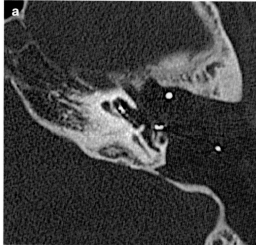

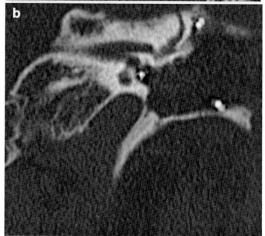

Fig. 8.79 Cochlear implant insertion via cochlear drill out. The patient had a diminutive basal turn of the cochlea. Axial (**a**) and coronal (**b**) CT images show the electrode of the cochlear implant passing through a drilled-out cochleostomy rather than through the round window and hypoplastic basal turn. The mastoid has been obliterated for perilymphatic fistula

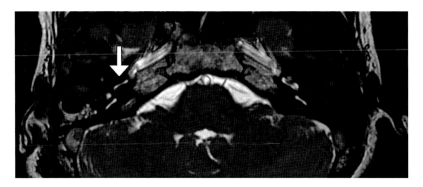

Fig. 8.80 Cochlear implant electrodes on MRI. Axial DRIVE image shows the low signal intensity electrodes in the right cochlea (*arrow*), with no significant artifacts. The subcutaneous magnet component of the implant was removed for the scan

8.18   Cochlear Implant Complications

8.18.1 Discussion

Complications related to cochlear implantation include infection, perilymphatic fistula from the round window or cochleostomy site with pneumolabyrinth, extrusion, erosion of the hardware into the intracranial compartment, device malposition, and extrusion of the electrode out of the cochlea. (Figs. 8.81, 8.82, 8.83, 8.84, 8.85, 8.86, 8.87, 8.88, and 8.89). Malposition of the electrode is a significant cause for cochlear implant malfunction and can be evaluated via dedicated radiographs or temporal bone CT. Potential malpositions to consider include "false insertion" of the electrode into hypotympanic air cells, Eustachian tube, or carotid canal, coiling or buckling of the electrode array within the cochlea, incomplete insertion into the cochlea, and "transcalar insertion" with violation of the basilar membrane and osseous spiral lamina such that the electrode extends from scala tympani into scala vestibuli. Transcalar insertion will result in loss of any residual natural hearing by damaging the delicate neurosensory elements and also will result in postoperative new bone formation that will require excessive high power settings/battery requirements to overcome resulting high impedance. If a congenital cochlear anomaly is present, it is possible for the electrode array to breach the deficient modiolus and extend into the internal auditory canal. A defect in the otic capsule can allow the electrodes to contact the labyrinthine segment of the facial nerve, which can result in unwanted stimulation of the facial nerve.

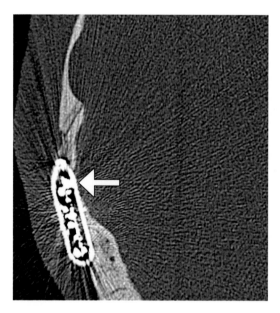

Fig. 8.81 Receiver-stimulator hardware erosion into the skull. Axial CT image shows a defect (*arrow*) in the squamous temporal bone under the receiver-stimulator hardware

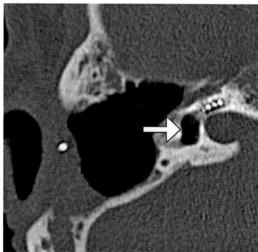

Fig. 8.82 Perilymphatic fistula. Axial CT image shows pneumolabyrinth (*arrow*) following cochlear implantation

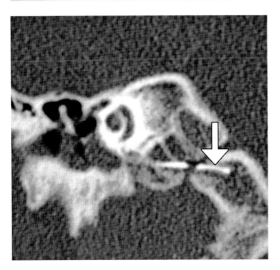

Fig. 8.83 Electrode malpositioning. Coronal CT image shows the "false insertion" of the electrode passing through hypotympanic air cells into the petrous apex and clivus (*arrow*)

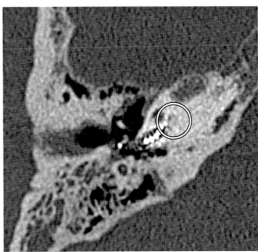

Fig. 8.85 Incomplete cochlear implant electrode insertion. Axial CT image shows the electrodes only partially inserted into the basal turn of the cochlea due to obstruction by labyrinthitis ossificans (*encircled*)

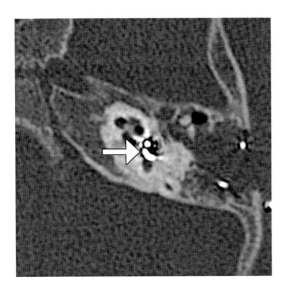

Fig. 8.84 Lateral cochlear implant electrode malpositioning. Axial CT image shows the distal end of the cochlear implant coiled on itself within the vestibule (*arrow*)

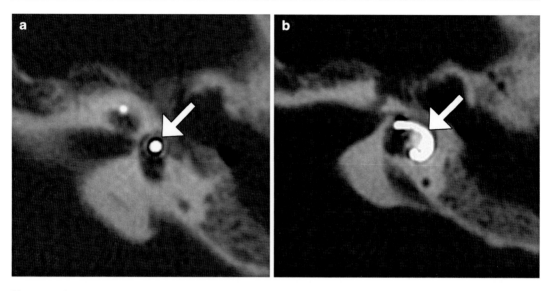

Fig. 8.86 Cochlear implant malpositioning within the vestibule. Axial CT images at two different levels (**a** and **b**) show that the electrodes enter the vestibule and lateral semicircular canal (*arrows*)

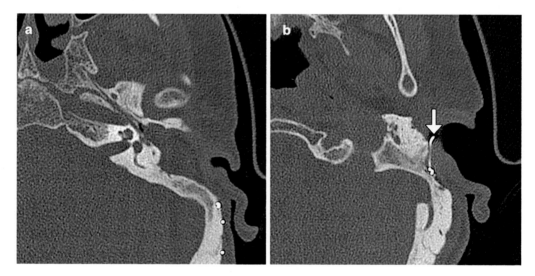

Fig. 8.87 Cochlear implant electrode extrusion. Serial axial CT images (**a–c**) show that the cochlear implant is absent from the cochlea and instead projects into the lumen of the external auditory canal (*arrows*)

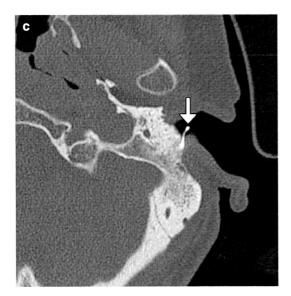

Fig. 8.87 (continued)

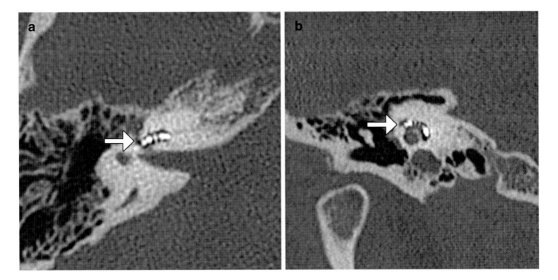

Fig. 8.88 Cochlear implant contact with facial nerve. Axial (**a**) and coronal (**b**) CT images show a defect in the otic capsule with electrodes in contact with the labyrinthine segment of the facial nerve (*arrows*)

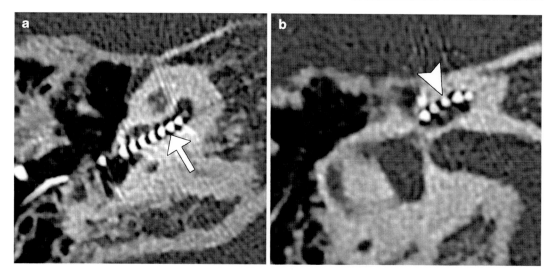

Fig. 8.89 Transcalar electrode array insertion. Axial CT images at two different levels (**a**, **b**) show that the cochlear implant is properly positioned within the scala tympani in the basal turn (*arrow*), but winds up in the scala vestibuli in the middle turn (*arrowhead*)

8.19 Auditory Brainstem Stimulator

8.19.1 Discussion

Auditory brainstem implants (ABIs) are used to provide some form for hearing capacity when the contralateral ear provides no hearing or if there is concern of contralateral hearing loss, such as in neurofibromatosis Type 2 patients. The components of the ABI are analogous to cochlear implants and include a receiver-stimulator and electrode array. The electrodes are implanted via the lateral recess of the fourth ventricle adjacent to the lateral aspect of the cochlear nucleus via a translabyrinthine or retrosigmoid approach (Fig. 8.90).

Complications related to ABI insertion include suboptimal production of auditory stimuli, cerebrospinal fluid leak along the course of the wire, and nonauditory stimuli, such as trigeminal neuralgia. Thin-section CT may be used to evaluate ABIs after implantation, although precise localization can be limited by metallic streak artifacts. Newer ABI models do not contain magnetic components and are MRI compatible.

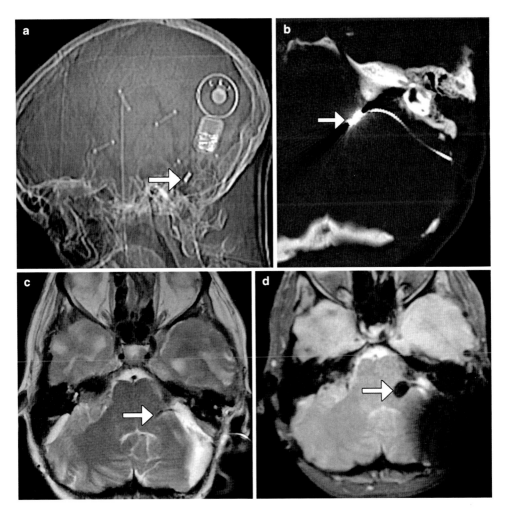

Fig. 8.90 Auditory brainstem stimulator. The patient has a history of neurofibromatosis Type 2 and left-sided hearing loss. Scout image (**a**) shows the receiver-stimulator and electrode tip (*arrow*) in the posterior fossa. Axial CT image (**b**) shows the auditory brain stimulator electrode (*arrow*) positioned in the left cerebellopontine angle. T2-weighted spin echo (**c**) and GRE (**d**) MRI sequences also show the tip of the electrode (*arrows*) in the left cerebellopontine angle, which is more conspicuous on GRE due to blooming effects

8.20   Repair of Perilymphatic Fistula

8.20.1 Discussion

Symptomatic perilymphatic fistulas can be treated via surgical repair. Closure can be obtained using packing materials such as temporalis fascia, which appears as soft tissue attenuation on CT (Fig. 8.91). The main complication is fistula recurrence, which occurs in 8–47% of cases. It is important to note that there may not be an imaging correlate for recurrent perilymphatic fistulas, although graft displacement can sometimes be observed. Temporal bone CT may be useful to evaluate recurrent symptoms following repair, whereby the presence of middle ear opacification beyond the round window niche may indicate recurrent fistula.

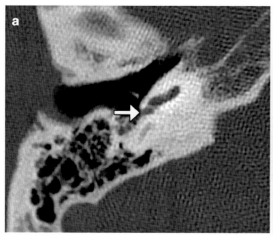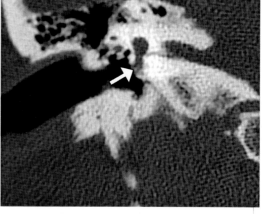

Fig. 8.91 Repair of perilymphatic fistula. The patient has a history of round window perilymphatic fistula repair, status post transcanal exploration and closure. Axial (**a**) and coronal (**b**) CT images demonstrate temporalis fascia packing in the round window niche (*arrows*)

8.21   Endolymphatic Sac Decompression and Shunting

8.21.1   Discussion

Endolymphatic sac decompression and shunting have been used for treating intractable vertigo in patients with Meniere's disease. The procedure consists of performing mastoidectomy and exposing the plate of the bone overlying the sigmoid sinus and posterior cranial fossa dura. These changes are readily depicted on temporal bone CT (Fig. 8.92). The surgery can be limited to decompression alone, in which the endolymphatic sac is not opened. Alternatively, the endolymphatic sac can be incised and drained into either the mastoid or subarachnoid space, whereby a communication is created between the sac and the basal cistern. Silicone shunt tubing or valves can also be inserted and are sometimes visible on temporal bone CT. It is also common to see the bone over the adjacent posterior semicircular canal to be intentionally thinned, but hopefully not violated, as a consequence of this surgery.

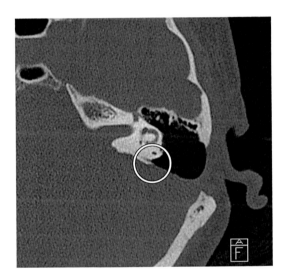

Fig. 8.92 Endolymphatic sac decompression. Axial CT image shows a left mastoidectomy with a defect in the region of the left vestibular aqueduct (*encircled*)

8.22 Labyrinthectomy

8.22.1 Discussion

Labyrinthectomy is a treatment option for Meniere's disease when preservation of hearing is not a consideration. The procedure can be performed via a transmastoid or transcanal approach. The transmastoid approach consists of a canal wall-up mastoidectomy removal of the semicircular canals and ablation of the vestibule (Fig. 8.93). On the other hand, the transcanal approach involves simply opening the vestibule so that the vestibular neurosensory elements can be eliminated via the middle ear by elevating the tympanic membrane and resecting a portion of the scutum, as well as the stapes and incus. A defect between the round and oval windows is created (Fig. 8.94). No matter which approach is used, vestibule defects are sometimes filled with Gelfoam or other packing material.

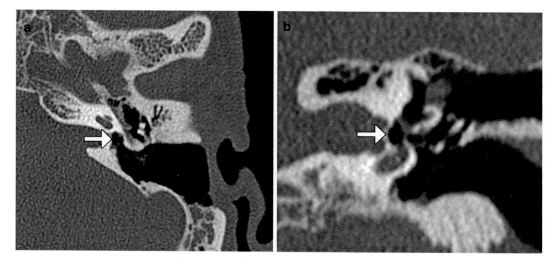

Fig. 8.93 Transmastoid labyrinthectomy. Axial (**a**) and coronal (**b**) CT images show an air-filled cavity (*arrows*) in the expected location of the vestibule, which communicates with the mastoid bowl. The ossicles remain intact

Fig. 8.94 Transcanal labyrinthectomy. Axial (**a**) and coronal (**b**) CT images show a defect that extends inferior to the oval window (*arrow*). There is also disruption of the ossicular chain

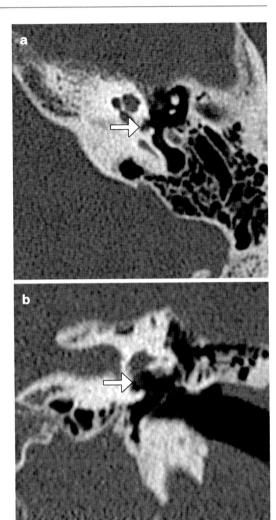

8.23　Vestibular Nerve Section

8.23.1 Discussion

Vestibular nerve sectioning (neurotomy) is another treatment option for intractable Meniere's disease if preservation of residual hearing is a consideration. Vestibular neurotomy consists of delicately severing the vestibular nerve fibers just distal to the division between cochlear and vestibular nerves. This procedure can be performed via a retrosigmoid, retrolabyrinthine, or middle cranial fossa approach, and changes associated with these surgical approaches can be identified on radiologic images (Fig. 8.95). In particular, thin-section steady state MRI sequences, can evaluate for residual vestibular nerve fibers that could be responsible for recurrent vertigo attacks.

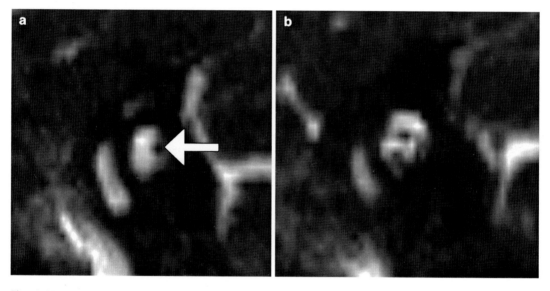

Fig. 8.95 Vestibular neurotomy. Sagittal CISS MRI image (**a**) shows the absence of the vestibular and cochlear nerves in the internal auditory canal. The remaining seventh cranial nerve (*arrow*) sags posteriorly in the internal auditory canal. Sagittal CISS of the normal contralateral side (**b**) shows intact internal auditory canal nerves for comparison

8.24 Superior Semicircular Canal Dehiscence Repair

8.24.1 Discussion

Repair of superior semicircular canal dehiscence is an option to treat associated vestibular and audiological symptoms. The procedure can be performed via a transmastoid or middle cranial fossa approach. Repair can be achieved via several techniques that aim to plug the dehiscent canal and/or resurface and repair the adjacent middle cranial floor. Materials used to accomplish this include bone pate, fascia, and bone wax (plugging), bone graft, cartilage graft, and hydroxyapatite cement (resurfacing and skull base repair). It is very common that these patients have diffuse thinning of the middle cranial fossa floor on both sides and sometimes cerebrospinal fluid leak or encephalocele may also be present. On CT, bone graft, hydroxyapatite, and bone putty are high attenuation (Fig. 8.96), while temporalis fascia and bone wax are generally imperceptible since they are used in small quantities and have imaging characterization that blend in with the surrounding soft tissues.

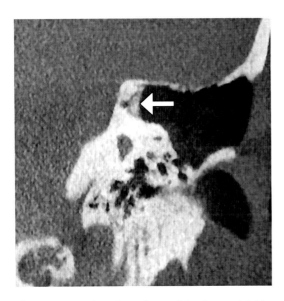

Fig. 8.96 Plugging of superior semicircular canal dehiscence. Coronal CT image demonstrates bone putty (*arrow*) filling the defect along the lateral aspect of the superior semicircular canal. The procedure was performed via a transmastoid approach

8.25 Tube Drainage of Petrous Apex Cholesterol Granuloma

8.25.1 Discussion

Drainage tube insertion can be performed for treating symptomatic petrous apex cholesterol cysts (granulomas). Silastic drainage tubes can be inserted into the lesion after drilling of the temporal bone and creating a drainage tract into the middle ear. Alternatively, the tube can be inserted into the cysts via the middle cranial fossa with drainage into the sphenoid sinus via sphenoidotomy (Fig. 8.97). The desired end result of treatment is permanent ventilation of the cyst cavity (Fig. 8.98). Potential complications of drainage include tube obstruction with cyst recurrence and damage to the labyrinthine structures and surrounding cranial nerves, particularly the facial and trigeminal nerves depending on the approach. Lesions that are not amenable to tube drainage can be treated by complete surgical resection.

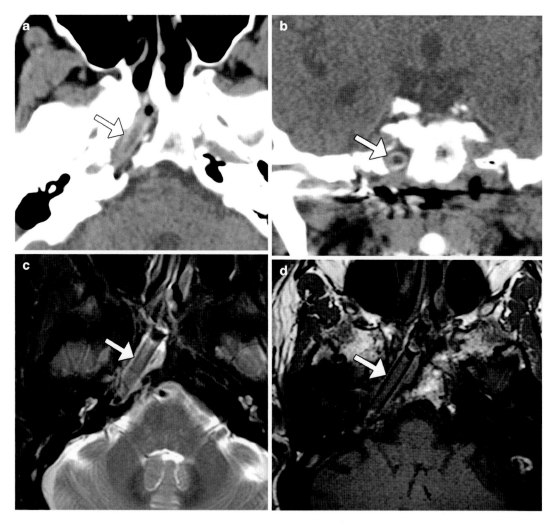

Fig. 8.97 Transsphenoidal tube drainage of cholesterol cyst. Axial (**a**) and coronal (**b**) CT images and axial T2-weighted (**c**) and T1-weighted (**d**) MR images show a Silastic drainage tube (arrows) that extends from the right petrous apex to the sphenoid sinus (Courtesy of Hugh Curtin, M.D.)

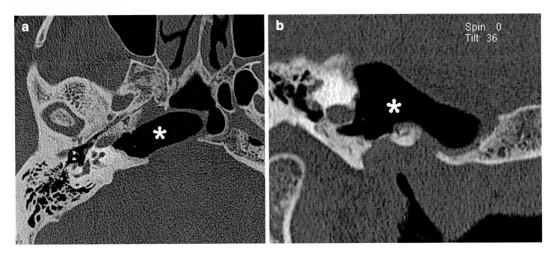

Fig. 8.98 Drained cholesterol cyst. Axial (**a**) and Stenver reformatted (**b**) CT images show an air-filled cavity in the right petrous apex (*), which has demineralized walls

Further Reading

BAHA Device

Azadarmaki R, Tubbs R, Chen DA, Shellock FG (2014) MRI information for commonly used otologic implants: review and update. Otolaryngol Head Neck Surg 150(4):512–519.

Scholz M, Eufinger H, Anders A, Illerhaus B, König M, Schmieder K, Harders A (2003) Intracerebral abscess after abutment change of a bone-anchored hearing aid (BAHA). Otol Neurotol 24(6):896–899

Stewart CM, Clark JH, Niparko JK (2011) Bone-anchored devices in single-sided deafness. Adv Otorhinolaryngol 71:92–102

Auriculectomy

Osborne RF, Shaw T, Zandifar H, Kraus D (2008) Elective parotidectomy in the management of advanced auricular malignancies. Laryngoscope 118(12):2139–2145

Pointer DT Jr, Friedlander PL, Amedee RG, Liu PH, Chiu ES (2010) Infratemporal fossa reconstruction following total auriculectomy: an alternative flap option. J Plast Reconstr Aesthet Surg 63(8):e615–e618

Auricular Reconstruction

Reinisch JF, Lewin S (2009) Ear reconstruction using a porous polyethylene framework and temporoparietal fascia flap. Facial Plast Surg 25(3):181–189

Romo T 3rd, Reitzen SD (2008) Aesthetic microtia reconstruction with Medpor. Facial Plast Surg 24(1):120–128

Canaloplasty and Meatoplasty

Lavy J, Fagan P (2001) Canalplasty: review of 100 cases. J Laryngol Otol 115(4):270–273

Mingkwansook V, Curtin HD, Kelly HR 2015 CT findings in the external auditory canal after transcanal surgery. AJNR Am J Neuroradiol 36(5):982–986.

Parisier SC, Bent JP 3rd (1999) Canalplasty. Otolaryngol Clin North Am 32(3):457–469

Atresiaplasty

De la Cruz A, Teufert KB (2003) Congenital aural atresia surgery: long-term results. Otolaryngol Head Neck Surg 129(1):121–127

Teufert KB, De la Cruz A (2004) Advances in congenital aural atresia surgery: effects on outcome. Otolaryngol Head Neck Surg 131(3):263–270

Myringotomy and Tympanostomy Tubes

Hajiioannou JK, Bathala S, Marnane CN (2009) Case of perilymphatic fistula caused by medially displaced tympanostomy tube. J Laryngol Otol 123(8):928–930

Klein MA, Kelly JK, Eggleston D (1988) Recognizing tympanostomy tubes on temporal bone CT: typical and atypical appearances. AJR Am J Roentgenol 150(6):1411–1414

Myringoplasty and Tympanoplasty

Alicandri-Ciufelli M, Marchioni D, Grammatica A, Soloperto D, Carpeggiani P, Monzani D, Presutti L (2012) Tympanoplasty: an up-to-date pictorial review. J Neuroradiol 39(3):149–157

Elmorsy SM, Amer HE (2011) Insertion of middle-ear silastic sheeting during tympanoplasty: hearing outcomes. J Laryngol Otol 125(5):445–448

Friedman AB, Gluth MB, Moore PC, Dornhoffer JL 2013 Outcomes of cartilage tympanoplasty in the pediatric population. Otolaryngol Head Neck Surg 148(2);297–301

Karaman E, Duman C, Isildak H, Enver O (2010) Composite cartilage island grafts in type 1 tympanoplasty: audiological and otological outcomes. J Craniofac Surg 21(1):37–39

Yetiser S, Hidir Y (2009) Temporalis fascia and cartilage-perichondrium composite shield grafts for reconstruction of the tympanic membrane. Ann Otol Rhinol Laryngol 118(8):570–574

Incus Interposition

O'Reilly RC, Cass SP, Hirsch BE, Kamerer DB, Bernat RA, Poznanovic SP (2005) Ossiculoplasty using incus interposition: hearing results and analysis of the middle ear risk index. Otol Neurotol 26(5):853–858

Stone JA, Mukherji SK, Jewett BS, Carrasco VN, Castillo M (2000) CT evaluation of prosthetic ossicular reconstruction procedures: what the otologist needs to know. Radiographics 20(3):593–605

Partial Ossicular Reconstruction Prosthesis (PORP), Total Ossicular Reconstruction Prosthesis (TORP), and Vibrating Ossicular Prosthesis (VORP)

Gluth, MB, Moore PC. Dornhoffer JL 2012 Method and reproducibility of a standardized technique of ossiculoplasty technique.Otol Neurotol 33(7);1207–1212

Kiefer J, Arnold W, Staudenmaier R (2006) Round window stimulation with an implantable hearing aid (Soundbridge) combined with autogenous reconstruction of the auricle – a new approach. ORL J Otorhinolaryngol Relat Spec 68(6): 378–385

Stone JA, Mukherji SK, Jewett BS, Carrasco VN, Castillo M (2000) CT evaluation of prosthetic ossicular reconstruction procedures: what the otologist needs to know. Radiographics 20(3):593–605

Stapedectomy, Stapedotomy, and Stapes Prosthesis

Fritsch MH (2007) MRI scanners and the stapes prosthesis. Otol Neurotol 28(6):733–738

Stone JA, Mukherji SK, Jewett BS, Carrasco VN, Castillo M (2000) CT evaluation of prosthetic ossicular reconstruction procedures: what the otologist needs to know. Radiographics 20(3):593–605

Ossicular Prosthesis Complications

Kösling S, Bootz F (2001) CT and MR imaging after middle ear surgery. Eur J Radiol 40(2):113–118

Stone JA, Mukherji SK, Jewett BS, Carrasco VN, Castillo M (2000) CT evaluation of prosthetic ossicular reconstruction procedures: what the otologist needs to know. Radiographics 20(3):593–605

Transcanal Atticotomy

Tarabichi M (2004) Endoscopic management of limited attic cholesteatoma. Laryngoscope 114(7):1157–1162

Tarabichi M (2010) Transcanal endoscopic management of cholesteatoma. Otol Neurotol 31(4):580–588

Eustachian Tube Occlusion Procedures

Hacein-Bey L, Conneely MF, Hijaz TA, Leonetti JP (2010) Radiologic appearance of chronic parapharyngeal Teflon granuloma. Am J Otolaryngol 31(5): 392–394

Kirsch CF, Suh JD, Lufkin RB, Canalis RF (2007) False-positive positron-emission tomography-CT of a Teflon granuloma in the parapharyngeal space occurring after treatment for a patulous Eustachian tube. AJNR Am J Neuroradiol 28(7):1371–1372

Sato T, Kawase T, Yano H, Suetake M, Kobayashi T (2005) Trans-tympanic silicone plug insertion for chronic patulous Eustachian tube. Acta Otolaryngol 125(11):1158–1163.

Mastoidectomy and Mastoid Obliteration

Gluth MB, Friedman AB, Atcherson SR, Dornhoffer JL (2013) Hearing aid tolerance after revision and obliteration of canal wall-down mastoidectomy cavities. Otol Neurotol 34(4);711–714

Bennett M, Warren F, Haynes D (2006) Indications and technique in mastoidectomy. Otolaryngol Clin North Am 39(6):1095–1113

Mehta RP, Harris JP (2006) Mastoid obliteration. Otolaryngol Clin North Am 39(6):1129–1142

Mukherji SK, Mancuso AA, Kotzur IM, Slattery WH 3rd, Swartz JD, Tart RP, Nall A (1994) CT of the temporal bone: findings after mastoidectomy, ossicular reconstruction, and cochlear implantation. AJR Am J Roentgenol 163(6):1467–1471

Mastoidectomy Complications

Gluth MB, Metrailer AM, Dornhoffer JL, Moore PC (2012) Patterns of failure in canal wall down mastoidectomy cavity instability. Otol Neurotol 33(6);998–1001

Kösling S, Bootz F (2001) CT and MR imaging after middle ear surgery. Eur J Radiol 40(2):113–118

Lloyd KM, DelGaudio JM, Hudgins PA (2008) Imaging of skull base cerebrospinal fluid leaks in adults. Radiology 248(3):725–736

Maheshwari S, Mukherji SK (2002) Diffusion-weighted imaging for differentiating recurrent cholesteatoma from granulation tissue after mastoidectomy: case report. AJNR Am J Neuroradiol 23(5):847–849

Nadol JB Jr (1985) Causes of failure of mastoidectomy for chronic otitis media. Laryngoscope 95(4):410–413

Neely JG, Kuhn JR (1985) Diagnosis and treatment of iatrogenic cerebrospinal fluid leak and brain herniation during or following mastoidectomy. Laryngoscope 95(11):1299–1300

Lateral Temporal Bone Resection

Barrs DM (2001) Temporal bone carcinoma. Otolaryngol Clin North Am 34(6):1197–1218, x

Gidley PW (2009) Managing malignancies of the external auditory canal. Expert Rev. Anticancer Ther 9(9):1277–1282

Metrailer AM, Gluth MB (2013) Lateral temporal bone resection. In: Kountakis SE (ed) Encyclopedia of otolaryngology, head & neck surgery, 1st edn. Heidelberg, Springer, pp 1458–1462.

Moore MG, Deschler DG, McKenna MJ, Varvares MA, Lin DT (2007) Management outcomes following lateral temporal bone resection for ear and temporal bone malignancies. Otolaryngol Head Neck Surg 137(6): 893–898

Willging JP, Pensak ML (1991) Temporal bone resection. Ear Nose Throat J 70(9):612–617

Cochlear Implants

Briggs RJ, Tykocinski M, Stidham K, Roberson JB (2005) Cochleostomy site: implications for electrode placement and hearing preservation. Acta Otolaryngol 125(8):870–876

Fischer N, Pinggera L, Weichbold V, Dejaco D, Schmutzhard J, Widmann G (2015) Radiologic and functional evaluation of electrode dislocation from the scala tympani to the scala vestibuli in patients with cochlear implants. AJNR Am J Neuroradiol 36(2):372–377.

Verbist BM, Frijns JH, Geleijns J, van Buchem MA (2005) Multisection CT as a valuable tool in the postoperative assessment of cochlear implant patients. AJNR Am J Neuroradiol 26(2):424–429

Witte RJ, Lane JI, Driscoll CL, Lundy LB, Bernstein MA, Kotsenas AL, Kocharian A (2003) Pediatric and adult cochlear implantation. Radiographics 23(5):1185–1200

Cochlear Implant Complications

Gluth, MB, Singh R, Atlas MD (2011) Prevention and management of cochlear implant infections Cochlear Implants Int 12(4):223–227

Sunde J, Webb JB, Moore PC, Gluth MB, Dornhoffer JL (2013) Cochlear implant failure, revision, and reimplantation. Otol Neurotol 34(9);1670–1674

Jain R, Mukherji SK (2003) Cochlear implant failure: imaging evaluation of the electrode course. Clin Radiol 58(4):288–293

Mecca MA, Wagle W, Lupinetti A, Parnes S (2003) Complication of cochlear implantation surgery. AJNR Am J Neuroradiol 24(10):2089–2091

Auditory Brainstem Stimulator

Lo WW (1998) Imaging of cochlear and auditory brain stem implantation. AJNR Am J Neuroradiol 19(6):1147–1154

Patel SH, Halpern CH, Shepherd TM, Timpone VM. Electrical stimulation and monitoring devices of the CNS: An imaging review. J Neuroradiol. 2017 Feb 6. pii: S0150-9861(17)30047-0

Repair of Perilymphatic Fistula

Black FO, Pesznecker S, Norton T, Fowler L, Lilly DJ, Shupert C, Hemenway WG, Peterka RJ, Jacobson ES (1991) Surgical management of perilymph fistulas.

A new technique. Arch Otolaryngol Head Neck Surg 117(6):641–648

Black FO, Pesznecker S, Norton T, Fowler L, Lilly DJ, Shupert C, Hemenway WG, Peterka RJ, Jacobson ES (1992) Surgical management of perilymphatic fistulas: a Portland experience. Am J Otol 13(3):254–262

Endolymphatic Sac Decompression and Shunting

Brinson GM, Chen DA, Arriaga MA (2007) Endolymphatic mastoid shunt versus endolymphatic sac decompression for Ménière's disease. Otolaryngol Head Neck Surg 136(3):415–421

Derebery MJ, Fisher LM, Berliner K, Chung J, Green K (2010) Outcomes of endolymphatic shunt surgery for Ménière's disease: comparison with intratympanic gentamicin on vertigo control and hearing loss. Otol Neurotol 31(4):649–655

Durland WF Jr, Pyle GM, Connor NP (2005) Endolymphatic sac decompression as a treatment for Meniere's disease. Laryngoscope 115(8):1454–1457

Lee IJ, Choi AL, Yie MY, Yoon JY, Jeon EY, Koh SH, Yoon DY, Lim KJ, Im HJ (2010) CT evaluation of local leakage of bone cement after percutaneous kyphoplasty and vertebroplasty. Acta Radiol 51(6):649–654

Teufert KB, Doherty J (2010) Endolymphatic sac shunt, labyrinthectomy, and vestibular nerve section in Meniere's disease. Otolaryngol Clin North Am 43(5):1091–1111

Labyrinthectomy

Berryhill WE, Graham MD (2002) Chemical and physical labyrinthectomy for Meniere's disease. Otolaryngol Clin North Am 35(3):675–682

Katzenell U, Gordon M, Page M (2010) Intratympanic gentamicin injections for the treatment of Ménière's disease. Otolaryngol Head Neck Surg 143(5 Suppl 3):S24–S29

Teufert KB, Doherty J (2010) Endolymphatic sac shunt, labyrinthectomy, and vestibular nerve section in Meniere's disease. Otolaryngol Clin North Am 43(5):1091–1111

Vestibular Nerve Sectioning

Aw ST, Magnussen JS, Todd MJ, McCormack S, Halmagyi GM (2006) MRI of the vestibular nerve after selective vestibular neurectomy. Acta Otolaryngol 126(10):1053–1056

Teufert KB, Doherty J (2010) Endolymphatic sac shunt, labyrinthectomy, and vestibular nerve section in

Meniere's disease. Otolaryngol Clin North Am 43(5):
1091–1111

Superior Semicircular Canal Dehiscence Repair

Agrawal SK, Parnes LS (2008) Transmastoid superior semicircular canal occlusion. Otol Neurotol 29(3):363–367
Fiorino F, Barbieri F, Pizzini FB, Beltramello A (2010) A dehiscent superior semicircular canal may be plugged and resurfaced via the transmastoid route. Otol Neurotol 31(1):136–139
Portmann D, Guindi S (2008) Surgery of the semicircular canals. Rev Laryngol Otol Rhinol (Bord) 129(1):3–9
Vlastarakos PV, Proikas K, Tavoulari E, Kikidis D, Maragoudakis P, Nikolopoulos TP (2009) Efficacy

assessment and complications of surgical management for superior semicircular canal dehiscence: a meta-analysis of published interventional studies. Eur Arch Otorhinolaryngol 266(2):177–186

Tube Drainage of Cholesterol Cysts

Jaramillo M, Windle-Taylor PC (2001) Large cholesterol granuloma of the petrous apex treated via subcochlear drainage. J Laryngol Otol 115(12):1005–1009
Sanna M, Dispenza F, Mathur N, De Stefano A, De Donato G (2009) Otoneurological management of petrous apex cholesterol granuloma. Am J Otolaryngol 30(6):407–414
Sincoff EH, Liu JK, Matsen L, Dogan A, Kim I, McMenomey SO, Delashaw JB Jr (2007) A novel treatment approach to cholesterol granulomas. Technical note. J Neurosurg 107(2):446–450

Imaging of Orthognathic, Maxillofacial, and Temporomandibular Joint Surgery

9

Daniel Thomas Ginat, Per-Lennart A. Westesson, and Russell Reid

9.1 Vertical Ramus Osteotomy

9.1.1 Discussion

Intraoral vertical ramus osteotomy is a treatment option for mandibular prognathism. In this technique, a vertically oriented cut made in the mandibular ramus allows the mandibular ramus to be lengthened and the temporomandibular joint disc to recapture (Fig. 9.1). The procedure yields satisfactory results and has fewer complications than intra-articular techniques. Expected changes following vertical ramus osteotomy that can be appreciated on imaging include cortical bone thickening, narrowing of the bone marrow space, medial tilting of the mandibular condyle, and masticator muscle atrophy (Fig. 9.2).

D.T. Ginat, M.D., M.S. (✉)
Department of Radiology, University of Chicago, Chicago, IL, USA
e-mail: dtg1@uchicago.edu

P.-L. A. Westesson, M.D., Ph.D., D.D.S.
Division of Neuroradiology, University of Rochester Medical Center, Rochester, NY, USA

R. Reid, M.D., Ph.D.
Department of Surgery, University of Chicago, Chicago, IL, USA

© Springer International Publishing Switzerland 2017
D.T. Ginat, P.-L.A. Westesson (eds.), *Atlas of Postsurgical Neuroradiology*,
DOI 10.1007/978-3-319-52341-5_9

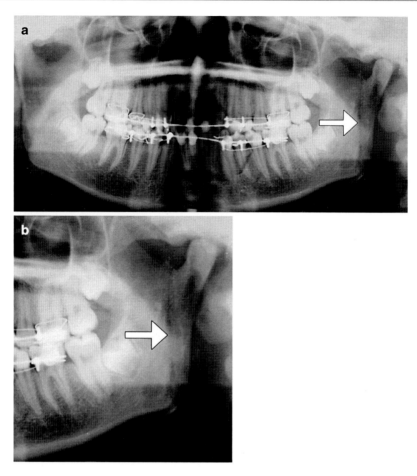

Fig. 9.1 Vertical ramus osteotomy. The patient has a history of temporomandibular joint disc dysfunction. Panorex (**a**) and lateral radiograph (**b**) show a unilateral left mandibular ramus vertical osteotomy (*arrows*)

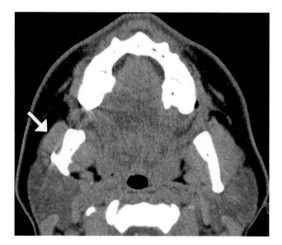

Fig. 9.2 Muscle atrophy after vertical ramus osteotomy. Axial CT image shows mildly decreased bulk of the masticator muscles on the right (*arrow*), ipsilateral to where vertical ramus osteotomy was performed

9.2   Sagittal Split Osteotomy

9.2.1   Discussion

The sagittal split osteotomy is a commonly performed procedure for correcting maxillofacial deformities, such as mandibular hypoplasia or hyperplasia. The surgery consists of bilateral osteotomies through the mandibular ramus with either advancement or setback of the mandibular body (Fig. 9.3). Once repositioned, the mandible is internally fixed using either position screws or plates and screws. Sagittal split osteotomies are sometimes combined with other types of maxillofacial procedures, such as the LeFort I osteotomy. Dysesthesia of the inferior alveolar nerve is one of the most common complications since the osteotomy is in the region of the inferior alveolar nerve. Facial nerve palsy and maxillary nerve pseudoaneurysm are rare complications of the sagittal split surgery.

Fig. 9.3 Sagittal split osteotomy. The patient has a history of maxillary hypoplasia and transverse discrepancy and mandibular hyperplasia. Coronal (**a**) and 3D CT (**b**) images show an osteotomy gap through the mandibular angle (*arrows*) and screw fixation

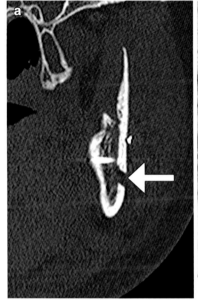
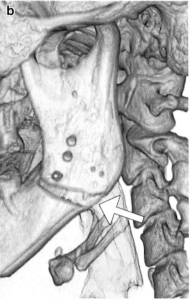

9.3   Genioplasty

9.3.1   Discussion

Genioplasty consists of altering the projection of the genial tubercle of the mandible. It can be performed via an osteotomy through the genial tubercle and can generally be described as shortening or lengthening genioplasty. The genial tubercle can be repositioned in all three planes to correct the sagittal, vertical, and transverse components of the chin deformity by sliding the bone fragment (Fig. 9.4). The osteotomy is performed well below the dental roots and mental foramina in order to avoid complications. Prostheses can be used for lengthening genioplasty, such as those composed of silicone, either alone or in conjunction with advancement osteotomy (Figs. 9.5 and 9.6).

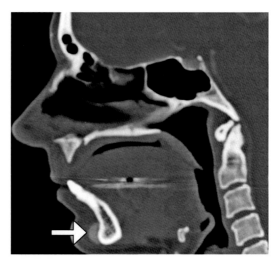

Fig. 9.5 Chin augmentation with implant. Coronal CT images show a silicone prosthesis (*arrow*) positioned anterior to the genial tubercle

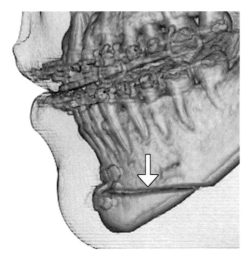

Fig. 9.4 Sliding genioplasty. 3D CT image shows anterior translation of the inferior portion of the mandibular body, producing a step-off (*arrow*)

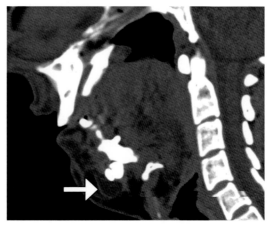

Fig. 9.6 Lengthening genioplasty with combined osteotomy and implant. The patient has a history of Nager's syndrome with severe micrognathia. Sagittal CT image shows the low attenuation porous polyethylene implant (*arrow*) and the advanced genial tubercle with fixation hardware

9.4   Mandibular Angle Augmentation

9.4.1   Discussion

Mandibular angle augmentation with alloplastic implants is an option for correcting hemifacial microsomia and other deformities (Fig. 9.7). The most commonly used materials for augmentation include silicone and porous polyethylene. The goal is to improve facial contours while maintaining the pterygomasseteric sling. Cross-sectional imaging can be useful for evaluating the position of the implants and assessing for complications, such as foreign body granulomas and infection.

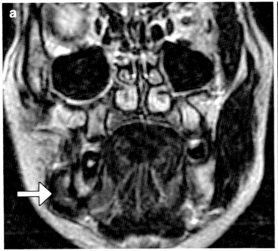 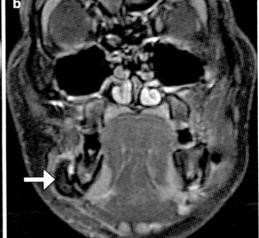

Fig. 9.7 Mandibular angle augmentation. The patient has a history of hypoplastic right mandible in a patient with hemifacial microsomia. The implant has a density intermediate between fat and fluid. The coronal T2-weighted (a) and contrast-enhanced T1-weighted (b) MR images show that the implant material has intermediate T2 and low T1 signal (*arrows*)

9.5   Mandibular Distraction

9.5.1   Discussion

Mandibular distraction devices are used for mandibular bone lengthening to treat both posttraumatic deformities and congenital mandibular deficiencies. The devices are available as single (Fig. 9.8) versus multivector/curvilinear (Fig. 9.9) and internal versus external designs. In addition, transport distractors can be used to shift bone fragments anteriorly or posteriorly (Fig. 9.10). The devices are usually composed of stainless steel or titanium and are therefore radiopaque and can be adjusted from the exterior. The devices are attached to the mandible after mandibular osteotomy has been performed. The goal of this technique is to promote gradual bone growth (osteogenesis) across the gap created by the corticotomy and distraction. Bone growth, alignment, and most complications can be evaluated via radiographs or CT. Complications of mandibular distraction osteogenesis include relapse, tooth injury, hypertrophic scarring, nerve injury, infection, inappropriate distraction vector, device failure, fusion error, and temporomandibular joint injury.

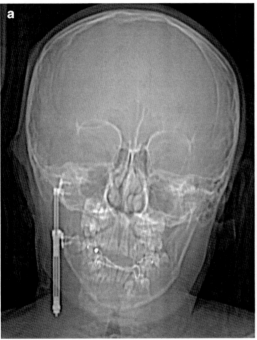
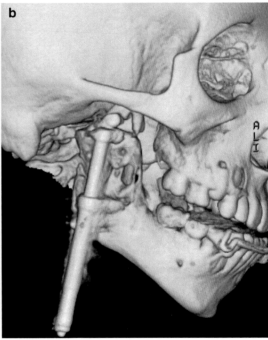

Fig. 9.8 Single-vector distraction device. The child has a history of congenital right mandibular deficiency. Scout (**a**) and 3D CT (**b**) images demonstrate a single-vector right mandibular device in position, which spans the osteotomy gap in the mandibular ramus

Fig. 9.9 Curvilinear distraction device. Sagittal CT images (**a**, **b**) obtained at different time points show interval inferior advancement of the lower foot of the device

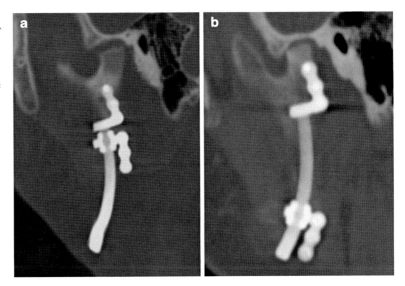

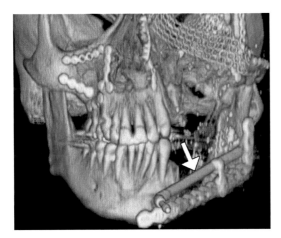

Fig. 9.10 Transport distraction device. The patient has extensive facial fractures secondary to a gunshot wound. 3D CT image shows the transport distractor device (*arrow*) positioned across the left mandibular body defect with satisfactory vector alignment

9.6   LeFort I Osteotomy

9.6.1   Discussion

The LeFort I osteotomy procedure and its modifications are commonly performed to correct malocclusion and maxillomandibular deformities. LeFort I osteotomies and modifications thereof are performed in conjunction with other procedures, such as sagittal split osteotomies and approaches to the skull base via a transoral route. The standard procedure involves separating and moving forward the anterolateral walls of the maxillary sinus, inferior portion of the nasal cavity, and pterygoid plates. Fixation of the osteotomy fragments can be accomplished using microfixation plates and screws. Alternatively, maxillary distractors can be used to gradually correct the deformity as osteogenesis progresses. Bone grafts can also be applied adjacent to the osteotomy site in order to promote healing. Diagnostic imaging may be used to assess postoperative alignment, for which high-resolution CT with 3D reformats is particularly insightful (Fig. 9.11). Anatomical complications occur in 2 to 3% of cases and include deviation of the nasal septum, nonunion of the osteotomy gap, and impingement upon the nasolacrimal duct (Fig. 9.12), while significant infections, such as abscesses or maxillary sinusitis, occur in approximately 1% of cases. Furthermore, perforation of the periosteum in the maxillary sinuses can lead to herniation of the buccal fat pad, which may not only obscure the surgical field but can lead to sinus obstruction (Fig. 9.13). Neurovascular injury involving the palatine canal can occur with pterygomaxillary disjunction when the osteotomy extends too far posteriorly beyond the piriform rim (Fig. 9.14).

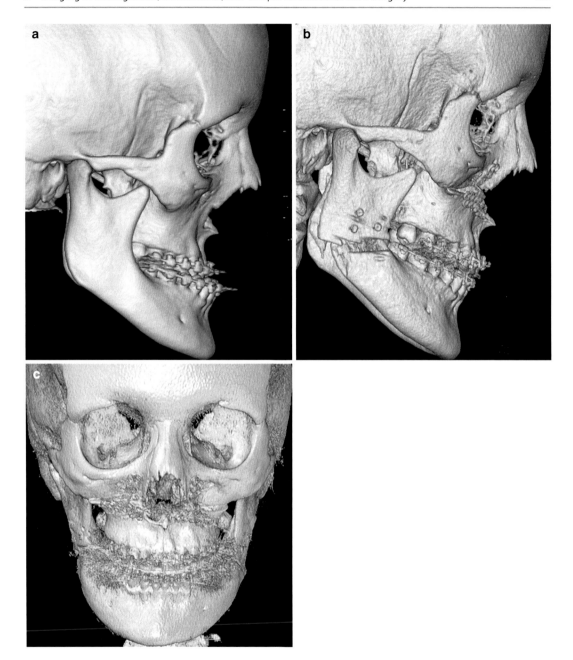

Fig. 9.11 LeFort I osteotomy with microfixation plate. Preoperative 3D CT image (**a**) shows maxillary underjet associated with midface hypoplasia. Postoperative 3D CT images (**b** and **c**) show bilateral LeFort I osteotomies secured with plates and screws, resulting in improved dental occlusion. Bilateral sagittal split osteotomies were also performed

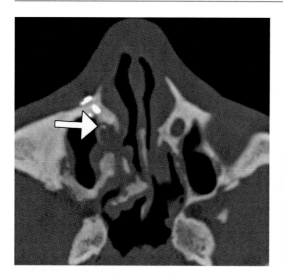

Fig. 9.12 Nasolacrimal duct obstruction following LeFort I osteotomy with internal fixation. Axial CT images show a bone fragment (*arrow*) displaced into the right nasolacrimal duct by the adjacent screw

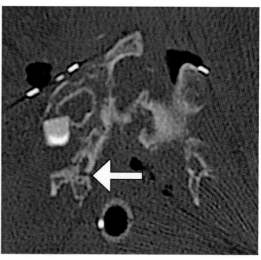

Fig. 9.14 Palatine canal disruption. Axial CT image shows the LeFort osteotomy traversing the right greater palatine canal (*arrow*)

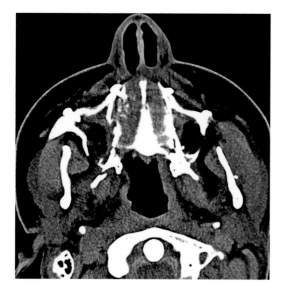

Fig. 9.13 LeFort I surgery with buccal fat herniation into the maxillary sinus. Axial CT image shows portions of buccal fat within the bilateral maxillary sinuses

9.7   LeFort III Osteotomy

9.7.1   Discussion

The LeFort III procedure is indicated for correcting midface hypoplasia involving the nasal and zygomatic complex and orbits, such as with Crouzon, Apert, and Pfeiffer syndromes. Indeed, LeFort III advancement can augment the orbital volume and surface area with correction of the ocular bulb proptosis in addition to correcting malocclusion. While variations exist, the LeFort III procedure essentially involves performing osteotomies through the frontozygomatic suture, floor of the orbit, and the nasion and separating the vomer and ethmoid from the cranial base in the midline and the pterygomaxillary junction. Mobilization of the midface is an extensive procedure, with a high risk of blood loss. In order to minimize morbidity, gradual advancement via distraction osteogenesis can be performed (Fig. 9.15). Once again, high-resolution craniofacial CT with 3D reconstructions can be used to assess the degree of anatomic changes after surgical treatment and evaluate certain complications. In addition to some of the complications that may be encountered with LeFort I osteotomy and distraction,

complications particular to LeFort III procedures include cerebrospinal fluid rhinorrhea, meningitis, and ocular and cerebral injury.

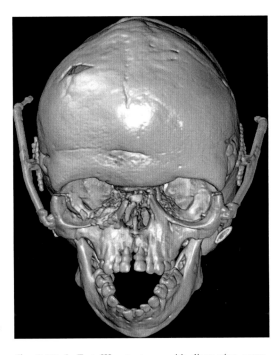

Fig. 9.15 LeFort III osteotomy with distraction osteogenesis. Postoperative 3D CT image shows bilateral transorbital and zygomatic osteotomies with distraction devices in position

9.8   Fixation of Mandible Fractures

9.8.1   Discussion

A variety of techniques can be used to treat mandible fractures, including maxillomandibular fixation (Figs. 9.16 and 9.17), open reduction and internal fixation using plates and screws with or without maxillomandibular fixation (Fig. 9.18), and external fixation device application (Fig. 9.19). Maxillomandibular fixation consists of applying circumdental wires, securing Erich arch bars or their derivatives to the mandible and maxilla, confirming appropriate reduction, and applying fixation wires.

Complications that may result from mandible fracture fixation include malunion/nonunion, hardware failure, and osteomyelitis. Imaging plays a role in evaluating these complications and planning a secondary operation. The panorex and 3D CT images are particularly useful for providing a complete view of the hardware and fractures. Most of the hardware fixation components are metallic, although sometimes stiff rubber bands are used to secure the maxilla to the mandible

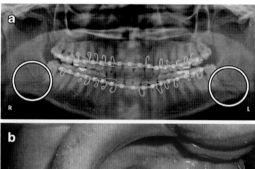
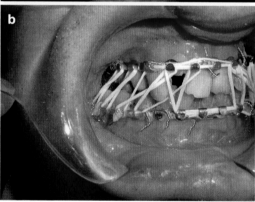

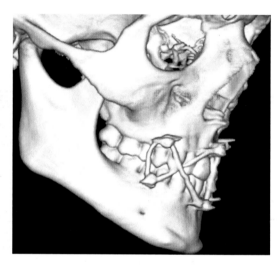

Fig. 9.17 Maxillomandibular fixation with intermaxillary fixation (IMF) screws and wire. 3D CT shows the screws securing the wire in a figure of eight configuration

Fig. 9.16 Maxillomandibular fixation with Erich arch bars. Panorex (**a**) shows bilateral mandibular fractures (*encircled*) and the metallic maxillomandibular fixation hardware at the level of the maxilla. Clinical photograph of maxillomandibular fixation with rubber bands (**b**) (Courtesy of Patrik Keshishian, DDS)

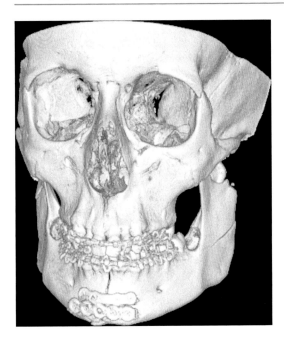

Fig. 9.18 Open reduction and internal fixation and maxillomandibular fixation. 3D CT image shows plate and screw fixation of a mandible body fracture. Bilateral displaced subcondylar fractures are also present without hardware fixation

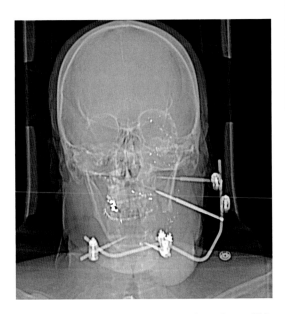

Fig. 9.19 External fixation of comminuted mandible fractures. Frontal radiographic image shows the external fixation device in position. Numerous other facial fractures treated via internal fixation and scattered metallic debris are also noted, which represent bullet fragments from a self-inflicted gunshot wound

9.9   Mandibulotomy

9.9.1   Discussion

The transcervical and transcervical-parotid approaches are routinely performed to resect tumors of the parapharyngeal space. Occasionally, the wider exposure necessary for large or malignant tumors can be provided by midline or parasymphyseal mandibulotomy (Fig. 9.20). An additional mandibular ramus osteotomy, or "double osteotomy," can be performed if additional exposure is required. These maneuvers allow for complete tumor resection without significant disruption of dentition, sensation, or occlusion.

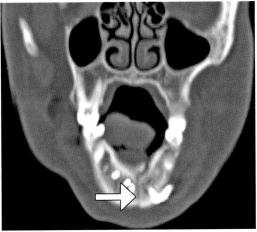

Fig. 9.20 Parasymphyseal mandibulotomy. The patient is status post tongue base carcinoma resection. Mandibulotomy was performed to gain access to the lesion. Coronal CT image shows a parasagittal defect in the body of the mandible (*arrow*), which is otherwise fixed via metal plate and screws

9.10 Enucleation

9.10.1 Discussion

Enucleation of tumors and cysts can produce irregular margins and periosteal reaction that appears aggressive and can resemble infection of tumor recurrence/progression (Fig. 9.21). Sometimes the cavities are filled with bone graft material. Nevertheless, healing and spontaneous filling of the residual cavities have been reported to occur in all cases of uncomplicated mandibular cyst enucleation. In particular, the cavities generally decrease in size by over 80% by 24 months. Similarly, bone density increases by over 90% by 24 months on average. Complications of these procedures include tumor recurrence or seeding, injury to the inferior alveolar nerve, osteomyelitis, and soft tissue infections.

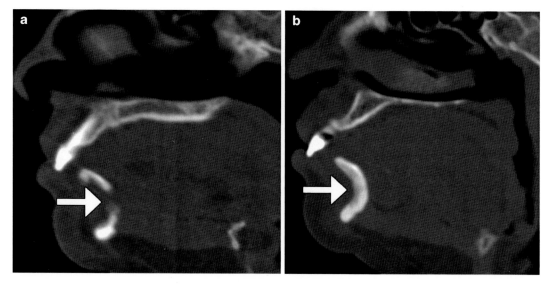

Fig. 9.21 Enucleation. The patient has a history of brown tumor of the mandible. Sagittal CT image obtained 3 weeks enucleation (**a**) shows a defect in the right mandibular body (*arrow*). Sagittal CT obtained 3 months later (**b**) demonstrates interval healing of the defect (*arrow*)

9.11 Cyst Decompression

9.11.1 Discussion

Decompression with stenting can be used to treat large mandibular cysts (Fig. 9.22). The stents typically remain in position for about 6–8 months, at which point the cysts decrease in size on average by 80%. The procedure consists of unroofing the cyst, irrigating the cyst cavity. The stents are inserted in the cavity and secured by the overlying mucosa and sutures. The stent appears as a high-attenuation tubular structure on CT.

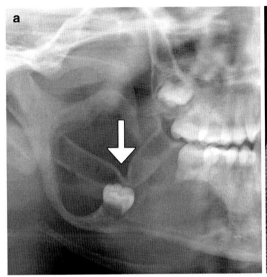 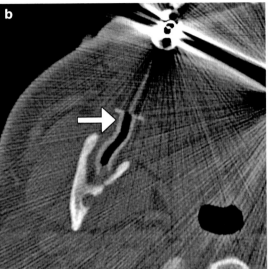

Fig. 9.22 Cyst drainage. Panoramic radiograph (**a**) in a patient with a right mandibular angle dentigerous cyst treated with fenestration and stent decompression (*arrow*). Axial image (**b**) in a different patient with a history of odontogenic keratocyst shows a stent (*arrow*) within a right mandibular cyst cavity

9.12 Coronoidectomy

9.12.1 Discussion

Excessively elongated coronoid processes of the mandible can result in trismus. Treatment consists of coronoidectomy, which can be performed endoscopically, and involves performing osteotomies across the base of the coronoid process but often leaving at least some portion of the coronoid process behind (Fig. 9.23). Alternatively, transzygomatic coronoidectomy performed for zygomaticocoronoid ankyloses or pseudoarthrosis typically involves resection of the abnormal section of the zygomatic arch and coronoid process (Fig 9.24).

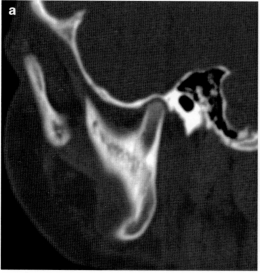 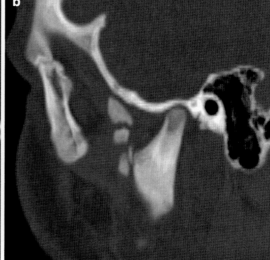

Fig. 9.23 Endoscopic coronoidectomy. The patient had a history of Hecht syndrome (trismus-pseudocamptodactyly syndrome). Preoperative sagittal CT image (**a**) shows an abnormally elongated coronoid process. Postoperative sagittal CT image (**b**) shows interval fragmentation of the coronoid process

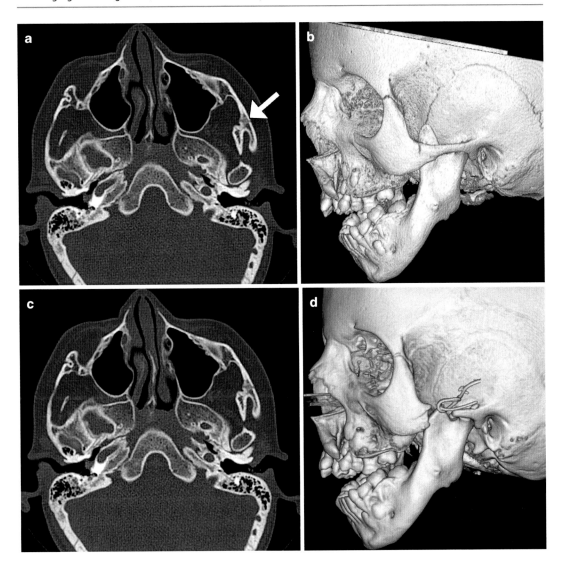

Fig. 9.24 Transzygomatic coronoidectomy. The patient has a history of arthrogryposis multiplex congenita. The preoperative axial (**a**) and 3D (**b**) CT images show left zygomaticocoronoid ankylosis (*arrow*). The postoperative axial (**c**) and 3D (**d**) CT images show interval resection of the fused zygomaticocoronoid segment

9.13 Mandibulectomy and Mandibular Reconstruction

9.13.1 Discussion

Various types of mandibulectomy can be performed for treating both developmental and neoplastic conditions. Marginal mandibulectomy consists of excising part of the surface of the mandible, usually the inner surface, and is mainly performed to minimal tumor extension into the mandible (Fig. 9.25). Segmental mandibulectomy consists of resecting the full thickness of a portion of the mandible, leaving a gap between segments of the mandible (Fig. 9.26). The mandible is often reconstructed using a variety of grafts, such as a free fibula osteocutaneous flap. Plates and screws are also incorporated for securing the

bone segments. Condylectomy consists of resecting the mandibular condyle, often along with the disc and joint capsule (Figs. 9.27 and 9.28). This procedure may be performed for resection of lesions that affect the temporomandibular joint such as pigmented villonodular synovitis or neoplasm of the mandible that extends to the condyle. Occasionally, transport distractors for osteogenesis are used in the reconstruction. Complications related to mandibulectomy and condylectomy include infection (Fig. 9.29), devascularization/osteonecrosis (Fig. 9.30), hardware failure (Fig. 9.31), dislocation/malocclusion that is often accompanied by accelerated degenerative disease of the temporomandibular joints secondary to the altered biomechanical stresses (Fig. 9.32), and tumor recurrence, which is often best depicted on MRI (Fig. 9.33).

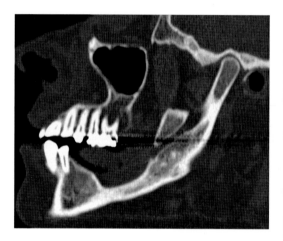

Fig. 9.25 Marginal mandibulectomy. Sagittal CT image shows right marginal mandibulectomy of right mandibular body following ameloblastoma resection several years before. The edges of the osteotomy have healed

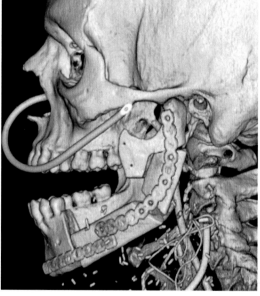

Fig. 9.26 Segmental mandibulectomy. 3D CT image demonstrates resection of a large portion of the right mandible with fibula bone graft and sideplate and screw reconstruction

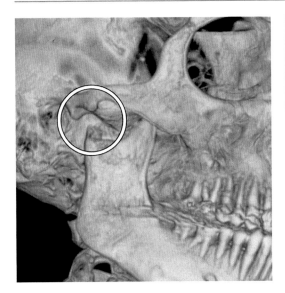

Fig. 9.27 Condylectomy. The 3D CT image demonstrates the absence of the right mandibular condyle leaving a gap between the healed mandibular ramus osteotomy and glenoid (*encircled*)

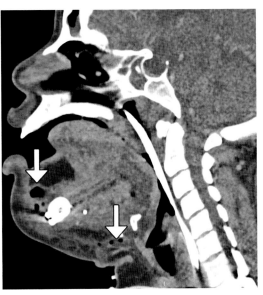

Fig. 9.29 Graft infection. Sagittal CT image shows gas and fluid collections (*arrows*) in the surgical bed

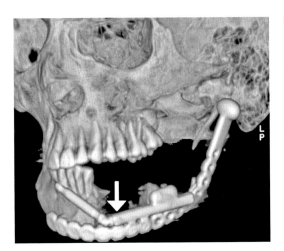

Fig. 9.28 Partial mandibulectomy and condylectomy with condylar prosthesis. 3D CT shows a left mandibular body and condyle prosthesis. There is also a custom bipolar transport distractor (*arrow*)

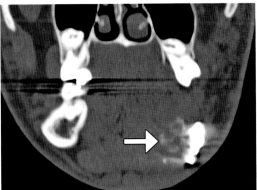

Fig. 9.30 Devitalized fibular graft. Coronal CT image shows demineralization of the right mandibular fibular bone graft (*arrow*)

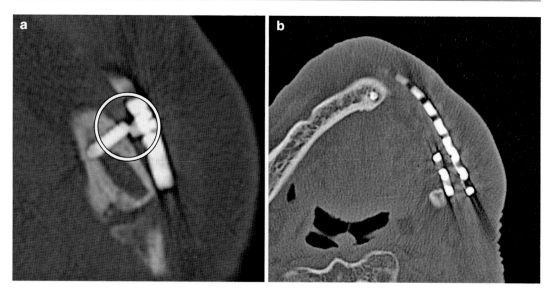

Fig. 9.31 Hardware fracture. Axial CT image (**a**) obtained after partial mandibulectomy and sideplate and screw reconstruction shows a displaced fracture of a screw (*encircled*). Axial CT image in a different patient (**b**) shows overlap of the fractured mandibular reconstruction plate

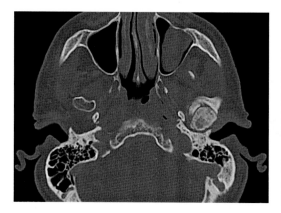

Fig. 9.32 Temporomandibular joint dislocation and accelerated arthritis. Axial CT image obtained after right partial mandibulectomy shows anterior dislocation of the right condyle due to the unopposed forces of the pterygoid muscles after surgery. There is also secondary degenerative change affecting the left temporomandibular joint related to the altered biomechanics

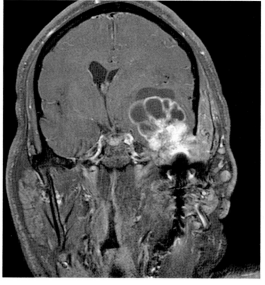

Fig. 9.33 Tumor recurrence. The patient has a history of ameloblastoma treated via left hemimandibulectomy. Coronal fat-suppressed post-contrast T1-weighted MRI shows a heterogeneous mass in the region of the left glenoid fossa with intracranial extension

9.14   Eminectomy and Meniscal Plication

9.14.1   Discussion

Eminectomy with or without meniscal plication is a treatment option of chronic, recurrent temporomandibular joint dislocation. The recurrent dislocations often result in pterygoid spasm and severe pain. Eminectomy consists of resecting the articular eminence of the glenoid (Fig. 9.34). For plication, the lateral pterygoid is detached from the meniscus, which is then rotated such that the disc from the posterior portion overlies the condylar head as a cap upon the condyle. Anchors can be placed to ensure stability of the construct. On MRI, the absence of the eminence and a thickened disc are apparent. In addition, MRI can show increased rotation and translation of the condylar head.

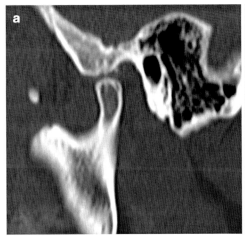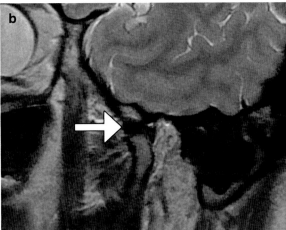

Fig. 9.34 Eminectomy. Both patients have a history of chronic left temporomandibular joint dislocation treated via eminectomy, temporomandibular joint meniscus plication, and lateral pterygoid myotomy. Sagittal CT (**a**) image shows reduction and flattening of the articular emi-nence with anterior translation of the condyle to remain in the appropriate range of motion. Sagittal proton density MRI in another patient (**b**) shows thickening of the folded disc (*arrow*) and flattening of the articular eminence

9.15   Temporomandibular Joint Discectomy

9.15.1 Discussion

Discectomy without disc replacement has been used as a treatment for painful temporomandibular joint internal derangement. Following tem- poromandibular joint discectomy, a narrow soft tissue interface normally forms between the mandibular condyle and the glenoid fossa, which effectively functions as a substitute for the resected disc. On MRI, this soft tissue has intermediate to high signal intensity (Fig. 9.35). The soft tissue normally mineralizes over time, resulting in a shallower glenoid fossa.

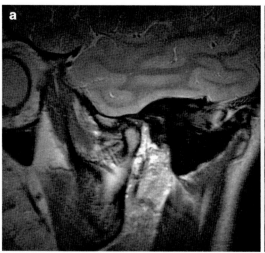 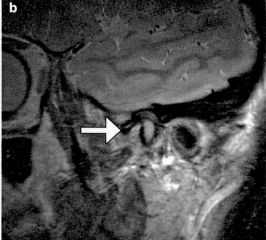

Fig. 9.35 Discectomy. The patient has a history of temporomandibular joint cyst treated via discectomy. Postoperative sagittal proton density MRI (**a**) shows the absence of the low-signal disc and an area of intermediate to high signal in the joint space. The contralateral sagittal proton density MRI (**b**) shows the normal disc (*arrow*) for comparison

9.16   Temporomandibular Joint Costochondral Graft Reconstruction

9.16.1 Discussion

The morphology and tissue components make rib costochondral grafts well suited for temporomandibular joint reconstruction, particularly in the pediatric population due to the graft's growth potential. The procedure generally consists of resecting the mandibular condyle, trimming the cartilaginous portion of the graft to match the normal contour of the articular surface, and affixing the osseous portion of the graft to the mandibular ramus (Fig. 9.36). This type of reconstruction provides satisfactory function in the majority of cases. However, complications include fracture, continued ankylosis, differential growth of the graft with respect to the contralateral side, degenerative disease (Fig. 9.37), and graft resorption (Fig. 9.38).

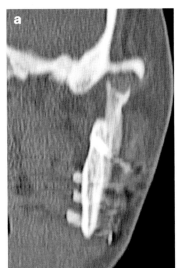
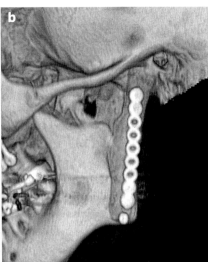

Fig. 9.36 Rib grafts. The patient has a history of hemifacial microsomia, status post costochondral reconstruction of the right temporomandibular joint. Coronal (**a**) and 3D (**b**) CT images show the cartilaginous portion of the right costochondral graft seated within the glenoid fossa. The osseous portion of the graft is attached to the mandibular ramus by plate and screw fixation

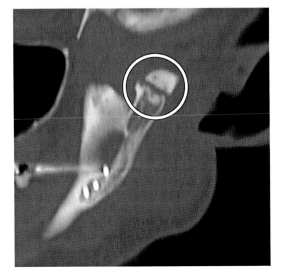

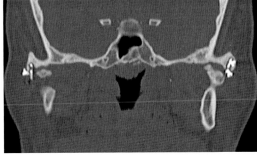

Fig. 9.38 Rib graft resorption. Coronal CT image demonstrates small inferior remnants of the bilateral rib grafts resulting in superior migration of the mandible and erosion of the fixation hardware into the zygomatic processes

Fig. 9.37 Rib graft degenerative disease. Sagittal CT image shows joint space narrowing between the left rib graft and the zygomatic arch (*encircled*) due to severe thinning of the cartilage

9.17 Temporomandibular Joint Disc Replacement Implants

9.17.1 Discussion

Two main types of alloplastic temporomandibular joint disc implants have been used: Proplast-Teflon and silicone rubber (Silastic). Proplast implants were intended to be permanent, but have been banned by the FDA. Silicone implants can be used either on a temporary or a permanent basis. Both types of implants appear as uniformly low-signal, linear structures on both T1-weighted and T2-weighted MRI sequences. On CT, both types of prostheses are hyperattenuating (Fig. 9.39).

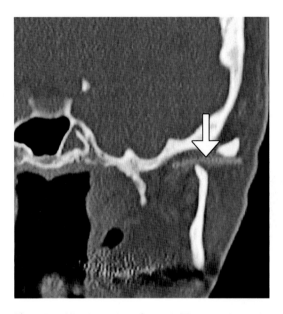

Fig. 9.39 Silastic implant. Coronal CT image shows the implant is well-seated in the temporomandibular joint space (*arrow*)

9.18 Temporomandibular Joint Hemiarthroplasty

9.18.1 Discussion

Hemiarthroplasty consists of resurfacing one side of the temporomandibular joint with either prosthesis for the fossa-eminence (Fig. 9.40) or ramus-condyle (Figs. 9.41 and 9.42), which directly contacts the opposing articular surface. Sometimes a fat graft is also applied adjacent to the prosthesis. Revision surgery is ultimately required in over 20% of cases without fat graft and about 6% of cases with fat graft.

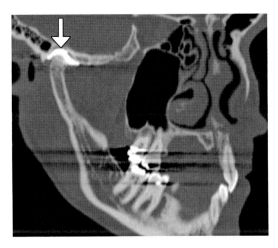

Fig. 9.40 Temporomandibular joint hemiarthroplasty glenoid implant. Sagittal CT image shows a metallic implant seated in the glenoid fossa (*arrow*) (Courtesy of Joel Curé, MD)

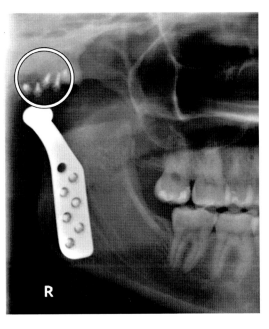

Fig. 9.42 Lorenz prosthesis. Lateral radiographs shows right mandibular ramus osteotomy and a prosthesis that includes a metallic condylar component and a radiolucent glenoid fossa component (*encircled*), both of which are secured via titanium screws

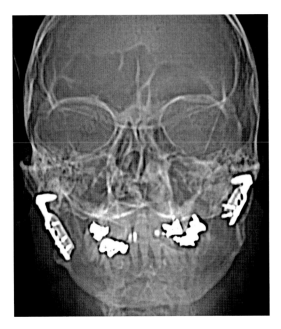

Fig. 9.41 Temporomandibular joint hemiarthroplasty with ramus-condyle unit implant. Frontal scout image shows bilateral ramus-condyle hardware

9.19   Temporomandibular Total Joint Arthroplasty

9.19.1 Discussion

Total temporomandibular joint resurfacing is performed in order to restore normal jaw motion and provide pain relief for a variety of conditions, such as neoplasms, arthritis, and ankylosis. The main types of temporomandibular prostheses include fossa-eminence, condylar, and total temporomandibular replacement. Although success rates of at least 90% have been achieved with some designs and materials, proper fitting of the prosthetic components to the skull is challenging. As a result, presurgical CT is often used to customize TMJ prostheses, thereby optimizing stability and function. The implants usually consist of radiopaque metallic condylar component and either radiolucent polymer components (plastic-on-metal) (Fig. 9.43) or metallic glenoid fossa components (metal-on-metal) (Fig. 9.44). In addition, three component prostheses have been introduced, such as the Concepts total temporomandibular joint prosthesis, which includes a plastic spacer positioned between the glenoid and condylar implants (Fig. 9.45).

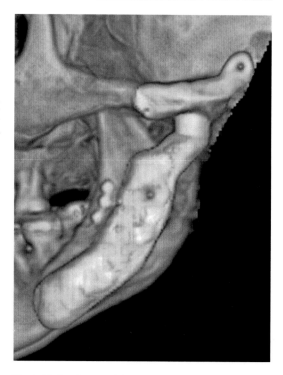

Fig. 9.43 Synthes total joint prosthesis. 3D CT image shows both metallic mandibular and glenoid fossa components

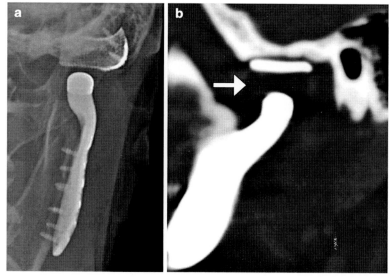

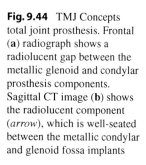

Fig. 9.44 TMJ Concepts total joint prosthesis. Frontal (**a**) radiograph shows a radiolucent gap between the metallic glenoid and condylar prosthesis components. Sagittal CT image (**b**) shows the radiolucent component (*arrow*), which is well-seated between the metallic condylar and glenoid fossa implants

9.20 Temporomandibular Joint Disc Implant and Prosthesis Failure

9.20.1 Discussion

Proplast-Teflon laminate implants were first used in temporomandibular joint meniscectomy (interpositional arthroplasty) for treatment of internal derangement in 1974 and became available as precut discs in 1983. However, Proplast-Teflon implants were prone to perforation, fragmentation, migration, and foreign body reaction, which can lead to severe condylar, glenoid fossa, and articular eminence erosion, as well as penetration into the middle cranial fossa (Figs. 9.45 and 9.46). Patients may present even after many years with temporomandibular joint pain, decreased joint range of motion, crepitus, preauricular swelling, regional lymphadenopathy, malocclusion, and facial deformity, often requiring implant removal and debridement of the joint. The degree of facial pain correlates with perforation and breakdown of the implants. Due to their high failure rate, Proplast-Teflon temporomandibular joint implants were removed from the market in 1993. Failed Proplast-Teflon temporomandibular joint implants often result in bony erosions, which could be poorly or well defined, with or without sclerotic margins. CT can reveal soft tissue mass corresponding to foreign body granuloma and accurately delineates migration and fragmentation of the hyperattenuating Proplast-Teflon implant, soft tissue calcifications, and destructive changes of the adjacent osseous structures. MRI is well suited for depicting the soft tissue changes, including the intermediate T1 and T2 signal-enhancing foreign body granuloma and the presence of associated avascular necrosis in the surrounding bone, which can appear as decreased marrow signal on T1. Ultimately, erosive change of the glenoid fossa and the mandibular condyle can result. The integrity of the glenoid fossa is critical since erosions can extend into the middle cranial fossa (Fig. 9.47). Osteolysis with loosening of temporomandibular joint prostheses is another complication that can be associated with pain and is recognized by the presence of lucency between the bone and the prosthesis that measures greater than 2 mm (Fig. 9.48). Loosening can be accompanied by dislocation of the prosthesis. Alternatively, new bone formation can result in ankylosis and limitation of mouth opening. Pseudoarthroses can sometimes form in the bony mass and can appear as linear lucencies on CT (Fig. 9.49). Evaluation of temporomandibular joint prosthetic complications often requires both MRI and CT. MRI readily shows the extent of infection, fragmentation of the implant material, and distension of the joint capsule, while CT is useful for evaluating the integrity of the implants and associated osseous structures.

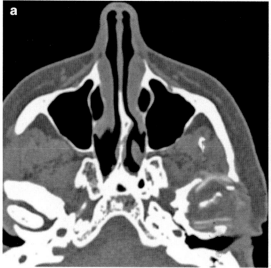

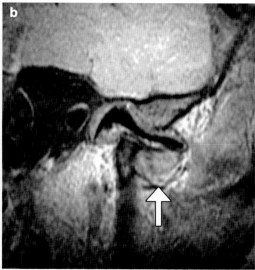

Fig. 9.45 Teflon granuloma. Axial CT image (**a**) shows the linear hyperattenuating implant in the temporomandibular joint space. The glenoid fossa is markedly expanded secondary to a soft tissue mass. Sagittal proton density MR image in a different patient (**b**) shows an expanded joint capsule and intermediate-signal-intensity material surrounding the low-signal-intensity implant (*arrow*)

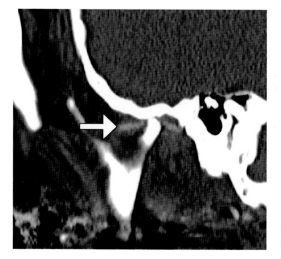

Fig. 9.46 Implant perforation. Sagittal CT image shows a fragmented silicone implant (*arrow*)

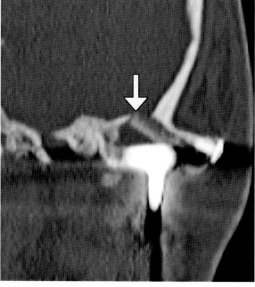

Fig. 9.47 Implant intracranial migration. Coronal sagittal CT image shows erosion of the Teflon portion of the implant into the middle cranial fossa (*arrow*)

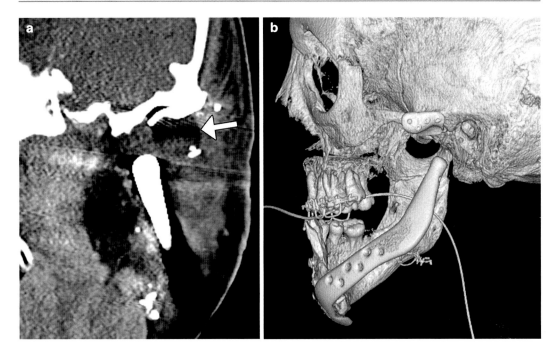

Fig. 9.48 Temporomandibular joint prosthesis dislocation. Coronal (**a**) and 3D (**b**) CT images show inferomedial dislocation of the left condylar prosthesis from the radiolucent component (arrow)

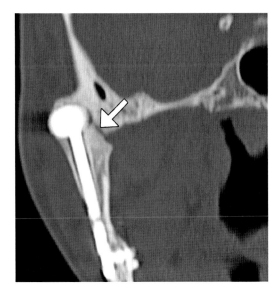

Fig. 9.49 Pseudoarthrosis. Coronal CT image shows superolateral migration of the right temporomandibular joint hemiarthroplasty hardware. The lucency (*arrow*) between the medial mandibular ramus and the skull base represents a pseudoarthrosis

Further Reading

Vertical Ramus Osteotomy

Chen CM, Lee HE, Yang CF, Shen YS, Huang IY, Tseng YC, Lai ST (2008) Intraoral vertical ramus osteotomy for correction of mandibular prognathism: long-term stability. Ann Plast Surg 61(1):52–55

Jung YS, Kim SY, Park SY, Choi YD, Park HS (2010) Changes of transverse mandibular width after intraoral vertical ramus osteotomy. Oral Surg Oral Med Oral Pathol Oral Radiol Endod 110(1):25–31

Westesson PL, Dahlberg G, Hansson LG, Eriksson L, Ketonen L (1991) Osseous and muscular changes after vertical ramus osteotomy. A magnetic resonance imaging study. Oral Surg Oral Med Oral Pathol 72(2):139–145

Sagittal Split Osteotomy

Patel PK, Novia MV (2007) The surgical tools: the LeFort I, bilateral sagittal split osteotomy of the mandible, and the osseous genioplasty. Clin Plast Surg 34(3):447–475

Rai KK, Shivakumar HR, Sonar MD (2008) Transient facial nerve palsy following bilateral sagittal split ramus osteotomy for setback of the mandible: a review of incidence and management. J Oral Maxillofac Surg 66(2):373–378

Silva AC, O'Ryan F, Beckley ML, Young HY, Poor D (2007) Pseudoaneurysm of a branch of the maxillary artery following mandibular sagittal split ramus osteotomy: case report and review of the literature. J Oral Maxillofac Surg 65(9):1807–1816

Genioplasty

Abrahams JJ (2001) Dental CT imaging: a look at the jaw. Radiology 219(2):334–345

Lindquist CC, Obeid G (1988) Complications of genioplasty done alone or in combination with sagittal split-ramus osteotomy. Oral Surg Oral Med Oral Pathol 66(1):13–16

Patel PK, Novia MV (2007) The surgical tools: the LeFort I, bilateral sagittal split osteotomy of the mandible, and the osseous genioplasty. Clin Plast Surg 34(3):447–475

Mandibular Angle Augmentation

Bastidas N, Zide BM (2010) The treachery of mandibular angle augmentation. Ann Plast Surg 64(1):4–6

Semergidis TG, Migliore SA, Sotereanos GC (1996) Alloplastic augmentation of the mandibular angle. J Oral Maxillofac Surg 54(12):1417–1423

Mandibular Distraction

Chopra S, Enepekides DJ (2007) The role of distraction osteogenesis in mandibular reconstruction. Curr Opin Otolaryngol Head Neck Surg 15(4):197–201

Goiato MC, Ribeiro AB, Dreifus Marinho ML (2009) Surgical and prosthetic rehabilitation of patients with hemimandibular defect. J Craniofac Surg 20(6):2163–2167

Master DL, Hanson PR, Gosain AK (2010) Complications of mandibular distraction osteogenesis. J Craniofac Surg 21(5):1565–1570

Lefort I Surgery

Buchanan EP, Hyman CH. LeFort I Osteotomy. Semin Plast Surg 2013;27(3):149–154.

Kramer FJ, Baethge C, Swennen G, Teltzrow T, Schulze A, Berten J, Brachvogel P. Intra- and perioperative complications of the LeFort I osteotomy: a prospective evaluation of 1000 patients. J Craniofac Surg 2004;15(6):971-977; discussion 978–9.

Li KK, Meara JG, Alexander A Jr. Location of the descending palatine artery in relation to the Le Fort I osteotomy. J Oral Maxillofac Surg 1996;54(7):822–825; discussion 826–7.

Lefort III Surgery

Festa F, Pagnoni M, Valerio R, Rodolfino D, Saccucci M, d'Attilio M, Caputi S, Iannetti G. Orbital volume and surface after Le Fort III advancement in syndromic craniosynostosis. J Craniofac Surg 2012;23(3):789–792.

Nout E, Cesteleyn LL, van der Wal KG, van Adrichem LN, Mathijssen IM, Wolvius EB. Advancement of the midface, from conventional Le Fort III osteotomy to Le Fort III distraction: review of the literature. Int J Oral Maxillofac Surg 2008;37(9):781–789.

Fixation of Mandible Fractures

Choi BH, Huh JY, Yoo JH (2003) Computed tomographic findings of the fractured mandibular condyle after open reduction. Int J Oral Maxillofac Surg 32(5):469–473

Fox AJ, Kellman RM (2003) Mandibular angle fractures: two-miniplate fixation and complications. Arch Facial Plast Surg 5(6):464–469

Gear AJ, Apasova E, Schmitz JP, Schubert W (2005) Treatment modalities for mandibular angle fractures. J Oral Maxillofac Surg 63(5):655–663

Yamamoto MK, D'Avila RP, de Cerqueira Luz JG (2013) Evaluation of surgical retreatment of mandibular fractures. J Craniomaxillofac Surg 41(1):42–46

Mandibulotomy

Amin MR, Deschler DG, Hayden RE (1999) Straight midline mandibulotomy revisited. Laryngoscope 109(9):1402–1405

Kolokythas A, Eisele DW, El-Sayed I, Schmidt BL (2009) Mandibular osteotomies for access to select parapharyngeal space neoplasms. Head Neck 31(1):102–110

Smith GI, Brennan PA, Webb AA, Ilankovan V (2003) Vertical ramus osteotomy combined with a parasymphyseal mandibulotomy for improved access to the parapharyngeal space. Head Neck 25(12):1000–1003

Enucleation

Chiapasco M, Rossi A, Motta JJ, Crescentini M (2000) Spontaneous bone regeneration after enucleation of large mandibular cysts: a radiographic computed analysis of 27 consecutive cases. J Oral Maxillofac Surg 58(9):942–948; discussion 949

Connor SE, Chaudhary N (2008) CT-guided percutaneous core biopsy of deep face and skull-base lesions. Clin Radiol 63(9):986–994

Pradel W, Eckelt U, Lauer G (2006) Bone regeneration after enucleation of mandibular cysts: comparing autogenous grafts from tissue-engineered bone and iliac bone. Oral Surg Oral Med Oral Pathol Oral Radiol Endod 101(3):285–290

Cyst Decompression

Cakarer S, Selvi F, Isler SC, Keskin C (2011) Decompression, enucleation, and implant placement in the management of a large dentigerous cyst. J Craniofac Surg 22(3):922–924

Enislidis G, Fock N, Sulzbacher I, Ewers R (2004) Conservative treatment of large cystic lesions of the mandible: a prospective study of the effect of decompression. Br J Oral Maxillofac Surg 42(6):546–550

Coronoidectomy

Lefaivre JF, Aitchison MJ (2003) Surgical correction of trismus in a child with Hecht syndrome. Ann Plast Surg 50(3):310–314

Ramalho-Ferreira G, Faverani LP, Fabris AL, Pastori CM, Magro-Filho O, Ponzoni D, Aranega AM, Garcia-Júnior IR (2011) Mandibular movement restoration through bilateral coronoidectomy by intraoral approach. J Craniofac Surg 22(3):988–991

Robiony M, Casadei M, Costa F. Minimally invasive surgery for coronoid hyperplasia: endoscopically assisted intraoral coronoidectomy. J Craniofac Surg 2012;23(6):1838–1840.

Talmi YP, Horowitz Z, Yahalom R, Bedrin L (2004) Coronoidectomy in maxillary swing for reducing the incidence and severity of trismus–a reminder. J Craniomaxillofac Surg 32(1):19–20

Miyamoto S, Takushima A, Momosawa A, Ozaki M, Harii K. Transzygomatic coronoidectomy as a treatment for pseudoankylosis of the mandible after transtemporal surgery. Scand J Plast Reconstr Surg Hand Surg. 2008;42(5):267–270

Mandibulectomy and Mandibular Reconstruction

Chana JS, Chang YM, Wei FC, Shen YF, Chan CP, Lin HN, Tsai CY, Jeng SF (2004) Segmental mandibulectomy and immediate free fibula osteoseptocutaneous flap reconstruction with endosteal implants: an ideal treatment method for mandibular ameloblastoma. Plast Reconstr Surg 113(1):80–87

Goiato MC, Ribeiro AB, Dreifus Marinho ML (2009) Surgical and prosthetic rehabilitation of patients with hemimandibular defect. J Craniofac Surg 20(6):2163–2167

Vayvada H, Mola F, Menderes A, Yilmaz M (2006) Surgical management of ameloblastoma in the mandible: segmental mandibulectomy and immediate reconstruction with free fibula or deep circumflex iliac artery flap (evaluation of the long-term esthetic and functional results). J Oral Maxillofac Surg 64(10):1532–1539

Eminectomy and Meniscal Plication

Baldwin AJ, Cooper JC (2004) Eminectomy and plication of the posterior disc attachment following arthrotomy for temporomandibular joint internal derangement. J Craniomaxillofac Surg 32(6):354–359

Cascone P, Ungari C, Paparo F, Marianetti TM, Ramieri V, Fatone M (2008) A new surgical approach for the treatment of chronic recurrent temporomandibular joint dislocation. J Craniofac Surg 19(2):510–512

Williamson RA, McNamara D, McAuliffe W (2000) True eminectomy for internal derangement of the temporomandibular joint. Br J Oral Maxillofac Surg 38(5):554–560

Temporomandibular Joint Discectomy

Hansson L-G, Eriksson L, Westesson PL (1992) Temporomandibular joint: magnetic resonance evaluation after discectomy. Oral Surg Oral Med Oral Pathol 74:801–810

Temporomandibular Joint Costochondral Graft Reconstruction

El-Sayed KM (2008) Temporomandibular joint reconstruction with costochondral graft using modified approach. Int J Oral Maxillofac Surg 37(10):897–902

Saeed NR, Kent JN (2003) A retrospective study of the costochondral graft in TMJ reconstruction. Int J Oral Maxillofac Surg 32(6):606–609

Siavosh S, Ali M (2007) Overgrowth of a costochondral graft in a case of temporomandibular joint ankylosis. J Craniofac Surg 18(6):1488–1491

Troulis MJ, Tayebaty FT, Papadaki M, Williams WB, Kaban LB (2008) Condylectomy and costochondral graft reconstruction for treatment of active idiopathic condylar resorption. J Oral Maxillofac Surg 66(1):65–72

Temporomandibular Joint Disc Replacement Implants

Ferreira JN, Ko CC, Myers S, Swift J, Fricton JR (2008) Evaluation of surgically retrieved temporomandibular joint alloplastic implants: pilot study. J Oral Maxillofac Surg 6(6):1112–1124

Heffez L, Mafee MF, Rosenberg H, Langer B (1987) CT evaluation of TMJ disc replacement with a Proplast-Teflon laminate. J Oral Maxillofac Surg 45:657–665

Kaplan PA, Ruskin JD, Tu HK, Knibbe MA (1988) Erosive arthritis of the temporomandibular joint caused by Teflon-Proplast implants: plain film features. AJR Am J Roentgenol 151(2):337–339

Kulber DA, Davos I, Aronowitz JA (1995) Severe cutaneous foreign body giant cell reaction after temporomandibular joint reconstruction with Proplast-Teflon. J Oral Maxillofac Surg 53(6):719–722; discussion 722–723

Schellhas KP, Wilkes CH, el Deeb M, Lagrotteria LB, Omlie MR (1988) Permanent Proplast temporomandibular joint implants: MR imaging of destructive complications. AJR Am J Roentgenol 151:731–735

Smith RM, Goldwasser MS, Sabol SR (1993) Erosion of a Teflon-Proplast implant into the middle cranial fossa. J Oral Maxillofac Surg 51(11):1268–1271

Wolford LM (1997) Temporomandibular joint devices: treatment factors and outcomes. Oral Surg Oral Med Oral Pathol Oral Radiol Endod 83(1):143–149

Temporomandibular Joint Hemiarthroplasty

Baltali E, Keller EE (2008) Surgical management of advanced osteoarthritis of the temporomandibular joint with metal fossa-eminence hemijoint replacement: 10-year retrospective study. J Oral Maxillofac Surg 66(9):1847–1855

Park J, Keller EE, Reid KI (2004) Surgical management of advanced degenerative arthritis of temporomandibular joint with metal fossa-eminence hemijoint replacement prosthesis: an 8-year retrospective pilot study. J Oral Maxillofac Surg 62(3):320–328

Temporomandibular Total Joint Arthroplasty

Park J, Keller EE, Reid KI (2004) Surgical management of advanced degenerative arthritis of temporomandibular joint with metal fossa-eminence hemijoint replacement prosthesis: an 8-year retrospective pilot study. J Oral Maxillofac Surg 62(3):320–328

van Loon JP, de Bont GM, Boering G (1995) Evaluation of temporomandibular joint prostheses: review of the literature from 1946 to 1994 and implications for future prosthesis designs. J Oral Maxillofac Surg 53(9):984–996; discussion 996–997

Westermark A, Hedén P, Aagaard E, Cornelius CP (2011) The use of TMJ concepts prostheses to reconstruct patients with major temporomandibular joint and mandibular defects. Int J Oral Maxillofac Surg 40(5):487–496

Wolford LM (1997) Temporomandibular joint devices: treatment factors and outcomes. Oral Surg Oral Med Oral Pathol Oral Radiol Endod 83(1):143–149

Temporomandibular Joint Disc Implant and Prosthesis Failure

Heffez L, Mafee MF, Rosenberg H, Langer B (1987) CT evaluation of TMJ disc replacement with a proplastteflon laminate. J Oral Maxillofac Surg 45(8):657–665

Kalamchi S, Walker RV (1987) Silastic implant as a part of temporomandibular joint arthroplasty. Evaluation of its efficacy. Br J Oral Maxillofac Surg 25(3):227–236

Schellhas KP, Wilkes CH, el Deeb M, Lagrotteria LB, Omlie MR (1988) Permanent proplast temporomandibular joint implants: MR imaging of destructive complications. AJR Am J Roentgenol 151(4):731–735

Wolford LM (2006) Factors to consider in joint prosthesis systems. Proc (Bayl Univ Med Cent) 19(3):232–238

Imaging the Postoperative Neck

10

Daniel Thomas Ginat, Elizabeth Blair,
and Hugh D. Curtin

10.1 Reconstruction Flaps

10.1.1 Discussion

Flap reconstruction is routinely performed for closing soft tissue, bone, and/or skin defects created by head and neck tumor resection. Many donor sites and types of flaps are available including local, regional, and free flaps (Figs. 10.1, 10.2, 10.3, 10.4, 10.5, 10.6, 10.7, 10.8, 10.9, 10.10, and 10.11 and Table 10.1).

The pectoralis major muscle flap is often used as a rotation flap for head and neck reconstruction surgery. Due to the highly vascular nature of the pedicled pectoralis major flap, it is desirable for repairing defects in previously radiated areas. The pedicled flap is brought over the clavicle with its vascular supply and is often used to provide coverage of the carotid arteries or to reinforce primary

pharyngeal closure. Pectoralis myocutaneous flaps can also be "tubed" to create a neopharynx, in which there is a deep core of fatty tissue, a more superficial area of the muscle, and overlying skin that forms the "pseudomucosa." Initially, the myocutaneous flaps maintain muscle bulk, but often gradually become atrophied and replaced by fat.

Osteomyocutaneous and bone grafts are mainly used to reconstruct mandibulectomy defects. The fibula is a common donor site, but the scapula, ribs, and other bones can be used as well. The bone grafts are often cut into smaller sections in order to reconstruct the curved contours of the mandible. The grafts are usually secured using plates and screws. The soft tissues attached to the bone flaps are useful for providing bulk to large surgical defects.

Colon interposition, gastric pull-through, and jejunal/ileal grafts have been used to reconstruct the upper aerodigestive tract after procedures that involve resection of part or all of the pharynx and/or esophagus, such as with pharyngolaryngoesophagectomy. On imaging, rugal folds and haustra can be identified with gastric and colon interposition, respectively. Alternatively, musculomucosal flaps, such as the FAMM flap, can be used to reconstruct relatively superficial upper aerodigestive tract defects.

Imaging with CT, MRI, and 18FDG-PET is routinely used for posttreatment imaging, particularly for tumor surveillance. Recurrence can be difficult to discern due to the altered anatomy of

D.T. Ginat, M.D., M.S. (✉)
Department of Radiology, University of Chicago,
Chicago, IL, USA
e-mail: dtg1@uchicago.edu

E. Blair, M.D.
Department of Surgery, Section of Otolaryngology-
Head and Neck Surgery, University of Chicago,
Chicago, IL, USA

H.D. Curtin, M.D.
Department of Radiology, Harvard Medical School,
Boston, MA, USA

Department of Radiology, Massachusetts Eye and Ear
Infirmary, Boston, MA, USA

© Springer International Publishing Switzerland 2017
D.T. Ginat, P.-L.A. Westesson (eds.), *Atlas of Postsurgical Neuroradiology*,
DOI 10.1007/978-3-319-52341-5_10

the surgical bed on CT or MRI ((Fig. 10.12), such as the soft tissue components of the flaps. 18FDG-PET/CT is particularly helpful in such instances, but is ideally performed no sooner than 12 weeks following surgery in order to minimize the rate of false-positive results. However, it is helpful to obtain a baseline CT or MRI soon after surgery for subsequent comparison and to correlate the findings with the operative note.

While serosanguinous fluid collections or seromas in the surgical bed after flap reconstruction are commonly encountered on early postoperative imaging, large perioperative hematomas are rare. However, these can lead to flap ischemia; therefore, prompt recognition and re-exploration can help salvage the flap. On CT, the hematomas can appear as mass-like heterogeneous lesions (Fig. 10.13).

Infection of the flap is a serious complication, which may require urgent debridement or revision. Diagnostic imaging is useful for delineating the extent of the infected fluid collections, which can contain gas, have peripheral enhancement, and surrounding fat stranding (Fig. 10.14). Infections in the surgical bed can be predisposed by the presence of fistulas with the skin and/or aerodigestive tract.

Anastomotic leaks are potential sources for infection. CT or fluoroscopic examinations with oral contrast administration can be useful for assessing the presence of leaks. The presence of hyperattenuation from the oral contrast material in extraluminal fluid collections is indicative of a leak (Fig. 10.15). A baseline CT without oral contrast can be useful for comparison, since surgically implanted hyperattenuating material can potentially be misinterpreted as contrast.

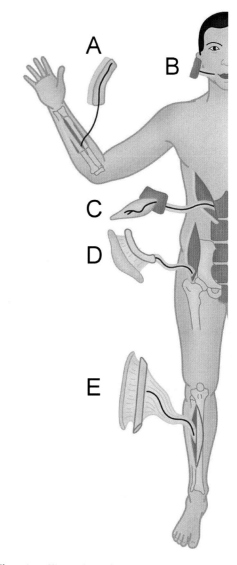

Fig. 10.1 Illustration of various types of tissue flaps. Fasciocutaneous (*A*). Musculomucosal (*B*). Myocutaneous (*C*). Bowel (*D*). Bone/osteomyocutaneous (*E*)

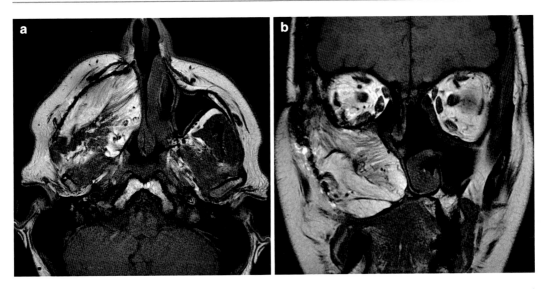

Fig. 10.2 Temporalis flap. Axial (**a**) and coronal (**b**) T1-weighted MR images show the characteristic fan-shaped appearance of the flap that fills the right nasal cavity, maxillectomy cavity, and masticator space

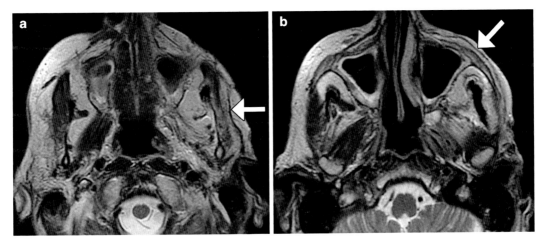

Fig. 10.3 Fasciocutaneous rotation advancement flap. The patient has a large defect following Mohs surgery for a cutaneous malignancy of the left cheek. Axial T2-weighted MR images (**a, b**) demonstrate the Scarpa's fascia component of the graft (*arrows*) as a low-signal-intensity band. The rest of the graft demonstrates normal fat signal intensity without evidence of recurrent disease. Atrophy of the left masticator muscles is noted

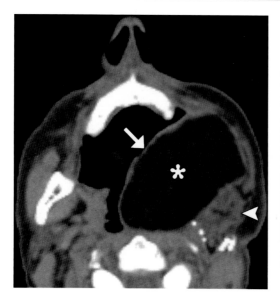

Fig. 10.4 Myocutaneous free flap. Axial CT image shows the skin (*arrow*), fat (***), and muscle (*arrowhead*) components of the thigh flap used to reconstruct the left oropharynx and oral cavity

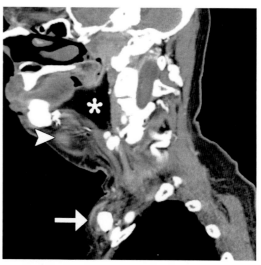

Fig. 10.5 Myocutaneous rotational flap. Axial CT image shows a pectoralis flap swung over the clavicle to fill a large surgical defect in the neck. The vascular pedicle is visible (*arrow*), as are the muscle (*arrowhead*) and adipose tissue (***) components of the flap. The muscle has undergone fatty degeneration

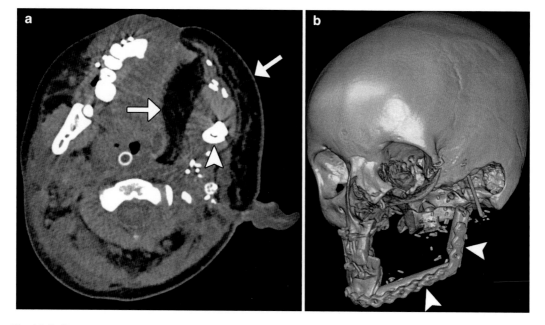

Fig. 10.6 Osteomyocutaneous flap. Axial (**a**) and 3D (**b**) CT images show left maxillofacial reconstruction using a fibular graft (*arrowheads*) with surrounding soft tissues (*arrows*)

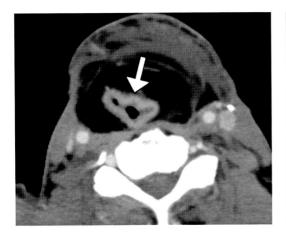

Fig. 10.7 Myocutaneous flap neopharynx. Axial CT image shows skin lining the neopharynx (*arrow*), which is surrounded by subcutaneous fat and muscle

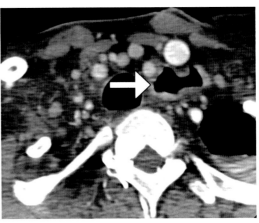

Fig. 10.9 Colonic interposition. Axial CT image shows a loop of large bowel (*arrow*) adjacent to the trachea

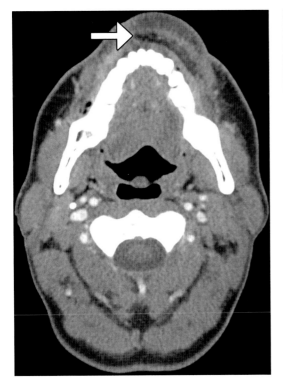

Fig. 10.8 Radial forearm free flap lip reconstruction. Axial CT image shows lower lip reconstruction utilizing radial forearm free flap and palmaris longus tendon (*arrow*), which provides near-anatomic contours

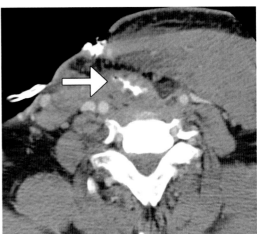

Fig. 10.10 Gastric transposition. Axial CT image shows the transposed stomach filled with barium, which outlines the rugal folds (*arrow*). Total pharyngolaryngoesophagectomy was also performed

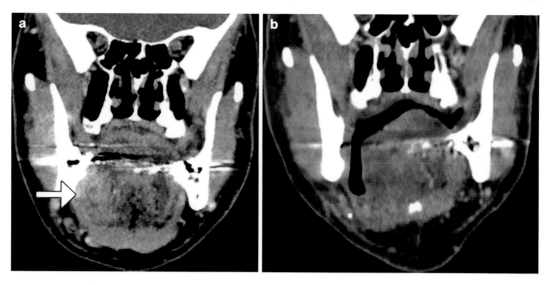

Fig. 10.11 Facial artery musculomucosal (FAMM) flap. Preoperative coronal CT image (**a**) shows an infiltrative mass in the right floor of the mouth (*arrow*). Postoperative coronal CT image (**b**) shows interval resection of the mass and reconstruction with a flap that closely approximately approximates the floor of the mouth

Table 10.1 Types of flap reconstruction

Components	Type	Description
Vascular supply	Random	Transected small vessels
	Free	Transected and reanastomosed large vessels
	Pedicle	Intact vascular supply with tissue rotated into position
Tissue	Fasciocutaneous	Composed of subcutaneous fat and fascia as well as dermal/epidermal tissue
	Myocutaneous	Composed of muscle, subcutaneous, and dermal/epidermal tissue. They are used to close large soft tissue defects and may sometimes also be used to reconstruct the aerodigestive tract. Common donor sites include pectoralis major and the anterolateral thigh
	Bone	Used to reconstruct mandible defects. Common donor sites include fibula, iliac crest, and scapula. May be used as part of an osteomyocutaneous flap
	Bowel	Used for upper aerodigestive tract reconstruction and includes jejunal and ilial grafts and gastric and colonic interpositions
	Musculomucosal	Used to close small to moderate upper aerodigestive tract mucosal defects, often using tissue supplied by the facial artery (FAMM flap)

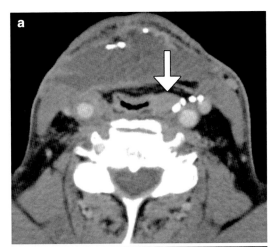

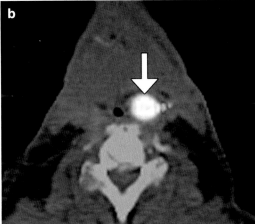

Fig. 10.12 Tumor recurrence. Axial CT image (**a**) shows a myocutaneous flap with subtle nodularity along the left aspect of the neopharynx (*arrow*) in a patient with history of head and neck squamous cell carcinoma, but no prior baseline exams available. 18FDG-PET/CT (**b**) was recommended and obtained 2 weeks later, which shows corresponding marked hypermetabolism (*arrow*)

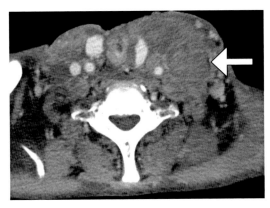

Fig. 10.13 Perioperative hematoma. Axial CT image obtained shortly after laryngectomy shows a heterogeneous mass-like hematoma (*arrow*) underlying the edematous left pectoralis flap

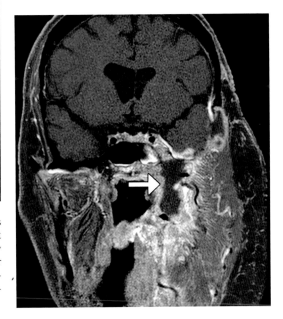

Fig. 10.14 Infected flap. Coronal fat-suppressed postcontrast T1-weighted MRI shows a fluid collection with surrounding enhancement (*arrow*) deep to the left neck myocutaneous flap, which represents an abscess

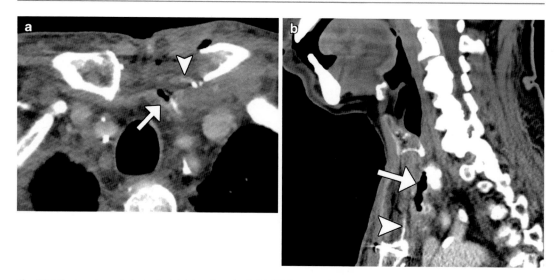

Fig. 10.15 Anastomotic leak. Axial (**a**) and sagittal (**b**) CT images obtained with intravenous and oral contrast show the presence of extraluminal oral contrast (*arrowheads*) in a collection adjacent to the jejunal graft (*arrows*)

10.2 Neck Dissection

10.2.1 Discussion

Neck dissection is performed to diagnose and/or remove at risk and/or diseased lymph nodes and, in some cases, surrounding structures. The main types of neck dissection include selective, modified, radical, and extended neck dissection (Table 10.2). Features of each of these can be appreciated on CT (Figs. 10.16, 10.17, 10.18, 10.19, and 10.20).

Postoperative imaging is usually performed with contrast-enhanced CT and serves to identify clinically occult disease, which occurs in 7.5–28% of cases. Per NCCN guidelines, a baseline study is usually obtained within about 6 months of surgery for comparison with subsequent studies, which are usually obtained depending on symptoms, physical exam, and findings from previous imaging. During the early postoperative period, local hemorrhage and edema are common findings for all types of neck dissection. These changes usually resolve by 6 weeks after surgery and have a reticular appearance on CT. Over time, there may be persistence of edema and development of fibrosis, particularly if radiotherapy is administered. The degree of retropharyngeal edema can be exacerbated by resection of the internal jugular vein. A stable postoperative appearance may not be attained until 12–18 months after surgery.

Following selective and modified radical neck dissection, atrophy of the sternocleidomastoid and strap muscles is also common. In addition, removal of the adipose tissue and lymph nodes around the carotid sheath decreases the space between the sternocleidomastoid and internal jugular veins. The presence of scarring may accentuate the degree of asymmetry and effacement of the fat planes. Nonvisualization of the ipsilateral internal jugular vein occurs in about 20% of cases of selective neck dissection and may be attributable to thrombosis and should be reported. Following removal of the ipsilateral submandibular gland with level I dissection, the remaining contralateral submandibular gland should not be misinterpreted as a lesion itself. Radical neck dis-

section results in more conspicuous flattening of the neck contour and blurring of the tissue planes than modified radical neck dissection. There may also be reduced flow in the carotid artery due to surgical manipulation and radiation therapy. Rarely, the common carotid artery is sacrificed during extended neck dissection. Myocutaneous flaps are usually required to reconstruct large defects resulting from radical and extended neck dissection. Tissue flaps are also sometimes used to provide coverage of the external carotid artery after modified radical neck dissection.

Potential pitfalls in the interpretation of imaging after neck dissection has been performed are cauterized adipose tissue and suture granulomas, which can be mistaken for lymphadenopathy. Cauterized adipose tissue can appear as nodular foci of soft tissue attenuation, but often conserve some degree of fat attenuation centrally (Fig. 10.21). Suture granulomas can also appear as soft tissue nodules, but the occasional presence of hyperattenuation centrally associated with the suture is a help clue (Fig. 10.22). In either case, these conditions tend to remain static on serial imaging, as opposed to recurrent neoplasm.

Complications depend on the extent of neck dissection. Denervation injury results in high T2 signal and enhancement within the first few months and fatty atrophy and laxity on a chronic basis. The more frequently encountered sites for denervation injury after neck dissection include the trapezius muscle and the tongue (Fig. 10.23). Extensive neck dissection can potentially impair lymphatic drainage and lead to cervicofacial edema, which appears as diffuse swelling and fat stranding (Fig. 10.24) and can be exacerbated by radiation therapy. Leakage of chyle from the lymphatic system can result in lymphoceles, which typically appear as unilocular fluid collections with thin walls (Fig. 10.25). Infections can occur in the skin and subcutaneous tissue as cellulitis and abscesses (Fig. 10.26). In addition, osteomyelitis of the clavicle can result from lower central compartment or supraclavicular lymph node dissection (Fig. 10.27). This should not be confused with degenerative changes and effusions of the sternoclavicular joint due to altered biomechanics and neuropathic joint (Fig. 10.28).

Table 10.2 Types of neck dissection

Type of neck dissection	Description
Selective (Fig. A) 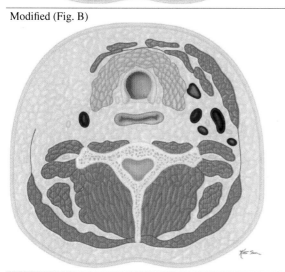	Removal of selected lymph nodes between levels I and V with preservation of the sternocleidomastoid, internal jugular vein, *and* spinal accessory nerve intact. There are four main types of SND: supraomohyoid, anterior, posterolateral, and lateral
Modified (Fig. B) 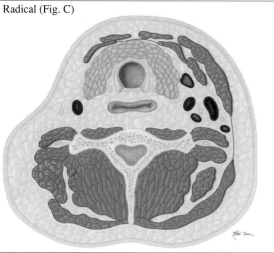	Removal of levels I and V lymph nodes with preservation of the sternocleidomastoid, internal jugular vein, *or* spinal accessory nerve intact
Radical (Fig. C)	Removal of selected lymph nodes from levels I and V, sternocleidomastoid, internal jugular vein, and spinal accessory nerve

Table 10.2 (continued)

Extended (Fig. D)	Same as radical neck dissection along with removal of another lymph node group (i.e., superior mediastinal) or nonlymphatic structure (i.e., carotid artery) or structure not normally included in neck dissection (i.e., salivary gland, thyroid)
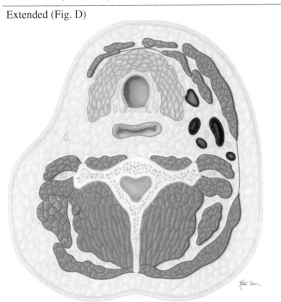	

CCA common carotid artery, *IJV* internal jugular vein, *LN* lymph node, *SCM* sternocleidomastoid

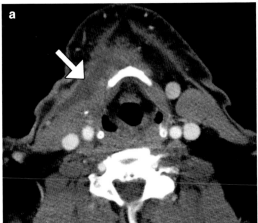
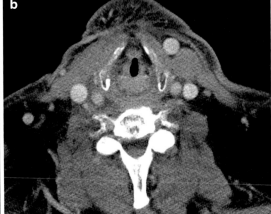

Fig. 10.16 Selective neck dissection. Axial CT image 4 weeks after lateral neck dissection (**a**) shows a seroma (*arrow*) overlying the right sternocleidomastoid muscle. There is loss of fat surrounding the carotid artery and subcutaneous tissues. Axial CT image obtained 2 years after right lateral neck dissection and radiotherapy (**b**) shows subcutaneous stranding. The sternocleidomastoid muscle and internal jugular vein are intact. Axial CT image (**c**) shows resection of the right submandibular gland and remaining left submandibular gland (*arrow*), producing an asymmetric appearance that should not be confused with a mass lesion

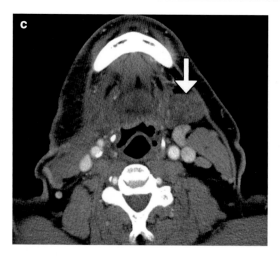

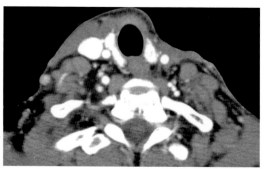

Fig. 10.18 Radical neck dissection. Axial CT image shows the absence of the left sternocleidomastoid and internal jugular vein as well as concavity of the left neck contour

Fig. 10.16 (continued)

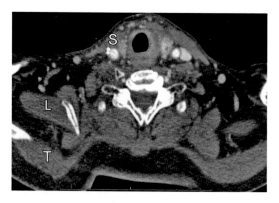

Fig. 10.17 Modified radical neck dissection. Axial CT image shows the absence of the right internal jugular vein and atrophy of the sternocleidomastoid (*S*) and trapezius (*T*) muscles but compensatory hypertrophy of the right levator scapulae (*L*). There is also mild edema in the right neck soft tissues

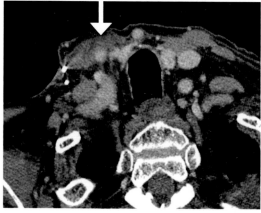

Fig. 10.19 Radical neck dissection with pectoralis rotational flap. Axial CT image shows right radical neck dissection, including resection of the right sternocleidomastoid. Instead, there is a pectoralis rotational flap (*arrow*) that covers the carotid artery

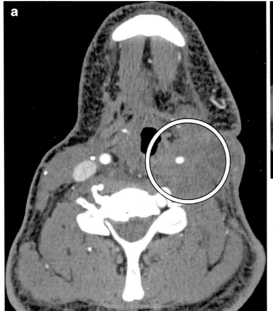

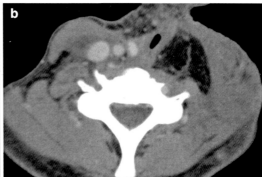

Fig. 10.20 Extended neck dissection. Preoperative axial CT image (**a**) shows an infiltrative tumor (*arrow*) that encases the left carotid artery. The patient had undergone prior radical neck dissection and radiation therapy.

Postoperative axial CT image (**b**) shows interval sacrifice of the left common carotid artery and myocutaneous flap reconstruction

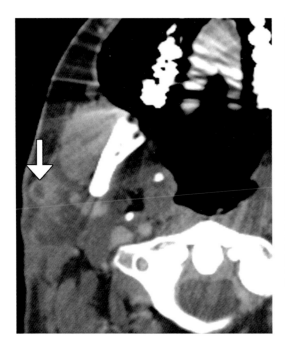

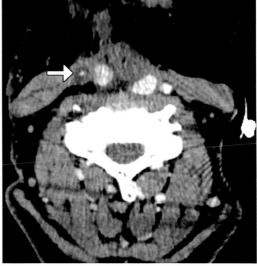

Fig. 10.22 Suture granuloma. AxialCT image after total laryngectomy shows a nodule with a central highattenuation focus (*arrow*)

Fig. 10.21 Cauterized adipose tissue. Axial CT image shows a nodular area with central hypoattenuation in the subcutaneous tissues of the right face (*arrow*), which represents biopsy-proven fibroadipose tissue

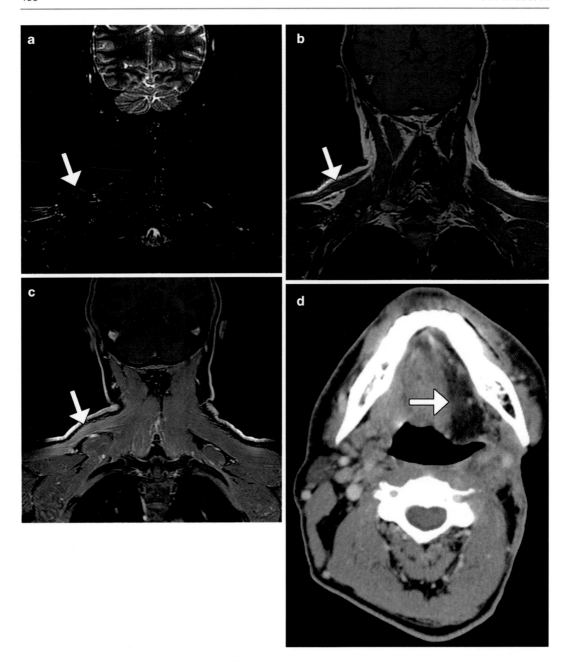

Fig. 10.23 Denervation related to neck dissection. Coronal STIR (**a**), T1-weighted (**b**), and post-contrast fat-suppressed T1-weighted (**c**) MR images show edema, and enhancement is an atrophic right trapezius muscle (*arrow*), ipsilateral to where neck dissection was performed. Axial CT image in a different patient (**d**) demonstrates fatty change in the left half of the tongue (*arrow*) after hypoglossal nerve sacrifice during neck dissection

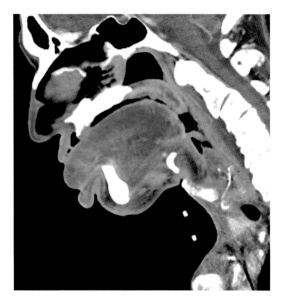

Fig. 10.24 Postoperative lymphedema. Sagittal CT image shows diffuse swelling of the cervicofacial soft tissues, particularly the tongue and lips, as well as diffuse fat stranding

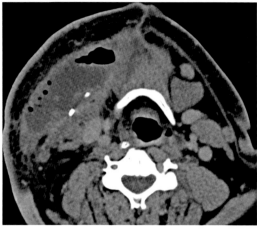

Fig. 10.26 Wound abscess. There is a large gas and fluid collection in the right neck surgical bed. There is also overlying subcutaneous fat stranding and skin thickening

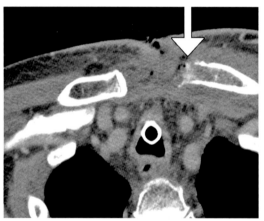

Fig. 10.27 Osteomyelitis. Axial CT image shows an open wound and sinus tract with regional subcutaneous fat stranding and erosion of the left medial clavicle (*arrow*)

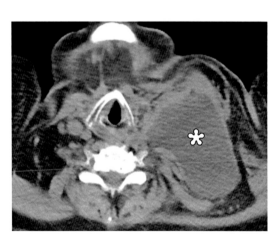

Fig. 10.25 Lymphocele. Axial CT image shows a large, unilocular fluid-attenuation collection (*) in the left neck that extends into the left chest subcutaneous tissues (Courtesy of John Wandtke, M.D.)

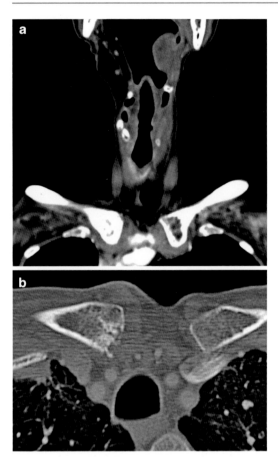

Fig. 10.28 Neuropathic joint. Coronal CT image (**a**) shows radical right neck dissection and flap reconstruction. Axial CT image (**b**) shows right proximal clavicle degenerative changes ipsilateral to the neck dissection

10.3   Parotidectomy

10.3.1   Discussion

Parotidectomy is most commonly performed for primary salivary neoplasm resection, but is also performed for oncologic management of skin cancers. Several types of parotidectomy can be implemented, including superficial parotidectomy and total parotidectomy with or without facial nerve preservation, depending on the type, size, and location of the tumor (Figs. 10.29, 10.30, and 10.31). The defects created by more extensive resections can be reconstructed using tissue flaps or synthetic materials. Furthermore, when the facial nerve is compromised, eyelid weights are often used to aid eye closure.

In general, complications and expected consequences related to parotidectomy may include cosmetic deformity, facial nerve deficits, sialocele, wound infection, hematoma, and tumor recurrence. In particular, recurrence of parotid pleomorphic adenoma has an incidence of 1–5% and most commonly occurs within the first 10 years following surgical resection. Recurrent lesions have fairly characteristic imaging features. On T2-weighted MRI, the majority of recurrent tumors have very high signal intensity due to myxoid contents. The presence of multiple subcentimeter nodules is a strong indicator of recurrence and is observed in about two-thirds of cases. This feature results in a "bunch of grapes" appearance (Fig. 10.32). Recurrent pleomorphic adenomas are sometimes located in the subcutaneous tissues or adjacent neck spaces perhaps due to spillage during surgery. The enhancement pattern is variable, depending upon the extent of cystic components, fibrosis, and necrosis.

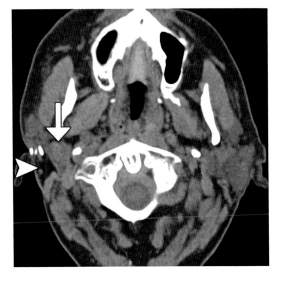

Fig. 10.29 Superficial parotidectomy with graft reconstruction. Axial CT image shows fat graft occupying the expected location of the right superficial parotid lobe (*arrowhead*). The deep lobe of the right parotid gland remains intact (*arrow*)

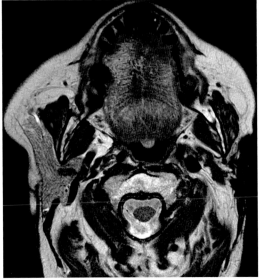

Fig. 10.30 Total parotidectomy. Axial T2-weighted MRI shows the absence of the left parotid gland, resulting in concavity of the overlying skin. The facial nerve could be spared along with the retromandibular vein, and the contralateral normal parotid gland is intact

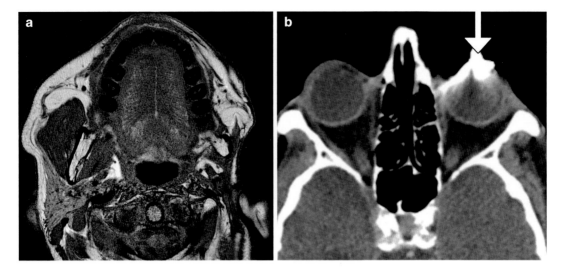

Fig. 10.31 Total parotidectomy with facial nerve sacrifice. Axial T1-weighted MRI (**a**) shows the absence of the left parotid gland and atrophy of the left facial muscles. Partial resection of the left masticator muscles and man- dibular ramus was also performed. The axial CT image (**b**) shows a left eyelid weight (*arrow*), with considerable metal streak artifact

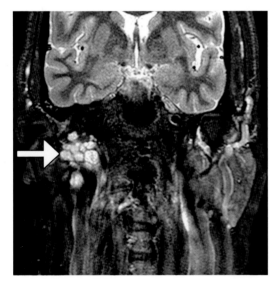

Fig. 10.32 Recurrent parotid pleomorphic adenoma. Coronal STIR MRI demonstrates a cluster of nodules with a "bunch of grapes" appearance (*arrow*)

10.4 Salivary Duct Stenting and Endoscopic Stone Removal

10.4.1 Discussion

Salivary duct stones can be managed by sialendoscopic extraction. Sometimes, plastic stents are inserted after stone removal in order to reduce the risk of subsequent stenosis (Fig. 10.33). These

appear as tubular hyperattenuating structures on CT and should not be misinterpreted as residual sialolithiasis. Occasionally, stone extraction can be complicated by sialocele or even cutaneous fistula formation due to the friability of the inflamed tissues in the setting of acute sialadenitis and sialodacryoadenitis. In such cases, imaging can be performed to assess for the extent of associated fluid collections and sinus tracts (Fig. 10.34).

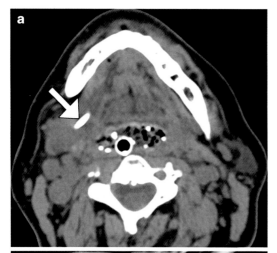
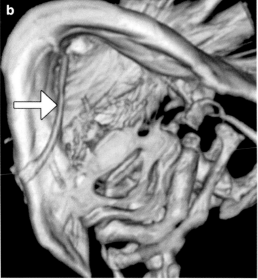

Fig. 10.33 Submandibular duct stent. Axial (**a**) and 3D CT (**b**) images show a hyperattenuating stent that passes through the right submandibular duct (*arrows*)

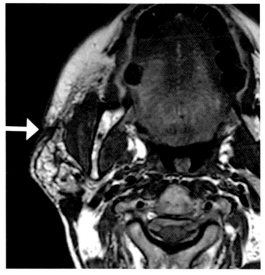

Fig. 10.34 Parotid cutaneous fistula after endoscopic stone extraction. Axial T1-weighted MRI shows a right face skin defect and sinus tract (*arrow*) extending to the underlying parotid gland

10.5 Facial Reanimation

10.5.1 Discussion

Facial reanimation can be performed for treating the effects of chronic facial nerve paralysis. This can be accomplished with techniques, such as functioning free muscle transfer or temporalis muscle transposition and suspension combined with suborbicularis oculi fat (SOOF) lift. Overall, these techniques successfully restore smiles and provide improvement in mouth function in most patients.

Functioning free gracilis microneurovascular muscle transfer is a form of dynamic facial reanimation that can help restore facial tone and movement. The free muscle flap is buried in the subcutaneous tissues of the face extending from the temporal fossa to the oral commissure region. CT and MRI can demonstrate the intact muscle fibers in the healthy grafts (Fig. 10.35). In addition, Doppler ultrasound is useful for evaluating the patency of the feeding artery and draining vein. Transfer of compound flaps containing muscle and other tissue, such as the skin, can be performed for cases of complex facial paralysis that involve skin or soft tissue deficits after tumor excision. Alternatively, tensor fascia lata and AlloDerm grafts can be used and also appear as soft tissue bands on imaging, but these do not offer dynamic facial animation (Figs. 10.36 and 10.37).

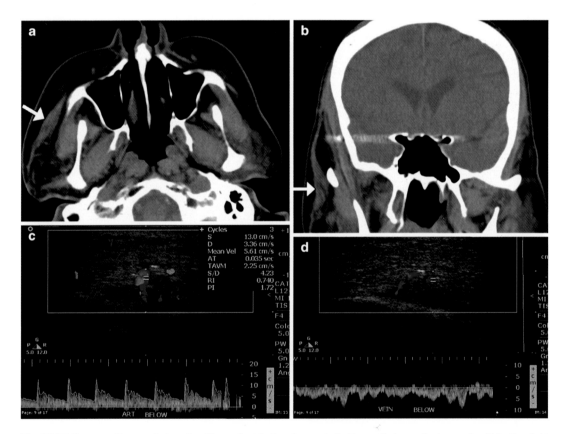

Fig. 10.35 Free gracilis muscle transfer. The patient had right facial paralysis after right cerebellopontine angle schwannoma resection. Axial (**a**) and coronal (**b**) CT images demonstrate the grafted muscle (*arrows*) within the right face subcutaneous tissues. Doppler ultrasound images of the graft artery (**c**) and vein (**d**) display normal waveforms

Temporoparietal fascia and temporalis muscle transposition and suspension procedures consist of detaching and repositioning the flap approximately 180° inferiorly toward the oral commissure and/or nasolabial folds via a tunnel through subcutaneous tissues (Figs. 10.38 and 10.39). The tissues superficial to the plane of dissection can be translated superomedially and sutured to the fascia of the temporalis muscle. If necessary, the

procedure can be augmented using Silastic prostheses to fill the defect. Alternatively, the muscle can be extended using polytetrafluoroethylene.

The suborbicularis oculi fat (SOOF) lift involves superior mobilization of midface structures, which are fastened to the orbital rim using a variety of approaches (Fig. 10.40). Often, the intraorbital fat pads are also released and sutured to the SOOF.

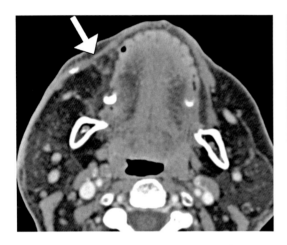

Fig. 10.36 Tensor fascia lata graft. Axial CT image shows the band-like graft positioned in the right face subcutaneous tissues, inserting into the oral commissure (*arrow*)

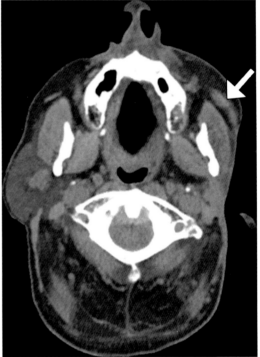

Fig. 10.37 AlloDerm graft. The patient is status post total left parotidectomy with facial nerve sacrifice. Axial CT image shows the soft tissue attenuation sling (*arrow*) in the left check subcutaneous tissues

Fig. 10.38 Temporoparietal fascia and muscle flap. The patient has a history of left facial paralysis. Coronal CT image shows the flap swung inferiorly over the zygomatic arch (*arrow*). There is considerable soft tissue swelling at the surgical site

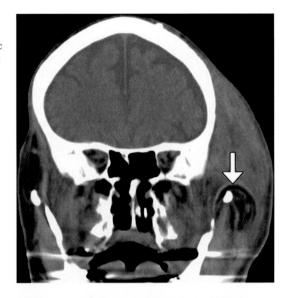

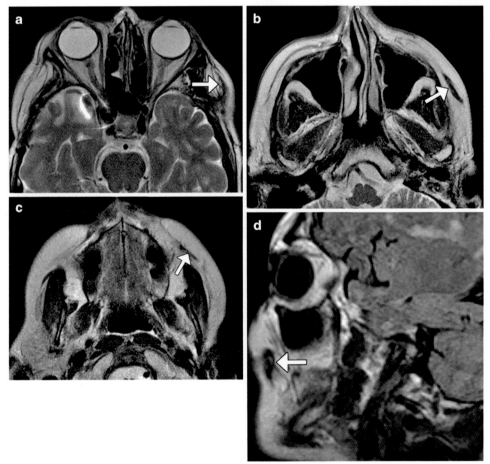

Fig. 10.39 Temporalis muscle transposition and suborbicularis oculi fat (*SOOF*) lift. The patient had left facial paralysis status post parotidectomy and facial nerve resection for adenoid cystic carcinoma. Serial axial T2-weighted MR images from superior to inferior (**a–c**) and a sagittal T2-weighted FLAIR image (**d**) show the left temporalis (*arrows*) turned inferomedially toward the mouth. The suborbicularis oculi fat pad has also been raised

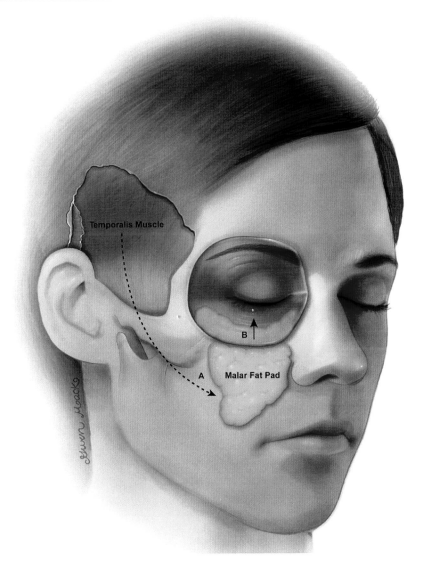

Fig. 10.40 Schematic of the temporalis transposition technique. In the temporalis transposition (*A*), the temporalis muscle is detached from the calvarium and brought inferomedially over the zygoma toward the oral commissure and nasolabial folds. In the SOOF lift (*B*), the suborbicularis oculi fat pad is repositioned superiorly

10.6 Oral Cavity Tumor Resection and Reconstruction

10.6.1 Discussion

Depending on the stage of oral tongue malignancies, such as squamous cell carcinomas, variable degrees of glossectomy may be performed, ranging from partial, subtotal, or total, with or without floor of the mouth resection, mandibulectomy, and laryngectomy (Figs. 10.41, 10.42, 10.43, 10.44, and 10.45). Of note, composite tumor resection consisting of glossectomy, mandibulectomy, and neck dissection known as "Commando," an acronym for combined mandibulectomy and neck dissection operation, can be performed for advanced cancers of the oral cavity. Furthermore, the submandibular gland may be removed with rerouting of the duct as part of the approach or as part of the combined suprahyoid neck dissection. Alternatively, the submandibular gland may be the main target of surgery when it is involved by primary salivary gland neoplasms. There are a variety of options for reconstructing surgical defects in the oral cavity region, including myocutaneous flaps, such as single or double bilobed

radial forearm flaps, FAMM flaps, submental island flaps, and acellular dermal matrix, or a combination of these.

The role of imaging after glossectomy is to evaluate complications, such as infection, sialocele, and tumor recurrence (Figs. 10.46, 10.47, and 10.48). Of note, one must be particularly vigilant for the presence of perineural tumor spread on imaging before and after surgery, especially following resection of salivary gland malignancies, which is often along the maxillary division branches of the trigeminal nerve for oral cavity tumors. Furthermore, since radiation often accompanies surgical treatment of oral cancers, the mandible is at risk for osteonecrosis. This complication tends to occur at least 1 year after radiation therapy and appears as areas of cortical irregularity and lucency (Fig. 10.49). There can be superimposed infection and pathological fracture.

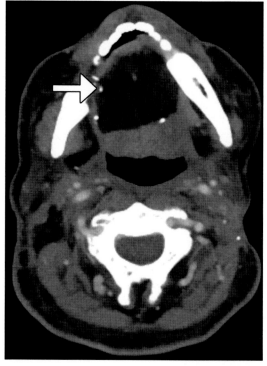

Fig. 10.42 Subtotal glossectomy. The patient had a history of squamous cell carcinoma of the tongue. Axial CT image shows that the majority of the oral tongue has been resected and reconstructed using a myocutaneous graft (*arrow*). Surgical clips are present along the margins of the graft

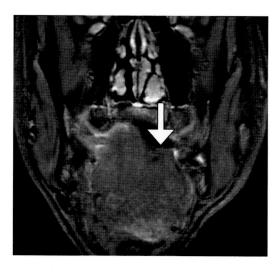

Fig. 10.41 Partial hemiglossectomy with primary closure. Coronal fat-suppressed post-contrast T1-weighted MRI shows a defect in the left lateral tongue (*arrow*), without graft reconstruction resulting in asymmetric prominence of the normal right side of the tongue

Fig. 10.43 Total glossectomy and laryngectomy. The patient had a history of chemoradiation for stage IV squamous cell carcinoma of the base of the tongue. Subsequently, total laryngectomy and total glossectomy with myocutaneous flap reconstruction were performed. Sagittal CT image demonstrates complete absence of the native tongue with placement of a myocutaneous flap with predominantly fat attenuation components (*arrow*). The flap provides near-anatomic contours for the reconstructed tongue

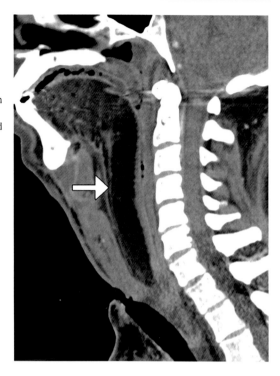

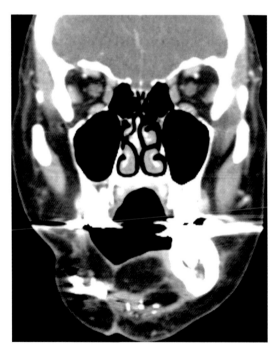

Fig. 10.44 Commando. Coronal CT image shows glossectomy, and right hemimandibulectomy with flap reconstruction. Neck dissection, which is not shown, was also performed

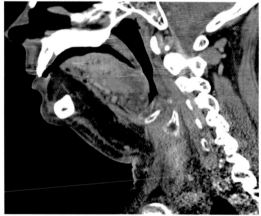

Fig. 10.45 Floor of mouth resection with marginal mandibulectomy. Sagittal CT image shows extensive resection of the floor of mouth contents along with the gingiva and alveolar portions of the mandible. The defect has been reconstructed using a myocutaneous flap

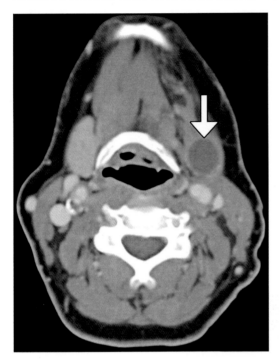

Fig. 10.46 Sialocele after floor of mouth resection and submandibular duct rerouting. Axial CT image shows a well-defined fluid collection in the right submandibular space (*arrow*)

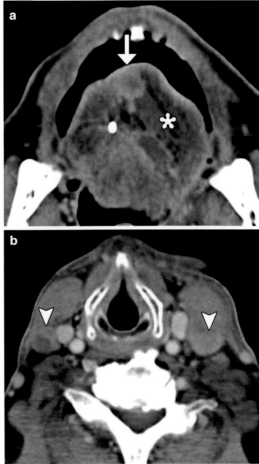

Fig. 10.47 Locoregional tumor recurrence. Axial CT images (**a**, **b**) show recurrent tumor (*arrow*) at the glossectomy site (*) as well as bilateral lymphadenopathy (*arrowheads*) from metastatic squamous cell carcinoma

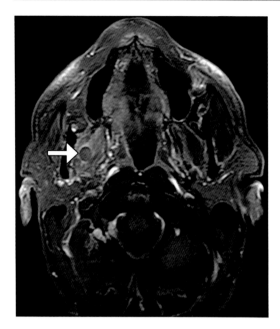

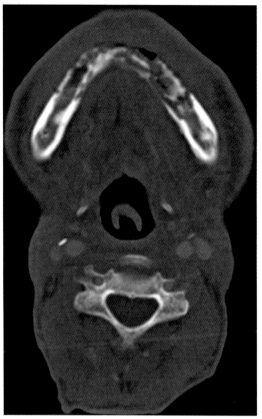

Fig. 10.48 Perineural tumor. Axial fat-suppressed post-contrast T1-weighted MRI shows marked expansion of a branch of the right maxillary division of the trigeminal nerve that represents perineural tumor (*arrow*) that remained after resection of a submandibular gland adenoid cystic carcinoma at another institution

Fig. 10.49 Mandibular osteonecrosis. Axial CT image shows extensive irregular lucency on the mandible after radiation and floor of mouth tumor resection

10.7 Tonsillectomy and Adenoidectomy

10.7.1 Discussion

Tonsillectomy and adenoidectomy are two of the most commonly performed pediatric surgical procedures. The main indications for tonsillectomy and adenoidectomy include adenotonsillar hyperplasia with obstructive sleep apnea, failure to thrive, or abnormal dentofacial growth; malignant neoplasms; and adenotonsillar hyperplasia with upper airway obstruction, dysphagia, or speech impairment and halitosis. Furthermore, otitis media and recurrent or chronic rhinosinusitis or adenoiditis are indications for adenoidectomy, but not tonsillectomy, while recurrent or chronic pharyngotonsillitis, peritonsillar abscess, and streptococcal carriage are indications for tonsillectomy, but not adenoidectomy. Frequently, the appearance on postoperative imaging is that of asymmetric absence of Waldeyer ring tissue, whereby the residual normal tissue can hypertrophy and should not be mistaken for a lesion (Fig. 10.50). Sometimes, the trace amounts of residual Waldeyer ring tissues can regrow over the course of years after tonsillectomy/adenoidectomy, such that the effects of surgery are not noticeable. As in many other parts of the head and neck, when more extensive surgeries are performed for tumor resection, the resulting defects may be reconstructed using soft tissue flaps (Fig. 10.51).

Among patients who underwent tonsillectomy for obstructive apnea, cine MRI is a useful modality for evaluating anatomy and function when there are recurrent symptoms. Potential causes include glossoptosis, hypopharyngeal collapse, recurrent and enlarged adenoids and lingual tonsils, and macroglossia. If lingual tonsils were greater than 10 mm in diameter and abutted both the posterior border of the tongue and the posterior

pharyngeal wall, they can be considered markedly enlarged (Fig. 10.52). On the other hand, patients can develop velopharyngeal insufficiency following excessive removal of adenoid tissues. This can manifest as a gap between the pharynx and soft palate on cine MRI, which can be treated via palatoplasty or pharyngeal augmentation with substances, such as hydroxyapatite filler (Fig. 10.53).

Among patients who underwent tonsillectomy/ adenoidectomy for neoplasm, 18FDG-PET/CT is useful for evaluating recurrent tumor. However, infection at the site of surgery can manifest as focal hypermetabolism (Fig. 10.54). Noninfectious inflammation and granulation tissue at the surgical site can also yield false-positive results on 18FDG-PET/CT. However, as opposed to tumor recurrence, activity on 18FDG-PET/CT should decrease over time with infection and inflammation.

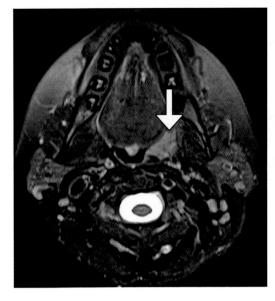

Fig. 10.50 Tonsillectomy. Axial fat-suppressed T2-weighted MRI shows the absence of the right lingual tonsil and a remaining hypertrophied left anterior palatine tonsil (*arrow*). The postoperative changes are otherwise virtually imperceptible

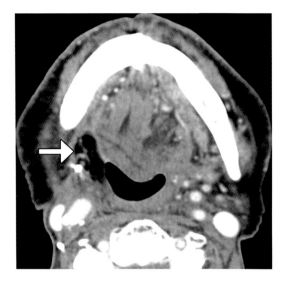

Fig. 10.51 Tonsillectomy with flap reconstruction. Axial CT images show flap reconstruction of the right tonsillectomy defect (*arrow*), after resection of an invasive squamous cell carcinoma. There is nevertheless a relative paucity of tissue on the right side

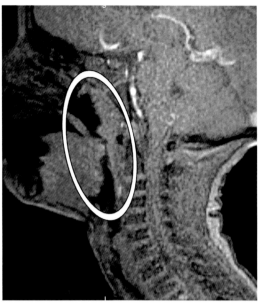

Fig. 10.52 Recurrent enlargement of adenoids and tonsils. Cine MRI in a child with obstructive apnea previously treated with adenotonsillectomy shows enlarged adenoid and lingual tonsils associated with airway narrowing (*encircled*)

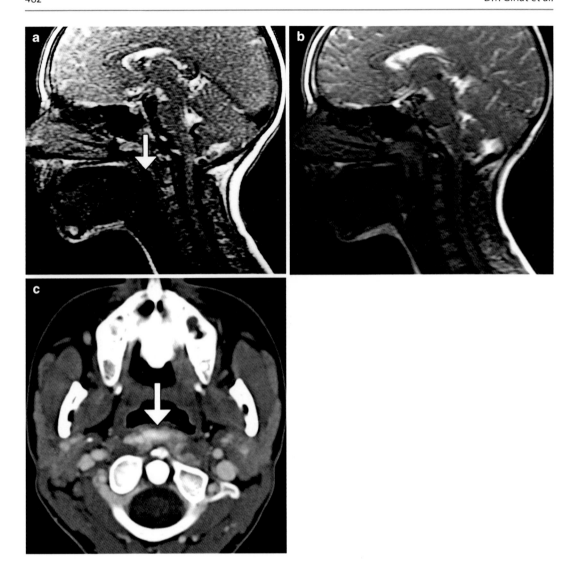

Fig. 10.53 Velopharyngeal insufficiency after adenoidectomy. The patient underwent a Furlow palatoplasty to repair a submucosal cleft with marked improvement but persistent velopharyngeal insufficiency with fatigue at the end of the day. Posterior pharyngeal wall pharyngoplasty with calcium hydroxyapatite filler injection augmentation was then performed. Sagittal cine MR image (**a**) after adenoidectomy and palatoplasty shows velopharyngeal gap that persists throughout the cycle (*arrow*). Sagittal MR image (**b**) obtained after adenoid augmentation shows increased bulk of the adenoids with no residual velopharyngeal gap. Axial CT image (**c**) in a different patient shows the high attenuation Radiesse within the retropharyngeal space at the level of the oro- and nasopharynx (*arrow*)

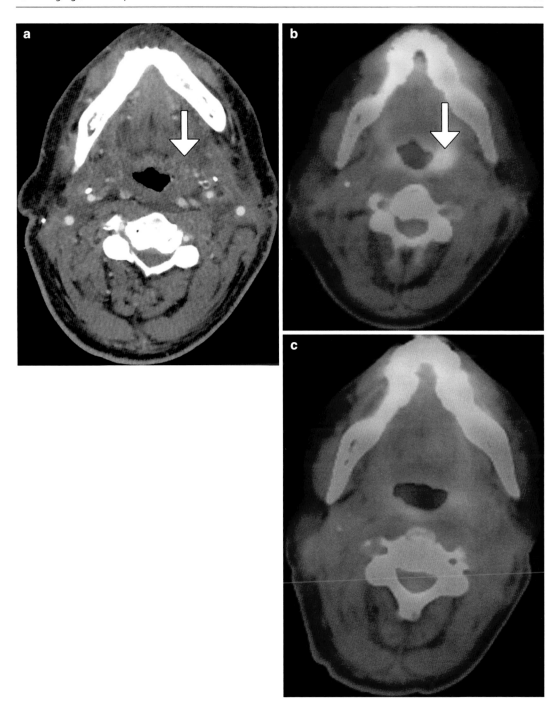

Fig. 10.54 Postoperative infection mimicking tumor recurrence. Contrast-enhanced CT (**a**) shows asymmetric edema of the pharyngeal mucosal and parapharyngeal spaces (*arrow*), but no distinct mass. 18FDG-PET/CT (**b**) obtained soon after shows focal hypermetabolism in the left oropharyngeal surgical bed (*arrow*). The lesion proved to be fungal pharyngitis, and follow-up 18FDG-PET/CT (**c**) obtained 6 months later showed resolution of the lesion

10.8   Transoral Robotic Surgery

10.8.1 Discussion

Transoral robotic surgery (TORS) is a minimally invasive technique that involves the use of endoscopic visualization and dexterous robotic arms and has been mainly implemented for resecting T1 and T2 squamous cell carcinomas of the oropharynx, although various other applications have been explored. TORS offers a high rate of preserved postoperative swallowing function, but low incidence of complications. The postoperative imaging findings to TORS generally differ from those related to open surgery. Tongue base tumor TORS resection typically includes approximately the half of the tongue base on the side of the tumor, with dissection to the circumvallate papillae and glossotonsillar sulcus. Consequently,

during the first weeks to months after surgery, retraction of the tongue base bed is apparent on postoperative imaging (Fig. 10.55), without evidence of solid enhancement. A radical tonsillectomy using a TORS approach involves the tonsil, anterior and posterior tonsillar pillars, portions of the soft palate, tongue base, to encompass the superior constrictor muscle as the depth of resection and the posterior pharyngeal wall are resected. Imaging during the first several postoperative weeks typically demonstrates distortion of the fat planes around the medial pterygoid muscle and retropharyngeal edema (Fig. 10.56), which can result from retraction or thermal injury during the surgery. Over the ensuing months, scar tissue formation leads to gradual retraction of the lateral oropharyngeal wall, with "tilting" of the soft palate toward the surgical bed.

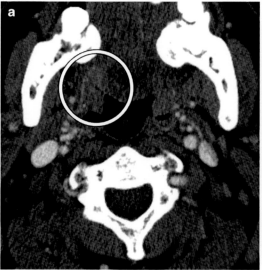
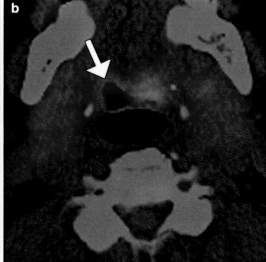
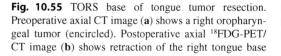

Fig. 10.55 TORS base of tongue tumor resection. Preoperative axial CT image (**a**) shows a right oropharyngeal tumor (encircled). Postoperative axial ¹⁸FDG-PET/CT image (**b**) shows retraction of the right tongue base surgical bed (*arrow*) without evidence of tumor, but residual normal hypermetabolic left lingual tissue, which should not be misinterpreted as tumor

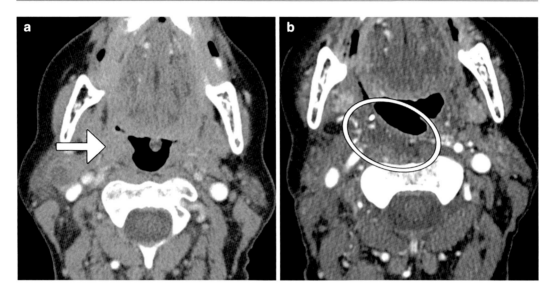

Fig. 10.56 TORS lateral oropharyngectomy. Preoperative axial CT image (**a**) shows a right palatine tonsil squamous cell carcinoma (*arrow*). Postoperative CT image (**b**) shows interval resection of the tumor and edema in the region of the surgical bed, with extension into the retropharyngeal space (*encircled*)

10.9   Sistrunk Procedure

10.9.1 Discussion

The Sistrunk procedure is performed for resection of thyroglossal duct cysts and neoplasms. The procedure includes removal of the variable amounts of the central portion of the hyoid bone, following the cyst tract to the base of the tongue (Fig. 10.57). This surgical technique has not significantly changed since it was first described in 1920. Complications occur in 7.5% of cases and mainly include cyst recurrence and infection (Figs. 10.58 and 10.59).

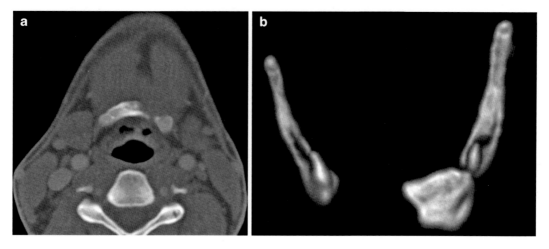

Fig. 10.57 Sistrunk procedure. Axial CT (**a**) and 3D (**b**) CT images show surgical defects in the midportion of the hyoid bone in two different patients

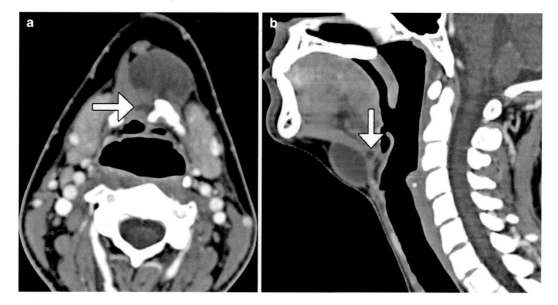

Fig. 10.58 Recurrent thyroglossal duct cyst. Axial (**a**) and sagittal (**b**) CT images show a midline fluid collection with a tract that extends from the Sistrunk resection site (*arrows*)

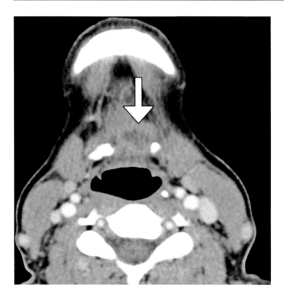

Fig. 10.59 Abscess after Sistrunk procedure. Axial CT image shows a rim-enhancing fluid collection at the site of hyoid bone resection (*arrow*)

10.10 Laryngectomy

10.10.1 Discussion

A wide variety of laryngectomy procedures can be performed, depending on the size and location of tumor within the larynx, ranging from conservative to radical. CT is often used to follow patients who underwent laryngectomy. The types of laryngectomy with their corresponding descriptions and imaging features are depicted in Figs. 10.60, 10.61, 10.62, 10.63, 10.64, 10.65, and 10.66 and listed in Table 10.3. There is an increasing trend towards laryngeal conservation procedures in order to preserve function. Laser photoangiolysis can effectively remove tumors of the vocal cords, which can then heal with near-anatomic configuration. In addition, reconstruction of the laryngeal framework can be performed during laryngectomy using materials such as aortic grafts.

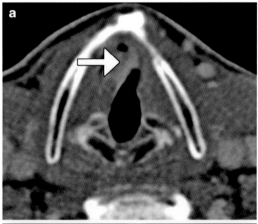
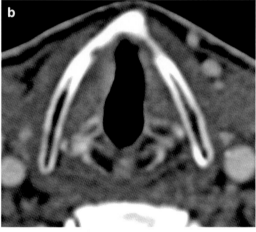

Fig. 10.60 Angiolytic laser cordectomy. Preoperative axial CT image (**a**) shows a right glottic carcinoma (*arrow*). Postoperative axial CT image (**b**) shows interval resection of the mass and minimal asymmetry of the neocord

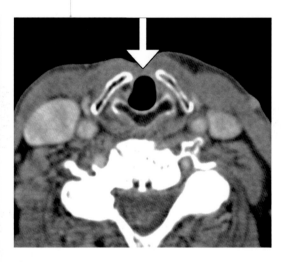

Fig. 10.61 Complex laryngectomy with aortic graft reconstruction. Axial CT image shows partial laryngectomy with soft tissue spanning the anterior tracheal cartilage defect, which represents the aortic graft (*arrow*)

Fig. 10.62 Vertical partial laryngectomy. Axial (**a**), coronal (**b**), and 3D (**c**) CT images show hemilaryngectomy with the absence of the right thyroid cartilage and thyroarytenoid (*arrowheads*). The neovestibule is asymmetric. The contralateral thyroid cartilage and thyroarytenoid remain intact

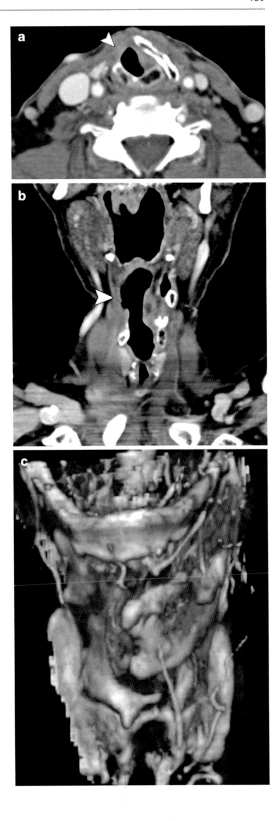

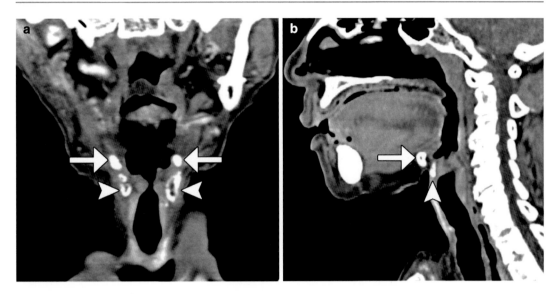

Fig. 10.63 Horizontal laryngectomy. Coronal (**a**) and sagittal (**b**) CT images show supraglottic laryngectomy with the absence of the epiglottis, absence of preepiglottic fat, and asymmetry of the neovestibule. The hyoid bone (*arrow*) abuts the residual thyroid cartilage (*arrowhead*)

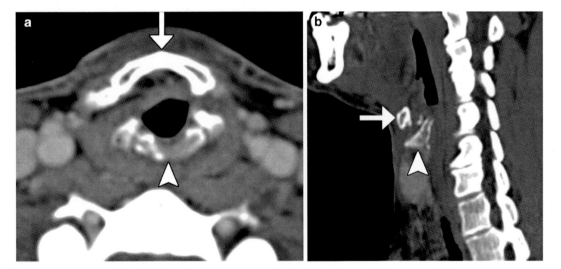

Fig. 10.64 Supracricoid laryngectomy with cricohyoidopexy. Axial (**a**) and sagittal (**b**) CT images show the hyoid (*arrows*) closely apposed to the cricoid (*arrowheads*) with absence of the thyroid cartilages

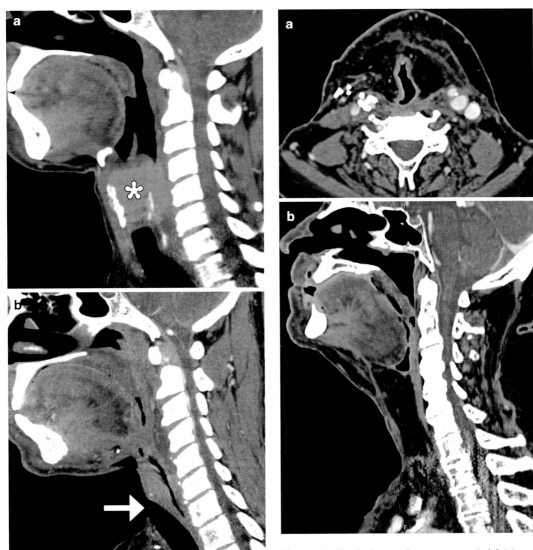

Fig. 10.65 Total laryngectomy. Preoperative sagittal CT image (**a**) shows a large laryngeal squamous cell carcinoma (*). Postoperative sagittal CT image (**b**) shows the absence of the laryngeal framework and hyoid bone. A tracheostomy has been created (*arrow*)

Fig. 10.66 Total pharyngolaryngectomy. Axial (**a**) and coronal (**b**) CT images show total resection of the larynx and hypopharynx with flap reconstruction, resulting in a neopharynx

Table 10.3 Types of laryngectomy

	Procedure	Description	Imaging features
Conservative	Microsurgery	Minimally invasive excision of small tumors using lasers. Mainly used for excision of vocal cord tumors and variable portions of the vocal cord (cordectomy)	CT may appear normal once vocal cord tissue regenerates. On CT, a defect in the vocal cord may be visible, but may appear normal once vocal cord tissue regenerates, resulting in a pseudocord
	Vertical partial laryngectomy	Frontolateral laryngectomy: resection of vertical segment of thyroid cartilage, one vocal cord, the laryngeal ventricle and false cord, anterior commissure, and small anterior portion of contralateral cord	Frontolateral laryngectomy: CT shows vertical defect in thyroid lamina, with irregular sclerotic border, absent aryepiglottic fold, paraglottic and preepiglottic fat, scar at site of excised true vocal cord that extends from the contralateral thyroid cartilage to the ipsilateral arytenoid area that forms pseudocord, tilting of neovestibule to the side of the major excision, and normal subglottic larynx
		Hemilaryngectomy: resection of same structures as in frontolateral laryngectomy and mucosa from the aryepiglottic fold to the upper border of the cricoid cartilage, arytenoid cartilage, and ipsilateral thyroid lamina	Hemilaryngectomy: CT shows similar findings as with frontolateral laryngectomy. Reconstruction with tissue grafts or prostheses may be identified
	Horizontal laryngectomy	Supraglottic laryngectomy: resection of epiglottis, aryepiglottic folds, false vocal cords, upper third of thyroid cartilage, and thyrohyoid membrane	Supraglottic laryngectomy: CT at the supraglottic level shows dilated cavity. The hyoid and remaining thyroid cartilage are visible in the same axial section. The glottic and subglottic structures are normal
		Supracricoid laryngectomy: resection of laryngeal structures from the cricoid cartilage to the hyoid bone with preservation of at least one arytenoid cartilage and cricohyoidopexy or cricohyoidoepiglottopexy reconstruction	Supracricoid laryngectomy: CT shows soft tissue replacing false and true vocal cords and surrounding the arytenoid cartilage. The neoglottis is asymmetric and has a pseudocord appearance
	Near-total laryngectomy	Resection of entire larynx except for portions of thyroid lamina, thyroarytenoid muscle, and entire arytenoid cartilage and recurrent laryngeal nerve on one side	CT can demonstrate the laryngeal remnants. A tracheostomy in lower neck is present

Table 10.3 (continued)

	Procedure	Description	Imaging features
Radical	Total laryngectomy	Removal of the epiglottis, aryepiglottic folds, true and false vocal cords, subglottic larynx, hyoid bone, thyroid cartilage, arytenoid cartilages, cricoid cartilage, and one or more tracheal rings. In addition, a partial or total thyroidectomy is often performed as well	CT shows the absence of entire larynx, hyoid, variable portions of the tracheal rings, and part or all of the thyroid glands. The neopharynx appears as a concentric layer of soft tissue. Excess tissue at the anastomosis can resemble the epiglottis ("pseudoepiglottis"). A tracheostomy is invariably present
	Pharyngolaryngectomy	In addition to total laryngectomy, there is more extensive resection of the pharynx, such that primary anastomosis between the esophagus and remaining portions of the pharynx is not feasible. Rather, flap or graft reconstruction is performed to create a neopharynx	The flap or graft material that spans the surgical defect can be visualized, connecting the esophagus inferiorly with the remaining pharyngeal mucosal tissue superiorly. The graft has a tubular configuration that forms a lumen (neopharynx). A tracheostomy is also present

Complications following laryngectomy include mass-like formations of granulation tissue, which can mimic tumor recurrence (Fig. 10.67); infection, which can lead to the carotid artery blow out (Fig. 10.68); tumor recurrence, which can be associated with development of pharyngocutaneous fistula (Fig. 10.69), particularly with concomitant radiation therapy; and laryngoceles in the setting of laryngeal framework conservation surgery (Fig. 10.70).

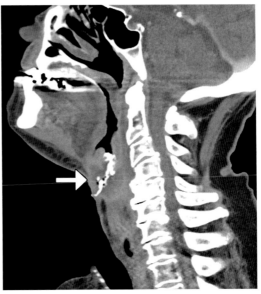

Fig. 10.68 Recurrent tumor with pharyngocutaneous fistula. Sagittal CT image shows a fistulous tract (*arrow*) that extends from the hypopharynx to the overlying skin filled with injected contrast, traversing necrotic recurrent tumor

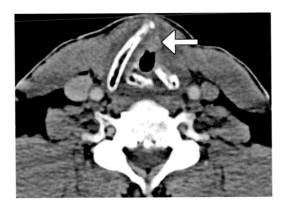

Fig. 10.67 Granulation tissue. Axial CT image shows a mildly enhancing soft tissue nodule (*arrow*) in the left anterior commissure where partial laryngectomy and aortic graft reconstruction were performed

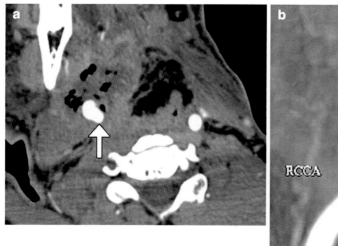
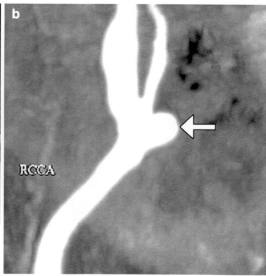

Fig. 10.69 Carotid blowout. Axial (**a**) and curved planar reformatted (**b**) CTA images show a fluid and gas collection surrounding the right carotid artery following laryngectomy and neck dissection with flap reconstruction, as well as radiation therapy. There is also an outpouching (*arrows*) at the right carotid bulb, compatible with pseudoaneurysm

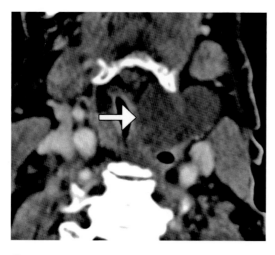

Fig. 10.70 Postoperative laryngocele. Axial CT image shows a lobulated fluid collection (*arrow*) extending laterally beyond the larynx following partial laryngectomy

10.11   Tracheoesophageal Puncture and Voice Prostheses

10.11.1   Discussion

Voice prostheses (tracheoesophageal puncture devices), such as Provox and Blom-Singer, are used to provide voice restoration following total laryngectomy (Figs. 10.71 and 10.72). These devices are implanted across a surgical tracheo-esophageal puncture or fistula created at the superior aspect of the tracheal stoma. Voice prostheses contain a one-way valve that prevents saliva from entering the trachea, but allow air to pass into the esophagus to enable "esophageal speech" (Fig. 10.73). The devices are usually changed after several months due to biofilm accumulation. Complications related to voice prostheses are uncommon, but migration/malposition, leakage around the valve, and valve incompetence can occur. In addition, they can become dislodged and aspirated into the trachea or swallowed, and may appear as a foreign body. CT with multiplanar reformations can be used effectively to evaluate position of the prosthesis, since the cylindrical plastic and metallic components are readily visible (Fig. 10.74).

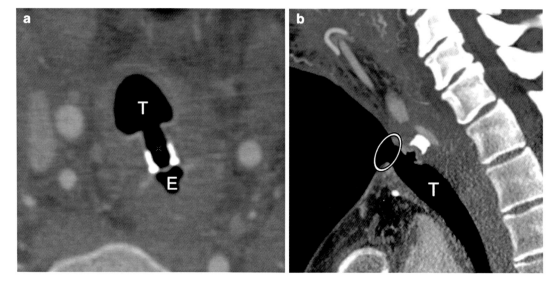

Fig. 10.71 Provox voice prosthesis. Axial (**a**) and sagittal (**b**) CT images show the voice prosthesis, the trachea (*T*), and the esophagus (*E*) at the level of the stoma (*oval*)

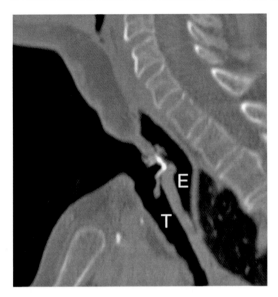

Fig. 10.72 Blom-Singer voice prosthesis. Sagittal CT image shows the prosthesis with its characteristic "duck-bill" in the tissue plane between the trachea (*T*) and esophagus (*E*)

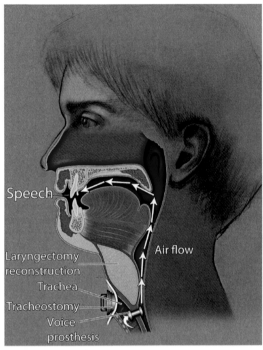

Fig. 10.73 Illustration depicts a voice prosthesis and relevant anatomy

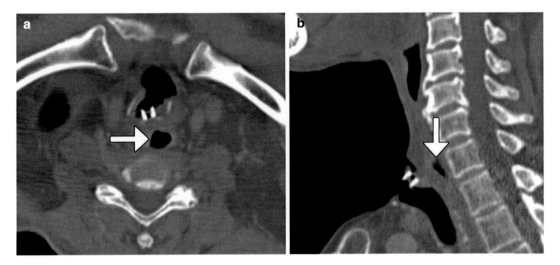

Fig. 10.74 Voice prosthesis migration. Oblique axial (**a**) and sagittal (**b**) CT images show anterior displacement of the device, which does not attain the esophageal lumen (*arrows*)

10.12   Montgomery T-Tubes

10.12.1   Discussion

Montgomery T-tubes are silicone tubes that have three limbs extending into the subglottic larynx, trachea, and tracheostomy (Fig. 10.75). T-tubes are used to manage complex laryngotracheal lesions, such as tracheal stenosis, tracheomalacia, and tracheal injury. Perhaps the main complication is subglottic granulation tissue formation, which can be treated by laser therapy. In addition, these tubes are at risk for mucus plugging and occlusion, which may not be recognized clinically in the emergency department.

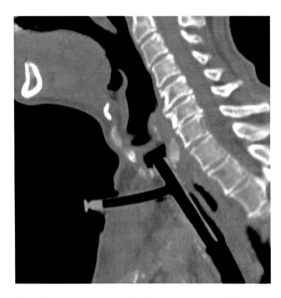

Fig. 10.75 Montgomery® T-tube. Sagittal CT image shows the limbs of the tube in the narrow subglottic larynx, trachea, and tracheostomy

10.13 Salivary Bypass Stent

10.13.1 Discussion

Salivary bypass stents, such as the Montgomery® salivary bypass tube, are long tubes composed of silicone with a flanged superior end, which are hyperattenuating on CT (Fig. 10.76). Salivary bypass stents serve as an effective way of diverting and excluding the oral-alimentary stream. The devices are also used as part of the repair of cervical esophageal and hypopharyngeal strictures and to facilitate the management of tracheoesophageal fistulae or esophageal disruption. Stents can be secured with sutures or left unsecured, which may predispose to migration into the intestinal tract.

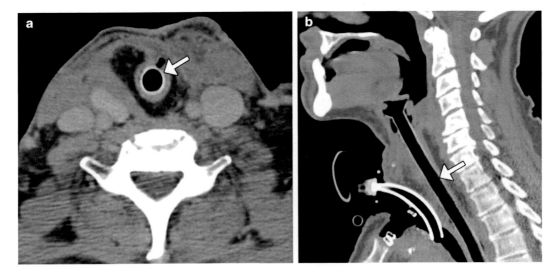

Fig. 10.76 Montgomery® salivary bypass tube. Axial (**a**) and sagittal (**b**) CT images show the salivary bypass stent (*arrows*) positioned within the neopharynx. A tracheostomy tube is also present

10.14 Laryngeal Stents

10.14.1 Discussion

The Montgomery® laryngeal stent is a molded silicone prosthesis that conforms to the endolaryngeal surface and that is firm enough to support the endolarynx postoperatively yet is soft and flexible enough to ensure a conforming fit while minimizing injury to soft tissues. These stents are radioattenuating on CT (Fig. 10.77). Montgomery stents can be used for laryngotracheal support or for the treatment of chronic aspiration. Laryngeal stenting requires concomitant tracheostomy.

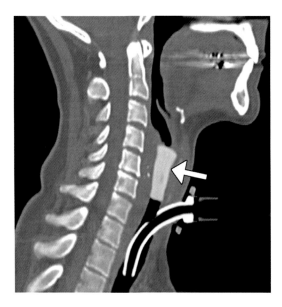

Fig. 10.77   Laryngeal stent. Sagittal CT image shows the hyperattenuating silicon stent within the neolarynx (*arrows*). A tracheostomy tube is also present

10.15 Laryngoplasty and Vocal Fold Injection

10.15.1 Discussion

Medialization laryngoplasty (thyroplasty) is a type of laryngeal framework surgery used to treat vocal cord paralysis. The procedure consists of creating a thyroid cartilage window and implanting devices such as silicone (Montgomery) prostheses. The Montgomery vocal cord positioning prosthesis is a triangular-shaped single block that is typically positioned deep to the thyroid cartilage (Fig. 10.78). However, the classic form of medialization laryngoplasty involves depressing the fragment thyroid cartilage at the window and implanting the prosthesis superficial to this (Fig. 10.79). Other implantable materials include cartilage grafts (Fig. 10.80) and hydroxyapatite prostheses (Fig. 10.81).

A variety of agents are used for vocal cord injection, including temporary, semipermanent, and permanent agents (Table 10.4). These materials are injected into the thyroarytenoid muscle or paraglottic space under laryngoscopic guidance. The imaging features vary depending upon the specific agent used (Figs. 10.82, 10.83, 10.84, 10.85, and 10.86). Polytetrafluoroethylene implants demonstrate heterogeneous hyperattenuation on CT and have irregular medial margins. Silicone implants are also hyperattenuating, similar to the adjacent thyroid cartilage. These materials are hypointense on T1 and T2 MRI sequences. Fat grafts are characteristically radiolucent and hyperintense on both T1 and T2.

Fig. 10.78 Medialization laryngoplasty with Montgomery prosthesis. Axial (**a**) and coronal (**b**) CT images demonstrate the triangular silicone prosthesis (*arrows*). There is rotation of the arytenoid and medialization of the vocal cord

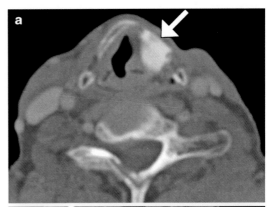

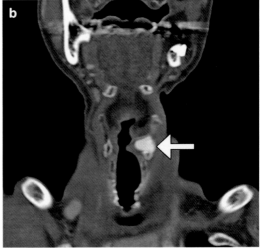

Complications of laryngoplasty include excessive or inadequate augmentation; foreign body granuloma formation, particularly with Teflon; implant rotation or lateralization; migration; and airway compromise (Figs. 10.87, 10.88, 10.89, 10.90, 10.91, and 10.92). Excess or inadequate medialization is mainly a clinical judgment, and imaging is used for planning revision surgery.

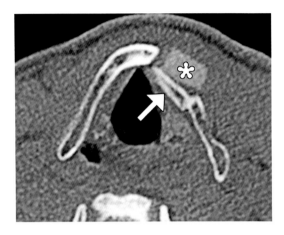

Fig. 10.79 "Classical" laryngoplasty. Axial CT image shows a silicone block implant (*) positioned superficial to the depressed left thyroid cartilage fragment (*arrow*)

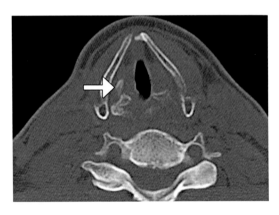

Fig. 10.80 Cartilage graft laryngoplasty. Axial CT image shows a partially calcified tragal cartilage graft in the right paraglottic space (*arrow*)

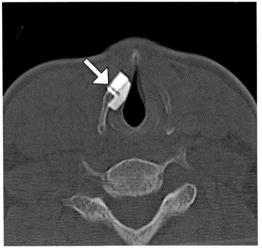

Fig. 10.81 Medialization laryngoplasty with hydroxyapatite prosthesis. Axial CT image shows a hyperattenuating right vocal cord implant (*arrow*) shaped to match the contours of a normal vocal cord

Table 10.4 Types of agents used for vocal cord injection

Category	Agents
Temporary	Freeze-dried acellular micronized human dermis (Cymetra), hyaluronic acid (Restylane), collagen, Gelfoam
Semipermanent	Calcium hydroxylapatite (Radiesse), autologous fat
Permanent	Silicone, Gore-Tex, Teflon

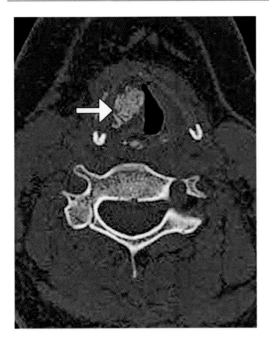

Fig. 10.82 Medialization laryngoplasty with polytetra-fluoroethylene. Axial CT image shows the high-density material with a cerebriform appearance (*arrow*) within the right vocal fold producing medialization of the right vocal fold

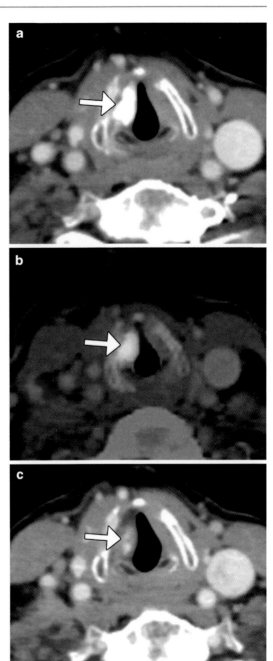

Fig. 10.83 Vocal fold augmentation with injectable calcium hydroxylapatite (Radiesse). Initial axial CT image (**a**) and PET/CT image (**b**) show the high attenuation material within the right vocal cord with corresponding hypermetabolism (*arrows*). Axial CT image (**c**) obtained 4 months later shows partial resorption of the filler material (*arrow*)

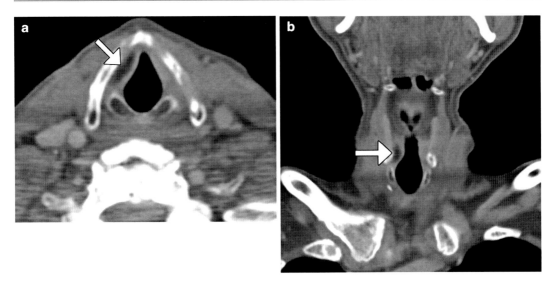

Fig. 10.84 Fat injection. Axial (**a**) and coronal (**b**) CT images show fat attenuation within the right vocal fold (*arrows*)

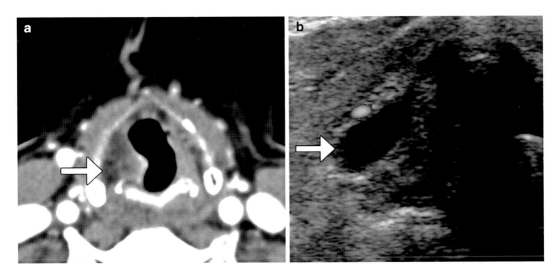

Fig. 10.85 Vocal fold injection with hyaluronic acid. Axial CT image (**a**) shows enlargement of the left vocal cord with nearly fluid-attenuation material (*arrow*). The Doppler ultrasound image (**b**) shows a corresponding anechoic area without internal vascular flow (*arrow*)

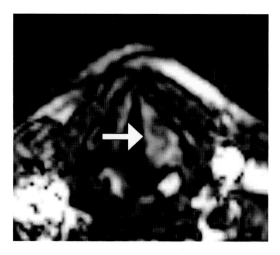

Fig. 10.86 Vocal fold injection with micronized acellular human dermis. Axial T2-weighted MRI shows curvilinear hypointensity surrounded by diffuse high signal in the enlarged left vocal fold (*arrow*)

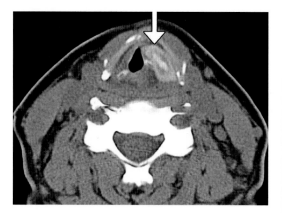

Fig. 10.87 Teflon foreign body granuloma. Axial CT image shows mass-like soft tissue material surrounding the left vocal cord implant (*arrow*)

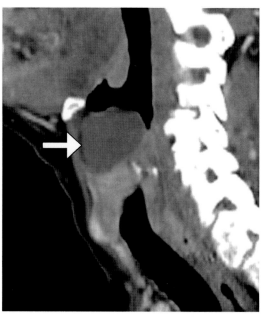

Fig. 10.88 Laryngocele. Sagittal CT image shows a fluid collection (*arrow*) above the vocal cord medialization material

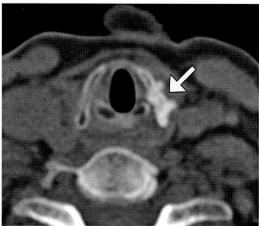

Fig. 10.89 Laryngoplasty material extrusion. The patient did not experience improvement after attempted laryngoplasty. Axial CT image shows lateral extrusion of the implant (*arrow*) through the cartilage window and concavity of the left vocal cord. The patient underwent subsequent revision laryngoplasty

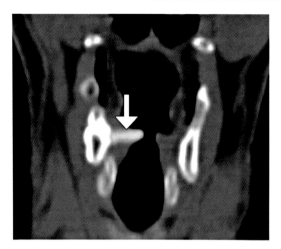

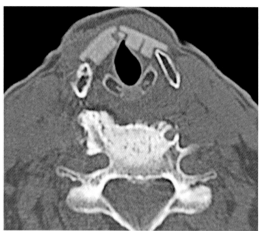

Fig. 10.90 Montgomery prosthesis rotated into airway. Coronal CT image shows that the prosthesis projects too far into the airway (*arrow*). The patient presented with hoarseness after trauma

Fig. 10.92 Insufficient medialization. The patient did not experience improvement in phonation after the surgery. Axial CT image shows bilateral implants in position, but the rima glottidis is relatively wide. Revision surgery was subsequently performed

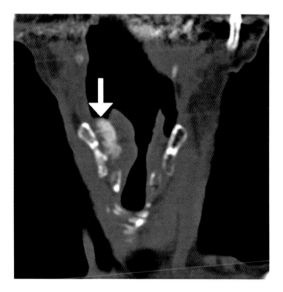

Fig. 10.91 Laryngoplasty material supraglottic migration. Coronal CT image demonstrates superior extension of the Gore-Tex (*arrow*) to the level of the right piriform sinus and thickened aryepiglottic fold

10.16 Arytenoid Adduction

10.16.1 Discussion

Arytenoid adduction was designed to enhance posterior glottal closure in patients with paralytic dysphonia and may be performed in addition to medialization laryngoplasty. The medially rotated arytenoid and associated narrowing of the posterior rima glottidis can be depicted on CT (Fig. 10.93) and should not be mistaken for unintended dislocation. Laryngeal edema is a common occurrence during the early postoperative period, with a peak at 3 days after surgery, although this does not generally result in airway compromise.

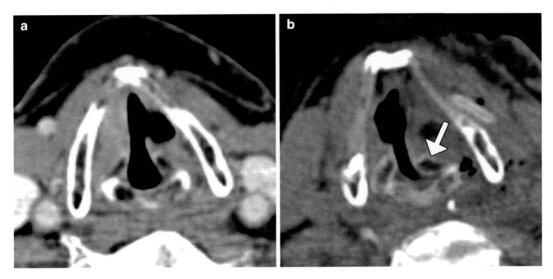

Fig. 10.93 Arytenoid adduction. Preoperative axial CT image (**a**) shows stigmata of left vocal cord paralysis. Postoperative axial CT image (**b**) shows interval medial repositioning of the left arytenoid (*arrow*) along with the vocal cord

10.17 Arytenoidectomy

10.17.1 Discussion

Arytenoidectomy consists of removing the arytenoid and is indicated for treating airway obstruction in patients with bilateral median vocal cord paralysis, ankylosis of the cricoarytenoid joint due to arthritis, and tumors of the arytenoid cartilage. This can be accomplished endoscopically via a submucosal approach or laser surgery. Unilateral arytenoidectomy results in asymmetric widening of the posterior airway (Fig. 10.94).

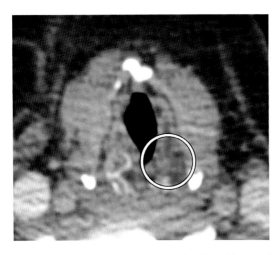

Fig. 10.94 Arytenoidectomy. The patient has a history of bilateral vocal cord paralysis. Axial CT image shows the absence of the left arytenoid (*circle*) resulting in asymmetric widening of the otherwise narrow airway on the left

10.18 Laryngeal Cartilage Remodeling

10.18.1 Discussion

Laryngeal cartilage remodeling surgery can be performed to treat deformities that result from trauma, laryngoplasty, or cancer and can be performed as part of sex change procedures. Miniplates are commonly used for reconstruction.

CT is a suitable modality for evaluating the results of the surgery and suspected complications, such as submucosal hematomas. Panorex and 3D CT are particularly useful for depicting the positioning of the hardware and alignment of the laryngeal cartilages (Fig. 10.95). Postoperative hematomas are among the more common complications of laryngeal framework surgery and can be problematic if there is compromise of the airway (Fig. 10.96).

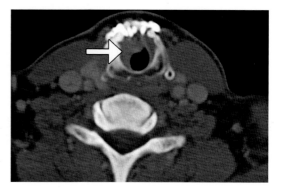

Fig. 10.96 Hematoma after cricoid cartilage repair. Axial CT shows miniplate and screw fixation of an anterior cricoid cartilage fracture. There is near-anatomic alignment, but there is underlying submucosal swelling that narrows the airway (*arrow*)

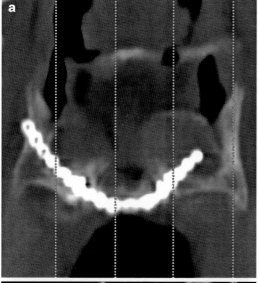

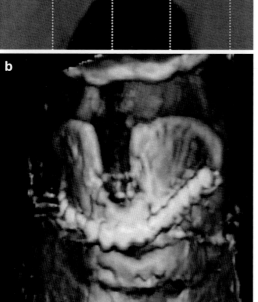

Fig. 10.95 Laryngeal framework reconstruction surgery. Panorex (**a**) and 3D (**b**) reformatted CT images demonstrate microfixation plates along the thyroid cartilage

10.19 Tracheotomy

10.19.1 Discussion

Tracheotomy is performed in order to secure the airway and consists of creating an opening between the skin and trachea, or tracheostomy, via open surgical or bronchoscopic techniques. Once the passage is created and dilated, a tracheostomy tube is inserted. There are various types of tracheotomy tubes, but these commonly consist of an obturator, curved inner and outer cannulas, and an inflatable cuff. CT with multiplanar reconstructions and volume renderings, such as tissue transition projection, is a suitable method for evaluating position of tube in relation to tracheal wall (Fig. 10.97), tracheal stenosis, and various complications. Early complications related to tracheotomy and tracheostomy tubes include hemorrhage, infection, tube obstruction, and placement into a false tract (Fig. 10.98), while late complications include tracheomalacia, tracheoesophageal fistula, tracheoinnominate artery erosion, and tracheal stenosis (Fig. 10.99).

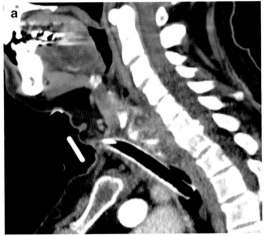
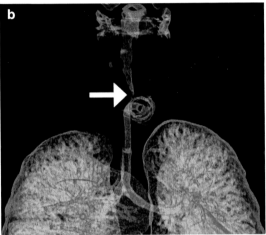

Fig. 10.97 Tracheostomy tube. Sagittal CT image (**a**) shows a tracheostomy tube in position for upper airway stenosis. The corresponding frontal tissue transition projection CT image (**b**) demonstrated the narrowing of the airway superior to the tracheostomy tube (*arrow*) to better advantage

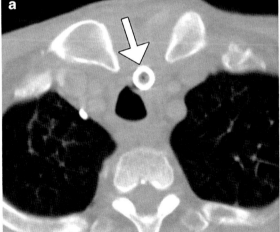
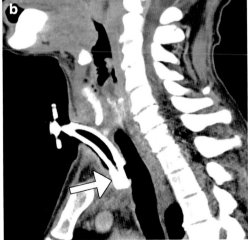

Fig. 10.98 Tracheostomy tube in a false tract. Axial (**a**) and sagittal (**b**) CT images show the tracheostomy tube tip (*arrows*) positioned anterolaterally to the tracheal lumen

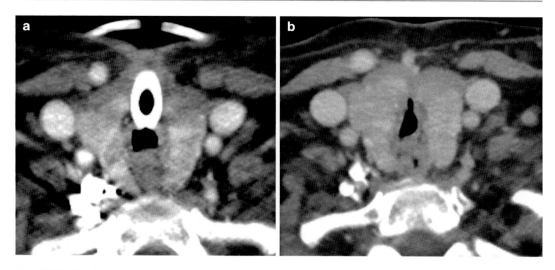

Fig. 10.99 Post-intubation tracheal stenosis. Axial CT image (**a**) obtained during intubation and axial CT image (**b**) obtained after removal of the endotracheal tube show interval narrowing of the tracheal lumen

10.20 Thyroidectomy

10.20.1 Discussion

Thyroidectomy consists of surgical resection of part or all of the thyroid glands for treating benign and malignant conditions. The basic types of thyroidectomy are listed in Table 10.5 and depicted in Figs. 10.100, 10.101, 10.102, and 10.103.

The traditional approach for thyroidectomy involves making a transverse incision several centimeters above the sternal notch. The use of robots and extracervical approaches, such as the axillary approach, has made minimally invasive thyroid surgery possible.

Perioperative tracheal perforation, recurrent laryngeal nerve injury, hematoma, and infection are potential early complications of thyroidec-tomy that can have correlate findings on diagnostic imaging (Figs. 10.104, 10.105, and 10.106). Furthermore, imaging plays an important role in the postoperative evaluation for thyroid cancer. Ultrasound is generally suitable for evaluating the region of the surgical bed region, whereby tumor typically appears as hypoechoic or cystic nodules that might contain microcalcifications, especially with papillary thyroid carcinoma (Fig. 10.107). However, CT, MRI, and in cases of dedifferentiated thyroid cancer 18FDG-PET/CT are more sensitive for identifying recurrent tumor that encroaches upon the trachea (Fig. 10.108), which is a relatively common site of recurrence due to the difficulty in completely resecting tumor in that area. Furthermore, these modalities are better suited for identifying retropharyngeal lymph node metastases (Fig. 10.109), which can

Table 10.5 Basic types of thyroidectomy

Type	Description
Hemithyroidectomy (lobectomy)	Removal of an entire lobe and isthmusectomy
Subtotal thyroidectomy	Traditional technique: removal of the gland except for approximately 2–3 g of tissue in the ipsilateral or bilateral lower poles adjacent to the ligament of Berry Hartley-Dunhill technique: ipsilateral total lobectomy and isthmusectomy and subtotal resection on the contralateral side, leaving up to approximately 5 g of tissue
Near-total thyroidectomy	Removal of the gland except for less than 1 g of tissue in the inferior poles adjacent to the ligament of Berry
Total thyroidectomy	Removal of the entire gland

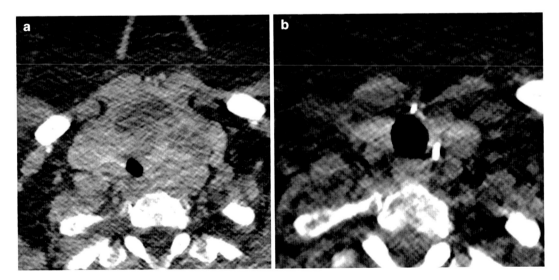

Fig. 10.100 Subtotal thyroidectomy. Initial axial CT image (**a**) shows a goiter compressing the trachea. Postoperative axial CT image (**b**) shows removal that the excess thyroid tissue has been removed and the trachea has re-expanded

be predisposed by altered lymphatic drainage following neck dissection.

Iodine 131 total body scans play an important role in the treatment and evaluation of local and distant tumor burden in patients with differentiated thyroid cancer after surgery has been performed (Fig. 10.110). High doses of I-131 are administered to ablate any residual thyroid tissue after thyroidectomy, since it is usually not feasible to remove all thyroid tissues during thyroidectomy. Activity in the region of the thyroid bed on the initial postsurgical scans is common. In particular, a thyroglossal duct remnant is apparent on postoperative I-131 scintigraphy in about one-third of patients after total thyroidectomy and appears as a midline linear band of increased activity superior to the thyroid bed. This finding should not be confused with metastases, since the presence of metastatic disease warrants even higher treatment doses. The expected end point after successful therapy is the absence of activity in the thyroid bed and other locations besides the salivary glands.

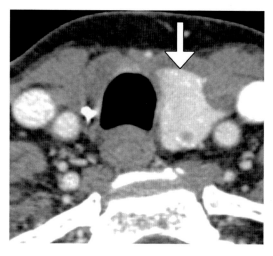

Fig. 10.101 Hemithyroidectomy. Axial CT image shows a residual left thyroid lobe containing cysts (*arrow*) and surgical clips in the right thyroidectomy bed

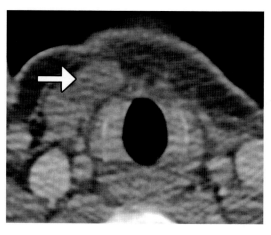

Fig. 10.103 Total thyroidectomy. Axial CT image shows complete absence of the thyroid gland as well as the left strap muscles. The remaining right strap muscles (*arrow*) should not be confused for tumor

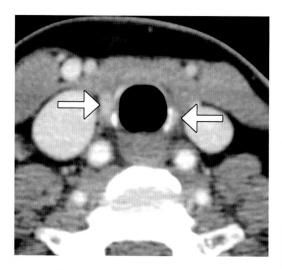

Fig. 10.102 Near-total thyroidectomy. Axial CT image shows a small amount of residual posterior thyroid tissue adjacent to the tracheoesophageal grooves, right greater than left (*arrows*)

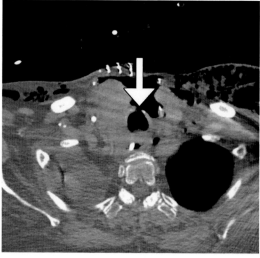

Fig. 10.104 Thyroidectomy complicated by tracheal perforation. Axial CT images show extensive anterior neck emphysema after recent thyroidectomy and a defect in the anterior wall of the trachea (*arrow*)

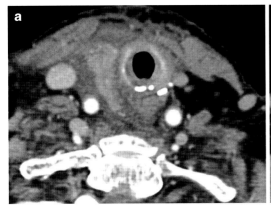
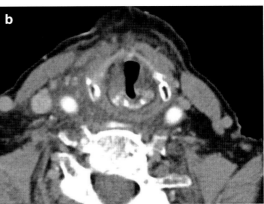

Fig. 10.105 Vocal cord paralysis. Axial CT image at the level of the thyroid bed (**a**) shows left hemithyroidectomy bed that extends into the left tracheoesophageal groove along the expected course of the recurrent laryngeal nerve.

Axial CT image at the level of the vocal cords (**b**) shows ipsilateral left vocal cord atrophy secondary to left recurrent laryngeal nerve injury

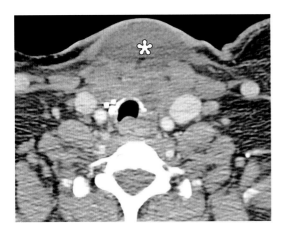

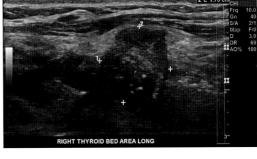

Fig. 10.107 Recurrent tumor in thyroidectomy bed. Ultrasound image shows a hypoechoic mass with microcalcifications in the thyroidectomy bed in a patient with a history of papillary thyroid carcinoma

Fig. 10.106 Abscess. Axial CT image shows a fluid collection in the anterior neck (*) extending from the thyroid bed. Secondary signs of infection, including skin thickening, subcutaneous fat stranding, and reactive lymph nodes are also apparent

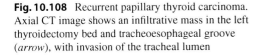

Fig. 10.108 Recurrent papillary thyroid carcinoma. Axial CT image shows an infiltrative mass in the left thyroidectomy bed and tracheoesophageal groove (*arrow*), with invasion of the tracheal lumen

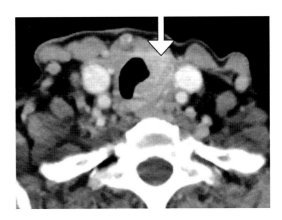

10.21 Neck Exploration and Parathyroidectomy

10.21.1 Discussion

Parathyroidectomy for parathyroid adenomas or hyperplasia is typically performed either as unilateral or bilateral neck exploration at the level of the thyroid gland. Normal portions of parathyroid gland that are encountered during exploration of a parathyroid adenoma can be reimplanted in the forearm, sternocleidomastoid, or subcutaneous tissues of the neck, such that function is maintained (Fig. 10.111). Parathyroid adenoma recurrence and adenomas in ectopic parathyroid glands are the main causes of failed neck exploration (Figs. 10.112 and 10.113). It is also important to be aware that adenomas can also arise in glands that have been surgically repositioned (Fig. 10.114). Options for imaging prior to re-exploration include technetium (^{99m}Tc) sestamibi scanning, ultrasound, and four-dimensional (4D) CT, or a combination of these. It has been reported that the sensitivity of 4D CT for localization is 88% compared with 54% for sestamibi imaging.

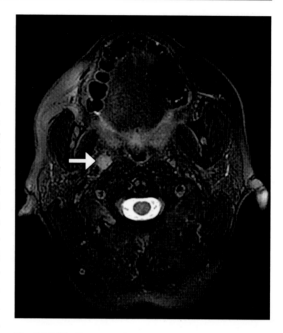

Fig. 10.109 Postoperative retropharyngeal lymph node metastasis. The patient has a history of papillary thyroid carcinoma, status post thyroidectomy and neck dissection. Axial fat-suppressed T2-weighted MRI shows an abnormal right retropharyngeal lymph node (*arrow*)

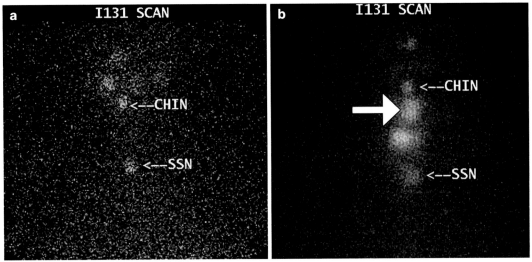

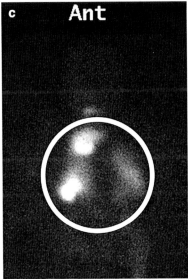

Fig. 10.110 I-131 total body scans after thyroidectomy and I-131 therapy. Normal scan without residual thyroid activity (**a**). Residual activity in the thyroid bed and thyroglossal duct remnant (*arrow*) (**b**). Pulmonary metastatic disease (*circle*) (**c**)

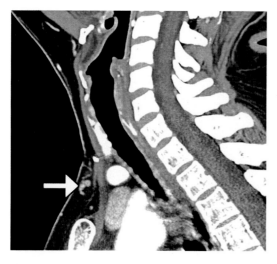

Fig. 10.111 Parathyroidectomy with parathyroid gland autotransplantation. Sagittal CT image shows a parathyroid gland (*arrow*) implanted in the midline subcutaneous tissues of the lower anterior neck

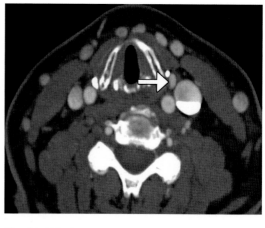

Fig. 10.112 Residual hyperplastic parathyroid. Axial CT image shows an avidly enhancing nodule (*arrow*) in the left neck adjacent to surgical clips

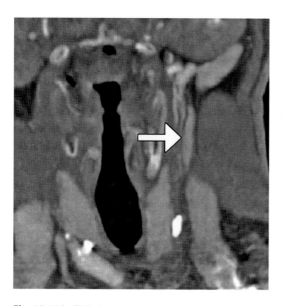

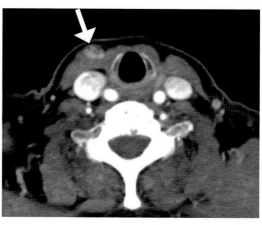

Fig. 10.114 Adenoma in a parathyroid gland previously surgically transplanted along the sternocleidomastoid muscle. Axial CT image shows a heterogeneous tumor along superficial aspect of the right sternocleidomastoid (*arrow*)

Fig. 10.113 Failed neck exploration due to ectopic parathyroid. The patient's hypercalcemia and related symptoms persisted following bilateral neck exploration. Coronal CT image shows a vertically elongated enhancing lesion along the carotid sheath superior to the thyroid gland (*arrow*). The initial surgical exploration was performed inferior and to the right of the lesion, as demarcated by the surgical clips

10.22 Brachytherapy

10.22.1 Discussion

Interstitial brachytherapy is sometimes performed for treating head and neck malignancies. A variety of devices are available, although the typical brachytherapy systems consist of radiation-emitting rods or needles that are inserted via stereotactic navigation. Imaging may be performed to assess placement and evaluate tumor response. The rods appear as transcutaneous metallic density linear structures in the region of the lesion or resection bed (Fig. 10.115).

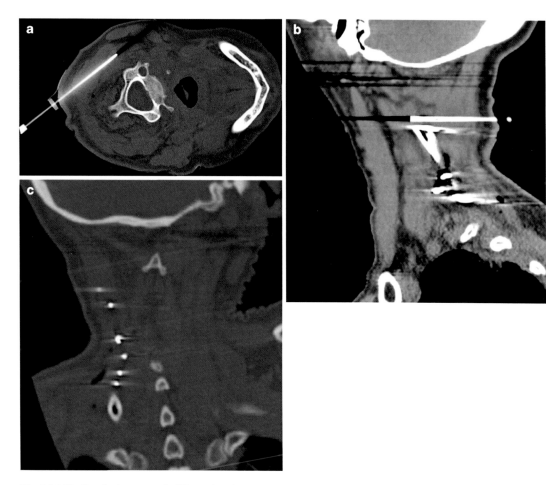

Fig. 10.115 Brachytherapy rods. The patient has a history of alveolar sarcoma of small parts in the right neck soft tissues, which was previously resected. Axial (**a**), sagittal (**b**), and coronal (**c**) CT images show an array of brachytherapy rods implanted in the region of the right neck resection cavity

10.23 Vagal Nerve Stimulation

10.23.1 Discussion

Vagus nerve stimulation is an effective method for controlling intractable seizures, with up to 50% reduction in seizure frequency. The device consists of two electrodes and an anchor loop implanted in the left neck at the midcervical level posterolateral to the internal and common carotid arteries and medial to the internal jugular vein. The electrodes are connected to a gen-erator that is implanted beneath the infraclavicular subcutaneous tissues. Unlike with the right vagus nerve, left vagal stimulation does not affect cardiac function. The most common side effects of vagus nerve stimulation include sore throat and voice changes. Radiographs or CT may be performed to delineate the position and integrity of the electrodes (Fig. 10.116). The vagal nerve stimulators are considered MRI conditional and output currents should be programmed to 0 mA before entering the MRI suite.

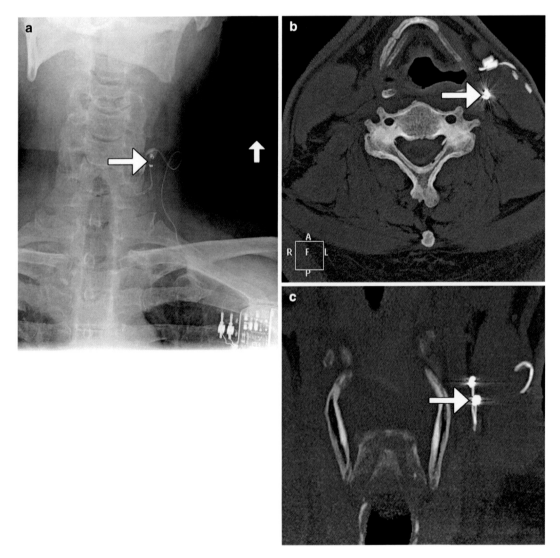

Fig. 10.116 Vagal nerve stimulator. Fontal neck radiograph (**a**) shows left vagus nerve lead in position (*arrow*). The pulse generator is partially shown in the left chest region. Axial (**b**) and coronal (**c**) CT images show the components of the stimulator electrodes (*arrows*)

Further Reading

Reconstruction Flaps

Ahmad FI, Gerecci D, Gonzalez JD, Peck JJ, Wax MK (2015) The role of postoperative hematoma on free flap compromise. Laryngoscope 125(8):1811–1815.

Blencowe NS, Hari CK, Porter GC (2010) Colonic diverticulitis in the neck: a late complication of laryngopha-ryngectomy surgery. Ann R Coll Surg Engl 92(6):W11–W13

Cansiz H, Cambaz B, Papila I, Tahami R, Güneş M (1998) Use of free composite graft for a large defect in the anterior skull base. J Craniofac Surg 9(1):76–78

Cordeiro PG, Disa JJ (2000) Challenges in midface reconstruction. Semin Surg Oncol 19(3):218–225

Futran ND, Mendez E (2006) Developments in reconstruction of midface and maxilla. Lancet Oncol 7(3):249–258

Hudgins PA (2002) Flap reconstruction in the head and neck: expected appearance, complications, and recurrent disease. Eur J Radiol 44(2):130–138

Hudgins PA, Burson JG, Gussack GS, Grist WJ (1994) CT and MR appearance of recurrent malignant head and neck neoplasms after resection and flap reconstruction. AJNR Am J Neuroradiol 15(9):1689–1694

Jackson IT, Webster HR (1994) Craniofacial tumors. Clin Plast Surg 21(4):633–648

Ji Y, Li T, Shamburger S, Jin J, Lineaweaver WC, Zhang F (2002) Microsurgical anterolateral thigh fasciocutaneous flap for facial contour correction in patients with hemifacial microsomia. Microsurgery 22(1):34–38

Moerman M, Fahimi H, Ceelen W, Pattyn P, Vermeersch H (2003) Functional outcome following colon interposition in total pharyngoesophagectomy with or without laryngectomy. Dysphagia 18(2):78–84

Tripathi M, Parshad S, Karwasra RK, Singh V (2015) Pectoralis major myocutaneous flap in head and neck reconstruction: an experience in 100 consecutive cases. Natl J Maxillofac Surg 6(1):37–41.

Tomura N, Watanabe O, Hirano Y, Kato K, Takahashi S, Watarai J (2002) MR imaging of recurrent head and neck tumours following flap reconstructive surgery. Clin Radiol 57(2):109–113

Wester DJ, Whiteman ML, Singer S, Bowen BC, Goodwin WJ (1995) Imaging of the postoperative neck with emphasis on surgical flaps and their complications. AJR Am J Roentgenol 164(4):989–993

Facial Reanimation

Bianchi B, Copelli C, Ferrari S, Ferri A, Bailleul C, Sesenna E (2010) Facial animation with free-muscle transfer innervated by the masseter motor nerve in unilateral facial paralysis. J Oral Maxillofac Surg 68(7):1524–1529

Chuang DC (2008) Free tissue transfer for the treatment of facial paralysis. Facial Plast Surg 24(2):194–203

Chuang DC, Mardini S, Lin SH, Chen HC (2004) Free proximal gracilis muscle and its skin paddle compound flap transplantation for complex facial paralysis. Plast Reconstr Surg 113(1):126–132; discussion 133–135

Ginat DT, Bhama P, Cunnane ME, Hadlock TA (2014) Facial reanimation procedures depicted on radiologic imaging. AJNR Am J Neuroradiol 35(9):1662–1666.

Horlock N, Sanders R, Harrison DH (2002) The SOOF lift: its role in correcting midfacial and lower facial asymmetry in patients with partial facial palsy. Plast Reconstr Surg 109(3):839–849; discussion 850–854

May M, Drucker C (1993) Temporalis muscle for facial reanimation. A 13-year experience with 224 procedures. Arch Otolaryngol Head Neck Surg 119(4):378–382; discussion 383–384

Shindo M (2000) Facial reanimation with microneurovascular free flaps. Facial Plast Surg 16(4):357–359

Tate JR, Tollefson TT (2006) Advances in facial reanimation. Curr Opin Otolaryngol Head Neck Surg 14(4):242–248

Oral Cavity Tumor Resection and Reconstruction

Bokhari WA, Wang SJ (2007) Tongue reconstruction: recent advances. Curr Opin Otolaryngol Head Neck Surg 15(4):202–207

Ko AB, Lavertu P, Rezaee RP (2010) Double bilobed radial forearm free flap for anterior tongue and floor-of-mouth reconstruction. Ear Nose Throat J 89(4):177–179

Murano EZ, Shinagawa H, Zhuo J, Gullapalli RP, Ord RA, Prince JL, Stone M (2010) Application of diffusion tensor imaging after glossectomy. Otolaryngol Head Neck Surg 143(2):304–306

Sinha UK, Chang KE, Shih CW (2001) Reconstruction of pharyngeal defects using AlloDerm and sternocleidomastoid muscle flap. Laryngoscope 111(11 Pt 1):1910–1916

Tonsillectomy and Adenoidectomy

Abou-Jaoude PM, Manoukian JJ, Daniel SJ, Balys R, Abou-Chacra Z, Nader ME, Tewfik TL, Schloss MD (2006) Complications of adenotonsillectomy revisited in a large pediatric case series. J Otolaryngol 35(3):180–185

Acar GO, Cansz H, Duman C, Oz B, Ciğercioğullar E (2011) Excessive reactive lymphoid hyperplasia in a child with persistent obstructive sleep apnea despite previous tonsillectomy and adenoidectomy. J Craniofac Surg 22(4):1413–1415

Archibald D, Lockhart PB, Sonis ST, Ervin TJ, Fallon BG, Miller D, Clark JR (1986) Oral complications of multimodality therapy for advanced squamous cell carcinoma of head and neck. Oral Surg Oral Med Oral Pathol 61(2):139–141

Darrow DH, Siemens C (2002) Indications for tonsillectomy and adenoidectomy. Laryngoscope 112(8 Pt 2 Suppl 100):6–10

Donnelly LF, Shott SR, LaRose CR, Chini BA, Amin RS (2004) Causes of persistent obstructive sleep apnea despite previous tonsillectomy and adenoidectomy in children with down syndrome as depicted on static and dynamic cine MRI. AJR Am J Roentgenol 183(1): 175–181

Fricke BL, Donnelly LF, Shott SR, Kalra M, Poe SA, Chini BA, Amin RS (2006) Comparison of lingual tonsil size as depicted on MR imaging between children with obstructive sleep apnea despite previous tonsillectomy and adenoidectomy and normal controls. Pediatr Radiol 36(6):518–523

Holsinger FC, McWhorter AJ, Ménard M, Garcia D, Laccourreye O (2005) Transoral lateral oropharyngectomy for squamous cell carcinoma of the tonsillar region: I. Technique, complications, and functional results. Arch Otolaryngol Head Neck Surg 131(7):583–591

Kapoor V, Fukui MB, McCook BM (2005) Role of 18FFDG PET/CT in the treatment of head and neck cancers: posttherapy evaluation and pitfalls. AJR Am J Roentgenol 184(2):589–597

Shott SR, Donnelly LF (2004) Cine magnetic resonance imaging: evaluation of persistent airway obstruction after tonsil and adenoidectomy in children with Down syndrome. Laryngoscope 114(10):1724–1729

Statham MM, Myer CM 3rd (2010) Complications of adenotonsillectomy. Curr Opin Otolaryngol Head Neck Surg 18(6):539–543

Transoral Robotic Surgery

Dziegielewski PT, Teknos TN, Durmus K, Old M, Agrawal A, Kakarala K, Marcinow A, Ozer E (2013) Transoral robotic surgery for oropharyngeal cancer: long-term quality of life and functional outcomes. JAMA Otolaryngol Head Neck Surg 139(11):1099–1108.

Loevner LA, Learned KO, Mohan S, O'Malley BW Jr, Scanlon MH, Rassekh CH, Weinstein GS (2013) Transoral robotic surgery in head and neck cancer: what radiologists need to know about the cutting edge. Radiographics 33(6):1759–1779.

Neck Dissection

Ferlito A, Robbins KT, Silver CE, Hasegawa Y, Rinaldo A (2009) Classification of neck dissections: an evolving system. Auris Nasus Larynx 36(2):127–134

Hamilton BE, Nesbit GM, Gross N, Andersen P, Sauer D, Harnsberger HR (2011) Characteristic imaging findings in lymphoceles of the head and neck. AJR Am J Roentgenol 197(6):1431–1435

Hudgins PA, Kingdom TT, Weissler MC, Mukherji SK (2005) Selective neck dissection: CT and MR imaging findings. AJNR Am J Neuroradiol 26(5):1174–1177

McGarvey AC, Osmotherly PG, Hoffman GR, Chiarelli PE (2014) Lymphoedema following treatment for head and neck cancer: impact on patients, and beliefs of health professionals. Eur J Cancer Care (Engl). 23(3):317–327

Robbins KT (1998) Classification of neck dissection: current concepts and future considerations. Otolaryngol Clin N Am 31(4):639–655

Seethala RR (2009) Current state of neck dissection in the United States. Head Neck Pathol 3(3):238–245

Som PM, Urken ML, Biller H, Lidov M (1993) Imaging the postoperative neck. Radiology 187(3):593–603

Parotidectomy

Leonetti JP, Marzo SJ, Petruzzelli GJ, Herr B (2005) Recurrent pleomorphic adenoma of the parotid gland. Otolaryngol Head Neck Surg 133(3):319–322

Moonis G, Patel P, Koshkareva Y, Newman J, Loevner LA (2007) Imaging characteristics of recurrent pleomorphic adenoma of the parotid gland. AJNR Am J Neuroradiol 28(8):1532–1536

Upton DC, McNamar JP, Connor NP, Harari PM, Hartig GK (2007) Parotidectomy: ten-year review of 237 cases at a single institution. Otolaryngol Head Neck Surg 136(5):788–792

Yasumoto M, Sunaba K, Shibuya H et al. (1999) Recurrent pleomorphic adenoma of the head and neck. Neuroradiology 41:300–304

Salivary Duct Stenting

Chu DW, Chow TL, Lim BH, Kwok SP (2003) Endoscopic management of submandibular sialolithiasis. Surg Endosc 17(6):876–879

Walvekar RR, Bomeli SR, Carrau RL, Schaitkin B (2009) Combined approach technique for the management of large salivary stones. Laryngoscope 119(6): 1125–1129

Laryngectomy

Alaani A, Hogg R, Minhas SS, Jennings C, Johnson AP (2005) Pseudoaneurysm after total pharyngolaryngectomy with jejunal graft insertion: two different presentations. Eur Arch Otorhinolaryngol 262(4): 255–258

Ferreiro-Argüelles C, Jiménez-Juan L, Martínez-Salazar JM, Cervera-Rodilla JL, Martínez-Pérez MM, Cubero-Carralero J, González-Cabestreros S, López-Pino MA, Fernández-Gallardo JM (2008) CT findings after laryngectomy. Radiographics 28(3):869–882; quiz 914

Ganly I, Patel S, Matsuo J, Singh B, Kraus D, Boyle J, Wong R, Lee N, Pfister DG, Shaha A, Shah J (2005) Postoperative complications of salvage total laryngectomy. Cancer 103(10):2073–2081

Iguchi H, Takayama M, Kusuki M, Nakamura A, Kanazawa A, Hachiya K, Yamane H (2006) Carotid artery pseudoaneurysm as a rare sequela of surgery for laryngeal cancer. Acta Otolaryngol 126(5):557–560

Maroldi R, Battaglia G, Nicolai P, Maculotti P, Cappiello J, Cabassa P, Farina D, Chiesa A (1997) CT appearance of the larynx after conservative and radical surgery for carcinomas. Eur Radiol 7(3):418–431

Zeitels SM, Burns JA, Lopez-Guerra G, Anderson RR, Hillman RE (2008) Photoangiolytic laser treatment of early glottic cancer: a new management strategy. Ann OtolRhinol Laryngol Suppl 199:3–24

Tracheoesophageal Puncture and Voice Prostheses

Callanan V, Gurr P, Baldwin D, White-Thompson M, Beckinsale J, Bennett J (1995) Provox valve use for post-laryngectomy voice rehabilitation. J Laryngol Otol 109(11):1068–1071

Chen HC, Tang YB, Chang MH (2001) Reconstruction of the voice after laryngectomy. Clin Plast Surg 28(2):389–402

Pawar PV, Sayed SI, Kazi R, Jagade MV (2008) Current status and future prospects in prosthetic voice rehabilitation following laryngectomy. J Cancer Res Ther 4(4):186–191

Montgomery T-Tubes

Liu HC, Lee KS, Huang CJ, Cheng CR, Hsu WH, Huang MH (2002) Silicone T-tube for complex laryngotracheal problems. Eur J Cardiothorac Surg 21(2): 326–330

Pinedo-Onofre JA, Tellez-Becerra JL, Patiño-Gallegos H, Miranda-Franco A, Lugo-Alvarez G (2010) Subglottic stenosis above tracheal stoma: technique for Montgomery T-tube insertion. Ann Thorac Surg 89(6): 2044–2046

Salivary Bypass Stents

Bitter T, Pantel M, Dittmar Y, Guntinas-Lichius O, Wittekindt C (2012) Stent migration to the ileum-A potentially lethal complication after montgomery salivary bypass tube placement for hypopharyngeal stenosis after laryngectomy. Head Neck 34(1): 135–137, Epub 2010 Jul 27

Kim AW, Liptay MJ, Snow N, Donahue P, Warren WH (2008) Utility of silicone esophageal bypass stents in the management of delayed complex esophageal disruptions. Ann Thorac Surg 85(6):1962–1967; discussion 1967

Lörken A, Krampert J, Kau RJ, Arnold W (1997) Experiences with the Montgomery Salivary Bypass Tube (MSBT). Dysphagia 12(2):79–83

Laryngeal Stents

Eliachar I, Stein J, Strome M (1995) Augmentation techniques in laryngotracheal reconstruction. Acta Otorhinolaryngol Belg 4:397–406

Mouney DF, Lyons GD (1985) Fixation of laryngeal stents. Laryngoscope 8:905–907

Weisberger EC, Huebsch SA (1982) Endoscopic treatment of aspiration using a laryngeal stent. Otolaryngol Head Neck Surg 2:215–222

Laryngoplasty and Vocal Fold Injection

Bock JM, Lee JH, Robinson RA, Hoffman HT (2007) Migration of Cymetra after vocal fold injection for laryngeal paralysis. Laryngoscope 117(12): 2251–2254

Kumar VA, Lewin JS, Ginsberg LE (2006) CT assessment of vocal cord medialization. AJNR Am J Neuroradiol 27(8): 1643–1646

Moonis G, Dyce O, Loevner LA, Mirza N (2005) Magnetic resonance imaging of micronized dermal graft in the larynx. Ann Otol Rhinol Laryngol 114(8): 593–598

Zeitels SM, Mauri M, Dailey SH (2003) Medialization laryngoplasty with Gore-Tex for voice restoration secondary to glottal incompetence: indications and observations. Ann Otol Rhinol Laryngol 112(2):180–184

Arytenoid Adduction

Narajos N, Toya Y, Kumai Y, Sanuki T, Yumoto E (2012) Videolaryngoscopic assessment of laryngeal edema after arytenoid adduction. Laryngoscope 122(5):1104–1108.

Vachha BA, Ginat DT, Mallur P, Cunnane M, Moonis G (2016) "Finding a voice": imaging features after phonosurgical procedures for vocal fold paralysis. AJNR Am J Neuroradiol 37:1574–1580.

Arytenoidectomy

Danino J, Goldenberg D, Joachims HZ (2000) Submucosal arytenoidectomy: new surgical technique and review of the literature. J Otolaryngol 29(1):13–16

Misiolek M, Namyslowski G, Warmuzinski K, Karpe J, Rauer R, Misiolek H (2003) The influence of laser arytenoidectomy on ventilation parameters in patients with bilateral vocal cord paralysis. Eur Arch Otorhinolaryngol 260(7):381–385

Szmeja Z, Wójtowicz JG (1999) Laser arytenoidectomy in the treatment of bilateral vocal cord paralysis. Eur Arch Otorhinolaryngol 256(8):388–389

Laryngeal Cartilage Remodeling

Isshiki N (2000) Progress in laryngeal framework surgery. Acta Otolaryngol 120(2):120–127

Woo P (1990) Laryngeal framework reconstruction with miniplates. Ann Otol Rhinol Laryngol 99(10 Pt 1):772–777

Tracheotomy

De Leyn P, Bedert L, Delcroix M, Depuydt P, Lauwers G, Sokolov Y, Van Meerhaeghe A, Van Schil P; Belgian Association of Pneumology and Belgian Association of Cardiothoracic Surgery (2007) Tracheotomy: clinical review and guidelines. Eur J Cardiothorac Surg 32(3):412–421.
Kaylie DM, Wax MK (2002) Massive subcutaneous emphysema following percutaneous tracheostomy. Am J Otolaryngol 23(5):300–302.
Kost KM (2005) Endoscopic percutaneous dilatational tracheotomy: a prospective evaluation of 500 consecutive cases. Laryngoscope 115(10 Pt 2):1–30.
Tsitouridis I, Michaelides M, Dimarelos V, Arvaniti M (2009) Endotracheal and tracheostomy tube-related complications: imaging with three-dimensional spiral computed tomography. Hippokratia 13(2):97–100.

Thyroidectomy

Alsanea O, Clark OH (2000) Treatment of Graves' disease: the advantages of surgery. Endocrinol Metab Clin N Am 29(2):321–337
Lang BH (2010) Minimally invasive thyroid and parathyroid operations: surgical techniques and pearls. Adv Surg 44:185–198
Langer JE, Luster E, Horii SC, Mandel SJ, Baloch ZW, Coleman BG (2005) Chronic granulomatous lesions after thyroidectomy: imaging findings. AJR Am J Roentgenol 185(5):1350–1354
Lee SW, Lee J, Lee HJ, Seo JH, Kang SM, Bae JH, Ahn BC (2007) Enhanced scintigraphic visualization of thyroglossal duct remnant during hypothyroidism after total thyroidectomy: prevalence and clinical implication in patients with differentiated thyroid cancer. Thyroid 17(4):341–346
Otsuki N, Nishikawa T, Iwae S, et al (2007) Retropharyngeal node metastasis from papillary thyroid carcinoma. Head Neck 29:508–511
Shin JH, Han BK, Ko EY, Kang SS (2007) Sonographic findings in the surgical bed after thyroidectomy: comparison of recurrent tumors and nonrecurrent lesions. J Ultrasound Med 26(10):1359–1366

Neck Exploration and Parathyroidectomy

Gross ND, Wax MK (2004) Unilateral and bilateral surgery for parathyroid disease. Otolaryngol Clin N Am 37(4):799–817, ix–x

Mortenson MM, Evans DB, Lee JE, Hunter GJ, Shellingerhout D, Vu T, Edeiken BS, Feng L, Perrier ND (2008) Parathyroid exploration in the reoperative neck: improved preoperative localization with 4D-computed tomography. J Am Coll Surg 206(5):888–895; discussion 895–896
Russell C (2004) Unilateral neck exploration for primary hyperparathyroidism. Surg Clin North Am 84(3): 705–716
Simental A, Ferris RL (2008) Reoperative parathyroidectomy. Otolaryngol Clin N Am 41(6): 1269–1274, xii

Sistrunk Procedure

Hirshoren N, Neuman T, Udassin R, Elidan J, Weinberger JM (2009) The imperative of the Sistrunk operation: review of 160 thyroglossal tract remnant operations. Otolaryngol Head Neck Surg 140(3):338–342
Josephson GD, Spencer WR, Josephson JS (1998) Thyroglossal duct cyst: the New York Eye and Ear Infirmary experience and a literature review. Ear Nose Throat J 77(8):642–644, 646–647, 651
Maddalozzo J, Venkatesan TK, Gupta P (2001) Complications associated with the Sistrunk procedure. Laryngoscope 111 (1): 119–123

Brachytherapy

Bale RJ, Freysinger W, Gunkel AR, Vogele M, Sztankay A, Auer T, Eichberger P, Martin A, Auberger T, Scholtz AW, Jaschke W, Thumfart WF, Lukas P (2000) Head and neck tumors: fractionated frameless stereotactic interstitial brachytherapy-initial experience. Radiology 214(2):591–595
Ding M, Newman F, Raben D (2005) New radiation therapy techniques for the treatment of head and neck cancer. Otolaryngol Clin N Am 38(2):371–395,vii–viii
Krempien RC, Grehn C, Haag C, Straulino A, Hensley FW, Kotrikova B, Hofele C, Debus J, Harms W (2005) Feasibility report for retreatment of locally recurrent head-and-neck cancers by combined brachy-chemotherapy using frameless image-guided 3D interstitial brachytherapy. Brachytherapy 4(2):154–162

Vagal Nerve Stimulation

Kotagal P (2011) Neurostimulation: vagus nerve stimulation and beyond. Semin Pediatr Neurol 18(3): 186–194
Ramani R (2008) Vagus nerve stimulation therapy for seizures. J Neurosurg Anesthesiol 20(1):29–35

Imaging of Postoperative Spine

11

Daniel Thomas Ginat, Ryan Murtagh,
Per-Lennart A. Westesson, Marc Daniel Moisi,
and Rod J. Oskouian

11.1 Overview

The main categories of spine surgery include stabilization, decompression, disc replacement, as well as percutaneous vertebral augmentation and other minimally invasive procedures (Table 11.1).

Postoperative imaging is generally obtained to evaluate the position of implants, adequacy of decompression, fusion status, and potential complications. The imaging findings of spine surgical procedures, devices and implants, and complications are depicted throughout the chapter.

D.T. Ginat, M.D., M.S. (✉)
Department of Radiology, University of Chicago,
Chicago, IL, USA
e-mail: dtg1@uchicago.edu

R. Murtagh, M.D., M.B.A.
Department of Radiology, Diagnostic Imaging
Moffitt Cancer Center, Tampa, FL, USA

P.-L. A. Westesson, M.D., Ph.D., D.D.S.
Division of Neuroradiology, University of Rochester
Medical Center, Rochester, NY, USA

M.D. Moisi, M.D., M.S. • R.J. Oskouian, M.D.
Department of Neurosurgery, Swedish Neuroscience
Institute, Seattle, WA, USA

© Springer International Publishing Switzerland 2017
D.T. Ginat, P.-L.A. Westesson (eds.), *Atlas of Postsurgical Neuroradiology*,
DOI 10.1007/978-3-319-52341-5_11

Table 11.1 Main types of spine surgery

Technique	Description
Stabilization	
Fusion (spondylodesis)	Uniting portions of the spine via instrumentation and/or graft materials. A variety of approaches can be implemented (anterior, lateral, posterior, etc.)
Distraction	Halo, traction, interfacet, or interspinous process devices to provide distractive force to vertebral column
Decompression	
Laminotomy	Partial removal of the lamina on one side
Hemilaminectomy (unilateral laminectomy)	Removal of a single lamina with exposure limited to one side of the interspinous ligament with decompression of one or both sides of the spinal canal
Total laminectomy	Removal of the bilateral lamina along with the spinous process
Laminoplasty	Expansion of the spinal canal while preserving the dorsal laminar arch
Corpectomy	Complete or partial removal of the vertebral body
Vertebrectomy (spondylectomy)	Complete or partial removal of the vertebra
Foraminotomy	Expansion of the neural foramen, usually via resection of part or all of the facet
Facetectomy	Resection of part or all of the facet
Discectomy/microdiscectomy	Removal of herniated disc material
Miscellaneous	
Disc and nucleus pulposus replacement	Dynamic reconstruction of the intervertebral disc with artificial disc or nucleus pulposus
Dynamic stabilization	Various devices inserted into the disc space, interspinous space, or facet joints
Vertebroplasty, kyphoplasty, skyphoplasty, Kiva implantation, and sacroplasty	Minimally invasive injection of cement or device into vertebrae, or sacrum, with or without balloon expansion
Nucleoplasty	Radiofrequency ablation of herniated disc
Epidural blood patch	Minimally invasive closure of dura for treatment of cerebrospinal fluid leaks

11.2   Spine Decompression

11.2.1 Laminotomy and Foraminotomy

11.2.1.1   Discussion

Laminotomy consists of removing the margins of lamina and can be unilateral or bilateral. The spinous process and interspinous ligaments are often preserved; however, a partial resection of the spinous process may be necessary in order to facilitate the approach to the lamina. This procedure can be performed to provide access for forami-

notomy or discectomy. On imaging, widening of interlaminar space can be identified, which is often best identified in the coronal plane (Fig. 11.1). These surgical defects often have geometric margins. Sclerosis of the remaining portions of the lamina can be observed, as healing progresses. Similarly, foraminotomy, which is performed for neural foraminal stenosis, can appear as a generously sized neural foramen with circular or rectilinear contours and irregular margins from shaving away of the surrounding cortical bone, which are best appreciated in the sagittal plane (Fig. 11.2).

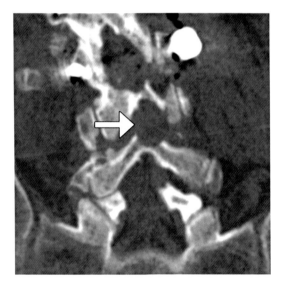

Fig. 11.1 Laminotomy. Coronal CT image demonstrates thinning and of the left L4 and L5 lamina (*arrows*) resulting in a widened interspinous space

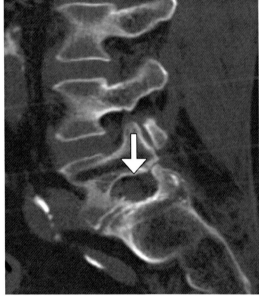

Fig. 11.2 Foraminotomy. Sagittal CT image shows an artificially widening L5–S1 neural foramen (*arrow*)

11.2.2 Laminectomy

11.2.2.1 Discussion

Hemilaminectomy or unilateral laminectomy consists of resecting the lamina via dissection on one side of the interspinous ligament. This procedure is mainly performed in order to gain access for foraminotomy or discectomy. The hemilaminectomy defect is readily apparent on CT and MRI, but can be of variable width (Fig. 11.3).

In some instances, when preservation of the interspinous ligament is necessary, after the unilateral hemilaminectomy is performed, the ligamentum flavum is removed bilaterally for bilateral decompression of the neural structures.

Bilateral laminectomy consists of removing the spinous process along with both laminae, thereby "unroofing" the posterior spinal canal. This procedure is commonly performed for spinal canal decompression, particularly related to degenerative disc disease, spinal stenosis, epidural infections, epidural or subdural hematomas, and tumor. Bilateral laminectomy can be performed in conjunction with other procedures such as discectomy, facetectomy, and/or fusion for restoring stability. Both CT and MRI can readily show changes related to laminectomy and are routinely used to assess patients after surgery, even in the presence of hardware (Fig. 11.4). If the dura is opened (durotomy) or resected during the procedure, duraplasty is often performed, in which artificial dural replacement materials are used (Fig. 11.5). Too tight closure of the dura or duraplasty material can lead to compression of the spinal canal contents. This can be evaluated via MRI, in which there is concavity of the dura or duraplasty material (Fig. 11.6). Spinal cord contusions can occur secondary to decompression of severe stenosis. Contusions lead to typically transient and rarely permanent neurological deficits, with severity depending on location, which can be delineated on MRI as T2 hyperintense lesions (Fig. 11.7). Spinal cord

infarct can result from disruption of the blood supply to the spinal cord and acutely appears as predominantly central high T2 signal with corresponding restricted diffusion on MRI (Fig. 11.8). This is due to hypoperfusion of the anterior spinal artery. Additional complications related to laminectomy are depicted in the "Failed Back Surgery" section.

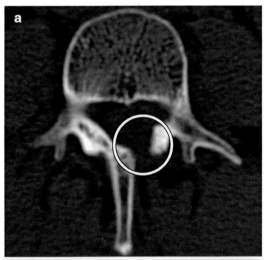
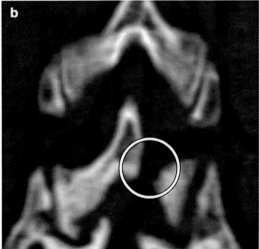

Fig. 11.3 Hemilaminectomy. Axial (**a**) and coronal (**b**) CT image demonstrates an opening in the left lamina (*encircled*)

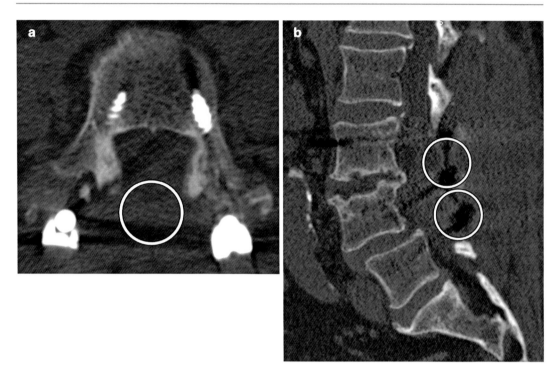

Fig. 11.4 Bilateral laminectomy. Axial (**a**) and sagittal (**b**) CT images show absence of the lamina and spinous processes at L3 and L4 (*encircled*). There is also posterior fusion hardware

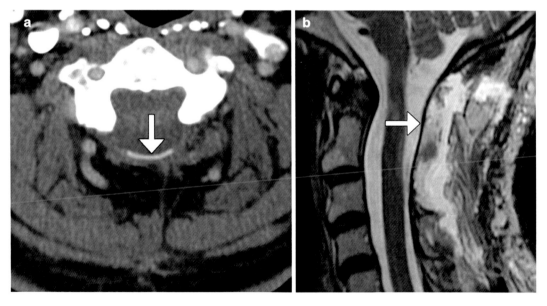

Fig. 11.5 Laminectomy and duraplasty. Axial CT image (**a**) shows hyperattenuating Gore-Tex duraplasty material that lines the posterior spinal canal at laminectomy site (*arrow*). The sagittal T2-weighted MRI (**b**) shows that the duraplasty material has low signal (*arrow*), similar to normal dura

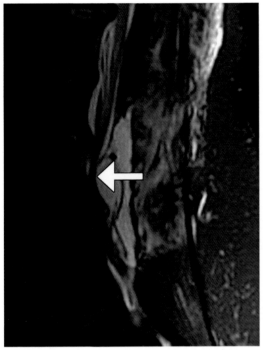

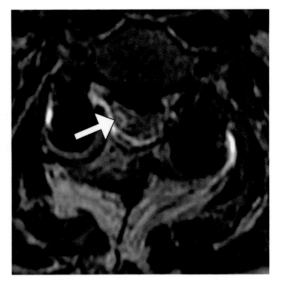

Fig. 11.7 Spinal cord contusion. The patient woke up with a right hemiparesis. Axial T2-weighted MRI shows edema in the right lateral cortical spinal tract after cervical laminectomy and fusion for cervical spine stenosis

Fig. 11.6 Tight durotomy closure. The patient experienced worsening radiculopathy after surgery. Sagittal T2-weighted MRI shows compression of the cauda equina nerve roots by the dura (*arrow*) after recent laminectomy. The patient returned to the operating room for release of the durotomy repair and duroplasty with immediate relief of symptoms

Fig. 11.8 Spinal cord infarct. The patient experienced paraplegia after surgery. Sagittal T2-weighted (**a**) and DWI (**b**) MR images show edema and restricted diffusion within the mid-cervical spinal cord at the same level of the laminectomies (*arrows*)

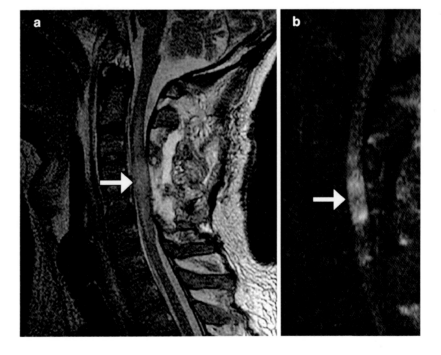

11.2.3 Facetectomy

11.2.3.1 Discussion

Facetectomy is mainly performed as part of treating far lateral disc herniations, facet hypertrophy, and limbus vertebral fractures. Facetectomy can essentially be performed as partial (usually medial) or total (Gil's procedure). At times, a partial lateral facetectomy would be performed if an extra-foraminal decompression and approach is required. Various approaches can be used, including endoscopic, intertransverse, extra-foraminal, and transpars techniques. The degree of bony resection is best appreciated on CT, while MRI is optimal for the assessment of nerve root decompression (Figs. 11.9 and 11.10). Scar tissue often fills the facetectomy defect.

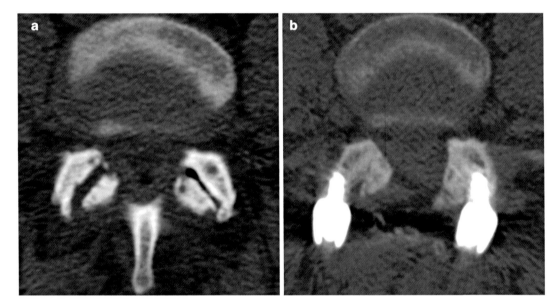

Fig. 11.9 Partial facetectomy. Preoperative axial CT image (**a**) shows bilateral facet degenerative changes. Postoperative axial CT image (**b**) shows resection of the medial aspects of the bilateral facet joints

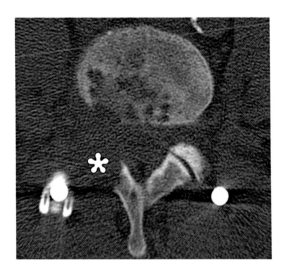

Fig. 11.10 Total facetectomy. Axial CT shows complete absence of the right facet joint (*)

11.2.4 Microdiscectomy

11.2.4.1 Discussion

Microdiscectomy is a minimally invasive technique for treating symptomatic disc herniations and consists of curettage of disc material under surgical microscope visualization typically done with a midline or paramedian approach (Fig. 11.11). Portions of ligamentum flavum are often removed (flavectomy) in order to provide adequate access to the disc and to contribute to decompression of the spinal canal (Fig. 11.12). The posterior elements otherwise remain intact,

thereby preserving stability of the spinal column. Clinical success of microdiscectomy is over 90% at 6 months and over 80% at 10 years. Complications are uncommon and include infection, dural tear, nerve root injury, and residual or re-herniation of disc fragments. Imaging is important for evaluating potential complications. Occasionally, hemostatic agents placed near the disc space can resemble a residual or re-herniated disc fragment, except these materials tend to have lower signal on T1-weighted and T2-weighted MRI sequences than does disc material (Fig. 11.13).

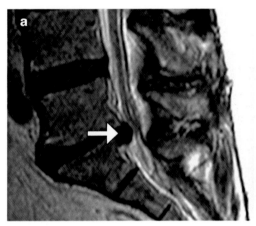
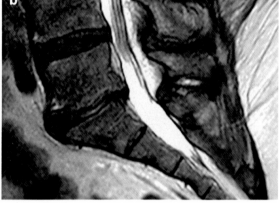

Fig. 11.11 Microdiscectomy. Preoperative sagittal T2-weighted MRI (**a**) shows a disc herniation at L5–S1 (*arrow*). Sagittal T2-weighted MRI (**b**) obtained after microdiscectomy shows interval resection of the herniated disc material, without significant alteration to the surrounding structures

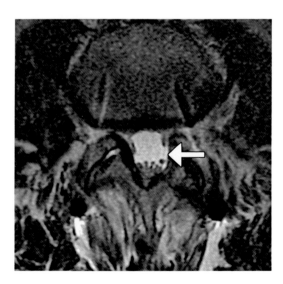

Fig. 11.12 Flavectomy. Axial T2-weighted MRI shows absence of a portion of the left ligamentum flavum (*arrow*)

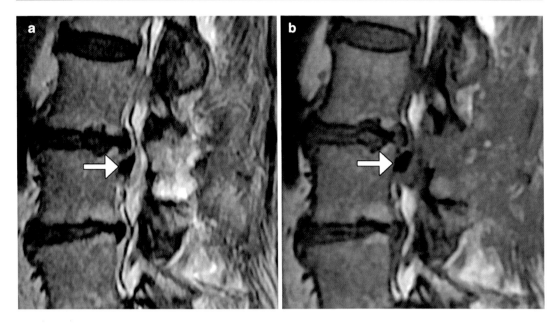

Fig. 11.13   Sagittal T2-weighted (**a**) and sagittal T1-weighted (**b**) MR images show low-intensity hemostatic material packed into the left lateral recess just inferior to the operated disc space (*arrows*)

11.2.5 Laminoplasty

11.2.5.1 Discussion

Laminoplasty is performed to widen the spinal canal while preserving as much of the anatomy as possible in order to conserve stability. Cervical laminoplasty is recommended for the treatment of cervical degenerative myelopathy or ossification of the posterior longitudinal ligament, with recovery rates of nearly 60% and improvement in about 80%. Commonly implemented surgical techniques consist of either performing bilaminar osteotomies and shifting the posterior elements backward or performing laminar osteotomy on one side and using a burr to thin the contralateral lamina in order to create a hinge and rotating the posterior elements posterolaterally and often trimming the spinous processes (Fig. 11.14). Alternatively, "French door" osteotomy can be performed in which a trough is drilled bilaterally in the lamina and the spinous process is split in half, opening up the spinal canal. The osteotomy gaps ("open door") can be filled using bone or hardware (laminar prosthesis). Imaging may be performed after laminoplasty in order to evaluate for patients with complications such as persistent neck pain and diminished cervical motion, which can manifest as canal restenosis and loss of cervical lordotic alignment.

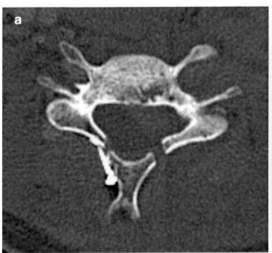
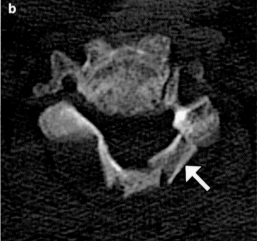

Fig. 11.14 Laminoplasty. Axial CT image (**a**) shows bilateral laminar osteotomies with posterior translation of the posterior elements, which are secured using a metal prosthesis on the right side. Axial CT image (**b**) in a dif- ferent patient shows a right laminar hinge and bone graft (*arrow*) interposed in the left laminar open door, In addition, there has been resection of the spinous process

11.2.6 Vertebrectomy

11.2.6.1 Discussion

Vertebrectomy is sometimes necessary to treat extensive spine, tumors, infections, or fracture-dislocations. Part (partial vertebrectomy) or all (total vertebrectomy) of a vertebra can be removed. In particular, corpectomy is a specific type of partial vertebrectomy in which the vertebral body is partially or completely resected. Extensive vertebrectomy operations are often performed in stages. For example, en bloc bone resection can be performed using a diamond threadwire saw (T-saw), osteotome, and/or Gigli saw. The threadwire is sometimes left in the surgical bed for staged operations, such that the device may sometimes be encountered on interval imaging (Fig. 11.15). Subsequently, the vertebra can be reconstructed using iliac crest, tibia, and fibula strut grafts or various types of synthetic cages. Interbody cages, such as the Harms cage, are interposed vertically between vertebral bodies after vertebral body resection in order to promote fusion and provide

mechanical support (Fig. 11.16). Expandable cage designs that can be adjusted to fit the length of the surgical defect are also available (Fig. 11.17). Morselized bone graft material is often packed inside the cage. The Harms cage is often used in combination with anterior or posterior fusion hardware, which yields fusion rates of over 90%. Carbon fiber cage systems can also be used for anterior column reconstruction following corpectomy, mainly in the setting of spine tumor and trauma surgery. Carbon fiber is a biocompatible material that can be used to make stackable cage systems. Except for the central metallic rod, on radiographs and CT, the carbon fiber components are radiolucent, while on MRI, the carbon fiber components are of low signal intensity on T1 and T2 sequences (Fig. 11.18). The role of imaging, particularly with CT, is to assess the progression of fusion and to evaluate for complications, such as graft or instrument displacement (Figs. 11.19 and 11.20). High-resolution CT with 3D renderings is particularly useful for assessing the position and integrity of the hardware.

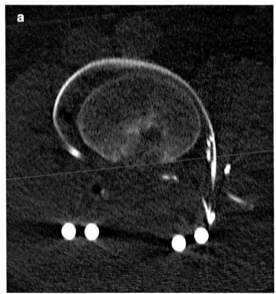
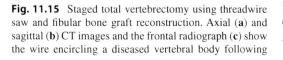
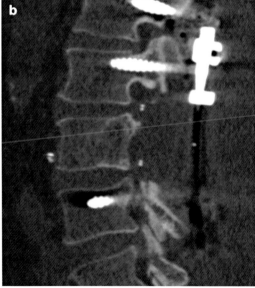

Fig. 11.15 Staged total vertebrectomy using threadwire saw and fibular bone graft reconstruction. Axial (**a**) and sagittal (**b**) CT images and the frontal radiograph (**c**) show the wire encircling a diseased vertebral body following laminectomy and posterior fusion. The follow-up sagittal CT image (**d**) shows interval corpectomy with fibular grafting and removal of the wire

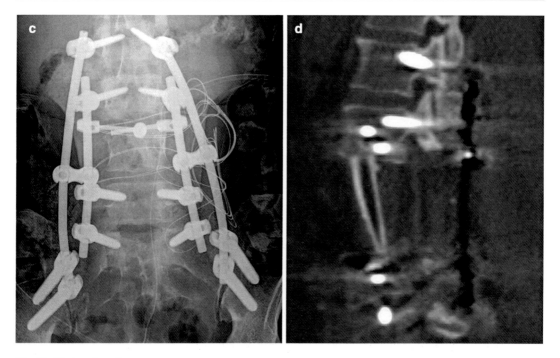

Fig. 11.15 (continued)

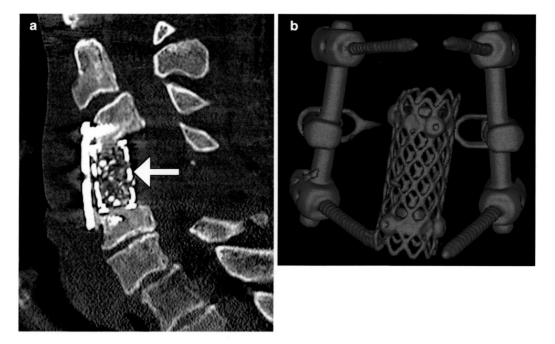

Fig. 11.16 Harms cage. Sagittal (**a**) CT image shows a cage filled with bone graft (*arrow*). There is also anterior fusion hardware. 3D CT image (**b**) in a different case shows a cylindrical metal mesh cage and adjacent posterior fusion hardware

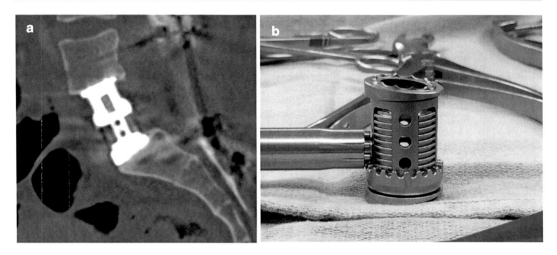

Fig. 11.17 Expandable cage. Sagittal CT image demonstrates the telescoping components of the metallic expandable cage (**a**). Photograph of an expandable cage (**b**)

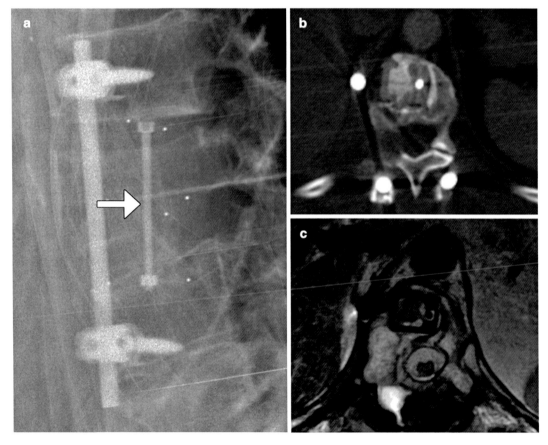

Fig. 11.18 Corpectomy with stackable carbon fiber reconstruction. Frontal (**a**) radiograph shows corpectomy and fusion with stackable carbon fiber-reinforced cages constrained by a central metallic rod (*arrow*). The cages are otherwise radiolucent except for tiny metallic markers. Axial CT image (**b**) shows the low attenuation rectangular stackable cages and constraining metallic rod. Axial T2-weighted MRI (**c**) shows the low signal intensity rectangular carbon fiber cage

Fig. 11.19 Slippage of expandable cage. Sagittal
CT image shows complete dislocation of the spine
from the corpectomy cage with associated angular
kyphosis of the cervical spine and compromise of
the spinal canal contents

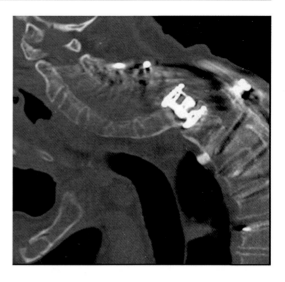

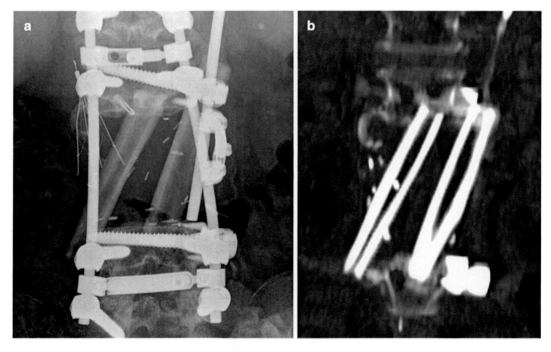

Fig. 11.20 Dislocated bone grafts. Frontal radiograph
(**a**) and coronal CT image (**b**) show lateral displacement
of the bilateral fibular grafts out of the corpectomy defect
such that the inferior end of the right graft and the superior
end of the left graft no longer contact the adjacent
endplates

11.2.7 Cordectomy

11.2.7.1   Discussion

Cordectomy involves resection of the spinal cord. This unusual procedure is reserved for selected patients with severe neurologic deficits and symptoms related to intramedullary tumors or extramedullary tumors that invade the spinal cord. Laminectomy, corpectomy, or vertebrectomy can be performed in conjunction with cordectomy. Therefore, materials used to stabilize the spine, such as methyl methacrylate, can safely extend into the spinal canal at the level of the cordectomy (Fig. 11.21).

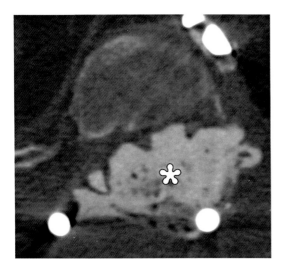

Fig. 11.21 Cordectomy. The patient is status post chordoma excision with recurrence, which required resection of the spinal cord and placement of posterior rods and methyl methacrylate for spinal stabilization. Axial CT image shows cement filling the spinal canal (*)

11.3 Spine Stabilization and Fusion

11.3.1 Halo and Traction Devices

11.3.1.1 Discussion

A variety of surgically affixed devices are available for immobilization and traction of unstable cervical spine fractures and dislocations, including halo vests and Gardner-Wells tongs (Figs. 11.22 and 11.23). Halo vests comprise a metallic ring secured to the skull via screws. The ring is attached to a padded fiberglass or plastic thoracic cast by metal struts. The Gardner-Wells device consists of two screws attached to both sides of the skull that support the tongs to which traction is applied. Both types of devices provide excellent long-term cervical spine fixation. Pullout of the screws is a rare, but potentially devastating complication. In addition to pullout, screw site infection or screw breaking through the inner cortex of the skull is a rare complication. In general, devices composed of aluminum or graphite-carbon composites and plastic joints are MRI compatible.

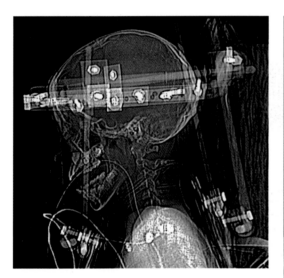

Fig. 11.22 Halo vest. Scout image shows the device secured to the skull and shoulder girdle

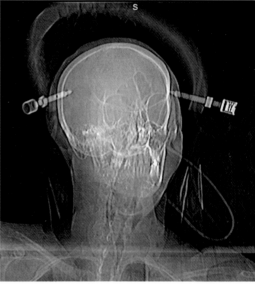

Fig. 11.23 Gardner-Wells device. Scout image shows the traction device with bilateral scalp screw fixation

11.3.2 Bone Graft Materials

11.3.2.1 Discussion

Several options are available for promoting bone fusion, including autologous, allograft, and synthetic bone grafts. Autologous bone grafts are often harvested from the iliac crest, rib, or local lamina, and spinous process (Fig. 11.24). Alternatively, a trephine system can be used to obtain a core of cancellous bone from an adjacent vertebral body, which leaves a cylindrical defect in the anterior portion of the vertebral body and pedicle (Fig. 11.25). Allografts are derived from cadavers and are available as bone chips or cylinders from fibula or rib and retain some bony structure (Fig. 11.26). Ultimately, an uninterrupted bony bridge should form across the vertebral bodies and facet joints as the bone graft fusion matures (Fig. 11.27).

The main types of synthetic bone graft substitutes that are used during spine surgery include ceramics, demineralized bone matrix, and composite materials. Demineralized bone matrix consists of non-collagenous proteins, bone growth factors, and collagen, which are intended to stimulate bone healing. These materials are radiolucent and difficult to visualize directly on imaging. Demineralized bone matrix is available in powder form or as putty that can be used to fill voids (Fig. 11.28). Sometimes demineralized bone

matrix is combined with bone grafts, which has attenuation intermediate between medullary and cortical bone. Ceramics include calcium sulfate, hydroxyapatite, tricalcium phosphate, or a combination of hydroxyapatite and tricalcium phosphate that are available in the form of pellets, pastes, or cement. These materials are denser than native bone. Composite materials such as moldable morsels contain mixtures of ceramic and collagen or other demineralized bone matrix components. The mineralized component (i.e., calcium phosphate) provides compressive strength and a substrate for bone formation, while the collagen contributes tensile strength and promotes hemostasis at the surgical site. On CT, such materials appear as grainy foci of heterogeneous attenuation (Fig. 11.29).

Recombinant bone morphogenic protein (BMP) is often added to bone graft agents in order to promote fusion. This substance promotes bone resorption or osteolysis. Despite this finding, fusion typically progresses and matures within 2 years. In fact, BMP expedites arthrodesis. On imaging, BMP-induced osteolysis appears as multiple cystic spaces in the endplate adjacent to the implant (Fig. 11.30). BMP is also known to form an excessive inflammatory response with excessive fluid collections in the early postoperative period, sometimes even leading to undesired bone formation within the spinal canal.

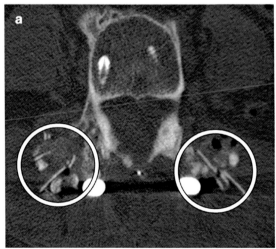
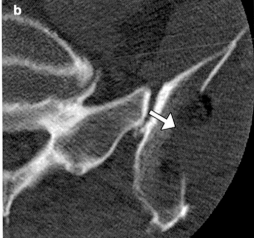

Fig. 11.24 Autologous bone graft harvested from the iliac crest. Axial CT of the spine (**a**) shows bilateral cortical and cancellous bone fragments with sharp edges (*encircled*). Demineralized bone matrix was also applied. Axial CT at a lower level (**b**) shows the iliac donor site packed with hemostatic agent (*arrow*)

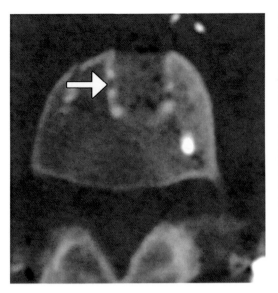

Fig. 11.25 Local vertebral body bone harvest. Axial CT image shows cylindrical defect in the anterior vertebral body (*arrow*)

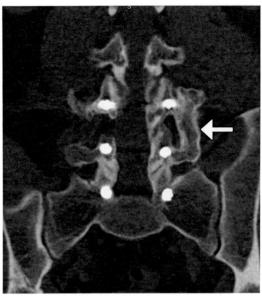

Fig. 11.27 Mature bone graft fusion. Coronal CT image shows a solid fusion mass that bridges the left L4 and L5 vertebrae from transverse process to transverse process (*arrow*)

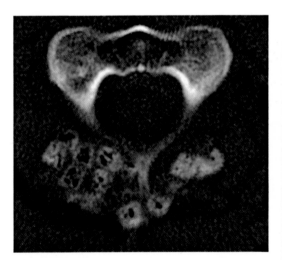

Fig. 11.26 Allograft bone chips. Axial CT image shows numerous cubes of cancellous cadaveric bone grafts within an adjacent to the laminectomy site. Many of the chips show a trabecular bone structure and contain air

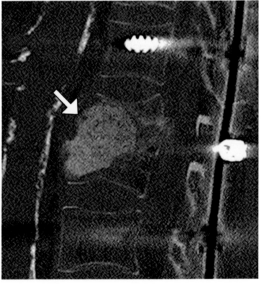

Fig. 11.28 Demineralized bone matrix. Sagittal CT image shows amorphous hyperattenuating material filling the space of partially collapsed vertebral bodies secondary to prior osteomyelitis (*arrow*)

Fig. 11.29 Composite Mozaik moldable morsels. Axial CT image shows the mixture of bone putty and moldable morsels as numerous tiny heterogeneously hyperattenuating foci (*encircled*) spanning the posterior surgical defect adjacent to the segmental instrumentation

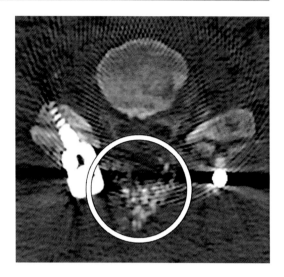

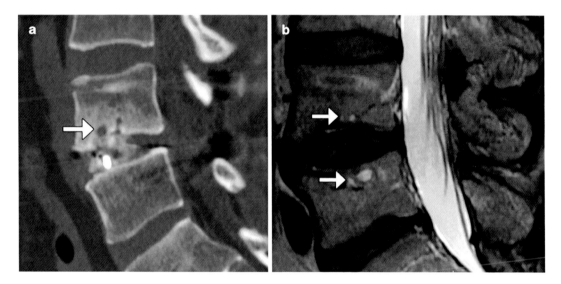

Fig. 11.30 Recombinant BMP-induced osteolysis. Sagittal (**a**) CT image shows rounded lucencies (*arrow*) along the inferior endplate of the vertebral body above the interbody fusion. Sagittal T2-weighted MRI (**b**) shows high-intensity foci (*arrows*) within the endplates adjacent to the interbody fusion material

11.3.3 Implantable Bone Stimulators

11.3.3.1 Discussion

Implantable (internal) bone stimulators are devices that deliver electrical currents to promote bone growth and healing and to expedite fusion. This device consists of electrodes that are positioned in contact with the site of spinal fusion and a small power source that is implanted in the subcutaneous tissues (Fig. 11.31). The role of imaging is to confirm proper positioning of the electrodes and assess progression of bony fusion or healing.

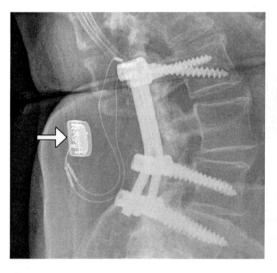

Fig. 11.31 Bone stimulator. Lateral radiograph shows the leads in contact with the fusion masses and the battery pack (*arrow*) implanted in the subcutaneous tissues

11.3.4 Odontoid Screw Fixation

11.3.4.1 Discussion

Anterior fixation of odontoid fractures consists of securing the fracture fragment with one or two lag or cortical screws depending on the diameter of the dens. A lag screw is used in order to help reduce the fracture. Complications of this procedure include hematomas, dysphagia, hoarseness, and vascular, spinal cord, or nerve root injuries. Radiographs and/or CT may be obtained for follow-up, especially in order to assess for union (Fig. 11.32). The tip of the screw can often safely project beyond the posterosuperior edge of the dens by several millimeters. Other options for treating odontoid fractures include posterior spinal fusion or halo-vest immobilization.

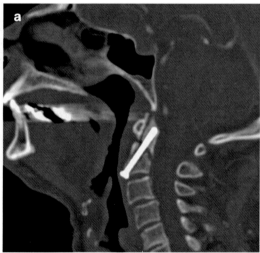

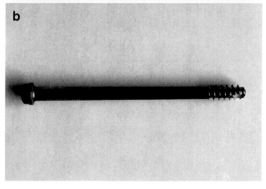

Fig. 11.32 Odontoid screw fixation. Sagittal CT (**a**) shows anterior fixation of the dens fracture via a single lag screw. The dens fracture fragments are well aligned, but remain unfused. Photograph of an odontoid lag screw (**b**)

11.3.5 Occipitocervical Fusion

11.3.5.1   Discussion

Indications for occipitocervical fusion include anterior and posterior bifid C1 arches with instability, absent occipital condyles, severe reducible basilar invagination, unstable dystopic os odontoideum, unilateral atlas assimilation, traumatic occipitocervical dislocation, complex craniovertebral junction fractures of C1 and C2, transoral craniovertebral junction decompression, cranial settling in Down's syndrome, tumors, and inflammatory disease such as Grisel's syndrome.

A variety of internal fixation methods have been developed for posterior craniocervical junction fusion including sublaminar wiring (Fig. 11.33) and occipital rods and plates (Fig. 11.34). Bone grafts are often added alongside the posterior elements in order to promote bony fusion. Interestingly, the degree of stabil-

ity does not seem to correlate with the presence or absence of radiographically evident bone graft fusion. Sublaminar wires have the potential to unravel, resulting in recurrent malalignment and instability (Fig. 11.35) and generally provide less stability than screw constructs. In addition, wire fracture can lacerate the spinal cord. The occipital screws can sometimes penetrate the inner table of the occipital bone (Fig. 11.36), which may not necessarily result in cerebellar injury, especially if it is only by a small extent. Transarticular screw fixation of the cervical spine can encroach upon the transverse foramina and potentially injure the vertebral arteries or even impinge upon the internal carotid arteries (Fig. 11.37). The incidence of nonunion or loosening is about 7% for occipitocervical fusion and atlantoaxial fusion, which appears as lucency around the hardware on CT (Fig. 11.38).

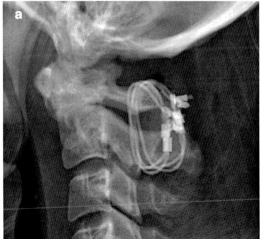
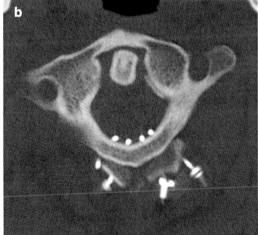
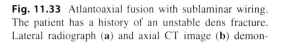

Fig. 11.33 Atlantoaxial fusion with sublaminar wiring. The patient has a history of an unstable dens fracture. Lateral radiograph (**a**) and axial CT image (**b**) demonstrate posterior atlantoaxial fixation with bilateral cables that pass into the spinal canal and around iliac crest bone grafts applied posterior to the C1 and C2 arches

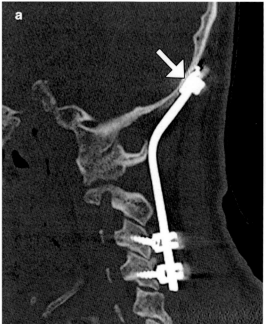

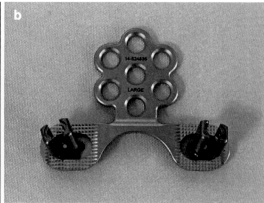

Fig. 11.34 Occipitocervical fusion with rods and screws. Sagittal CT image (**a**) shows the curvilinear posterior rod (*arrow*) attached to the occipital bone via plate (*arrow*) and screws and to the upper cervical spine via lateral mass screws. Photograph of an occipital plate (**b**)

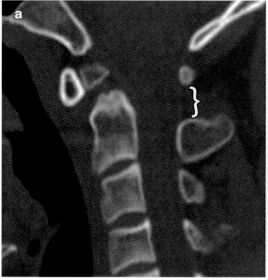

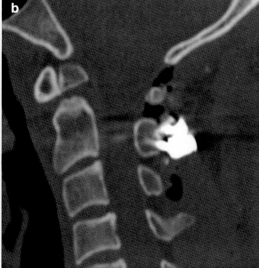

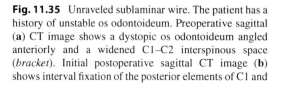

Fig. 11.35 Unraveled sublaminar wire. The patient has a history of unstable os odontoideum. Preoperative sagittal (**a**) CT image shows a dystopic os odontoideum angled anteriorly and a widened C1–C2 interspinous space (*bracket*). Initial postoperative sagittal CT image (**b**) shows interval fixation of the posterior elements of C1 and C2 with sublaminar wires and application of bone graft. There is resulting decreased C1–C2 interspinous distance and angulation of the os odontoideum. Subsequent sagittal CT image (**c**) shows interval widening of the C1–C2 interspinous distance and angulation of the os odontoideum similar to the configuration before surgery

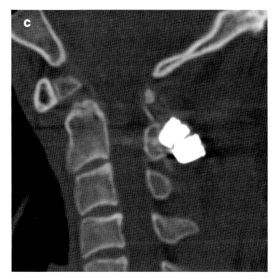

Fig. 11.35 (continued)

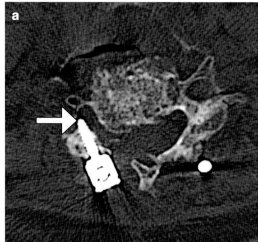

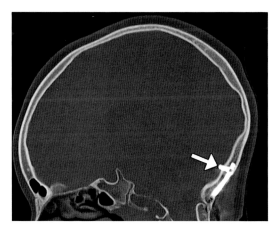

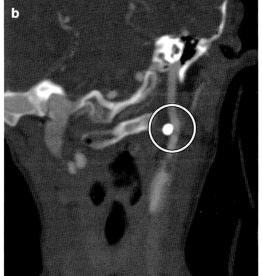

Fig. 11.36 Occipital screw intracranial penetration. Sagittal CT image shows penetration of the inner table with intracranial extension of a lateral occipital plate screw (*arrow*)

Fig. 11.37 Vascular compromise by screw malposition. Axial CT image (**a**) shows a right lateral mass screw within the right foramen transversarium (*arrow*). Coronal CTA image in another patient (**b**) shows impingement of the left internal carotid artery (*encircled*)

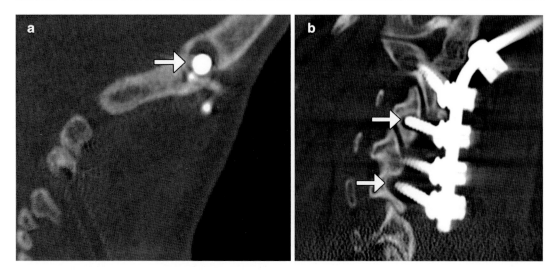

Fig. 11.38 Hardware loosening. Sagittal CT image (**a**) shows lucency surrounded the hardware in the occipital bone (*arrow*). Sagittal CT image (**b**) shows lucencies surrounding multiple lateral mass screws (*arrows*), which have begun to pull out

11.3.6 Anterior Cervical Fusion

11.3.6.1 Discussion

Anterior cervical plates are commonly used for fusion to treat degenerative conditions, as well as fractures, infections, and tumors. The hardware most commonly spans two or three vertebral body levels, but can be as many as five vertebral bodies. The plates are affixed to the vertebral bodies via screws (Fig. 11.39). The screws should not transgress the adjacent disc space. The plates and screws are most often metallic, although some biodegradable devices have been developed. Another technique for anterior cervical fusion is the use of interbody devices without the use of plate (stand-alone). These devices are typically composed of polyether ether ketone (PEEK) and are fixed to the vertebral body either with two or three screws or fins (Fig. 11.40). For example, Zero P is a Synthes device used as a stand-alone implant in cervical interbody fusion and incorporates both the interbody cage and fixation plate. The device has a low profile anteriorly, resulting in decreased soft tissue and esophageal irritation. Zero P and all similar devices are designed to reduce adjacent level ossification, since the plate does not irritate the adjacent disc.

Complications of anterior cervical fusion include hardware infection, dysphagia, hematoma, esophageal perforation, subsidence, spinal cord injury in the cervical spine, and bowel, or vascular injury in the lumbar spine. A fluid collection and foci of gas can be identified in the prevertebral space on CT with hardware infection (Fig. 11.41). MRI is used to evaluate for an associated epidural abscess.

Subsidence of the hardware or graft material is a chronic process in which the materials penetrate into the adjacent vertebral bodies or disc spaces. This can lead to postoperative deformity and sclerosis, which can be assessed on CT (Fig. 11.42).

Cervical spinal cord injury can rarely occur during screw placement, potentially creating a transecting spinal cord injury (Fig. 11.43). Dysphagia and dysphonia are common following anterior cervical fusion due to injury to the pharyngeal plexus and recurrent laryngeal nerve. CT can be used to assess the neck soft tissue in such cases, which may reveal supraglottic edema (Fig. 11.44). Otolaryngology consultation should be obtained for patients with postoperative dysphagia or dysphonia, particularly if that persists longer than 1–2 months.

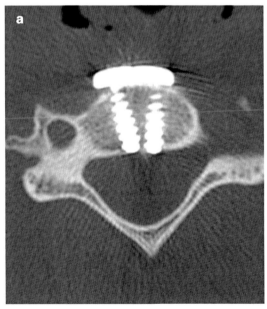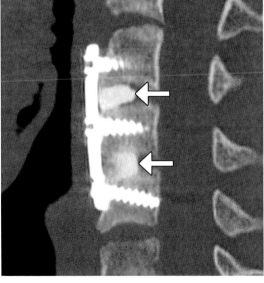

Fig. 11.39 Anterior cervical discectomy and fusion (ACDF). Axial (**a**), sagittal (**b**), and 3D (**c**) CT images show an anterior cervical plate secured flush against the vertebral bodies via screws. Anterior discectomy and placement of intervertebral allografts was also performed (*arrows*)

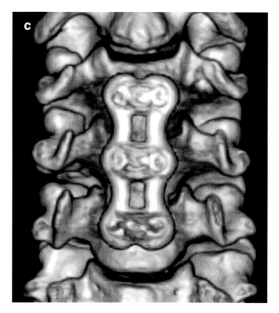

Fig. 11.39 (continued)

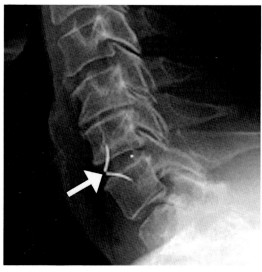

Fig. 11.40 Stand-alone anterior cervical discectomy and fusion. Lateral radiograph shows the LDR ROI-C cage and fins C6-7 (*arrow*)

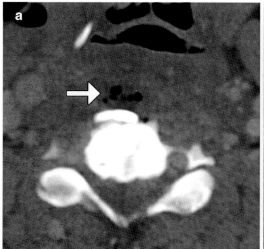

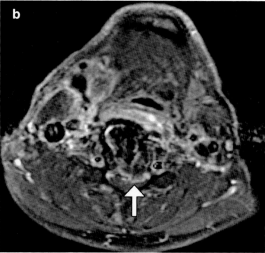

Fig. 11.41 Infection. Axial CT image (**a**) demonstrates a fluid collection containing foci of gas anterior to the anterior cervical spine hardware (*arrow*). Axial fat-suppressed post-contrast T1-weighted MRI (**b**) shows extensive enhancement in the prevertebral space as well as extension into the anterior epidural space (*arrow*)

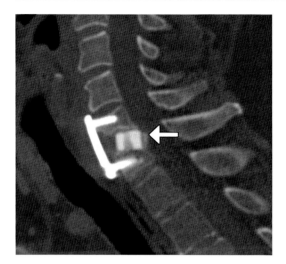

Fig. 11.42 Bone graft subsidence and retropulsion. Sagittal CT image shows the bone graft dowel (*arrow*) protruding into the spinal canal and adjacent vertebral bodies

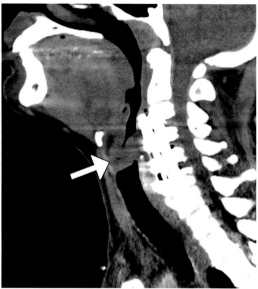

Fig. 11.44 Supraglottic swelling after anterior cervical fusion. The patient experiences difficulty breathing after cervical spine surgery. Sagittal CT image shows multiple level cervical anterior fusion with surgical hardware and swelling of the supraglottic soft tissues (*arrow*)

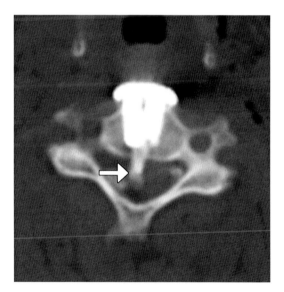

Fig. 11.43 Iatrogenic spinal cord transection from anterior cervical fusion. Axial CT image of the cervical spine shows a cylindrical bone fragment (*arrow*) within the central spinal canal. There is anterior fusion hardware and soft tissue air from the recent surgery (Courtesy of Richard White, MD)

11.3.7 Anterior Approach Thoracolumbar Spine Stabilization Devices

11.3.7.1 Discussion

Anterior surgical approach short-segment stabilization systems, such as the Kaneda device (DePuy Spine, Raynham, Mass) and the Vantage plate (Medtronic, Sofamor Danek, Memphis TN), are adjustable devices that can provide rigid fixation of the thoracolumbar vertebral column in the setting of burst fracture stabilization or corpectomy via anterior approaches. The Kaneda device consists of a rod and screws with additional staples, which reinforce the purchase of the screws in the vertebrae, resulting in robust fixation (Fig. 11.45). The Vantage plate features several slots for selecting the optimal level of the screws that are secured to adjacent vertebral bodies (Fig. 11.46). The device is inserted by using an anterior approach.

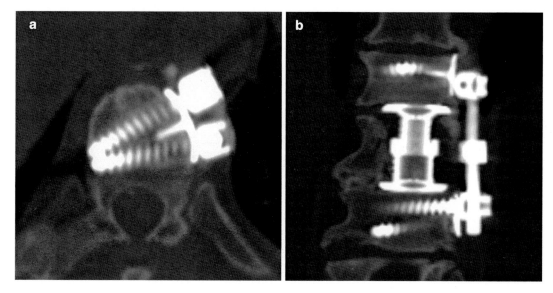

Fig. 11.45 Kaneda device. Axial (**a**) and coronal (**b**) CT images show the rod and screw system positioned along the left lateral aspect of the vertebrae. An expandable cage is also present in the intervening space

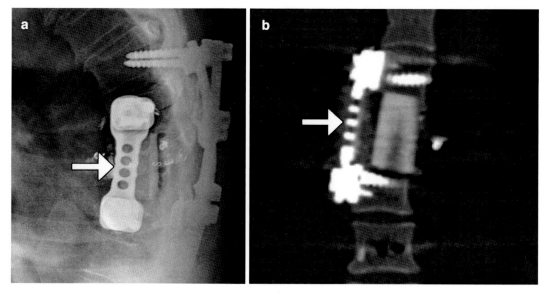

Fig. 11.46 Adjustable plate system. Lateral thoracic spine radiograph (**a**) and coronal CT image (**b**) show the adjustable plate (*arrow*) spanning the corpectomy site, where there is a tibial structural allograft

11.3.8 Posterior Fusion

11.3.8.1 Discussion

Most thoracic and lumbar spine fixation is performed via a posterior approach, most commonly using rods and pedicle screws. Pedicle screws attach posteriorly to rods or plates via clamps or bolts and have shallow cancellous threads that pass through the pedicle and into the vertebral body. The screw should enter 50–80% of the vertebral body and be parallel to the endplates with at least 2 mm of separation. The screws can produce considerable beam-hardening artifacts on CT, which can be minimized through the use of metal artifact reduction software (Fig. 11.47). On MRI, the pedicle screws can produce variable degrees of metal susceptibility artifact that can obscure adjacent structures, which is more pronounced at higher magnetic field strength (Fig. 11.48). Imaging via CT is sometimes performed in order to assess whether the screws are malpositioned (Fig. 11.49). Medial malpositioning is a potentially devastating complication that can result in spinal cord or nerve injury. Laterally malpositioned screws can injure exiting nerve roots. Pedicle screws can also potentially cause vascular injury, such as the aorta or inferior vena cava, if they are too long and exit the anterior vertebral body. Although transdiscal screws are sometimes used for fixation in scoliosis surgery, penetration into the disc space is generally avoided. Another option for securing rods is through lateral mass screws, which are situated between the superior and inferior articular processes, thereby lowering the likelihood of the types of malpositioning associated with pedicle screws (Fig. 11.50).

Instead of screws, rods can also be secured to the vertebrae via sublaminar wires or cables (Fig. 11.51). Sublaminar wires or cables pass around the lamina and rods and are twisted or clamped at their ends. Alternatively, laminar or sublaminar hooks can be used for compression or distraction. Hooks that pass below the lamina are termed up-going, while those that pass above the lamina are termed down-going (Fig. 11.52). These two configurations are usually applied simultaneously for optimal stability. The hooks are connected to the rods via screws, bolts, or washers. Facet screw fixation is an alternative to pedicle screw fixation whereby the articular facets are fused. The screws are not attached to rods but may be used in conjunction with interbody fusion or anterior plating (Fig. 11.53).

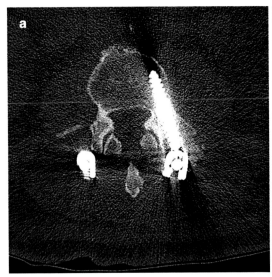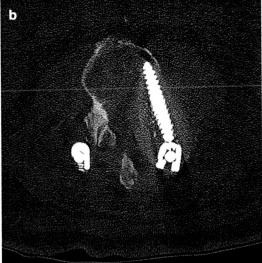

Fig. 11.47 Metal artifact reduction software. Axial CT image (**a**) shows extensive metal artifact associated with the surgical hardware. The corresponding axial CT image with metal artifact reduction software (**b**) shows much less artifact

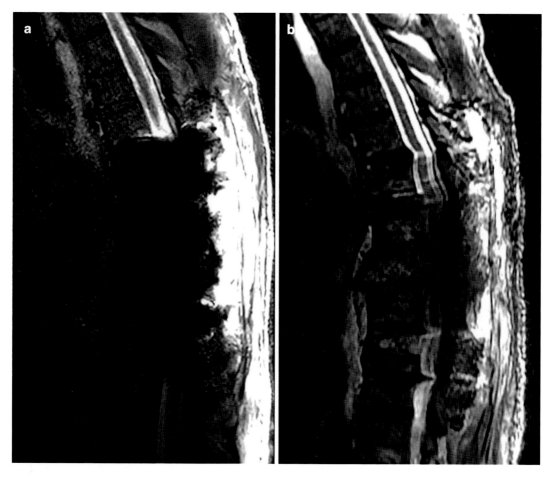

Fig. 11.48 Spine hardware artifacts at 3 T versus 1.5 T. Sagittal T2-weighted MRI performed on a 3 T scanner (**a**) shows extensive susceptibility artifact related to the pedicle screws, which obscures the surrounding anatomy. Sagittal T2-weighted MRI performed on a 1.5 T scanner (**b**) shows much less artifact from the hardware

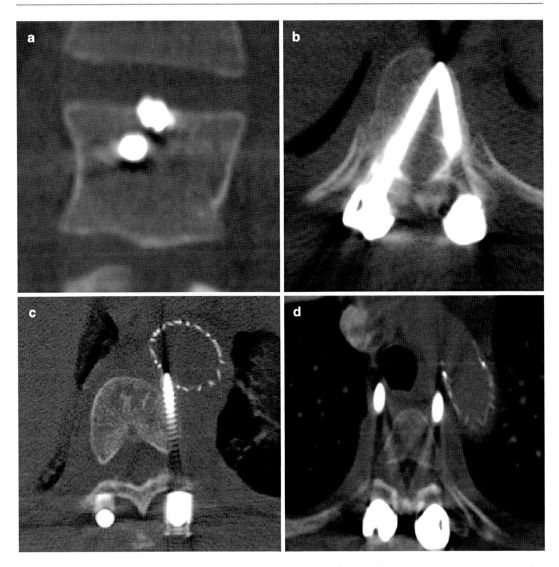

Fig. 11.49 Malpositioned screws. Coronal CT image (**a**) shows a screw that breaches the superior endplate and enters the intervertebral disc space. Axial CT image (**b**) in another patient shows medial malposition of the right tho- racic pedicle screw into the spinal canal (*arrow*), resulting in paraplegia. Axial CT images (c and d) in another patient show screws impinging upon the aorta, which contains an endograft and impinging upon the trachea

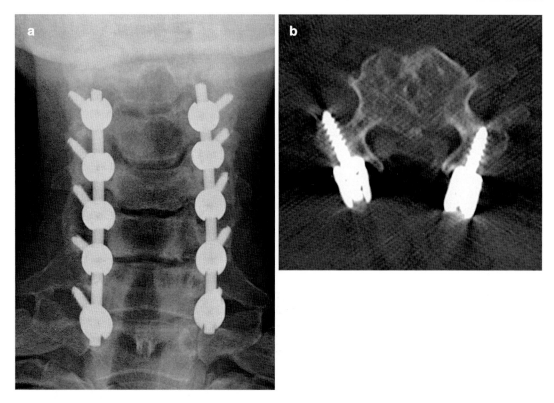

Fig. 11.50 Lateral mass screws and rods. Frontal radiograph (**a**) and axial CT image (**b**) show bilateral screws traversing the lateral mass. Unlike transpedicular screws, lateral mass screws are directed laterally

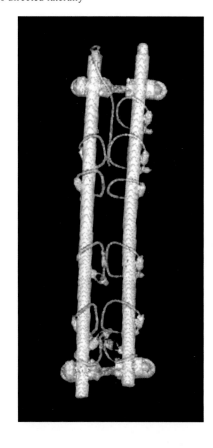

Fig. 11.51 Wire fixation. 3D CT image shows sublaminar wires attached to the rods

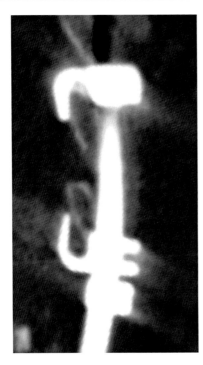

Fig. 11.52 Pedicle hooks. Sagittal CT image shows upgoing and down-going hooks secured to the laminae and attached to a rod

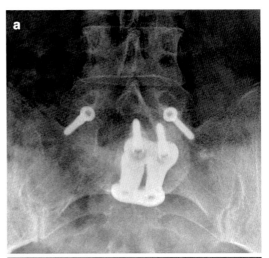

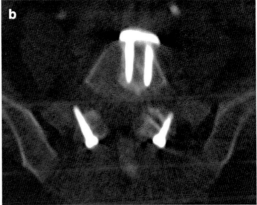

Fig. 11.53 Facet screws. Frontal radiograph (**a**) and axial CT image (**b**) demonstrate bilateral L5–S1 facet screws. Anterior fusion was also performed

11.3.9 Scoliosis Rods

11.3.9.1 Discussion

A variety of rods are used for posterior spinal fixation in the treatment of scoliosis, including Harrington, Knodt, and Luque (Figs. 11.54, 11.55, and 11.56). In contrast to threaded Knodt rods, Harrington rods feature flanged ends, which can attach to laminar hooks. Harrington rods are usually paired and interconnected by segmental wires for added stability. Luque rods are spinopelvic fixation devices that can be used to treat scoliosis, among other applications. The apparatus has a characteristic L shape in which the inferior angled portion can be affixed to the ilium. Depending on the direction in which the hooks

are placed, the rods can provide either compression or distraction. Perhaps the most common usage of these rods is for treatment of severe scoliosis, which can sometimes be partially corrected.

Complications include rod fracture or dislocation and screw pullout, which can be predisposed by the high torque inherent to the length of the hardware (Figs. 11.57, 11.58, and 11.59). The thoracolumbar fixation hardware may also lead to "flat-back" syndrome, in which there is loss of lumbar lordosis (Fig. 11.60). Scout and 3D CT reconstructions are particularly helpful for evaluating mechanical complications, while MRI might be more useful for assessing spinal canal involvement.

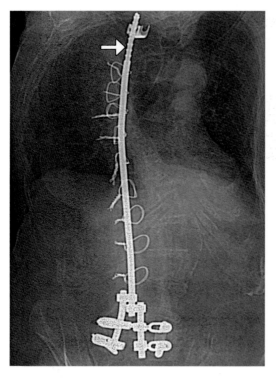

Fig. 11.54 Harrington rod. Frontal radiograph shows a metallic rod with flanged end (*arrow*) spanning the thoracolumbar spine in a patient with scoliosis

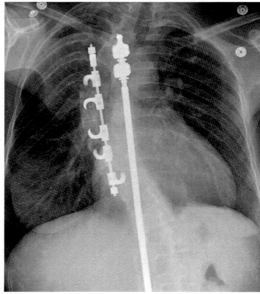

Fig. 11.55 Knodt rods. Frontal radiograph shows two rods with threaded ends

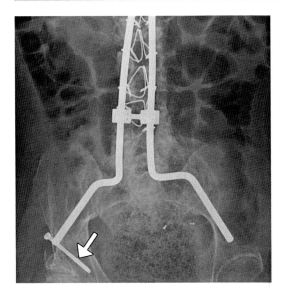

Fig. 11.56 Luque rods. Frontal radiograph shows instrumentation with pelvic fixation using the Galveston technique (*arrow*)

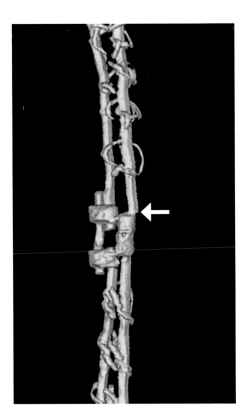

Fig. 11.57 Rod fracture. 3D CT image shows a displaced fracture of one of the Harrington rods (*arrow*)

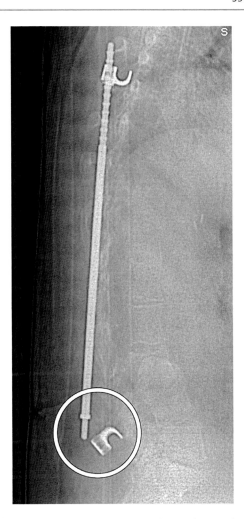

Fig. 11.58 Rod dislocation. Lateral scout images show posterior displacement of the inferior end of the Harrington rod (*encircled*) with separation from the hook

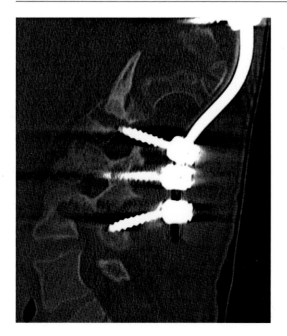

Fig. 11.59 Screw pullout. Sagittal CT image shows multiple screws that are posteriorly displaced along with the inferior end of the scoliosis rod

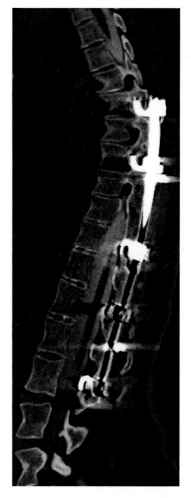

Fig. 11.60 Flat-back syndrome. The patient presents with chronic low back pain and poor posture. Sagittal CT image demonstrates straightening vertebral alignment with loss of lumbar lordosis along the same levels as the rods

11.3.10   Vertebral Stapling

11.3.10.1   Discussion

Vertebral body stapling is a minimally invasive, fusionless alternative to reduce curvature progression in patients with mild idiopathic scoliosis. Vertebral staples are composed of shape memory alloys that can be custom fit to the size of the vertebral body. The staples are inserted into the lateral aspects of the vertebral bodies across the disc spaces unilateral to the convex side of the scoliosis (Fig. 11.61). A thoracoscopic approach can be used for thoracic curves and a mini-open retroperitoneal approach for lumbar curves. Initial success rates are high and with few associated complications, although long-term follow-up is not yet available.

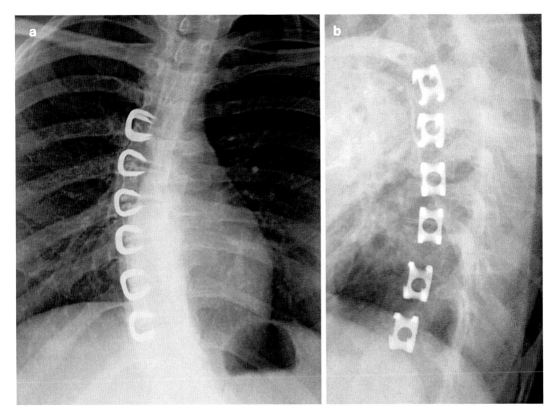

Fig. 11.61 Vertebral staples. Frontal (**a**) and lateral (**b**) radiographs show the C-shaped staples positioned in multiple contiguous vertebral bodies along the convex side of the thoracic scoliosis

11.3.11 Vertical Expandable Prosthetic Titanium Rib (VEPTR)

11.3.11.1 Discussion

VEPTR is used to gradually correct chest wall deformity and scoliosis in selected pediatric patients, with repeated lengthening sessions. The devices are typically implanted at the time of wedge thoracostomy and consist of an adjustable metal rod that is interposed vertically between ribs on the concave side of the scoliosis for distraction (Fig. 11.62). Most patients with VEPTR maintain near-normal thoracic spine growth rates and satisfactory lung volumes. Complications include device migration, infection, and brachial plexus injury.

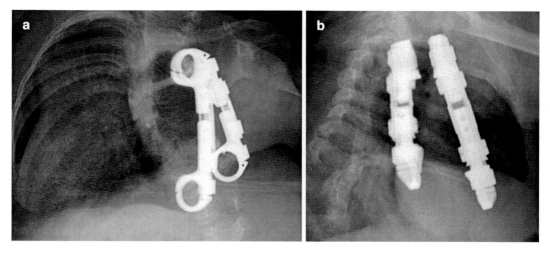

Fig. 11.62 Vertical expandable prosthetic titanium rib. The patient is a child with a history of severe scoliosis and associated chest wall deformity. Frontal (**a**) and lateral (**b**) radiographs show two metallic devices interposed between the right ribs

11.3.12   Interbody Fusion

11.3.12.1   Discussion

The goal of lumbar interbody fusion with prosthetic devices is to provide stability while promoting bony ingrowth. Many materials and devices have been used for this purpose, including bone threaded bone graft dowels or femoral rings, metal cages, and polymer cages. Femoral ring grafts are cylindrically shaped and inserted into the intervertebral disc space via anterior lumbar interbody fusion, posterior lumbar interbody fusion, or transforaminal lumbar interbody fusion approach (Fig. 11.63). A major disadvantage of such allograft device is the risk of disease transmission. Wide varieties of metal cages have been and continue to be developed. The first-generation Bagby and Kulich (BAK) and second-generation Ray threaded fusion cages are cylindrical, hollow, porous, threaded, titanium alloy cages that can be screwed into position in the intervertebral disc space (Fig. 11.64). The more recent third-generation LT-CAGE has been widely used in North America and has a trapezoidal, tapered configuration that provides increased surface area for bone growth and facilitates restoration of lumbar lordosis (Fig. 11.65).

More recent interbody fusion devices are mainly composed of polyether ether ketone (PEEK) or bio-compatible high-density carbon fiber. These materials are radiolucent, which facilitates visualization of the bone graft-vertebral body endplate interface. The devices also contain press-fit titanium markers in order to demarcate the boundaries of the device on radiographs. Many designs are in use, but generally are rectangular with grooves in order to promote vertebral body attachment. There are a variety of approaches that can be used for interbody fusion (Figs. 11.66, 11.67, 11.68, 11.69, 11.70, and 11.71 and Table 11.2).

Imaging can be used to assess the position of the implants, which should be located at least 2 mm anterior to the posterior wall of the vertebral body. Another role of imaging following interbody fusion surgery is to assess fusion versus pseudarthrosis. Radiographs with lateral flexion and extension views can be used for this purpose, although the accuracy is highly dependent upon precise positioning and the type of implant. Rather, CT is the modality of choice for evaluating interbody fusion, although the streak artifact from the early stainless devices can obscure adjacent bone formation. Early bone healing can often be appreciated at 3 months and is usually nearly complete at 6 months after surgery.

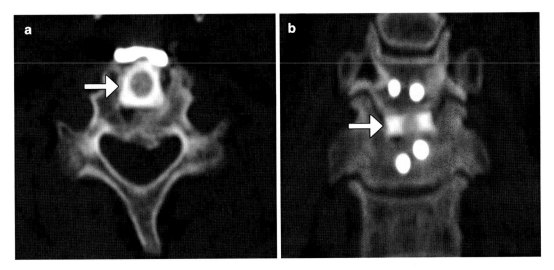

Fig. 11.63 Femoral ring allograft. Axial (**a**) and coronal (**b**) CT images show a cylindrical bone fragment inserted into the intervertebral disc space (*arrows*)

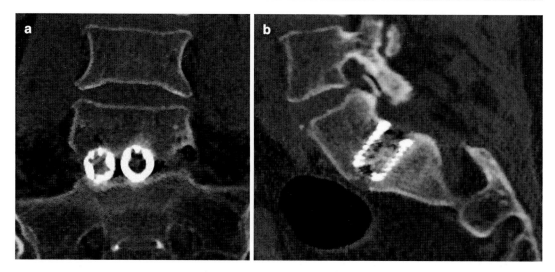

Fig. 11.64 Threaded cage. Sagittal (**a**) and coronal (**b**) CT images show two cylindrical hollow cages screwed into the intervertebral disc space

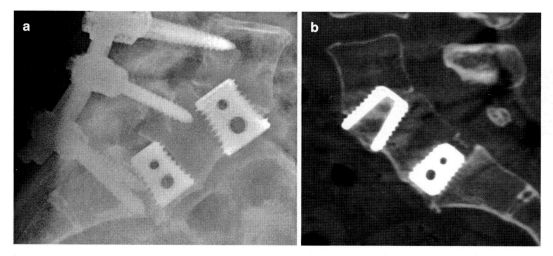

Fig. 11.65 Tapered LT-CAGE. Lateral radiograph (**a**) and sagittal CT image (**b**) show two metallic cages fitted into the intervertebral disc spaces. Mature bony fusion is most apparent on the CT

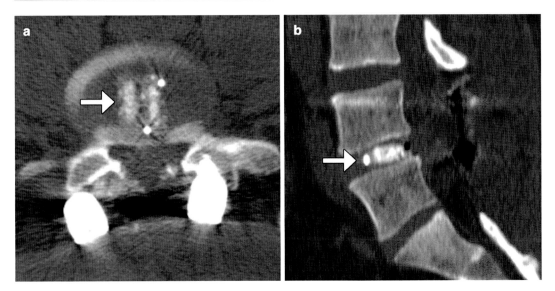

Fig. 11.66 PLIF. Axial (**a**) and sagittal CT (**b**) images show the radiolucent PEEK cage with metallic markers and filled with bone graft (*arrows*) in the midline of the intervertebral disc space. Laminectomy and posterior fusion hardware is also present

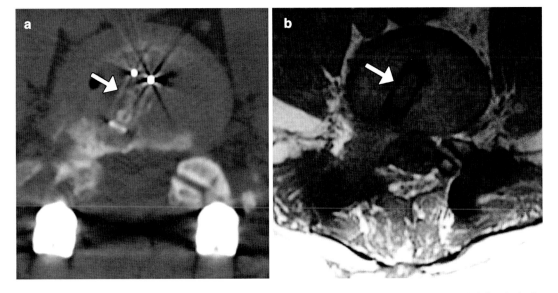

Fig. 11.67 TLIF. Axial CT (**a**) and axial T1-weighted (**b**) show the PEEK cage (*arrows*) positioned obliquely in the intervertebral space at nearly a 45° angle with respect to the sagittal plane

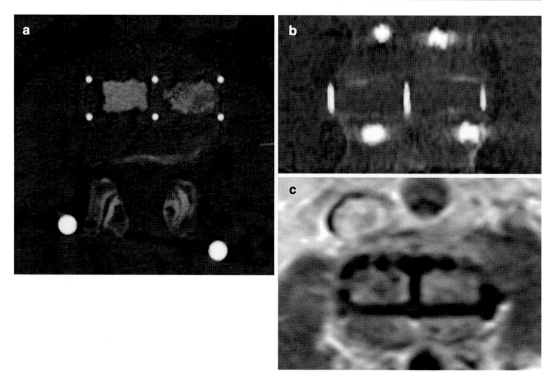

Fig. 11.68 XLIF. Axial (**a**) and coronal (**b**) CT images show the metallic markers of the XLIF device, which is positioned in the intervertebral space. There is bone graft material within the device. Axial T1-weighted (**c**) MRI shows the XLIF device as low signal intensity with a "figure of 8" shape

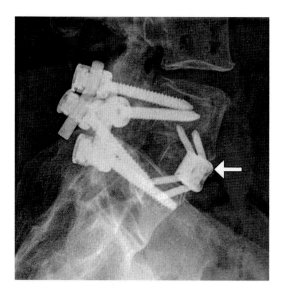

Fig. 11.69 ALIF. Lateral radiograph shows a Synfix device implanted in the L5–S1 anterior disc space (*arrow*). Posterior stabilization hardware is also present

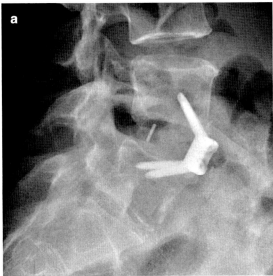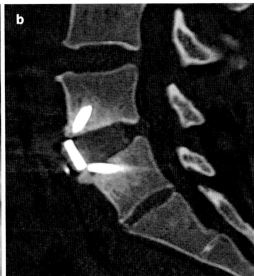

Fig. 11.70 Stalif. Frontal radiograph (**a**) and sagittal CT image (**b**) show that the device composed of both radiolucent and metallic parts, including titanium screws that enter the anterior vertebrae above and below. Note the absence of additional hardware. As such, the device "stands alone"

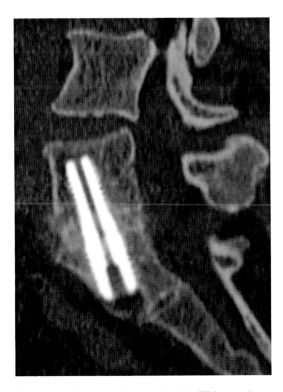

Fig. 11.71 Transsacral fusion. Sagittal CT image shows the vertically oriented axial lumbar interbody fusion hardware and mature bony bridging across the L5–S1 disc space

Table 11.2 Types of interbody fusion

Device	Description	Photographs of various types of interbody fusion devices
PLIF (posterior lumbar interbody fusion)	Consists of a posterior midline approach to the disc space. The interbody cage is inserted into the intervertebral disc space via a laminectomy or hemilaminectomy defect. As a result, the long axis of the device is typically positioned nearly parallel to the sagittal plane. Concurrent facetectomy is often performed	
TLIF (transforaminal lumbar interbody fusion)	Modification of the PLIF procedure, in which the interbody fusion prosthesis is more lateral. The long axis of the cage tends to be positioned obliquely (approximately 45°) with respect to the sagittal plane. This procedure can be performed via a midline approach as a PLIF or a minimally invasive approach with two paramedian incisions. Full facetectomy (unilateral or bilateral) is also performed. Fixed-size or expandable cages can be inserted into the disc space	
XLIF (extreme lateral interbody fusion; NuVasive, Inc., San Diego, CA)	Proprietary PEEK implant that is inserted laterally into the intervertebral space through a minimally invasive retroperitoneal approach. These implants have a characteristic of long, rectangular shape, designed to maximize surface area on which the epiphyseal ring can rest. There are also slots for packing bone graft. Other vendors endorse this approach and have different variations on the lateral cage	
OLIF (oblique lumbar interbody fusion; Medtronic, Minneapolis, MN)	A variant on the XLIF where the lateral spine is approached obliquely instead of orthogonally. The cages are placed in a similar fashion to the XLIF technique	
ALIF (anterior lumbar interbody fusion)	Consists of anterior discectomy and insertion of the interbody prosthesis via a retroperitoneal approach. The procedure can be performed with or without posterior stabilization. However, the addition of pedicle screw fixation with ALIF results in a significant increase in the rate of interbody fusion	
Stalif (stand-alone lumbar interbody fusion)	Can absorb energy, handle the normal weight of the body, and minimize stress on adjacent levels. Thus, the devices do not require additional fusion procedures, such as posterior pedicle screw and rod fixation	
AxiaLif (transsacral fusion)	Can be performed using the AxiaLif® system (TranS1, Inc., Wilmington, NC). Initially, a series of guide pins and dilator tubes are inserted under fluoroscopic guidance and used to obtain access to the L5–S1 disc space. Subsequently, a discectomy is performed percutaneously. Finally, a threaded titanium pin is placed across the disc space. This procedure is often combined with posterior fixation with facet or pedicle screws introduced through a minimally invasive technique	Photograph of AxiaLif device. (Courtesy of Quandary Medical)

11.4   Dynamic Stabilization Devices of the Spine

11.4.1 Total Disc Replacement

11.4.1.1   Discussion

Total disc replacement is an option for treating degenerative disc disease, in which motion at the operated level is preserved. In theory, this technique results in less load transfer to adjacent levels compared with fusion. Several types of disc replacement are available, including one-piece implants and implants with single- or double-gliding articulations with metal-on-metal or metal-on-polymer bearing surfaces (Figs. 11.72, 11.73, and 11.74). For example, the Charite® device is a three-part device consisting of two cobalt-chromium-molybdenum (CoCrMo) alloy endplates and a radiolucent ultra-high-molecular-weight polyethylene core. The radiolucent core is delineated by a small radiopaque metal wire. There are small "teeth" along the device endplates in an attempt to anchor the device in the vertebral endplates and limit migration. The endplates are coated with porous plasma-sprayed titanium and with calcium phosphate to promote bony ingrowth. ProDisc is also a three-part disc arthroplasty device with two metallic endplates and a radiolucent inlay that snaps onto the lower endplate to prevent extrusion. The device is secured in the adjacent vertebral bodies by ridged keels along both of the endplates (Fig. 11.75).

Migration of the disc prosthesis is not uncommon and usually occurs in the anterior direction (Fig. 11.76). Oversizing and positioning the prosthesis too far anteriorly in the disc space are risk factors for migration. Extrusion of the polyethylene inlay in the Charite device is a similar complication and can occur if the wire surrounding the core fractures in three-component prostheses. It is important to obtain cross-sectional imaging

for these complications in order to exclude impingement upon the adjacent great vessels.

Subsidence of total disc prostheses into the adjacent vertebral body occurs in about 3% of cases in the lumbar spine and can be asymptomatic or cause recurrence of pain. Risk factors include osteopenia, an oblique approach versus an anterior approach, removal of too much of the endplate, and the use of an undersized prosthesis. Total disc subsidence is most readily identified on lateral radiographs and sagittal or coronal CT reconstructions (Fig. 11.77).

The frequency of heterotopic ossification after total disc replacement ranges from 1.7% to 7.7%. Heterotopic ossification along the lateral aspect of the device often leads to ankylosis and limited range of motion, while the heterotopic bone anterior to the device is usually of no significance. Annular ossification can also occur, and this actually decreases the risk of device dislocation. On imaging, partial or complete bone formation across the disc space can be identified (Fig. 11.78).

Vertebral body fracture has been reported in less than 1% of cases with the Charite device and tends to involve the endplate (Fig. 11.79). In contrast, devices with a keel, such as ProDisc, are prone to the characteristic vertical split fractures. Short vertebral body heights predispose to fracture with these models. Prosthesis-associated fractures should be evaluated with CT to assess for spinal canal stenosis and associated findings, such as device migration.

Finally, it is important to consider disease at adjacent levels when patients present with pain following total disc replacement. Adjacent-level disc degeneration is perhaps the most common explanation in such situations. This outcome may result from increased stress on, or hypermobility of, adjacent segments. If nothing is apparent, MRI should be performed to evaluate the discs, although susceptibility effects from the hardware can degrade detail of the adjacent levels as well (Fig. 11.80).

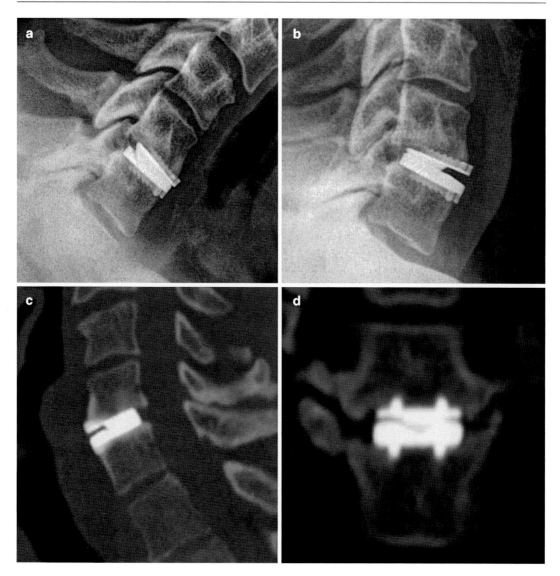

Fig. 11.72 Prestige cervical spine total disc prosthesis. Flexion (**a**) and extension (**b**) views of the cervical spine show the range of motion of the device. Sagittal (**c**) and coronal (**d**) CT images show the device positioned within the disc space, secured by two rows of corrugated keels

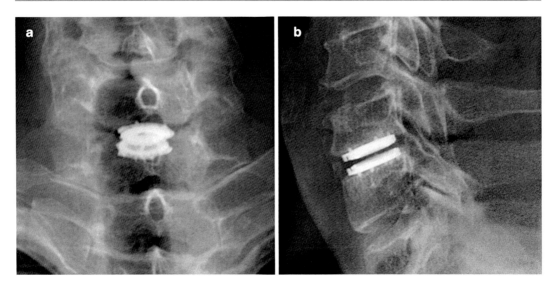

Fig. 11.73 Advent cervical spine total disc prosthesis. Frontal (**a**) and lateral (**b**) radiographs show the total disc replacement prosthesis in the lower cervical spine

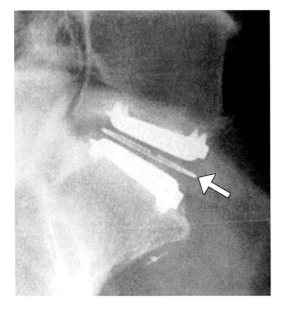

Fig. 11.74 Charite lumbar spine total disc prosthesis. Lateral radiograph shows the components, which comprises metallic endplates and a radiolucent polyethylene core and metallic wire ring (*arrow*)

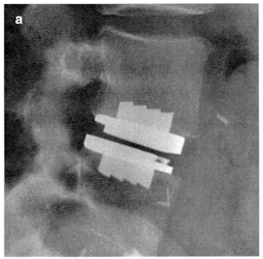

Fig. 11.75 ProDisc-L total disc prosthesis. Lateral view of the lumbar spine (**a**) demonstrates proper positioning of ProDisc-L, which features serrated keels perpendicular to the endplates. Photograph of ProDisc-L (**b**) (Courtesy of Synthes, West Chester, PA)

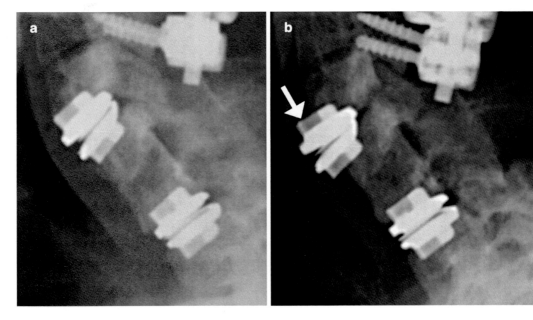

Fig. 11.76 Total disc prosthesis anterior migration. Initial postoperative lateral radiograph (**a**) shows satisfactory positioning of the C3–C4 total disc prosthesis. Lateral radiograph obtained at 4 postoperative months (**b**) shows interval anterior migration of the C3–C4 device (*arrow*)

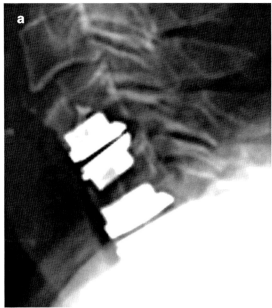

Fig. 11.77 Total disc prosthesis subsidence. Initial postoperative lateral radiograph (**a**) shows satisfactory positioning of the total disc prosthesis at C5–C6. Routine follow-up imaging at 6 weeks (**b**) shows that the superior endplate of the C5–C6 device has subsided into the inferior endplate of C5 (*arrow*)

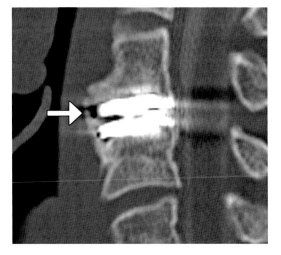

Fig. 11.78 Total disc prosthesis with heterotopic ossification and ankylosis. Sagittal CT image shows bone (*arrow*) spanning the disc space at the level of the prosthesis

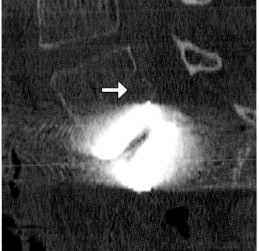

Fig. 11.79 Total disc replacement vertebral fracture. The patient presented to the emergency department with severe back pain. The patient underwent implantation of Charite® at L5–S1 about 6 months earlier. Sagittal CT image shows a small fracture involving the posterior-inferior corner of the L5 vertebral body (*arrow*)

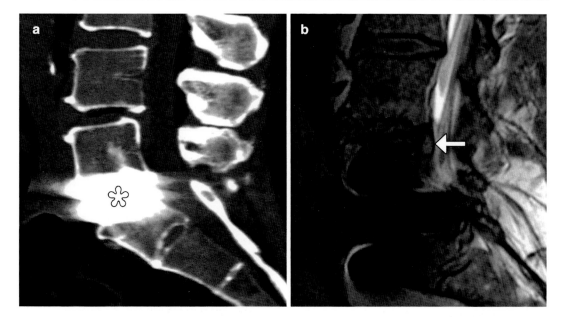

Fig. 11.80 Adjacent-level disc herniation after total disc replacement. The patient presented approximately 1 year after implantation of Charite® at the L5–S1 disc space level with persistent back pain. Sagittal CT image (**a**) shows degenerative disc disease at L4–L5 with vacuum disc phenomenon. The CT is otherwise limited at the level of the prosthesis due to the beam-hardening artifact from the device (*). However, axial sagittal T2-weighted MR image (**b**) shows a central and right subarticular recess disc extrusion resulting in right L5 nerve root compression (*arrow*) despite the susceptibility artifact from the hardware. This was new from an MRI of the lumbar spine obtained 6 months earlier

11.4.2 Nucleus Pulposus Replacement

11.4.2.1 Discussion

Nucleus pulposus (partial disc) replacement surgery is a minimally invasive technique that is indicated for younger patients with persistent disc herniation and prior discectomy. The two main types of nucleus replacement devices include elastomeric and mechanical nuclei. Elastomeric nuclei can be composed either of hydrogel or nonhydrogel materials and preformed or injectable. The mechanical nuclei can be either one- or two-piece.

The NUBAC is a mechanical two-piece nucleus pulposus replacement device that is composed of two endplates of PEEK-OPTIMA with an inner ball-and-socket articulation. The large contact area results in low subsidence risk. The device is radiolucent because of PEEK (polyether ether ketone), but has a characteristic of radiopaque makers (Fig. 11.81).

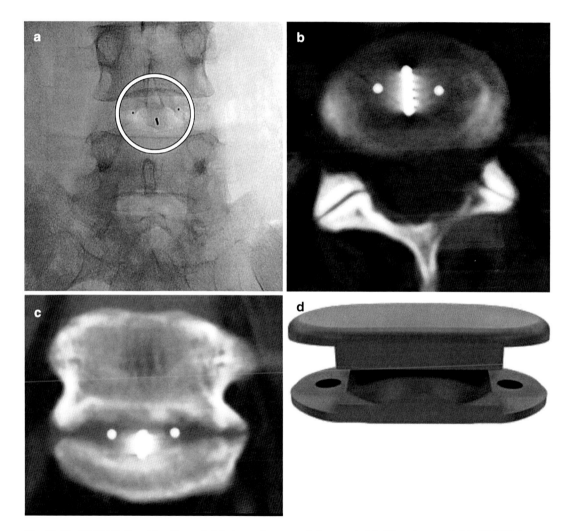

Fig. 11.81 NUBAC. Frontal radiograph (**a**) shows three radiopaque markers from the nucleus pulposus in the L4–L5 disc space (*encircled*). The remainder of the device is radiolucent. Axial (**b**) and coronal (**c**) CT MIP images show the device centered within the disc space. Photograph of NUBAC (**d**)

11.4.3 Posterior Dynamic Stabilization Devices

11.4.3.1 Discussion

Interspinous spacers are designed for minimally invasive treatment of neurogenic claudication. In this condition, symptoms like radicular pain, sensation disturbance, and loss of strength in the legs are relieved with flexion, presumably by decreasing epidural pressure and increasing the cross-sectional area of the spinal canal. The devices are typically placed into the interspinous space at the affected level. The implantation is less invasive than spinal fusion procedures, leaves the ALL and PLL intact, and does not preclude removal and additional spinal surgery.

Various designs for interspinous spacers are commercially available, including the Isobar, X-Stop, DIAM, and coflex, among others.

The Isobar incorporates radiopaque metallic posterior pedicle screws with limited motion provided by either a mobile screw head or mobile rods (Fig. 11.82). The mobile portion of this particular device consists of a stack of metal rings that allow for flexion and extension and a dampener that allows for limited axial loading. The dampener and rings are contained in a bell-shaped structure on the rod.

The X-Stop has an H-shaped configuration consisting of two metal plates positioned lateral to the spinous processes (Fig. 11.83). The interspinous ligament is conserved in order for this device to be effective.

The DIAM (device for intervertebral assisted motion) spinal stabilization system consists of a silicone core covered by a polyester sleeve. Three mesh bands hold the core in place. Two of the bands encircle the adjacent spinous processes, while a third encases the supraspinous ligament. The silicone device and bands are radiolucent, but radiopaque markers are placed along the superior-lateral aspect of the device (Fig. 11.84). As with other interspinous devices, loss of correction ensues over time, although this does not appear to affect clinical outcome.

The coflex is a saddle-shaped device composed of titanium that requires resection of the interspinous and supraspinous ligaments (Fig. 11.85). The wings are crimped onto the adjacent spinous processes. This device is inserted in conjunction with the central laminectomy.

Reported complications specific to interspinous prosthesis implantation include overcorrection, spinous process fractures (Fig. 11.86), and device dislocation (Fig. 11.87). These complications are not very common and may be predisposed by underlying anatomic variations.

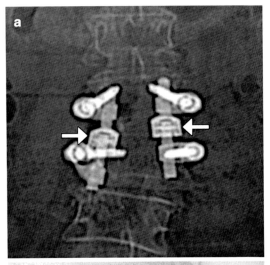

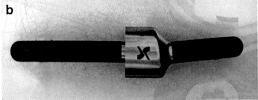

Fig. 11.82 Isobar. Frontal scout image (**a**) shows bilateral Isobar rods with mobile joints (*arrows*). Photograph of the Isobar (**b**) (Courtesy of Alphatec Spine, Carlsbad, CA, USA)

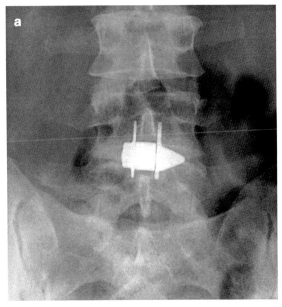

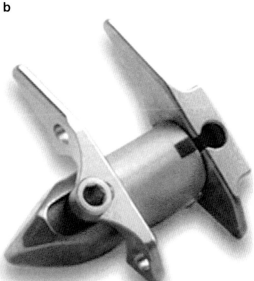

Fig. 11.83 X-Stop. Frontal radiograph (**a**) shows an X-Stop device in position L4–L5, which appears as H-shaped metallic hardware interposed between the spinous processes. Photograph X-Stop (**b**) (Courtesy of Medtronic Sofamor Danek USA)

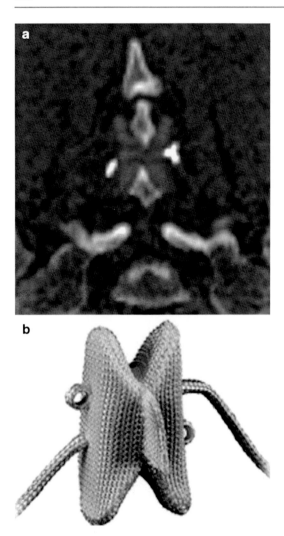

Fig. 11.84 DIAM. Coronal CT image (**a**) shows the DIAM interspinous spacer device with bilateral high attenuation markers on the sides. Photograph of the DIAM device (**b**) (Courtesy of Medtronic Sofamor Danek USA)

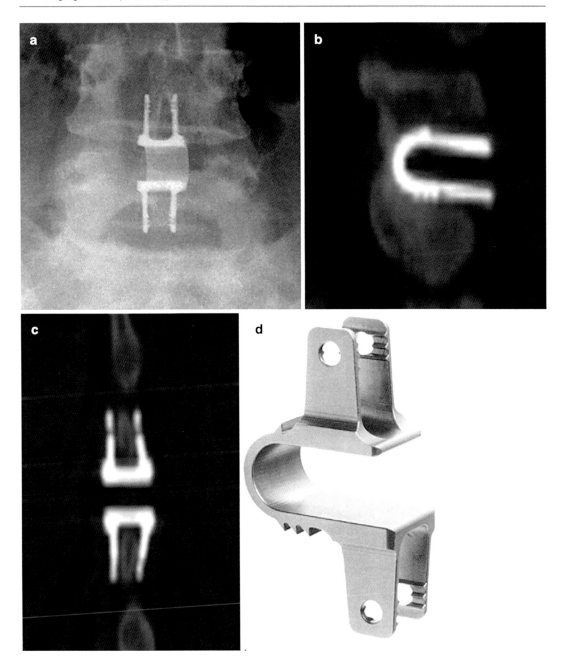

Fig. 11.85 Coflex. Frontal (**a**) radiograph and coronal (**b**) and sagittal (**c**) CT images show a coflex device positioned in the interspinous space. Photograph of Coflex (**d**) (Courtesy of Paradigm Spine, New York, NY)

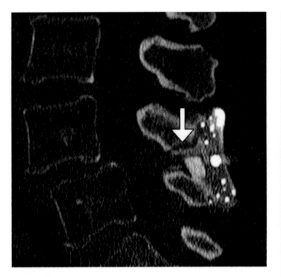

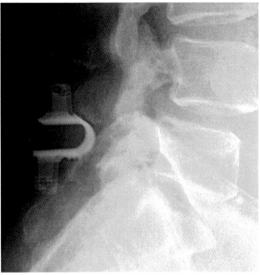

Fig. 11.86 Periprosthetic fracture. Sagittal CT image shows lucency (*arrow*) in the spinous process to which the interspinous prosthesis is attached. The bones are diffusely osteopenic and there is anterolisthesis at the operated level

Fig. 11.87 Dislocated device. Lateral radiograph shows disengagement of the device from the interspinous space into the soft tissues posterior to the spinous processes

11.4.4 Dynamic Facet Replacement

11.4.4.1 Discussion

Facet replacement devices have been created in an attempt to replace only the diseased elements in patients with facet arthropathy and spinal stenosis while maintaining normal or near-normal biomechanics of the spine. The total posterior facet replacement and dynamic motion segment stabilization system (TOPS) includes two titanium endplates on either side of a layer of radiolucent, compressible polycarbonate urethane. This polycarbonate acts as a shock absorber and allows for motion between the endplates, providing rotation, bending, flexion, and extension to the patient. The device is held in place by pedicle screws. On imaging, the screws and plates are radiopaque, and the central polycarbonate urethane layer is radiolucent (Fig. 11.88). Other devices used for facet replacement include TFAS (Total Facet Arthroplasty System) and Zyre.

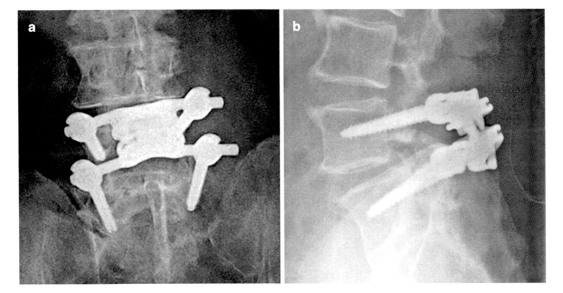

Fig. 11.88 Dynamic facet replacement device. Frontal (**a**) and lateral (**b**) radiographs show total posterior facet replacement and dynamic motion segment stabilization system at L4–L5

11.4.5 Dynamic Rods

11.4.5.1 Discussion

Dynamic posterior stabilization with pedicle fixation, such as Dynesys, consists of a semirigid fixation system that allows minimal movement between two segmental pedicle screws compared to a rigid metal rod and is used to treat lumbar spinal stenosis and degenerative spondylosis. Dynesys comprises and employs two titanium

pedicle screws at each treated level. The screws at adjacent levels are connected by rods comprised of radiolucent polyethylene terephthalate cord surrounded by a polycarbonate urethane spacer, which appears as a two concentric rings, slightly more hyperattenuating centrally (Fig. 11.89). Complications include screw loosening, screw breakage, and degeneration in the adjacent levels in up to approximately 50% of cases.

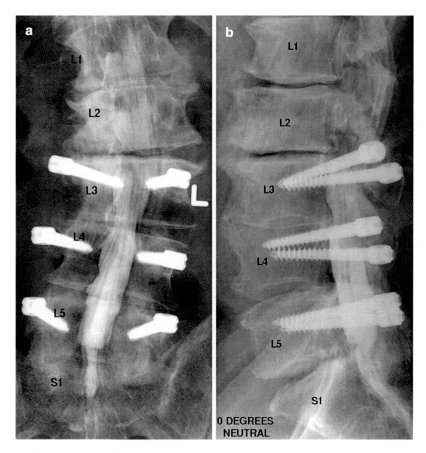

Fig. 11.89 Dynesys. Frontal (**a**) and lateral (**b**) radiographs show bilateral metallic pedicle screws at L3–L5, which are secured to radiolucent rods. Axial (**c**) and sagittal (**d**) CT myelogram images show the bilateral rods (*arrows*), which are nearly iso-attenuating to the sur-

rounding soft tissues, but slightly higher attenuation centrally, corresponding to the polyethylene terephthalate cord. Photograph of Dynesys Dynamic Stabilization System (**e**) (Courtesy of Zimmer Spine, Minneapolis, MN)

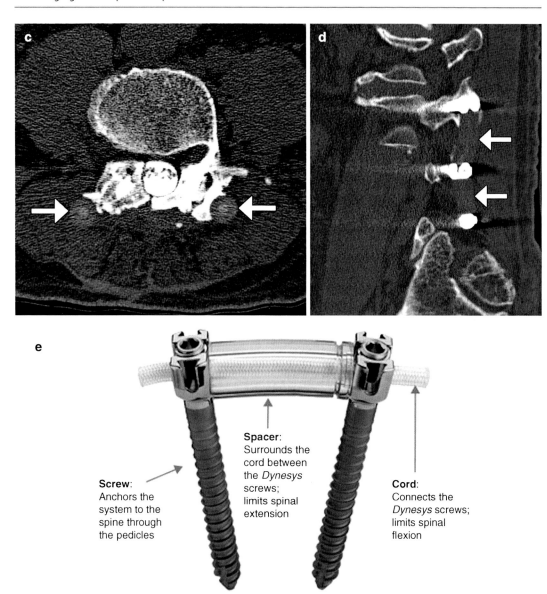

Screw:
Anchors the
system to the
spine through
the pedicles

Spacer:
Surrounds the
cord between
the *Dynesys*
screws;
limits spinal
extension

Cord:
Connects the
Dynesys screws;
limits spinal
flexion

Fig. 11.89 (continued)

11.5   Failed Back Surgery Syndrome and Related Spine Surgery Complications

11.5.1 Overview

Failed back surgery syndrome (FBSS) is a clinical entity that describes the persistence of lumbosacral pain following surgical intervention. Etiologies include structural abnormalities in the back, psychosocial influences, or a combination of these. Imaging plays an important role in eval-uating patients with FBSS. In particular, a comprehensive and systematic assessment of the postoperative spine includes a review of the neural and vascular structures, including the neural foramina, thecal sac, spinal cord and cauda equina, hardware, and adjacent structures such as the major abdominal vessels, psoas musculature, posterior mediastinum, and prevertebral soft tissues. Some of the causes of FBSS and related complications of spine surgery in general that can be identified on imaging are summarized in Fig. 11.90 and in the following sections.

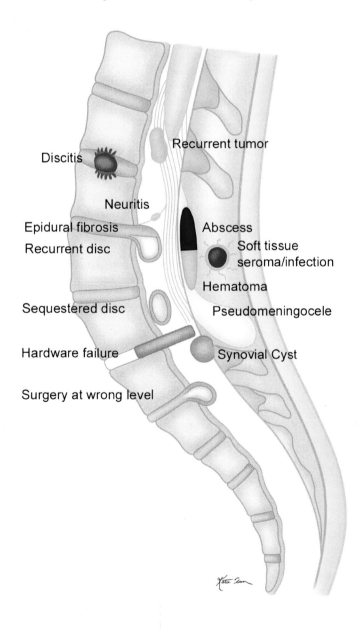

Fig. 11.90 Schematic of some of the potential causes of failed back surgery

11.5.2 Hardware Malpositioning and Migration

11.5.2.1 Discussion

The incidence of malpositioned pedicle screws ranges from 4% to 16%. Medial malpositioning of the screw can result in spinal cord or nerve root injury, while screws that extend too far beyond the vertebral body can injure the great vessels (Figs. 11.49 and 11.91). However, clinically significant sequelae of screw malpositioning, such as dissection, rupture, or pseudoaneurysm formation, are rare. CT with multiplanar reformats is useful for initial evaluation of screw position. CTA can be used to evaluate for significant vascular injury, and MRI or CT myelogram can help assess for nerve root compression.

Postoperative spinal hardware displacement can be a significant complications that can produce pain and new neurological symptoms. Retropulsion of interbody fusion devices and grafts most commonly occurs at L5–S1 and is associated with a wide disc space and multilevel fusion surgery. However, these devices can also become displaced anteriorly, especially if there has been a disruption of the anterior longitudinal ligament. Radiographs or CT can often adequately demonstrate the displacement of these materials into the spinal canal (Fig. 11.92).

Spinal rods can potentially become dissociated from the screws and migrate out of position. The rods have been reported to migrate into the spinal canal, retroperitoneum, and lower extremities. Radiographs can be used to screen for rod displacement (Fig. 11.93).

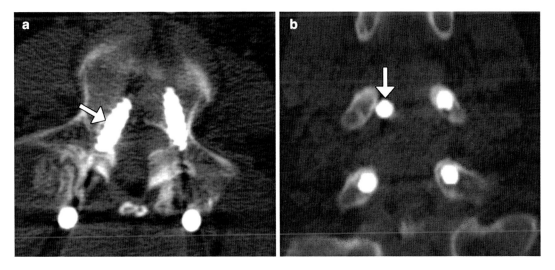

Fig. 11.91 Malpositioned screw. Axial (**a**) and coronal (**b**) CT images show the right pedicle screw (*arrows*) positioned too far medially, penetrating the spinal canal

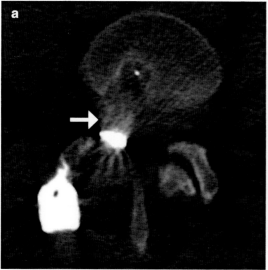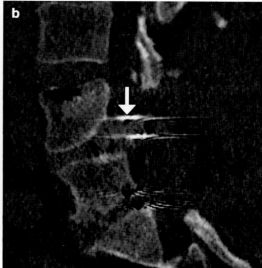

Fig. 11.92 Interbody fusion device retropulsion. The patient is status post anterior-posterior lumbar fusion arthrodesis at L4–L5 and L5–S1 with placement of bio-mechanical prosthetic interbody fusion device (Pioneer bullet-tip). Axial (**a**) and sagittal (**b**) images of the lumbar spine show retropulsion of the interbody box prosthesis into the spinal canal (*arrow*)

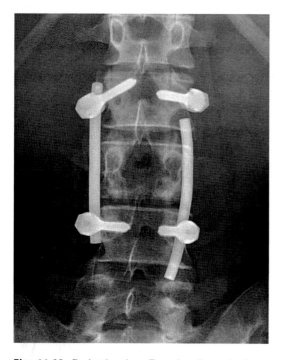

Fig. 11.93 Rod migration. Frontal radiograph shows inferior translation of the left posterior fusion rod, leaving a gap between the superior end of the rod and the superior pedicle screw

11.5.3 Hardware Loosening and Pseudarthrosis

11.5.3.1 Discussion

Spine hardware loosening is a fairly frequent finding on imaging, occurring in nearly 20% of patients and 5% of pedicle screws. Iliac screws followed by sacral screws are most commonly affected, perhaps related to torque. Loosening appears as a gap between the hardware and the bone greater than 2 mm (Fig. 11.94). Although loosening can be related to the presence of particulate debris activates phagocytes that release enzymes that result in osteolysis, it can be also a sign of underlying hardware infection. Furthermore, there can be associated pseudarthrosis (Fig. 11.95), which can be suggested by the following imaging findings:

1. Low to intermediate signal intensity defect between vertebral bodies or bone graft on T1-weighted MRI or lucency surrounding the fusion area on radiographs or CT
2. Progressive spondylolisthesis
3. Bone graft migration
4. Broken screws or lucency surrounding hardware
5. Bone graft resorption
6. Motion between flexion and extension radiographs

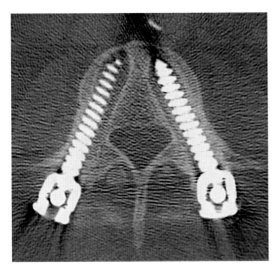

Fig. 11.94 Loosening. Axial CT image shows lucency surrounding the bilateral screws

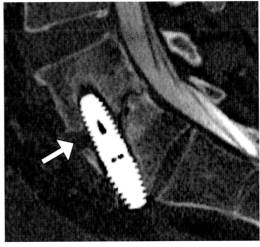

Fig. 11.95 Transsacral interbody fusion loosening and pseudarthrosis. Sagittal CT cisternogram image shows lucency surrounding the device and across the previously fused disc space (*arrow*)

11.5.4 Hardware and Periprosthetic Fractures

11.5.4.1 Discussion

Pedicle screw fracture has an incidence of 0.5–2.5%. CT can readily demonstrate hardware fracture, particularly if there is displacement (Fig. 11.96). The presence of a broken screw is strongly associated with loosening and pseudarthrosis, which should be sought on imaging. In addition, hardware can alter the stresses on the surrounding bone and predispose to fractures. The pedicle is a common location for hardware-related fracture (Fig. 11.97).

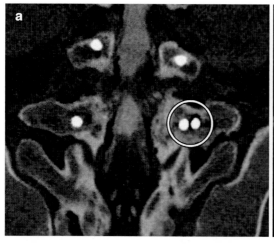
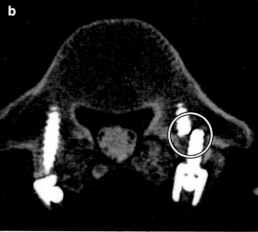

Fig. 11.96 Screw fracture. The patient has a history of three prior lumbar spine surgeries and presents with mechanical back pain. Axial (**a**) and coronal (**b**) CT myelogram images show a displaced fracture (*encircled*) of the left L5 pedicle screw

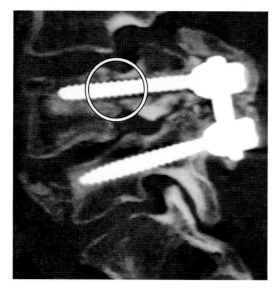

Fig. 11.97 Periprosthetic fracture. Sagittal CT image shows a lucency that traverses the left pedicle surrounding the screw (*encircled*)

11.5.5 Cerebrospinal Fluid Leak

11.5.5.1   Discussion

Cerebrospinal fluid leakage occurs in about 2% of patients after spine surgery and results from dural and arachnoid defects, allowing cerebrospinal fluid to escape the thecal sac and infiltrate the paraspinal surgical bed. In particular, pseudomeningoceles represent a form of cerebrospinal fluid leak contained by a capsule of fibrous tissue and have been reported to occur in over 5% of discectomy cases (Fig. 11.98). Nerve roots can herniate into and become entrapped within pseudomeningoceles. Thus, patients typically present with orthostatic hypotension, but may also have associated focal neurological deficits. Imaging options for cerebrospinal fluid leakage after spine surgery include conventional MRI to delineate the presence of the fluid collections, although the exam can be limited by surgical hardware artifacts and there is a differential diagnosis for the extradural fluid, including abscess and seroma/hematoma. Secondary findings that might be present on post-contrast images related to spinal hypotension include dilatation of the epidural venous plexus and diffuse dural thickening and enhancement. CT or MR myelography can provide a dynamic assessment that can help confirm the presence and site of cerebrospinal fluid leakage with high accuracy. Nuclear medicine spinal cisternograms are most suitable for detecting slow, intermittent leaks.

The diagnosis and localization of cerebrospinal fluid leak and pseudomeningoceles can be elusive. A variety of imaging techniques are available to evaluate the site of leakage, including MRI/MR myelography and CT myelography. MRI in spinal cerebrospinal fluid leak syndrome usually reveals cerebrospinal fluid signal intensity extradural fluid collections, spinal meningeal enhancement, and dilation of the epidural venous plexus. However, the actual site of cerebrospinal fluid leak is often not detectable with MRI. On the other hand, CT myelography can provide evidence delineate meningeal defects, the location of extradural collections, and their relationship to bony structures. However, CT myelography results in radiation exposure and it is a slightly invasive procedure.

Initial management of cerebrospinal fluid leak consists of cerebrospinal fluid diversion and epidural blood patch. If the leak or pseudomeningocele persists, dural repair and even flap reconstruction may be warranted.

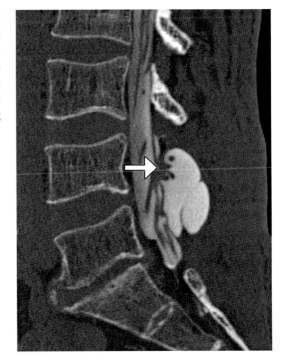

Fig. 11.98 Pseudomeningocele. Sagittal CT myelogram image shows a collection containing contrast material and herniated nerve roots (*arrow*)

11.5.6 Postoperative Seromas and Hematomas

11.5.6.1 Discussion

Aseptic fluid collections are commonly found on early postoperative imaging along the surgical approach after spine operations, including seromas and hematomas. Seromas consists of plasma from disrupted vessels and inflammation from injured soft tissues. There is an increased incidence of sterile seromas and painful edema in the lumbar region after posterolateral fusion with rhBMP-2. Seromas typically appear as simple fluid collections on imaging (Fig. 11.99).

Postoperative spinal epidural hematomas are clinically significant in up to 1% of cases, attrib-utable to mass effect upon the spinal cord or nerve roots. The majority of postoperative spinal hematomas occur at the operated level and rarely at a remote site. Prompt diagnosis and decompression of symptomatic epidural hematomas is important for averting an adverse outcome. Imaging diagnosis and assessment of the extent of spinal canal stenosis can be made via CT myelography or MRI. On MRI, epidural hematomas can be heterogeneous with a marbled appearance and of variable signal depending on the age of the hematoma. For example, hyperacute hematomas tend to have intermediate signal on T1 and bright on T2-weighted sequences (Fig. 11.100).

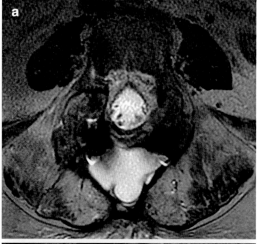

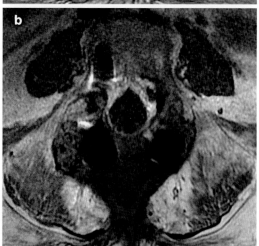

Fig. 11.99 Seroma. Axial T2-weighted (**a**) and T1-weighted (**b**) MR images show a simple fluid collection in the posterior paraspinal soft tissue surgical bed

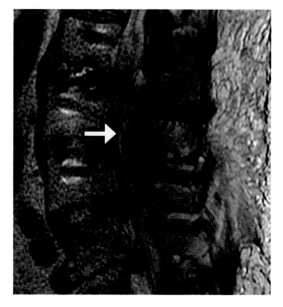

Fig. 11.100 Epidural hematoma. The patient underwent laminectomy and developed new lower extremity deficits caused by a large epidural hematoma confirmed on emergent decompression. Sagittal T2-weighted MRI shows a posterior epidural fluid collection (*arrow*) that severely narrows the spinal canal in conjunction with underlying degenerative disease

11.5.7 Surgical Site Infections

11.5.7.1 Discussion

Infection related to spine surgery has an overall incidence of 1.9% and is defined as occurring within 30 days of surgery or within 12 months of placement of foreign bodies and can be categorized by the depth of surgical tissue involvement, including superficial, deep incisional, or organ and surrounding space. *Staphylococcus aureus* is the most common causative organism. MRI with contrast is generally the modality of choice for evaluating postoperative infections. Rim-enhancing fluid collections, bony erosions and enhancing, and paraspinal inflammation are suggestive of infection (Figs. 11.101 and 11.102). Hardware removal is often necessary in cases of postoperative spine infection (Fig. 11.103). Other than removing old hardware and washout, antibiotic-impregnated methyl methacrylate beads are sometimes left in the surgical cavity for direct site treatment (Fig. 11.104).

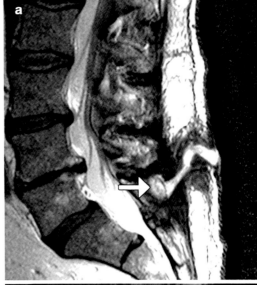

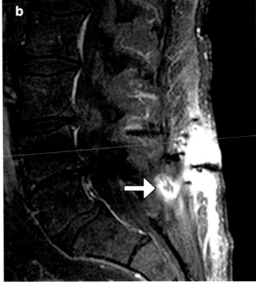

Fig. 11.102 Wound infection. Sagittal (**a**) T2-weighted and post-contrast fat-suppressed T1-weighted (**b**) MR images show a fluid collection (*arrows*) with surrounding enhancement and a draining sinus to the overlying skin in the posterior paraspinal soft tissues along the surgical approach following minimally invasive microdiscectomy

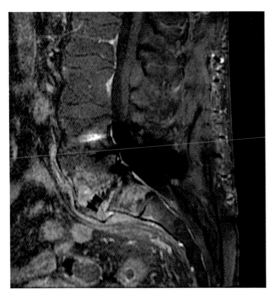

Fig. 11.101 Discitis-osteomyelitis. Sagittal post-contrast T1-weighted MRI shows enhancement in the vertebral bone marrow and prevertebral soft tissues at L5–S1 surrounding the intervertebral disc prosthesis

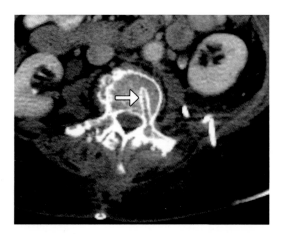

Fig. 11.103 Hardware removal and abscess drainage. Axial CT shows the site of pedicle screw removal (*arrow*) and paraspinal muscle abscess with drainage catheter from hardware infection

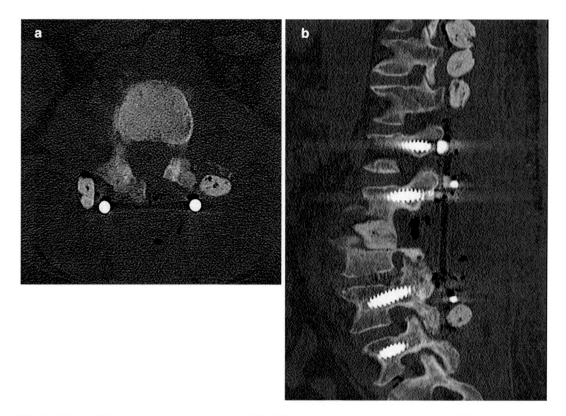

Fig. 11.104 Antibiotic beads. Axial (**a**) and sagittal (**b**) CT images show the hyperattenuating antibiotic-impregnated methyl methacrylate beads at multiple levels adjacent to the surgical hardware

11.5.8 Postoperative Neuritis

11.5.8.1 Discussion

Aseptic inflammatory neuritis can occur following lumbar spine surgery due to mechanical factors, such as compression, stretching, contusion, or transection. Diagnostic imaging is useful for excluding a mechanical etiology, such as impingement by screws or disc material. Furthermore, MRI may demonstrate enhancement of the nerve roots (Fig. 11.105). This finding has a 94% positive predictive value for residual or recurrent clinical symptoms. Furthermore, there may be an association between nerve root changes, postoperative epidural fibrosis, and the development of sciatica.

11.5.9 Arachnoiditis

11.5.9.1 Discussion

Postoperative arachnoiditis is an inflammatory process affecting the nerve roots that may be associated with anesthetics, chemotherapy, certain contrast agents, intradural hemorrhage, substances released from the intervertebral discs, the surgery itself, and infection. This condition produces symptoms in 6–16% of spine surgery cases. Three imaging patterns of arachnoiditis have been described, which can be well delineated on MRI:

1. "Empty sac" appearance in which the nerve roots are peripherally distributed (Fig. 11.106)
2. "Clumped" nerve roots centrally within the dural sac
3. "Mass" comprised of the dural-based aggregated nerve roots

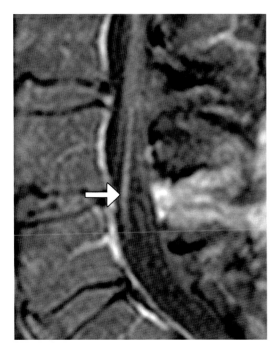

Fig. 11.105 Neuritis. The patient presented with left lower extremity weakness after surgery. Sagittal postcontrast T1-weighted MRI shows cauda equina nerve root enhancement (*arrow*)

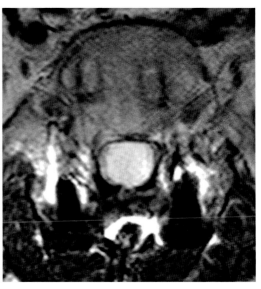

Fig. 11.106 Arachnoiditis with "empty sac" sign. Axial T2-weighted MRI shows that the cauda equina nerve roots are adherent to the margins of the thecal sac. Laminectomy posterior fusion and interbody fusion were performed

The presence and degree of contrast enhancement is variable for any of these patterns of arachnoiditis. A rare form of arachnoiditis is arachnoiditis ossificans, which is characterized by calcified plaques or ossification forms along the leptomeninges. On MRI, arachnoiditis ossificans appears as linear or mass-like intrathecal lesions that have high signal on T1-weighted sequences and variable signal on T2-weighted sequences. CT with multiplanar reformats is helpful for confirming the presence of arachnoiditis ossificans, which shows linear bone attenuation structures along the nerve roots (Fig. 11.107).

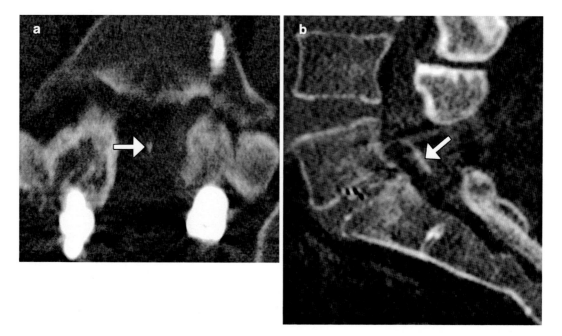

Fig. 11.107 Arachnoiditis ossificans. Axial (**a**) and sagittal (**b**) CT images show linear intrathecal calcification/ossification (*arrows*). There is evidence of prior laminectomy at the same level

11.5.10 Residual/Recurrent Disc Material Versus Epidural Scar

11.5.10.1 Discussion

Both postoperative epidural fibrosis (scar) and residual or recurrent disc material are rather common occurrences that can produce symptoms. Both disc material and epidural fibrosis can be hypo- or isointense on T1-weighted sequences and hyperintense on T2-weighted sequences relative to the annulus. However, scar enhances early and diffusely after contrast administration on MRI (Fig. 11.108). Scar can also encase and retract the thecal sac and nerve roots. On the other hand, disc material enhances peripherally but can fill with contrast on delayed imaging and tends to displace or compress the nerve roots or thecal sac (Fig. 11.109). The size of the scar decreases or remains the same after 6 months in the majority of cases. Similarly, residual disc material can also involute over time. MRI has an accuracy of 96–100% for differentiating between scar and disc.

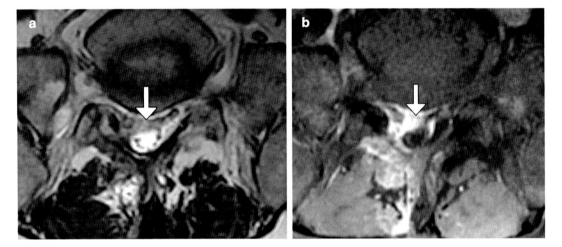

Fig. 11.108 Epidural fibrosis. Axial T2-weighted (**a**) and post-contrast T1-weighted (**b**) MR images show homogeneously enhancing soft tissue surrounding the right L5 nerve root (*arrow*)

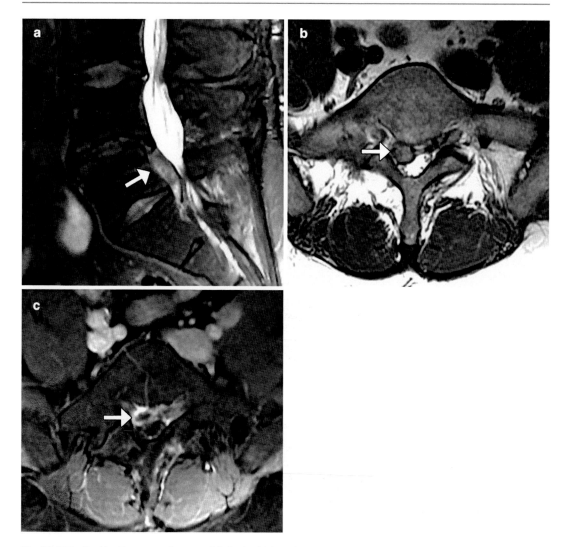

Fig. 11.109 Residual/recurrent disc material. Sagittal (**a**) and axial (**b**) T2-weighted MR images show a sequestered disc fragment that compresses the thecal sac at the level of the L5 vertebral body (*arrows*). Post-contrast fat-suppressed T1-weighted MRI (**c**) show enhancement surrounding the disc fragment (*arrow*)

11.5.11   Postoperative Synovial Cyst

11.5.11.1   Discussion

Synovial (juxtafacet) cysts are responsible for about 1% of cases of failed back surgery syndrome. These can form as a consequence of altered biomechanics on the facet joints and may also be predisposed by disruption of the facet capsule. Patients tend to present with ipsilateral leg pain that may or may not be accompanied by back pain. MRI can readily demonstrate synovial cysts and the associated mass effect (Fig. 11.110). These lesions are contiguous with the facet joint, and their contents generally follow fluid signal, although these may contain hemorrhage and solid components. Peripheral enhancement can also be observed. Cyst puncture and aspiration can provide symptomatic relief.

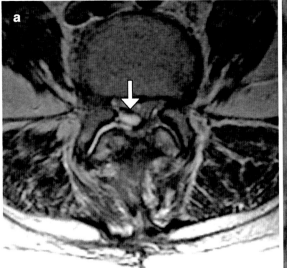
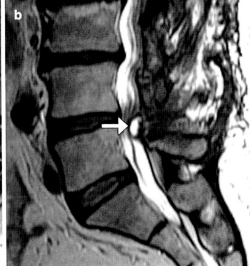

Fig. 11.110 Postoperative de novo synovial cyst. The patient underwent L3 and L4 laminectomy for decompression 6 months prior. There was no synovial cyst prior to surgery, and the patient initially did well after surgery, but a few months after, the patient began to develop back and right leg pain. Axial (**a**) and sagittal (**b**) T2-weighted MR images show a juxtafacet cyst (*arrows*) arising from the right L4–L5 facet joint, where there is an effusion and compression of the adjacent nerve roots

11.5.12   Residual/Recurrent Tumors

11.5.12.1   Discussion

The risk of residual or recurrent spinal tumor depends largely on the type of tumor and treatment. In general, postoperative imaging evaluation should cover the entire length of the surgical approach, since recurrence can occur anywhere along this path, especially at the original tumor margins. Gross total resection is often feasible for schwannomas, meningiomas, paragangliomas, myxopapillary ependymomas, ependymomas, and hemangioblastomas. Although astrocytomas are typically infiltrative neoplasms, radical resection can result in long progression-free survival. Nevertheless, follow-up imaging is often performed to monitor for residual/recurrent tumor. MRI with contrast is generally the modality of choice for evaluating residual/recurrent spinal tumor (Fig. 11.111). Initial postoperative changes with enhancement can sometimes mimic residual tumors. Follow-up MRI can help differentiate between these two processes, whereby residual tumor may persist and even grow. Comparison with prior imaging is also very useful. It is important to image along the entire length of the surgical approach for assessment of tumor recurrence, which may include the abdomen or chest if an anterior approach has been implemented.

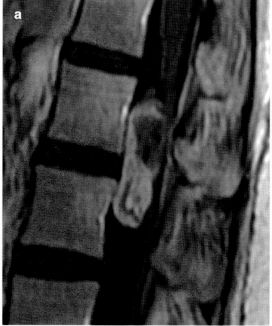 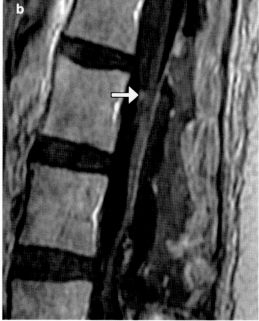

Fig. 11.111 Residual tumor. The patient has a history of conus medullaris schwannoma resected via a posterior approach. Preoperative sagittal post-contrast T1-weighted MRI (**a**) shows a heterogeneously enhancing mass that involves the proximal cauda equina. Postoperative sagittal post-contrast T1-weighted MRI (**b**) obtained 1 week after surgery shows a tiny focus of enhancement adjacent to the conus medullaris (*arrow*). Sagittal post-contrast T1-weighted MRI obtained 6 months later (**c**) shows interval increase in size of the enhancing nodule adjacent to the conus medullaris (*arrow*), but resolution of the cauda equina nerve root enhancement

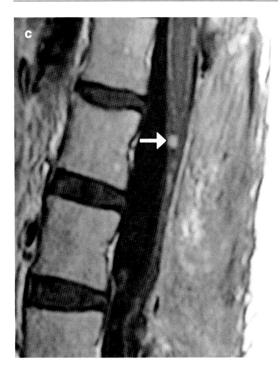

11.5.13 Inclusion Cysts

11.5.13.1 Discussion

Cutaneously derived inclusion cysts or epidermoids can occasionally form within the spinal canal and cause pain and neurological deficits following a spine procedure. Most cases have been reported following myelomeningocele repair, although this complication can presumably result from any other procedure, including lumbar punctures, in which fragments of skin are introduced into the spinal canal. The cysts can grow and exert mass effect upon the nerve roots. MRI typically reveals low T1 and high T2 signal (Fig. 11.112). The presence of high signal on diffusion-weighted imaging can be helpful in distinguishing epidermoid from arachnoid cyst.

Fig. 11.111 (continued)

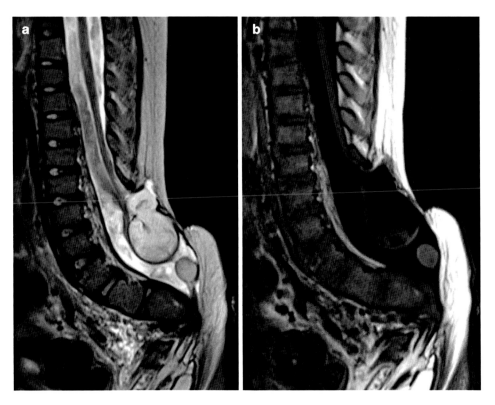

Fig. 11.112 Inclusion cysts. The patient has a history of prior myelomeningocele repair and presents with a lump at the surgical site. Sagittal T2-weighted (**a**) and T1-weighted (**b**) MR images show two well-defined, ovoid cystic masses in the posterior spinal canal at the site of prior myelomeningocele repair. Sagittal DWI (**c**) and ADC map (**d**) show that the lesions display restricted diffusion

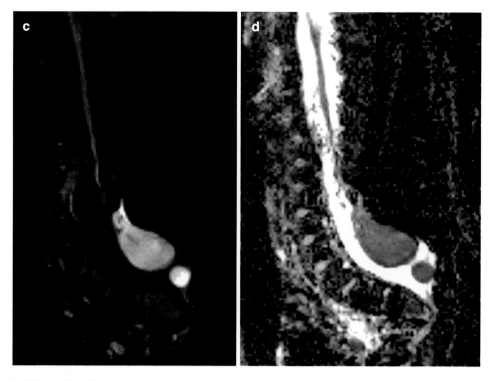

Fig. 11.112 (continued)

11.5.14   Retained Bone Fragments and New Bone Formation

11.5.14.1   Discussion
Residual bone fragments after spine surgery can migrate and impinge upon neural structures. The bony fragments are readily depicted on CT (Fig. 11.113). Facet and pedicle fractures after laminectomy can produce similar findings. Alternatively, bone can regrow after surgery and cause stenosis.

11.5.15   Retained Surgical Tools

11.5.15.1   Discussion
Various tools are used during spine surgery. In particular, drilling procedures are commonly performed during spine surgeries, which involve the use of drill bits. Rarely, the drill bits can break and become retained or even migrate. The small-diameter bits are more likely to break during surgery. Small retained drill bit fragments can initially go unnoticed, although patients may present with recurrent or new symptoms after surgery. CT is the modality of choice for evaluating possible retained drill bit fragments, which appear as linear metallic attenuation structures on CT (Fig. 11.114).

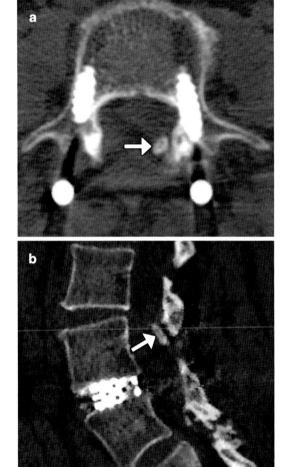

Fig. 11.113 Retained bone fragment. Axial (**a**) and sagittal (**b**) CT images demonstrate sequela of prior lumbar laminectomy and a portion of retained lamina within the spinal canal (*arrows*). There is also an interbody fusion cage at L4–L5

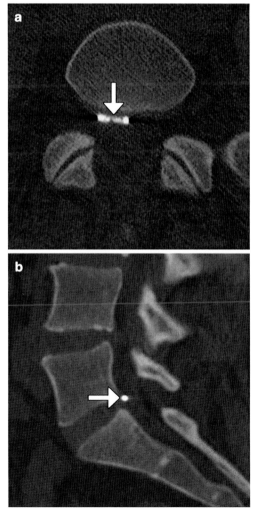

Fig. 11.114 Broken drill bit fragment. Axial (**a**) and sagittal (**b**) CT images show a cylindrical metallic object (*arrows*) posterior to the L5–S1 disc

11.5.16   Gossypiboma

11.5.16.1   Discussion

Retained surgical sponges can form gossypibomas, which are masses of cotton surrounded
by foreign-body reaction. These are uncommon

after spine surgery. Most gossypibomas reside in
the paraspinal soft tissues in the vicinity of the
surgical site (Fig. 11.115). These usually range in
size from 3.5 to 5.0 cm. Patients often present
with nonspecific back pain. On MRI, gossypibomas characteristically display hyperintense

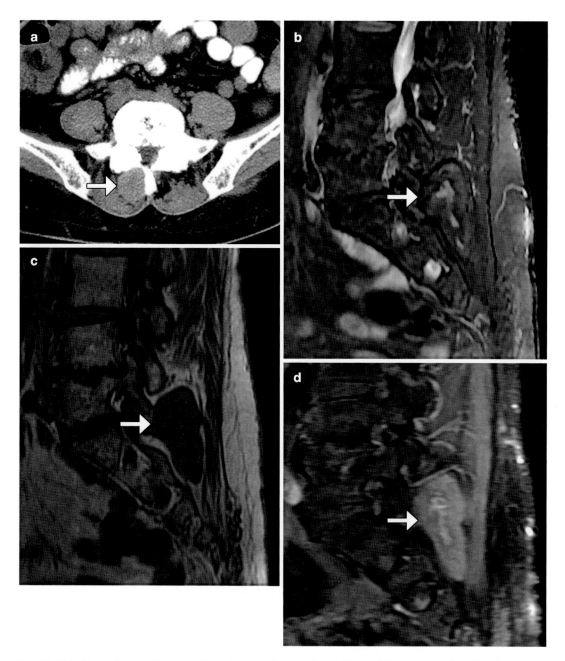

Fig. 11.115 Gossypiboma. The patient has a history of
spine surgery for lumbar stenosis many years prior in an
underdeveloped country. Axial CT (**a**) shows well-defined
right paravertebral mass (*arrow*). No radiopaque marker
was found. Sagittal T2-weighted (**b**), T1-weighted (**c**),
and post-contrast T1-weighted (**d**) MR images demonstrate a mass in the right paraspinal muscles with peripheral enhancement and a hyperintense core on T2 (*arrows*)

centers surrounded by low signal intensity on T2-weighted images and peripheral enhancement on post-contrast T1-weighted sequences. Most sponges contain radiopaque markers that can be recognized on CT and radiographs. However, some institutions may use sponges without radiopaque markers. On CT, gas bubbles or calcifications may be apparent, depending on the age of the gossypiboma.

11.5.17   Adjacent Segment Degenerative Disease

11.5.17.1   Discussion

Adjacent segment disease is a process related to spinal fusion in which degenerative change may develop at an accelerated pace at the mobile level next to fused level. This can lead to symptoms that can require additional surgical intervention. Radiographic signs of degenerative change adjacent to a fuse level are not uncommon. Potential findings include facet hypertrophy, disc herniation, loss of disc space height, and endplate changes (Fig. 11.116). The incidence of symptomatic adjacent degenerative disease is higher with pedicle instrumented fusion than other types of instrumented fusion.

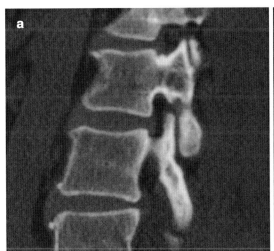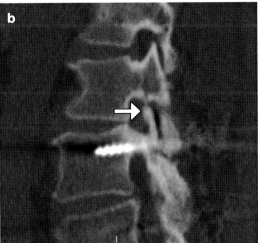

Fig. 11.116 Development of adjacent level degenerative disease. The patient underwent transforaminal lumbar interbody fusion at L3–L4 and L4–L5 and posterior lumbar arthrodesis L2–L5. Two years later, the patient began to experience symptoms consistent with cauda equina and conus medullaris compression. Preoperative sagittal CT image (**a**) shows no significant degenerative disease at L1–L2. Postoperative sagittal CT image (**b**) obtained 2 years later shows new facet hypertrophy (*arrow*), disc space narrowing, and endplate sclerosis at L1–L2. Spinal fusion hardware is partially visible

11.5.18   Postoperative Deformity

11.5.18.1   Discussion

Postoperative deformity can manifest as kyphosis and flat-back syndrome. Flat-back syndrome is an iatrogenic loss of lumbar lordosis due to the presence of thoracolumbar lordosis. Clinically, this condition consists of forward inclination of the spine, back pain, and inability to stand erect. Imaging plays an important role in the work-up of patients with flat-back syndrome. Sagittal CT or MRI and full-length lateral views of the spine with the knee and hips flexed are particularly useful for confirming the diagnosis. In addition, these studies are necessary for planning corrective procedures when conservative therapy fails. Several techniques are available to correct lumbar spine sagittal plane deformities, including pedicle subtraction (Fig. 11.117) and wedge osteotomies (Fig. 11.118).

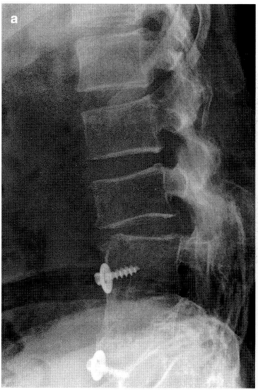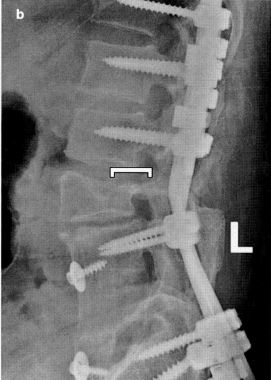

Fig. 11.117 Postoperative deformity treated with pedicle subtraction osteotomy. The patient presented with long-standing focal kyphosis following fusion from L4 to the sacrum. Lateral radiograph (**a**) shows straightening of L4 to the sacrum and kyphosis at the level above the surgically fused levels. Lateral radiograph after osteotomy (**b**) shows resection of a portion of the pedicles and posterior vertebral body with correction of lumbar lordosis (*bracket*)

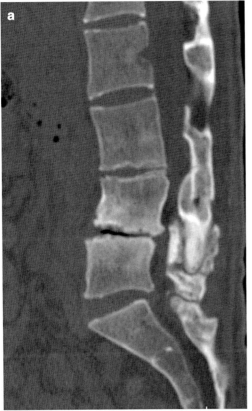

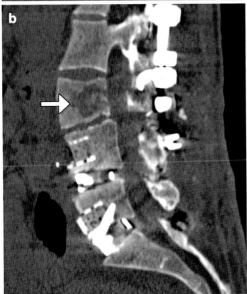

Fig. 11.118 Postoperative deformity treated with vertebral wedge osteotomy. Sagittal CT image (**a**) shows loss of the normal lumbar lordosis after previous lumbar surgeries. Sagittal (**b**) CT image obtained after wedge osteotomy shows a surgical defect in the posterior L3 vertebral body for wedge osteotomy (*arrow*). This vertebral body is now taller anteriorly than posteriorly, thereby restoring lumbar lordosis

11.6   Intrathecal Spinal Infusion Pump

11.6.1   Discussion

Intrathecal spinal infusion pump systems have been used to manage patients with intractable pain related to metastatic disease as well as those with spasms related to stroke, multiple sclerosis, or cerebral palsy. These devices resemble spinal stimulators on imaging, but the pump tends to be bulkier than the pulse generator (Fig. 11.119). Implanted infusion pumps are generally MRI compatible. Similar to spinal stimulators, patients may experience complications such as infection, device malposition, and spinal hypotension, which can result in diffuse meningeal enhancement and prominence of the epidural venous plexus (Fig. 11.120). Other complications include epidural hematoma, catheter breakage to spinal cord compression secondary to fibrotic mass formation, which is uncommon.

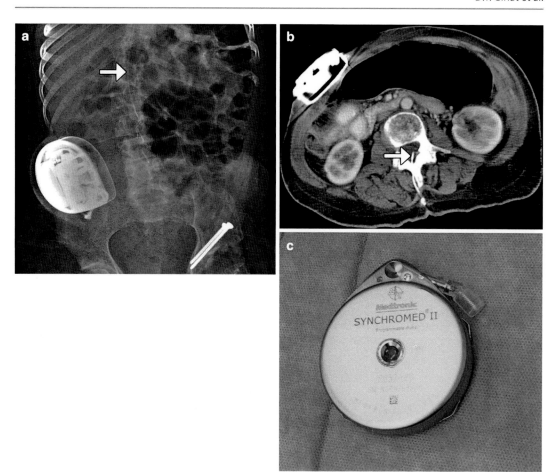

Fig. 11.119 Baclofen pump components. The patient has a history of cerebral palsy with a baclofen pump for spastic quadriparesis. Scout image (**a**) and axial CT image (**b**) show the pump mechanism in the subcutaneous tissues and the infusion catheter (*arrows*) within the spinal canal. Photograph of the pump device (**c**)

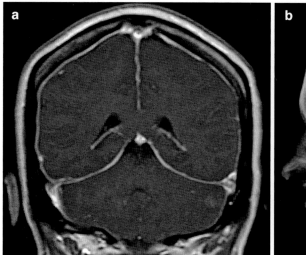
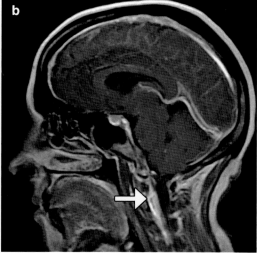

Fig. 11.120 Spinal hypotension syndrome. The patient presented with postural headaches after baclofen pump insertion. Coronal (**a**) and sagittal (**b**) post-contrast T1-weighted MR images show diffuse pachymeningeal thickening and enhancement, as well as prominence of the anterior spinal venous epidural plexus (*arrow*)

11.7   Spinal Cord Stimulators

11.7.1   Discussion

Spinal cord stimulators are used to treat patients with intractable pain and are positioned against the dorsal column. The models that consist of paddle electrodes require laminectomy for electrode positioning, while strip electrode models can be inserted percutaneously essentially at any level of the spine (Fig. 11.121). Spinal cord stimulators consist of a battery pack and pulse generator either kept externally or buried in the subcutaneous tissues, connected to an electrode that is inserted into the epidural space adjacent to the dorsal column or dorsal root ganglion. About 50% of patients experience pain relief. Complications related to spinal cord stimulators include intracranial/spinal hypotension secondary to cerebrospinal fluid leakage, migration or malposition, decreased effectiveness over time secondary to the formation of scar tissue, epidural hematoma, and infection (Fig. 11.122).

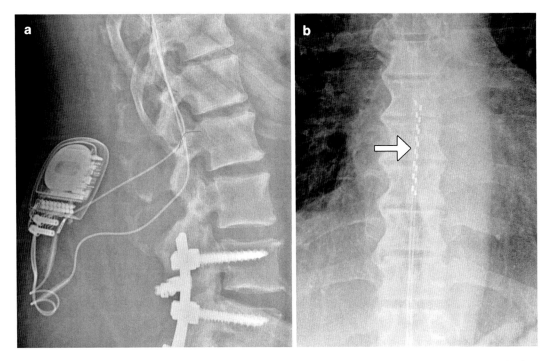

Fig. 11.121 Thoracic spinal cord stimulator. Lateral (**a**) and frontal (**b**) radiographs show the battery pack in the lower back and the electrodes in the thoracic spinal canal (*arrow*). Photographs of the battery packs on the left and various models of spinal cord stimulators, with strip electrodes shown on top right and paddle electrodes shown on the bottom right (**c**)

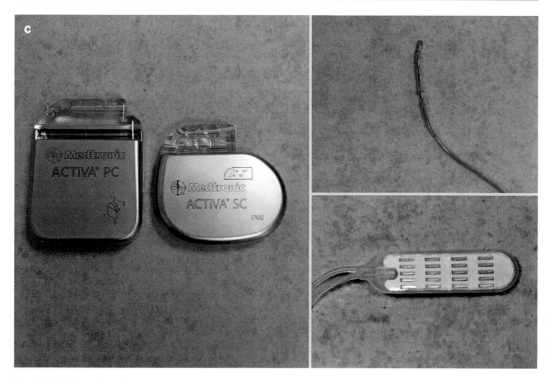

Fig. 11.121 (continued)

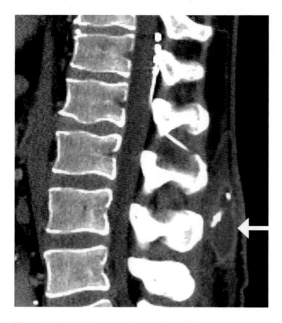

Fig. 11.122 Infected spine stimulator lead. Sagittal CT image shows a subcutaneous fluid collection (*arrow*) surrounding the spinal stimulator wire

11.8   Filum Terminale Sectioning

11.8.1   Discussion

Detethering of a tethered spinal cord by transecting or resecting a fatty filum terminale is performed to alleviate associated neurological symptoms. Postoperative MRI of the lumbar spine following detethering is generally performed if patients develop new symptoms suggestive of retethering or to assess associated conditions in patients with dysraphism that could otherwise explain the clinical deterioration. Discontinuity, along with thickening of the upper and lower remnants of the sectioned filum, constitutes evidence of a detethered filum (Fig. 11.123). The presence of conus relaxation, indicated by elevation or a more ventral position, is also reassuring, but is not consistently observed. Obtaining prone and supine imaging during the MRI exam can also be useful, in which no appreciable translation of the conus medullaris is observed when rethethering has occurred (Fig. 11.124).

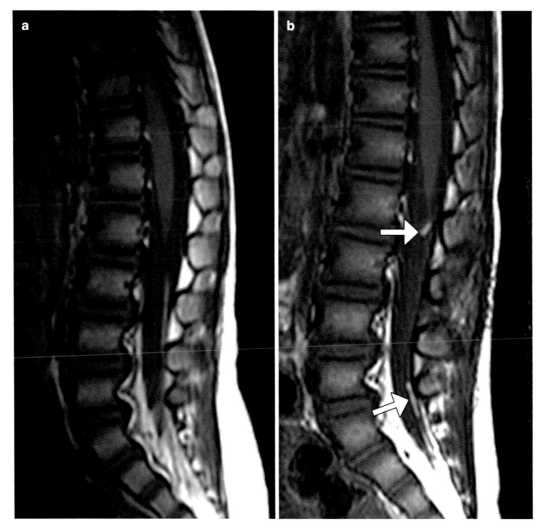

Fig. 11.123 Filum terminale sectioning. Preoperative sagittal T1-weighted MRI (**a**) shows a low-lying conus medullaris and fibrofatty filum terminate. Postoperative sagittal T1-weighted MRI (**b**) shows a wide gap in of the fibrofatty filum with retraction and slight thickening of both remaining segments (*arrows*)

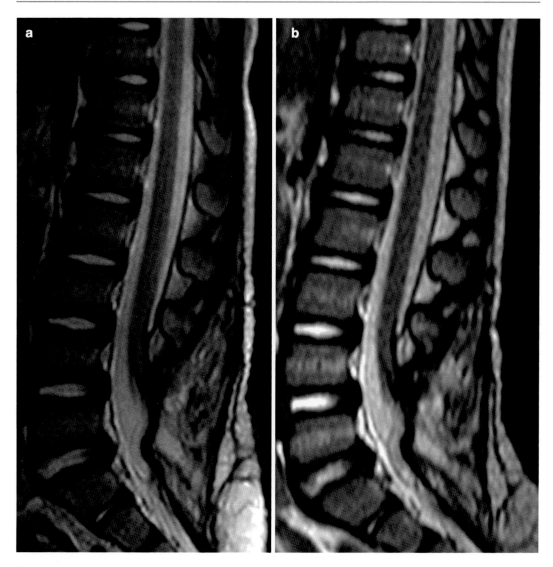

Fig. 11.124 Rethethering. Supine (**a**) and prone (**b**) sagittal T2-weighted MR images show findings related to prior detethering surgery, but no shift in the position of the conus medullaris, which is low-lying and posteriorly deviated alongside the dura

11.9 Percutaneous Spine Treatments

11.9.1 Vertebral Augmentation

11.9.1.1 Discussion

Kyphoplasty and vertebroplasty are percutaneous interventions that have been used to treat a variety of conditions including of osteoporotic vertebral compression fractures, certain spine tumors, and selected traumatic fractures. Vertebroplasty consists of injecting polymethylmethacrylate cement into the affected vertebral body, while kyphoplasty involves the use of a balloon that is first inflated in the vertebral body and then deflated prior to cement injection. Skyphoplasty is another cement vertebral augmentation technique that is no longer implemented. The procedure involves the use of SKy bone expander (Disc Orthopaedic Technology/ Disc-O-Tech, Monroe Township, New Jersey), which enlarges like an accordion into a popcorn-like crenulated configuration. Compared with kyphoplasty device, skyphoplasty generates higher pressures, expands more predictably, requires a larger cannula, and cannot be repositioned once it is deployed.

The imaging features for vertebroplasty and kyphoplasty are similar: cement should be confined to the intramedullary space of the vertebral body with disruption and compaction of the trabeculae (Fig. 11.125). However, the cement deposits from vertebroplasty tend to have a more diffuse and granular appearance, while cement deposits from kyphoplasty tend to be more localized and globular, filling the cavity produced by balloon dilatation. A small increase in vertebral body height is sometimes observed following vertebral augmentation (Fig. 11.126). The cement is hyperattenuating on radiographs and CT and very low signal intensity on all MRI sequences. Skyphoplasty produces the characteristic configuration of cement deposition that is often present on post-procedure imaging (Fig. 11.127).

During vertebral augmentation, cement can leak outside of the vertebral body and into the neural foramen and spinal canal (Figs. 11.128, 11.129, and 11.130), which can result in neurological deficits and predisposes to degenerative spondylosis. Overall, this type of complication occurs in 30–75% of cases, whether or not an intravertebral cleft exist. The heat generated from the exothermic reaction as the cement hardens can burn the spinal cord or nerve roots. However, significant neurological symptoms result in only a minority of cases. In addition, if there is preexisting spinal canal stenosis and the amount of cement is large, extravasation can be a major complication of vertebroplasty or kyphoplasty. Radiographs and CT can readily depict the hyperattenuating cement extending outside the vertebral body. MRI or CT myelography are useful for evaluating whether the cement impinges upon the spinal cord and nerve roots.

Cement embolization to the pulmonary arteries occurs in 4.6–6.8% of cases of kyphoplasty/ vertebroplasty. Leakage of cement into the paravertebral veins is a strong risk factor for cement embolization to the lungs. Underlying multiple myeloma may also be a risk factor. However, the incidence of this complication is the same for kyphoplasty as for vertebroplasty. On chest imaging, pulmonary artery cement emboli characteristically appear as high attenuation tubular or branching structures in the distribution of the pulmonary arteries (Fig. 11.131). The cement fragments can range widely in size, and small fragments are most readily identified on non-contrast CT.

The incidence of new compression fractures following vertebroplasty or kyphoplasty ranges from 5% in patients with idiopathic osteoporosis and up to about 45% in patients with steroid induced or secondary osteoporosis. Over two-thirds of new fractures occur in the adjacent vertebral body and present within 3 months of the procedure (Fig. 11.132). Extrusion of cement into the disc space appears to increase the risk for adjacent vertebral body fracture, likely as a result of altered biomechanics. Other factors associated with adjacent vertebral body fracture include a thoracolumbar junction location and greater height restoration.

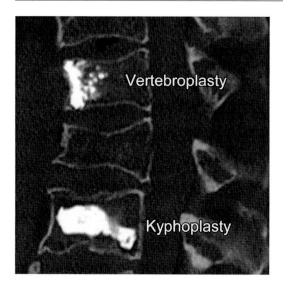

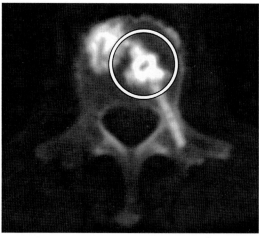

Fig. 11.125 Kyphoplasty and vertebroplasty. Sagittal CT image shows the granular deposits of vertebroplasty cement and the more globular deposits of cement from kyphoplasty, all of which are confined to the vertebral bodies

Fig. 11.127 Skyphoplasty. Axial CT image shows cement with characteristic lobulated margins in the vertebral body (*encircled*). There is also cement in the cannula insertion path across the left pedicle

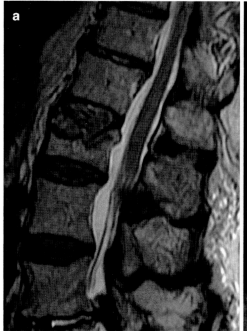

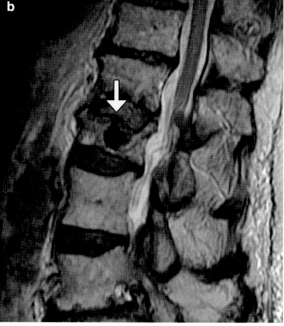

Fig. 11.126 Increased vertebral body height after vertebral augmentation. Initial sagittal T2-weighted MRI (**a**) shows a thoracic compression fracture. Sagittal T2-weighted MRI after vertebral augmentation (**b**) shows interval elevation of the superior endplate of the treated vertebral body (*arrow*)

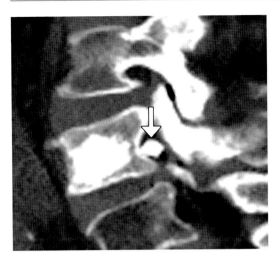

Fig. 11.128 Neural foramen cement leakage. Sagittal CT image of the lumbar spine shows cement within filling a neural foramen (*arrow*)

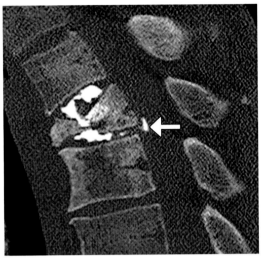

Fig. 11.129 Disc space and spinal canal cement leakage. Sagittal CT image shows cement extending into the adjacent intervertebral disc spaces, even extending into the spinal canal (*arrow*)

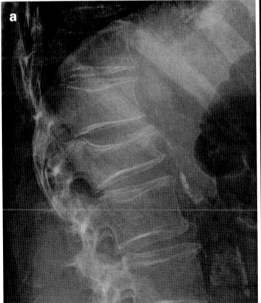

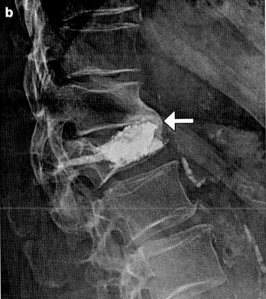

Fig. 11.130 Degenerative disc disease related to cement extravasation. Prevertebroplasty lateral radiograph (**a**) shows a thoracic vertebral compression fracture. Post-vertebroplasty lateral radiograph (**b**) shows cement within the adjacent disc space and interval development of end-plate sclerosis, worsening kyphosis and formation of a bridging osteophyte (*arrow*)

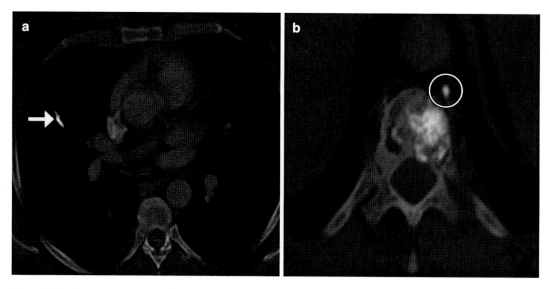

Fig. 11.131 Cement intravasation and pulmonary embolism. The patient has a history of multiple myeloma with compression fractures, for which the patient was treated with vertebral augmentation in the thoracic spine. After the procedure, the patient experienced shortness of breath.

Axial CT image (**a**) shows the presence of pulmonary artery cement embolism (*arrow*). Axial CT image at another level (**b**) shows intravasation of cement into the left paravertebral veins (*encircled*)

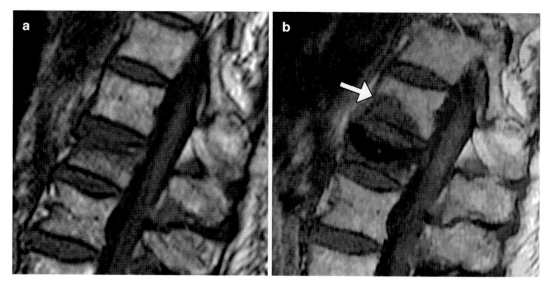

Fig. 11.132 Adjacent vertebral body fracture. The patient has a history of osteoporosis and presented with new pain 3 weeks after L2 kyphoplasty. Initial sagittal T1-weighted MRI (**a**) shows an acute compression fracture of the L2, but the L1 vertebral body is normal at this time. T1-weighted MRI after kyphoplasty (**b**) show cement in the L2 and an acute L1 vertebral body compression fracture as evidenced by edema and mild loss of height (*arrow*)

11.9.2 Kiva Device

11.9.2.1 Discussion

The Kiva VCF (vertebral compression fracture) system flexible implant is designed to provide structural support to the vertebral body and enables injection of bone cement during vertebral augmentation from T6 to L5. The implant appears as a spiral-shaped structure comprised of PEEK, which is visible on x-ray imaging modalities (Fig. 11.133).

11.9.3 Sacroplasty

11.9.3.1 Discussion

Analogous to kyphoplasty and vertebroplasty, sacroplasty is a minimally invasive procedure that involves percutaneous injection of polymethylmethacrylate cement into the sacral ala for treatment of sacral insufficiency fractures (Fig. 11.134). The rate of symptomatic improvement ranges from 50% immediately after the procedure to 90% at 1 year. Complications of sacroplasty include premature hardening, leakage of cement into the sacral neural foramina and into the sacroiliac joint, which can limit range of motion, and venous intravasation of cement with the risk of pulmonary embolism.

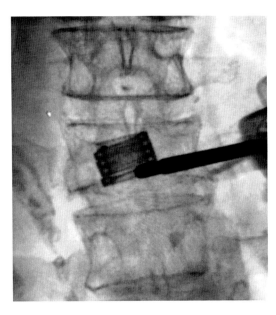

Fig. 11.133 Kiva device. Frontal radiograph obtained during percutaneous delivery of the device shows the helical structure within the fractured vertebral body (Courtesy of Benvenue Medical, Inc.)

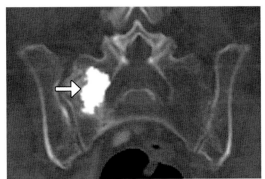

Fig. 11.134 Sacroplasty. The patient has a history of right sacral insufficiency fracture. Coronal CT image shows cement within the right sacral ala (*arrow*)

11.9.4 Percutaneous Interbody Fusion

11.9.4.1 Discussion

Percutaneous interbody fusion is a minimally invasive method for providing structural support to the level being fused. This can be accomplished using contained bone graft implant, such as OptiMesh. The device consists of an expandable polyethylene terephthalate meshed bag or pouch that is inserted into a voided disc space and then filled with bone graft material. The implant can be used as stand-alone or in combination with facet or pedicle screws. On imaging, the implant appears as an ovoid hyperattenuating mass within the disc space (Fig. 11.135). Overtime, solid bony fusion should form across the disc space. Potential complications include but are not limited to extrusion and failed fusion.

Another type of percutaneous disc intervention is nucleoplasty in which radiofrequency ablation is performed for treatment of disc herniation. This does not have any significant imaging correlates other than decrease in the disc herniation if successful.

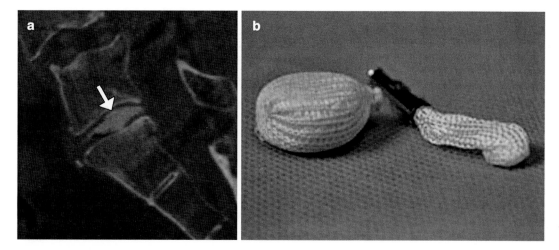

Fig. 11.135 Sagittal CT image (**a**) shows hyperattenuating material within the L5–S1 disc space (*arrow*). Photograph of OptiMesh (**b**)

11.9.5 CT-Guided Epidural Blood Patch

11.9.5.1 Discussion

CT-guided percutaneous patching targeted to the dural defect is a minimally invasive alternative to surgery for the treatment of spinal cerebrospinal fluid leaks. The procedure essentially consists of injecting a small amount of contrast material and autologous blood into the epidural space in the region of the suspected location of the dural defect. The distribution of the injected contrast and blood can be observed on CT and MRI soon after the procedure (Fig. 11.136).

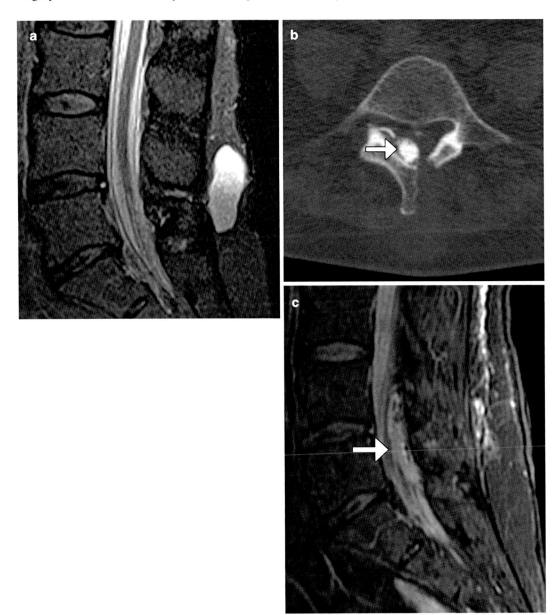

Fig. 11.136 CT-guided epidural blood patch. Initial sagittal STIR MRI (**a**) shows a fluid collection in the posterior subcutaneous tissues related to cerebrospinal fluid leakage and postoperative findings related to microdiscectomy in the lower lumbar spine. Axial CT image (**b**) obtained at the completion of the epidural blood patch procedure shows the contrast containing fluid in the right posterior epidural space (*arrow*). The blood patch appears as a fluid collection (*arrow*) along the dorsolateral epidural space related to recent blood patch with mild local mass effect on the thecal on the sagittal STIR MRI obtained 1 day later (**c**), but the fluid posterior subcutaneous fluid collection has diminished

11.9.6 Percutaneous Perineural Cyst Decompression

11.9.6.1 Discussion

Perineural cysts can occasionally cause symptoms that warrant treatment, such as radicular pain. Percutaneous cyst drainage is a minimally invasive treatment option that can be performed under image guidance. The cyst contents can be aspirated, thereby relieving the mass effect. Catheters that drain the cyst into the subarachnoid space can also be inserted (Fig. 11.137). The resulting decrease in size of the cyst and position of the drainage catheter can be assessed on MRI or CT myelography.

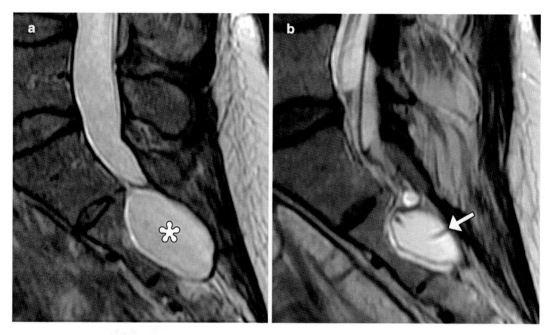

Fig. 11.137 Percutaneous sacral perineural cyst decompression with drainage catheter. Preoperative sagittal T2-weighted MRI (**a**) show a large intrasacral perineural cyst (*) with remodeling of the surrounding bone. Postoperative sagittal T2-weighted MR image (**b**) shows a drainage catheter (*arrow*) inserted within the cyst and interval decrease in size of the cyst

Further Reading

Overview

Allouni AK, Davis W, Mankad K, Rankine J, Davagnanam I (2013) Modern spinal instrumentation. Part 2: multi-modality imaging approach for assessment of complications. Clin Radiol 68(1):75–81

Davis W, Allouni AK, Mankad K, Prezzi D, Elias T, Rankine J, Davagnanam I (2013) Modern spinal instrumentation. Part 1: normal spinal implants. Clin Radiol 68(1):64–74

Thakkar RS, Malloy JP 4th, Thakkar SC, Carrino JA, Khanna AJ (2012) Imaging the postoperative spine. Radiol Clin N Am 50(4):731–747

Spine Decompression: Laminotomy and Foraminotomy

Genevay S, Atlas SJ (2010) Lumbar spinal stenosis. Best Pract Res Clin Rheumatol 24(2):253–265

Yuan PS, Booth RE Jr, Albert TJ (2005) Nonsurgical and surgical management of lumbar spinal stenosis. Instr Course Lect 54:303–312

Laminectomy

Angevine PD, Kellner C, Haque RM, McCormick PC (2011) Surgical management of ventral intradural spinal lesions. J Neurosurg Spine 15(1):28–37

Mall JC, Kaiser JA (1987) The usual appearance of the postoperative lumbar spine. Radiographics 7(2):245–269

Mathews HH, Long BH (2002) Minimally invasive techniques for the treatment of intervertebral disk herniation. J Am Acad Orthop Surg 10(2):80–85

Park J, Lee JB, Park JY, Lim DJ, Kim SD, Chung YK (2007) Spinal cord infarction after decompressive laminectomy for spontaneous spinal epidural hematoma–case report. Neurol Med Chir (Tokyo) 47(7):325–327

Turker RJ, Slack C, Regan Q (1995) Thoracic paraplegia after lumbar spinal surgery. J Spinal Disord 8(3):195–200

Facetectomy

Epstein NE (2002) Foraminal and far lateral lumbar disc herniations: surgical alternatives and outcome measures. Spinal Cord 40(10):491–500

Frizzell RT, Hadley MN (1993) Lumbar microdiscectomy with medial facetectomy. Techniques and analysis of results. Neurosurg Clin N Am 4(1):109–115

Microdiscectomy

Casey KF, Chang MK, O'Brien ED, Yuan HA, McCullen GM, Schaffer J, Kambin P (1997) Arthroscopic microdiscectomy: comparison of preoperative and postoperative imaging studies. Arthroscopy 13(4):438–445

Findlay GF, Hall BI, Musa BS, Oliveira MD, Fear SC (1998) A 10-year follow-up of the outcome of lumbar microdiscectomy. Spine (Phila Pa 1976) 23(10):1168–1171, Walton Centre for Neurology and Neurosurgery, Liverpool, United Kingdom

Kambin P, Zhou L (1997) Arthroscopic discectomy of the lumbar spine. Clin Orthop Relat Res 337:49–57

Nygaard OP, Jacobsen EA, Solberg T, Kloster R, Dullerud R (1999) Nerve root signs on postoperative lumbar MR imaging. A prospective cohort study with contrast enhanced MRI in symptomatic and asymptomatic patients one year after microdiscectomy. Acta Neurochir 141(6):619–622; discussion 623

Laminoplasty

Hale JJ, Gruson KI, Spivak JM (2006) Laminoplasty: a review of its role in compressive cervical myelopathy. Spine J 6(6 Suppl):289S–298S

Matz PG, Anderson PA, Groff MW, Heary RF, Holly LT, Kaiser MG, Mummaneni PV, Ryken TC, Choudhri TF, Vresilovic EJ, Resnick DK (2009) Joint section on disorders of the spine and peripheral nerves of the American Association of Neurological Surgeons and Congress of Neurological Surgeons. Cervical laminoplasty for the treatment of cervical degenerative myelopathy. J Neurosurg Spine 11(2):157–169

Ratliff JK, Cooper PR (2003) Cervical laminoplasty: a critical review. J Neurosurg 98(3 Suppl):230–238

Vertebrectomy

Boriani S, Biagini R, Bandiera S, Gasbarrini A, De LF (2002) Reconstruction of the anterior column of the thoracic and lumbar spine with a carbon fiber stackable cage system. Orthopedics 25(1):37–42

Douglas AF, Cooper PR (2007) Cervical corpectomy and strut grafting. Neurosurgery 60(1 Supp 1):S137–S142

Dickman CA, Rosenthal D, Karahalios DG, Paramore CG, Mican CA, Apostolides PJ, Lorenz R, Sonntag VK (1996) Thoracic vertebrectomy and reconstruction using a microsurgical thoracoscopic approach. Neurosurgery 38(2):279–293

Klezl Z, Bagley CA, Bookland MJ, Wolinsky JP, Rezek Z, Gokaslan ZL (2007) Harms titanium mesh cage fracture. Eur Spine J 16(Suppl 3):306–310

Krepler P, Windhager R, Bretschneider W, Toma CD, Kotz R (2002) Total vertebrectomy for primary malignant tumours of the spine. J Bone Joint Surg Br 84(5):712–715

Miyamoto K, Shimizu K, Nozawa S, Sakaguchi Y, Toki M, Hosoe H (2003 May 15) Kyphectomy using a surgical threadwire (T-saw) for kyphotic deformity in a child with myelomeningocele. Spine (Phila Pa 1976) 28(10):E187–E190

Obeid I, Guerin P, Gille O, Gangnet N, Aurouer N, Pointillart V, Vital JM (2011) Total vertebrectomy and spine shortening in the management of acute thoracic spine fracture dislocation: technical note and report of 3 cases. J Spinal Disord Tech 24(5):340–345

Rutherford EE, Tarplett LJ, Davies EM, Harley JM, King LJ (2007) Lumbar spine fusion and stabilization: hardware, techniques, and imaging appearances. Radiographics 27(6):1737–1749

Tomita K, Kawahara N (1996) The threadwire saw: a new device for cutting bone. J Bone Joint Surg Am 78(12):1915–1917

van der Haven I, van Loon PJ, Bartels RH, van Susante JL (2005) Anterior cervical interbody fusion with radiolucent carbon fiber cages: clinical and radiological results. Acta Orthop Belg 71(5):604–609

Zdeblick TA, Phillips FM (2003) Interbody cage devices. Spine (Phila Pa 1976) 28(15 Suppl):S2–S7

Cordectomy

Ewelt C, Stummer W, Klink B, Felsberg J, Steiger HJ, Sabel M (2010) Cordectomy as final treatment option for diffuse intramedullary malignant glioma using 5-ALA fluorescence-guided resection. Clin Neurol Neurosurg 112(4):357–361

Kyoshima K, Ito K, Tanabe A, Iwashita T, Goto T, Sato A, Nakayama J (2002) Malignant astrocytoma of the conus medullaris treated by spinal cordectomy. J Clin Neurosci 9(2):211–216

Raza SM, Anderson WS, Eberhart CG, Wolinsky JP, Gokaslan ZL (2005) The application of surgical cordectomy in the management of an intramedullary-extramedullary atypical meningioma: case report and literature review. J Spinal Disord Tech 18(5):449–454

Spine Stabilization and Fusion: Halo and Traction Devices

Clayman DA, Murakami ME, Vines FS (1990) Compatibility of cervical spine braces with MR imaging: a study of nine nonferrous devices. AJNR Am J Neuroradiol 11(2):385–390

Hunter TB, Yoshino MT, Dzioba RB, Light RA, Berger WG (2004) Medical devices of the head, neck, and spine. Radiographics 24(1):257–285

Lerman JA, Haynes RJ, Koeneman EJ, Koeneman JB, Wong WB (1994) A biomechanical comparison of Gardner-Wells tongs and halo device used for cervical spine traction. Spine (Phila Pa 1976) 19(21):2403–2406

Bone Graft Materials

Beaman FD, Bancroft LW, Peterson JJ, Kransdorf MJ, Menke DM, DeOrio JK (2006) Imaging characteristics of bone graft materials. Radiographics 26(2):373–388

Khanna G, Lewonowski K, Wood KB (2006) Initial results of anterior interbody fusion achieved with a less invasive bone harvesting technique. Spine (Phila Pa 1976) 31(1):111–114

Moore ST, Katz JM, Zhukauskas RM, Hernandez RM, Lewis CS, Supronowicz PR, Gill E, Grover SM, Long NS, Cobb RR (2011) Osteoconductivity and Osteoinductivity of Puros(R) DBM Putty. J Biomater Appl 26(2):151–171

Sethi A, Craig J, Bartol S, Chen W, Jacobsen M, Coe C, Vaidya R (2011) Radiographic and CT evaluation of recombinant human bone morphogenetic protein-2-assisted spinal interbody fusion. AJR Am J Roentgenol 197(1):W128–W133

Implantable Bone Stimulators

Hughes MS, Anglen JO (2010) The use of implantable bone stimulators in nonunion treatment. Orthopedics 10:151–157

Rogozinski A, Rogozinski C (1996) Efficacy of implanted bone growth stimulation in instrumented lumbosacral spinal fusion. Spine (Phila Pa 1976) 21(21):2479–2483

Victoria G, Petrisor B, Drew B, Dick D (2009) Bone stimulation for fracture healing: what's all the fuss? Indian J Orthop [serial online] 43:117–120, Cited 2012 Jan 13

Odontoid Screw Fixation

Daher MT, Daher S, Nogueira-Barbosa MH, Defino HL (2011) Computed tomographic evaluation of odontoid process: implications for anterior screw fixation of odontoid fractures in an adult population. Eur Spine J 20(11):1908–1914

Hsu WK, Anderson PA (2010) Odontoid fractures: update on management. J Am Acad Orthop Surg 18(7):383–394

Anterior Cervical Fusion

Akutsu H, Yanaka K, Sakamoto N, Matsumura A, Nose T (2004) Transient long segment spinal cord hyperintensity after anterior cervical discectomy. J Clin Neurosci 11(8):932–934

Blumenthal SL, Baker J, Dossett A, Selby DK (1988) The role of anterior lumbar fusion for internal disc disruption. Spine (Phila Pa 1976) 13(5):566–569

Bose B (1998) Anterior cervical fusion using Caspar plating: analysis of results and review of the literature. Surg Neurol 49(1):25–31

Freudenberger C, Lindley EM, Beard DW, Reckling WC, Williams A, Burger EL, Patel VV (2009) Posterior versus anterior lumbar interbody fusion with anterior tension band plating: retrospective analysis. Orthopedics 32(7):492

Kraus DR, Stauffer ES (1975) Spinal cord injury as a complication of elective anterior cervical fusion. Clin Orthop Relat Res 112:130–141

Winslow CP, Meyers AD (1999) Otolaryngologic complications of the anterior approach to the cervical spine. Am J Otolaryngol 20(1):16–27

Yonenobu K, Hosono N, Iwasaki M, Asano M, Ono K (1991) Neurologic complications of surgery for cervical compression myelopathy. Spine (Phila Pa 1976) 16(11):1277–1282

Anterior Approach Thoracolumbar Spine Stabilization Devices

Cardenas RJ, Javalkar V, Patil S, Gonzalez-Cruz J, Ogden A, Mukherjee D, Nanda A (2010) Comparison of allograft bone and titanium cages for vertebral body replacement in the thoracolumbar spine: a biomechanical study. Neurosurgery 66(6 Suppl Operative):314–318; discussion 318

Kanayama M, Ishida T, Hashimoto T, Shigenobu K, Togawa D, Oha F, Kaneda K (2010) Role of major spine surgery using Kaneda anterior instrumentation for osteoporotic vertebral collapse. J Spinal Disord Tech 23(1):53–56

Posterior Fusion

Amato V, Giannachi L, Irace C, Corona C (2010) Accuracy of pedicle screw placement in the lumbosacral spine using conventional technique: computed tomography postoperative assessment in 102 consecutive patients. J Neurosurg Spine 12(3):306–313

Bransford RJ, Lee MJ, Reis A (2011) Posterior fixation of the upper cervical spine: contemporary techniques. J Am Acad Orthop Surg 19(2):63–71

Hicks JM, Singla A, Shen FH, Arlet V (2010) Complications of pedicle screw fixation in scoliosis surgery: a systematic review. Spine (Phila Pa 1976) 35(11):E465–E470

Horn EM, Theodore N, Crawford NR, Bambakidis NC, Sonntag VK (2008) Transfacet screw placement for posterior fixation of C-7. J Neurosurg Spine 9(2):200–206

Kang HY, Lee SH, Jeon SH, Shin SW (2007) Computed tomography-guided percutaneous facet screw fixation in the lumbar spine. Technical note. J Neurosurg Spine 7(1):95–98

Kim DJ, Yun YH, Moon SH, Riew KD (2004) Posterior instrumentation using compressive laminar hooks and anterior interbody arthrodesis for the treatment of tuberculosis of the lower lumbar spine. Spine (Phila Pa 1976) 29(13):E275–E279

Slone RM, MacMillan M, Montgomery WJ, Heare M (1993) Spinal fixation. Part 2. Fixation techniques and hardware for the thoracic and lumbosacral spine. Radiographics 13(3):521–543

Zampolin R, Erdfarb A, Miller T (2014) Imaging of lumbar spine fusion. Neuroimaging Clin N Am 24(2):269–286

Occiptiocervical Fusion

Ahmed R, Traynelis VC, Menezes AH (2008) Fusions at the craniovertebral junction. Childs Nerv Syst 24(10):1209–1224

Blacklock JB (1994) Fracture of a sublaminar stainless steel cable in the upper cervical spine with neurological injury. Case report. J Neurosurg 81(6):932–933

Inamasu J, Kim DH, Klugh A (2005) Posterior instrumentation surgery for craniocervical junction instabilities: an update. Neurol Med Chir (Tokyo) 45(9):439–447

Lall R, Patel NJ, Resnick DK (2010) A review of complications associated with craniocervical fusion surgery. Neurosurgery 67(5):1396–1402; discussion 1402–1403

Stock GH, Vaccaro AR, Brown AK, Anderson PA (2006) Contemporary posterior occipital fixation. J Bone Joint Surg Am 88(7):1642–1649

Scoliosis Rods

Mohaideen A, Nagarkatti D, Banta JV, Foley CL (2000) Not all rods are Harrington - an overview of spinal instrumentation in scoliosis treatment. Pediatr Radiol 30(2):110–118

Nectoux E, Giacomelli MC, Karger C, Herbaux B, Clavert JM (2010) Complications of the Luque-Galveston scoliosis correction technique in paediatric cerebral palsy. Orthop Traumatol Surg Res 96(4):354–361

Steinmetz MP, Rajpal S, Trost G (2008) Segmental spinal instrumentation in the management of scoliosis. Neurosurgery 63(3 Suppl):131–138

Vertebral Stapling

Betz RR, Ranade A, Samdani AF, Chafetz R, D'Andrea LP, Gaughan JP, Asghar J, Grewal H, Mulcahey MJ (2010) Vertebral body stapling: a fusionless treatment option for a growing child with moderate idiopathic scoliosis. Spine (Phila Pa 1976) 35(2):169–176,

Shriners Hospitals for Children, Philadelphia, PA, USA. rbetz@shrinenet.org

Guille JT, D'Andrea LP, Betz RR (2007) Fusionless treatment of scoliosis. Orthop Clin North Am 38(4):541–545. vii

Trobisch PD, Samdani A, Cahill P, Betz RR (2011) Vertebral body stapling as an alternative in the treatment of idiopathic scoliosis. Oper Orthop Traumatol 23(3):227–231

Vertical Expandable Prosthetic Titanium Rib (VEPTR)

Emans JB, Caubet JF, Ordonez CL, Lee EY, Ciarlo M (2005) The treatment of spine and chest wall deformities with fused ribs by expansion thoracostomy and insertion of vertical expandable prosthetic titanium rib: growth of thoracic spine and improvement of lung volumes. Spine (Phila Pa 1976) 30(17 Suppl):S58–S68

Interbody Fusion

Anjarwalla NK, Morcom RK, Fraser RD (2006) Supplementary stabilization with anterior lumbar intervertebral fusion–a radiologic review. Spine (Phila Pa 1976) 31(11):1281–1287

Blumenthal SL, Ohnmeiss DD, NASS (2003) Intervertebral cages for degenerative spinal diseases. Spine J 3(4):301–309

Botolin S, Agudelo J, Dwyer A (2010) High rectal injury during trans-1 axial lumbar interbody fusion L5–S1 fixation. Spine 35(4):E144–E148

Cauthen JC, Theis RP, Allen AT (2003) Anterior cervical fusion: a comparison of cage, dowel and dowel-plate constructs. Spine J 3(2):106–117; discussion 117

Kim KS, Yang TK, Lee JC (2005) Radiological changes in the bone fusion site after posterior lumbar interbody fusion using carbon cages impacted with laminar bone chips: follow-up study over more than 4 years. Spine (Phila Pa 1976) 30(6):655–660

Murtagh RD, Quencer RM, Castellvi AE, Yue JJ (2011) New techniques in lumbar spinal instrumentation: what the radiologist needs to know. Radiology 260:317–330

Ozgur BM, Aryan HE, Pimenta L, Taylor WR (2006) Extreme Lateral Interbody Fusion (XLIF): a novel surgical technique for anterior interbody fusion. Spine 6:435–443

Rutherford EE, Tarplett LJ, Davies EM, Harley JM, King LJ (2007) Lumbar spine fusion and stabilization: hardware, techniques, and imaging appearances. Radiographics 27(6):1737–1749

Williams AL, Gornet MF, Burkus JK (2005) CT evaluation of lumbar interbody fusion: current concepts. AJNR Am J Neuroradiol 26(8):2057–2066

Zdeblick TA, Phillips FM (2003) Interbody cage devices. Spine (Phila Pa 1976) 28(15 Suppl):S2–S7

Dynamic Stabilization and Miscellaneous Devices of the Spine: Total Disc Replacement

Cinotti G, David T, Postacchini F (1996) Results of disc prosthesis after a minimum follow-up period of 2 years. Spine (Phila Pa 1976) 21(8):995–1000

David T (2007) Long-term results of one-level lumbar arthroplasty: minimum 10-year follow-up of the CHARITE artificial disc in 106 patients. Spine (Phila Pa 1976) 32(6):661–666

Lemaire JP, Skalli W, Lavaste F, Templier A, Mendes F, Diop A, Sauty V, Laloux E (1997) Intervertebral disc prosthesis. Results and prospects for the year 2000. Clin Orthop Relat Res 337:64–67

Lemaire JP, Carrier H, Sariali el H, Skalli W, Lavaste F (2005) Clinical and radiological outcomes with the Charité artificial disc: a 10-year minimum follow-up. J Spinal Disord Tech 18(4):353–359

Marnay T (2002) Lumbar disc replacement: 1–11 years results with ProDisc. Presented at the fourth annual meeting of the Spine Society of Europe, Nantes, 2002

Marshman LA, Friesem T, Rampersaud YR, Le Huec JC, Krishna M (2008) Subsidence and malplacement with the Oblique Maverick Lumbar Disc Arthroplasty: technical note. Spine J 8(4):650–655

Mayer HM (2005) Total disc replacement. J Bone Joint Surg Am 87(8):1029–1037

Murtagh RD, Quencer RM, Cohen DS et al (2009) Normal and abnormal imaging findings in lumbar total disk replacement: devices and complications. Radiographics 29:105–118

Phillips FM, Garfin SR (2005) Cervical disc replacement. Spine (Phila Pa 1976) 30(17 Suppl):S27–S33

Shim CS, Lee S, Maeng DH, Lee SH (2005) Vertical split fracture of the vertebral body following total disc replacement using ProDisc: report of two cases. J Spinal Disord Tech 18(5):465–469

van den Eerenbeemt KD, Ostelo RW, van Royen BJ, Peul WC, van Tulder MW (2010) Total disc replacement surgery for symptomatic degenerative lumbar disc disease: a systematic review of the literature. Eur Spine J 19(8):1262–1280

van Ooij A, Oner FC, Verbout AJ (2003) Complications of artificial disc replacement: a report of 27 patients with the SB Charite disc. J Spinal Disord Tech 16(4):369–383

Nucleus Pulposus Replacement

Coric D, Mummaneni PV (2008) Nucleus replacement technologies. J Neurosurg Spine 8(2):115–120

Murtagh RD, Quencer RM, Castellvi AE, Yue JJ (2011) New techniques in lumbar spinal instrumentation: what the radiologist needs to know. Radiology 260:317–330

Posterior Dynamic Stabilization Devices

Barbagallo GM, Olindo G, Corbino L, Albanese V (2009) Analysis of complications in patients treated with the X-Stop Interspinous Process Decompression System: proposal for a novel anatomic scoring system for patient selection and review of the literature. Neurosurgery 65(1):111–119; discussion 119–120

Chiu JC (2006) Interspinous process decompression (IPD) system (X-STOP) for the treatment of lumbar spinal stenosis. Surg Technol Int 15:265–275

Christie SD, Song JK, Fessler RG (2005) Dynamic interspinous process technology. Spine (Phila Pa 1976) 30(16 Suppl):S73–S78

Ha AS, Petscavage-Thomas JM (2014) Imaging of current spinal hardware: lumbar spine. AJR Am J Roentgenol 203(3):573–581

Kuchta J, Sobottke R, Eysel P, Simons P (2009) Two-year results of interspinous spacer (X-Stop) implantation in 175 patients with neurologic intermittent claudication due to lumbar spinal stenosis. Eur Spine J 18(6):823–829

Lindsey DP, Swanson KE, Fuchs P et al (2003) The effects of an interspinous implant on the kinematics of the instrumented and adjacent levels in the lumbar spine. Spine 28(19):2192–2197

Sangiorgio SN, Sheikh H, Borkowski SL, Khoo L, Warren CR, Ebramzadeh E (2011) Comparison of three posterior dynamic stabilization devices. Spine (Phila Pa 1976) 36(19):E1251–E1258

Dynamic Facet Replacement

Murtagh RD, Quencer RM, Castellvi AE, Yue JJ (2011) New techniques in lumbar spinal instrumentation: what the radiologist needs to know. Radiology 260:317–330

Wilke HJ, Schmidt H, Werner K et al (2006) Biomechanical evaluation of a new total posterior-element replacement system. Spine 31(24):2790–2796

Dynamic Rods

Bothmann M, Kast E, Boldt GJ, Oberle J (2008) Dynesys fixation for lumbar spine degeneration. Neurosurg Rev 31(2):189–196

Schwarzenbach O, Berlemann U, Stoll TM, Dubois G (2005) Posterior dynamic stabilization systems: DYNESYS. Orthop Clin North Am 36(3):363–372

Failed Back Surgery Syndrome and Related Complications

Hayashi D, Roemer FW, Mian A, Gharaibeh M, Müller B, Guermazi A (2012) Imaging features of postoperative complications after spinal surgery and instrumentation. AJR Am J Roentgenol 199(1):W123–W129

Malhotra A, Kalra VB, Wu X, Grant R, Bronen RA, Abbed KM (2015) Imaging of lumbar spinal surgery complications. Insights Imaging 6(6):579–590

Hardware Malpositioning and Migration

Foxx KC, Kwak RC, Latzman JM, Samadani U (2010) A retrospective analysis of pedicle screws in contact with the great vessels. J Neurosurg Spine 13(3):403–406

Hicks JM, Singla A, Shen FH, Arlet V (2010) Complications of pedicle screw fixation in scoliosis surgery: a systematic review. Spine (Phila Pa 1976) 35(11):E465–E470

Kimura H, Shikata J, Odate S, Soeda T, Yamamura S (2012) Risk factors for cage retropulsion after posterior lumbar interbody fusion: analysis of 1070 cases. Spine (Phila Pa 1976) 37(13):1164–1169

Lonstein JE, Denis F, Perra JH, Pinto MR, Smith MD, Winter RB (1999) Complications associated with pedicle screws. J Bone Joint Surg Am 81(11):1519–1528

Shem KL (2005) Late complications of displaced thoracolumbar fusion instrumentation presenting as new pain in individuals with spinal cord injury. J Spinal Cord Med 28(4):326–329

Hardware Loosening and Pseudarthrosis

Ko CC, Tsai HW, Huang WC, Wu JC, Chen YC, Shih YH, Chen HC, Wu CL, Cheng H (2010) Screw loosening in the Dynesys stabilization system: radiographic evidence and effect on outcomes. Neurosurg Focus 28(6):E10

Lu WW, Zhu Q, Holmes AD, Luk KD, Zhong S, Leong JC (2000) Loosening of sacral screw fixation under in vitro fatigue loading. J Orthop Res 18(5):808–814

Uzi EA, Dabby D, Tolessa E, Finkelstein JA (2001) Early retropulsion of titanium-threaded cages after posterior lumbar interbody fusion: a report of two cases. Spine (Phila Pa 1976) 26(9):1073–1075

Van Goethem JW, Parizel PM, Jinkins JR (2002) Review article: MRI of the postoperative lumbar spine. Neuroradiology 44(9):723–739

Hardware and Periprosthetic Fractures

Lonstein JE, Denis F, Perra JH, Pinto MR, Smith MD, Winter RB (1999) Complications associated with pedicle screws. J Bone Joint Surg Am 81:1519–1528

Sewell MD, Woodacre T, Clarke A, Hutton M (2016) Broken pedicle screw thread extraction from within the pedicle. Ann R Coll Surg Engl 98(4):285–286

Cerebrospinal Fluid Leak

Hadani M, Findler G, Knoler N, Tadmor R, Sahar A, Shacked I (1986) Entrapped lumbar nerve root in pseudomeningocele after laminectomy: report of three cases. Neurosurgery 19(3):405–407

Lee KS, Hardy IM (1992) Postlaminectomy lumbar pseudomeningocele: report of four cases. Neurosurgery 30(1):111–114

Murayama S, Numaguchi Y, Whitecloud TS, Brent CR (1989) Magnetic resonance imaging of post-surgical pseudomeningocele. Comput Med Imaging Graph 13(4):335–339

Phillips CD, Kaptain GJ, Razack N (2002) Depiction of a postoperative pseudomeningocele with digital subtraction myelography. AJNR Am J Neuroradiol 23(2):337–338

Teplick JG, Peyster RG, Teplick SK, Goodman LR, Haskin ME (1983) CT identification of postlaminectomy pseudomeningocele. AJR Am J Roentgenol 140(6):1203–1206

Tomoda Y, Korogi Y, Aoki T, Morioka T, Takahashi H, Ohno M, Takeshita I (2008) Detection of cerebrospinal fluid leakage: initial experience with three-dimensional fast spin-echo magnetic resonance myelography. Acta Radiol 49(2):197–203

Yoo HM, Kim SJ, Choi CG, Lee DH, Lee JH, Suh DC, Choi JW, Jeong KS, Chung SJ, Kim JS, Yun SC (2008) Detection of CSF leak in spinal CSF leak syndrome using MR myelography: correlation with radioisotope cisternography. AJNR Am J Neuroradiol 29(4):649–654

Seromas and Hematomas

Garrett MP, Kakarla UK, Porter RW, Sonntag VK (2010) Formation of painful seroma and edema after the use of recombinant human bone morphogenetic protein-2 in posterolateral lumbar spine fusions. Neurosurgery 66(6):1044–1049; discussion 1049

Martin CT, Kebaish KM (2010) Postoperative spinal epidural hematoma at a site distant from the main surgical procedure: a case report and review of the literature. Spine J 10(4):e21–e25

Postoperative Infection

Boody BS, Jenkins TJ, Hashmi SZ, Hsu WK, Patel AA, Savage JW (2015) Surgical site infections in spinal surgery. J Spinal Disord Tech 28(10):352–362

Katonis P, Tzermiadianos M, Papagelopoulos P, Hadjipavlou A (2007) Postoperative infections of the thoracic and lumbar spine: a review of 18 cases. Clin Orthop Relat Res 454:114–119

Weinstein MA, McCabe JP, Cammisa FP Jr (2000) Postoperative spinal wound infection: a review of 2,391 consecutive index procedures. J Spinal Disord 13(5):422–426

Postoperative Neuritis

Lee YS, Choi ES, Song CJ (2009) Symptomatic nerve root changes on contrast-enhanced MR imaging after surgery for lumbar disk herniation. AJNR Am J Neuroradiol 30(5):1062–1067

Arachnoiditis

Frizzell B, Kaplan P, Dussault R, Sevick R (2001) Arachnoiditis ossificans: MR imaging features in five patients. AJR Am J Roentgenol 177(2):461–464

Khosla A, Wippold FJ II (2002) CT myelography and MR imaging of extramedullary cysts of the spinal canal in adult and pediatric patients. AJR Am J Roentgenol 178:201–207

Revilla TY, Ramos A, González P, Alday R, Millán JM (1999) Arachnoiditis ossificans. Diagnosis with helical computed tomography. Clin Imaging 23(1):1–4

Sanders WP, Truumees E (2004) Imaging of the postoperative spine. Semin Ultrasound CT MR 25(6):523–535

Van Goethem JW, Parizel PM, Jinkins JR (2002) Review article: MRI of the postoperative lumbar spine. Neuroradiology 44(9):723–739

Residual/Recurrent Disc Material Versus Epidural Scar

Bundschuh CV, Modic MT, Ross JS, Masaryk TJ, Bohlman H (1988) Epidural fibrosis and recurrent disk herniation in the lumbar spine: MR imaging assessment. AJR Am J Roentgenol 150(4):923–932

Bundschuh CV, Stein L, Slusser JH, Schinco FP, Ladaga LE, Dillon JD (1990) Distinguishing between scar and recurrent herniated disk in postoperative patients: value of contrast-enhanced CT and MR imaging. AJNR Am J Neuroradiol 11(5):949–958

Ross JS (2000) Magnetic resonance imaging of the post-operative spine. Semin Musculoskelet Radiol 4(3):281–291

Ross JS, Obuchowski N, Modic MT (1999) MR evaluation of epidural fibrosis: proposed grading system with intra- and inter-observer variability. Neurol Res 21(Suppl 1):S23–S26

Suk KS, Lee HM, Moon SH, Kim NH (2001) Recurrent lumbar disc herniation: results of operative management. Spine (Phila Pa 1976) 26(6):672–676

Postoperative Synovial Cyst

Schofferman J, Reynolds J, Herzog R, Covington E, Dreyfuss P, O'Neill C (2003) Failed back surgery: etiology and diagnostic evaluation. Spine J 3(5):400–403

Slipman CW, Shin CH, Patel RK, Isaac Z, Huston CW, Lipetz JS, Lenrow DA, Braverman DL, Vresilovic EJ Jr (2002) Etiologies of failed back surgery syndrome. Pain Med 3(3):200–214; discussion 214–217

Walcott BP, Coumans JV (2012) Postlaminectomy synovial cyst formation: A possible consequence of ligamentum flavum excision. J Clin Neurosci 19(2):252–254. Epub 2011 Nov 1

Residual/Recurrent Tumors

Boriani S, Saravanja D, Yamada Y, Varga PP, Biagini R, Fisher CG (2009) Challenges of local recurrence and cure in low grade malignant tumors of the spine. Spine (Phila Pa 1976) 34(22 Suppl):S48–S57

Boström A, von Lehe M, Hartmann W, Pietsch T, Feuss M, Bostrom JP, Schramm J, Simon M (2011) Surgery for spinal cord ependymomas: outcome and prognostic factors. Neurosurgery 68(2):302–308; discussion 309

Inclusion Cysts

Danzer E, Adzick NS, Rintoul NE, Zarnow DM, Schwartz ES, Melchionni J, Ernst LM, Flake AW, Sutton LN, Johnson MP (2008) Intradural inclusion cysts following in utero closure of myelomeningocele: clinical implications and follow-up findings. J Neurosurg Pediatr 2(6):406–413

Mazzola CA, Albright AL, Sutton LN, Tuite GF, Hamilton RL, Pollack IF (2002) Dermoid inclusion cysts and early spinal cord tethering after fetal surgery for myelomeningocele. N Engl J Med 347(4):256–259

Tang L, Cianfoni A, Imbesi SG (2006) Diffusion-weighted imaging distinguishes recurrent epidermoid neoplasm from postoperative arachnoid cyst in the lumbosacral spine. J Comput Assist Tomogr 30(3):507–509

Retained Bone Fragments and New Bone Formation

Javid MJ, Hadar EJ (1998) Long-term follow-up review of patients who underwent laminectomy for lumbar stenosis: a prospective study. J Neurosurg 89(1):1–7

Rosen C, Rothman S, Zigler J, Capen D (1991) Lumbar facet fracture as a possible source of pain after lumbar laminectomy. Spine (Phila Pa 1976) 16(6 Suppl):S234–S238

Retained Surgical Tools

Lee CS, Chung SS, Park JC, Shin SK, Park YS, Kang KC (2011) A broken drill-bit fragment causing severe radiating pain after cervical total disc replacement: a case report. Asian Spine J 5(2):125–129

Wolfson KA, Seeger LL, Kadell BM, Eckardt JJ (2000) Imaging of surgical paraphernalia: what belongs in the patient and what does not. Radiographics 20(6):1665–1673

Gossypiboma

Is M, Karatas A, Akgul M, Yildirim U, Gezen F (2007) A retained surgical sponge (gossypiboma) mimicking a paraspinal abscess. Br J Neurosurg 21(3):307–308

Kim HS, Chung TS, Suh SH, Kim SY (2007) MR imaging findings of paravertebral gossypiboma. AJNR Am J Neuroradiol 28(4):709–713

Van Goethem JW, Parizel PM, Perdieus D, Hermans P, de Moor J (1991) MR and CT imaging of paraspinal textiloma (gossypiboma). J Comput Assist Tomogr 15(6):1000–1003

Adjacent Segment Degenerative Disease

Okuda S, Iwasaki M, Miyauchi A, Aono H, Morita M, Yamamoto T (2004) Risk factors for adjacent segment degeneration after PLIF. Spine (Phila Pa 1976) 29(14):1535–1540

Park P, Garton HJ, Gala VC, Hoff JT, McGillicuddy JE (2004) Adjacent segment disease after lumbar or lumbosacral fusion: review of the literature. Spine (Phila Pa 1976) 29(17):1938–1944

Postoperative Deformity

Jagannathan J, Sansur CA, Shaffrey CI (2008) Iatrogenic spinal deformity. Neurosurgery 63(3 Suppl):104–116

Noun Z, Lapresle P, Missenard G (2001) Posterior lumbar osteotomy for flat back in adults. J Spinal Disord 14(4):311–316

Wang MY, Berven SH (2007) Lumbar pedicle subtraction osteotomy. Neurosurgery 60(2 Suppl 1):ONS140–ONS146; discussion ONS146

Wiggins GC, Ondra SL, Shaffrey CI (2003) Management of iatrogenic flat-back syndrome. Neurosurg Focus 15(3):E8

Intrathecal Spinal Infusion Pump

Diehn FE, Wood CP, Watson RE Jr, Mauck WD, Burke MM (2011) Hunt CH (2011) Clinical safety of magnetic resonance imaging in patients with implanted SynchroMed EL infusion pumps. Neuroradiology 53(2):117–122

Langsam A (1999) A case of spinal cord compression syndrome by a fibrotic mass presenting in a patient with an intrathecal pain management pump system. Pain 83(1):97–99

Spinal Cord Stimulators

Hunter TB, Yoshino MT, Dzioba RB, Light RA, Berger WG (2004) Medical devices of the head, neck, and spine. Radiographics 24(1):257–285

North RB, Kidd DH, Zahurak M, James CS, Long DM (1993) Spinal cord stimulation for chronic, intractable pain: experience over two decades. Neurosurgery 32(3):384–394; discussion 394–395

Filum Terminale Sectioning

Kim AH, Kasliwal MK, McNeish B, Silvera VM, Proctor MR, Smith ER (2011) Features of the lumbar spine on magnetic resonance images following sectioning of filum terminale. J Neurosurg Pediatr 8(4):384–389

Ogiwara H, Lyszczarz A, Alden TD, Bowman RM, McLone DG, Tomita T (2011) Retethering of transected fatty filum terminales. J Neurosurg Pediatr 7(1):42–46

Percutaneous Spine Treatments: Vertebral Augmentation

Anselmetti GC, Muto M, Guglielmi G, Masala S (2010) Percutaneous vertebroplasty or kyphoplasty. Radiol Clin N Am 48(3):641–649

Anselmetti GC, Bonaldi G, Carpeggiani P, Manfre L, Masala S, Muto M (2011) Vertebral augmentation: 7 years experience. Acta Neurochir Suppl 108:147–161

Buchbinder R, Osborne RH, Ebeling PR, Wark JD, Mitchell P, Wriedt C, Graves S, Staples MP, Murphy B (2009) A randomized trial of vertebroplasty for painful osteoporotic vertebral fractures. N Engl J Med 361(6):557–568

Choe DH, Marom EM, Ahrar K, Truong MT, Madewell JE (2004) Pulmonary embolism of polymethyl methacrylate during percutaneous vertebroplasty and kyphoplasty. AJR Am J Roentgenol 183(4):1097–1102

Cyteval C et al (1999) Acute osteoporotic vertebral collapse: open study on percutaneous injection of acrylic surgical cement in 20 patients. AJR Am J Roentgenol 173(6):1685–1690

Duran C, Sirvanci M, Aydoğan M, Ozturk E, Ozturk C, Akman C (2007) Pulmonary cement embolism: a complication of percutaneous vertebroplasty. Acta Radiol 48(8):854–859

Garfin SR et al (2001) New technologies in spine: kyphoplasty and vertebroplasty for the treatment of painful osteoporotic compression fractures. Spine 26(14):1511–1515

Kim SH, Kang HS, Choi JA, Ahn JM (2004) Risk factors of new compression fractures in adjacent vertebrae after percutaneous vertebroplasty. Acta Radiol 45:440–445

Lazáry A, Speer G, Varga PP, Balla B, Bácsi K, Kósa JP, Nagy Z, Takács I, Lakatos P (2008) Effect of vertebroplasty filler materials on viability and gene expression of human nucleus pulposus cells. J Orthop Res 26(5):601–607

Lee IJ, Choi AL, Yie MY, Yoon JY, Jeon EY, Koh SH, Yoon DY, Lim KJ, Im HJ (2010) CT evaluation of local leakage of bone cement after percutaneous kyphoplasty and vertebroplasty. Acta Radiol 51(6):649–654

Lin EP, Ekholm S, Hiwatashi A, Westesson PL (2004) Vertebroplasty: cement leakage into the disc increases the risk of new fracture of adjacent vertebral body. AJNR Am J Neuroradiol 25:175–180

Lin WC, Cheng TT, Lee YC, Wang TN, Cheng YF, Lui CC, Yu CY (2008) New vertebral osteoporotic compression fractures after percutaneous vertebroplasty: retrospective analysis of risk factors. J Vasc Interv Radiol 19(2 Pt 1):225–231

Martin JB (1999) Vertebroplasty: clinical experience and follow-up results. Bone 25(2 Suppl):11S–15S

Peh WC, Munk PL, Rashid F, Gilula LA (2008) Percutaneous vertebral augmentation: vertebroplasty, kyphoplasty and skyphoplasty. Radiol Clin N Am 46(3):611–635. vii

Rashid R, Munk PL, Heran M, Malfair D, Chiu O (2009) SKyphoplasty. Can Assoc Radiol J 60(5):273–278

Tong SC, Eskey CJ, Pomerantz SR, Hirsch JA (2006) "SKyphoplasty": a single institution's initial experience. J Vasc Interv Radiol 17(6):1025–1030

Trout AT, Kallmes DF, Kaufmann TJ (2006) New fractures after vertebroplasty: adjacent fractures occur significantly sooner. AJNR Am J Neuroradiol 27(1):217–223

Kiva Device

Berjano P, Damilano M, Pejrona M, Consonni O, Langella F, Lamartina C (2014) KIVA VCF system in the treatment of T12 osteoporotic vertebral compression fracture. Eur Spine J 23(6):1379–1380

Tutton SM, Pflugmacher R, Davidian M, Beall DP, Facchini FR, Garfin SR (2015) KAST study: the Kiva system as a vertebral augmentation treatment-a safety and effectiveness trial: a randomized, noninferiority trial comparing the Kiva system with balloon kyphoplasty in treatment of osteoporotic vertebral compression fractures. Spine (Phila Pa 1976) 40(12):865–875

Sacroplasty

Frey ME, DePalma MJ, Cifu DX, Bhagia SM, Daitch JS (2007) Efficacy and safety of percutaneous sacroplasty for painful osteoporotic sacral insufficiency fractures: a prospective, multicenter trial. Spine (Phila Pa 1976) 32(15):1635–1640

Frey ME, Depalma MJ, Cifu DX, Bhagia SM, Carne W, Daitch JS (2008) Percutaneous sacroplasty for osteoporotic sacral insufficiency fractures: a prospective, multicenter, observational pilot study. Spine J 8(2):367–373

Heron J, Connell DA, James SL (2007) CT-guided sacroplasty for the treatment of sacral insufficiency fractures. Clin Radiol 62(11):1094–1100; discussion 1101–1103

Strub WM, Hoffmann M, Ernst RJ, Bulas RV (2007) Sacroplasty by CT and fluoroscopic guidance: is the procedure right for your patient? AJNR Am J Neuroradiol 28(1):38–41

Percutaneous Spine Fusion

Chiu JC, Stechison MT (2005) Percutaneous vertebral augmentation and reconstruction with an intravertebral mesh and morcelized bone graft. Surg Technol Int 14:287–296

Inamasu J, Guiot BH, Uribe JS (2008) Flexion-distraction injury of the L1 vertebra treated with short-segment posterior fixation and Optimesh. J Clin Neurosci 15(2):214–218

Lam S, Khoo LT (2005) A novel percutaneous system for bone graft delivery and containment for elevation and stabilization of vertebral compression fractures. Technical note. Neurosurg Focus 18(3):e10

Welch WC, Gerszten PC (2002) Alternative strategies for lumbar discectomy: intradiscal electrothermy and nucleoplasty. Neurosurg Focus 13(2):E7

Zheng X, Chaudhari R, Wu C, Mehbod AA, Erkan S, Transfeldt EE (2010) Biomechanical evaluation of an expandable meshed bag augmented with pedicle or facet screws for percutaneous lumbar interbody fusion. Spine J 10(11):987–993

CT-Guided Epidural Blood Patch

Karst M, Hollenhorst J, Fink M, Conrad I (2001) Computerized tomography-guided epidural blood patch in the treatment of spontaneous low cerebrospinal fluid pressure headache. Acta Anaesthesiol Scand 45(5):649–651

Mihlon F, Kranz PG, Gafton AR, Gray L (2014) Computed tomography-guided epidural patching of postoperative cerebrospinal fluid leaks. J Neurosurg Spine 21(5):805–810

Percutaneous Perineural Cyst Decompression

Landers J, Seex K (2002) Sacral perineural cysts: imaging and treatment options. Br J Neurosurg 16(2):182–185

Paulsen RD, Call GA, Murtagh FR (1994) Prevalence and percutaneous drainage of cysts of the sacral nerve root sheath (Tarlov cysts). AJNR Am J Neuroradiol 15(2):293–297; discussion 298–299

Imaging of Vascular and Endovascular Surgery

Daniel Thomas Ginat, Javier M. Romero,
and Gregory Christoforidis

12.1 Vascular Surgery

12.1.1 Direct Extracranial-Intracranial Revascularization

12.1.1.1 Discussion

Extracranial-intracranial (EC-IC) bypass is a revascularization option for complex cerebrovascular disease such as moyamoya in adults and flow replacement prior to planned vessel sacrifice for treatment of complex and fusiform aneurysms that are not amenable to coiling or clipping. Usually in EC-IC bypass, the superficial temporal artery is anastomosed to a middle cerebral artery branch (Fig. 12.1). Alternatively, saphenous vein grafts can be used, in which the venous graft normally appears relatively patulous with respect to the artery (Fig. 12.2). If these options fail, the occipital artery can be anastomosed to the middle cerebral artery (Fig. 12.3), or it can be used to supply the posterior cerebral artery. Regardless of the particular vessels used, EC-IC bypass is performed via a small craniectomy in the temporal region, so as to expose the Sylvian fissure and the right temporal lobe. On follow-up angiography, increase in caliber of the recipient and donor arteries can be observed. On the other hand, basal collateral vessels often regress. Graft patency can be readily assessed via MRA or CTA. Stenosis or occlusion of the bypass typically occurs at or near the anastomosis (Fig. 12.4). Correlation with pre-contrast images is recommended, since early clot can appear hyperattenuating, mimicking graft patency on CTA. A pitfall with time-of-flight MRA in particular is the loss of signal associated with the presence of adjacent surgical clips, which can obscure the bypass, mimicking a stenosis (Fig. 12.5). However, the presence of flow-related enhancement distally suggests that the vessel is indeed patent.

D.T. Ginat, M.D., MS (✉) • G. Christoforidis, M.D.
Department of Radiology, Pritzker School of
Medicine, University of Chicago, Chicago, IL, USA
e-mail: dtg1@uchicago.edu

J.M. Romero, M.D.
Department of Radiology, Harvard Medical School,
Massachusetts General Hospital, Boston, MA, USA

© Springer International Publishing Switzerland 2017
D.T. Ginat, P.-L.A. Westesson (eds.), *Atlas of Postsurgical Neuroradiology*,
DOI 10.1007/978-3-319-52341-5_12

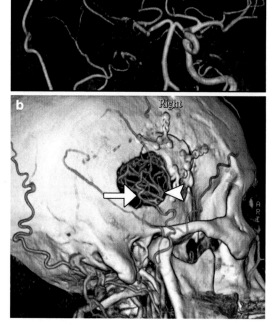

Fig. 12.1 MCA-STA bypass. The 3D MIP MRA (**a**) and 3D reformatted CTA image (**b**) show the superficial artery (*arrows*) entering the craniotomy and anastomosing with the prominent right superficial temporal artery (*arrowheads*) and M3 segment of the right middle cerebral artery

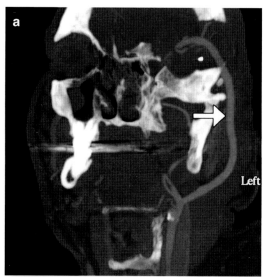

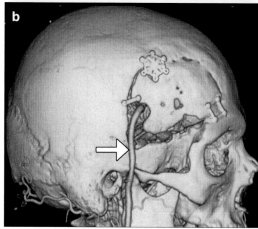

Fig. 12.2 EC-IC bypass with saphenous vein graft. Curved planar reformatted CT (**a**) and 3D CT (**b**) images show a large caliber saphenous vein graft (*arrows*) that connects the proximal ECA to the MCA

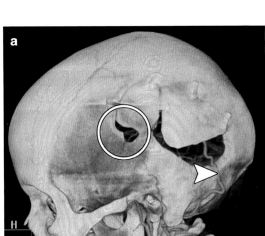

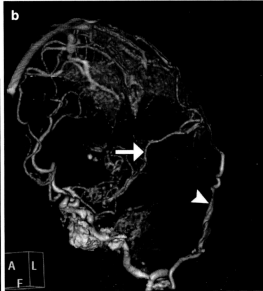

Fig 12.3 Occipital artery-MCA bypass. The patient has a history of failed left STA-MCA bypass. The 3D reformatted CTA image (**a**) shows the microcraniotomy (*encircled*) for the failed STA-MCA bypass and the left occipital artery (arrowhead) entering an additional craniotomy. The 3D reformatted CTA image (**b**) shows a patent anastomosis between the left occipital artery (*arrowhead*) and left middle cerebral artery (*arrow*)

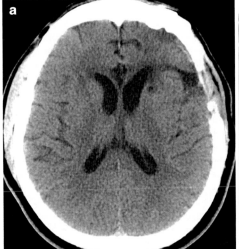

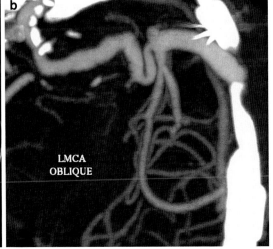

Fig. 12.4 EC-IC bypass occlusion. The patient has a history of complex left MCA aneurysm requiring left ICA occlusion and EC-IC bypass. Initial axial CT image (**a**) shows a small amount of encephalomalacia in the left temporal lobe and insula. The corresponding axial CTA MIP image (**b**) shows a patent bypass. Follow-up axial CT image (**c**) obtained 11 months later shows increased encephalomalacia. The corresponding axial CTA MIP image (**d**) now shows occlusion of the bypass near the anastomosis (*encircled*)

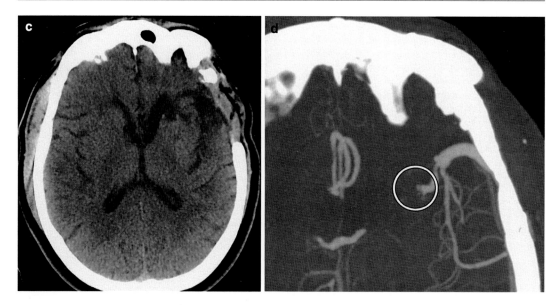

Fig. 12.4 (continued)

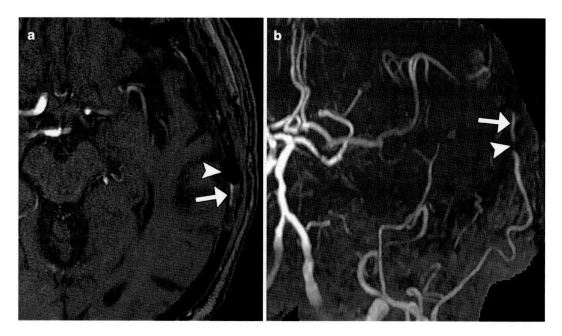

Fig. 12.5 Metal artifact simulating steno-occlusive disease of the STA-MCA bypass. Axial time-of-flight MRA image (**a**) shows susceptibility effect from a metallic clip (arrow) adjacent to the left superficial temporal artery branch (*arrowhead*). The corresponding MRA MIP image

(**b**) shows focal loss of signal (*arrow*) along the course of the left superficial temporal artery, but there intact flow-related enhancement distally (*arrow*), indicating patency of the vessel

12.1.2 Indirect Extracranial-Intracranial Revascularization

12.1.2.1 Discussion

Indirect surgical revascularization can be performed as part of complex aneurysm obliteration and moyamoya disease primarily in adults. There are several methods for establishing indirect revascularization, including multiple burr holes, encephaloduromyosynangiosis, and encephaloduroarteriosynangiosis/pial synangiosis, among others.

Creating burr multiple holes (Fig. 12.6) can promote neovascularization to the brain surface. On post-contrast images, enhancement across the burr holes can be appreciated and ADC maps can show increased diffusivity. Depending on the particular technique, favorable results are achieved in nearly 90% of cases. However, in some cases, the delicate anastomoses may not provide sufficient revascularization, and cerebral infarction may result as the underlying disease process ensues.

Encephaloduroarteriomyosynangiosis (EDAMS) consists of creating a linear craniotomy, narrow dural opening, and placing temporalis muscle flaps directly upon the exposed pial surface to stimulate collateral development (Fig. 12.7). The superficial temporal artery and attached flap are then sutured to the dura. Alternatively, encephalomyosynangiosis (EMS) can be performed for increasing both intracranial and extracranial collateral circulation by

inserting the temporal muscle deep to the craniotomy flap directly upon surface of the brain. During the early postoperative period, the swollen muscle can exert mild mass effect upon the underlying brain parenchyma (Fig. 12.8). Postoperative angiography reveals good revascularization in the majority of cases.

Encephaloduroarteriosynangiosis (EDAS)/pial synangiosis consists of creating a defect in the dura and arachnoid to enable direct suturing of the superficial temporal artery to the pia (Fig. 12.9). Following successful synangiosis, angiography shows progressive reduced flow in the moyamoya vessels and increase in size of the superficial temporal artery.

Angiography is well suited for monitoring the effects of synangiosis. Indeed, the angiographic findings of synangiosis are characteristic and include early filling of the middle cerebral artery branches via ECA injection, enlargement of the superficial temporal artery and middle meningeal artery, and the presence of transpial or transdural collateral vessels. Progression of proximal MCA or ICA stenosis is often apparent despite a successful surgical and clinical outcome, presumably due to diverted blood flow through the ECA circulation. In fact, the lack of MCA or ICA stenosis is associated with a relatively poor outcome. CT and MRI can be used to assess for complications, which include recurrence of ischemic events and chronic subdural hematomas.

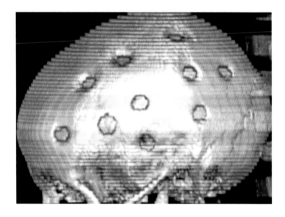

Fig. 12.6 Multiple burr holes for encephalogaleoperiosteal synangiosis. 3D CT image shows multiple left calvarial burr holes

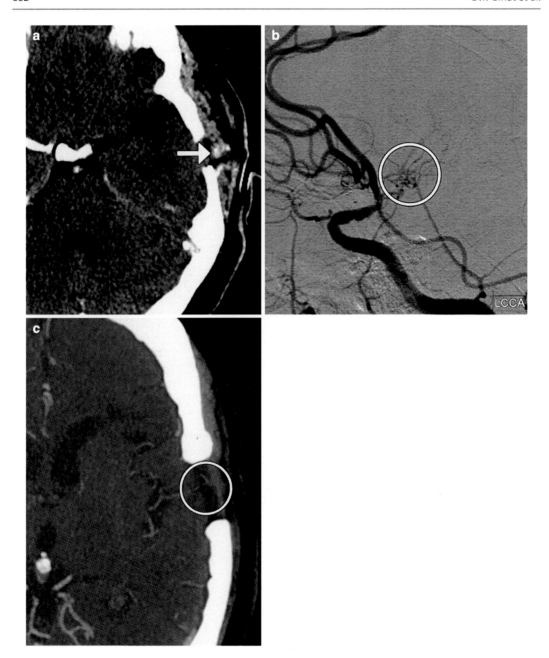

Fig. 12.7 Encephaloduromyosynangiosis. The patient has a history of left MCA occlusion as well as right MCA and ACA stenosis. The patient was managed medically but recently developed repeated episodes of transient ischemic attacks to the left hemisphere. Consequently, an onlay external to internal carotid artery bypass with myosynangiosis was performed. Specifically, a direct anastomosis was not feasible due to lack of adequately patent cortical branches. Rather, the superficial temporal artery branch was placed over the brain surface along with its fascial cuff. This was done after multiple openings were made in the arachnoid to allow for percolation of cerebrospinal fluid. In addition, the temporalis muscle flaps were placed on the exposed brain surface to allow for additional synangiosis. Axial CTA image (**a**) performed shortly after surgery shows a left temporal microcraniotomy and temporalis muscle flap with a superficial temporal artery branch and fascial cuff (*arrow*) juxtaposed against the brain surface. Lateral digital subtraction angiography imaged obtained by injection through the left common carotid artery 3 months after surgery (**b**) demonstrates small collateral vessels (*encircled*) communicating between the intracranial and extracranial arteries. Axial CTA obtained 9 months after surgery (**c**) also shows formation of small collateral vessels (*encircled*) that bridge the temporal lobe cortex and temporalis muscle

Fig 12.8 Encephalomyosynangiosis. Coronal CT image obtained during the early postoperative period shows the left temporalis muscle (*arrow*) tunneled under the left craniotomy flap, where it exerts mild mass effect upon the brain parenchyma

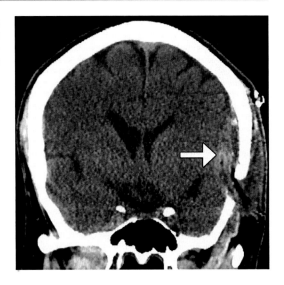

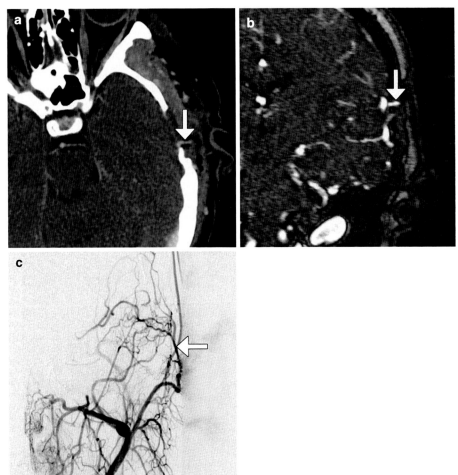

Fig. 12.9 Encephaloduroarteriosynangiosis/pial synangiosis. Axial CTA image (**a**) and coronal (**c**) contrast-enhanced MRA image (**b**) show the left superficial temporal artery (*arrows*) passing through the small craniotomy defect to contact the pial surface of the brain. The prominent left superficial temporal artery (*arrow*) supplying the pial surface of the brain is also well depicted on the digital subtraction angiogram (**c**) from an external carotid artery injection

12.1.3 Intracranial Aneurysm Wrapping

12.1.3.1 Discussion

The concept of wrapping aneurysms with strips of muscle tissue was first introduced by Cushing as a treatment of ruptured aneurysms. The temporalis muscle is an accessible source of the necessary tissue. Alternatively, muslin has also been used as a wrapping material. Since the 1980s, the practice of wrapping aneurysms has declined in popularity. Nevertheless, muscle wrapping is still used as a last resort for treatment of aneurysms when endovascular stenting/embolization or surgical clipping is not feasible.

Following aneurysm wrapping surgery, the aneurysm will typically appear about the same size or perhaps slightly smaller, since the main goal of the procedure is to prevent further expansion. Although the muscle wrap itself is often inconspicuous, it should not be confused with tumor or other abnormalities, such as hemorrhage, on imaging (Fig. 12.10). However, the wrap can resorb and allow aneurysm expansion and bleeding. Other complications include infection or foreign body reaction, if synthetic materials are used. Thus, the role of imaging following aneurysm wrapping is to evaluate for integrity of the wrap, aneurysm expansion or hemorrhage, and abscess or muslinoma formation.

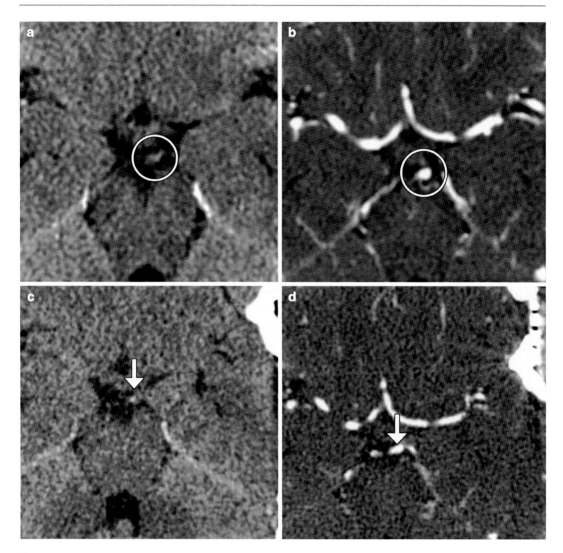

Fig. 12.10 Muscle wrap. The patient had a history of a growing left P1 segment aneurysm. Although aneurysm clipping was planned, muscle wrap was instead performed because clipping posed significant risk of occlusion of the thalamic perforator or constriction of the left P1 segment. Temporalis muscle was harvested. Preoperative axial CT (**a**) and CTA (**b**) images demonstrate an aneurysm arising from the posterosuperior aspect of the left P1 segment (*encircled*). Postoperative axial CT (**c**) and CTA (**d**) images show left temporal craniotomy and interval placement of the muscle wrap, which appears as soft tissue attenuation material surrounding the aneurysm and partially filling the left quadrigeminal plate cistern (*arrows*). The aneurysm is slightly less prominent than before surgery

12.1.4 Aneurysm Clipping and Hemostatic Ligation Clips

12.1.4.1 Discussion

Aneurysm clips are used to occlude the neck of aneurysms in order to prevent or cease hemorrhage due to rupture. These devices are available in a variety of shapes and sizes. They consist of a hinged wire with parallel ends that are straight or curved. In the past, aneurysm clips were composed of stainless steel or tungsten. Although these materials are biocompatible, they are not MRI compatible. These clips also produce considerable beam-hardening artifact that can obscure surrounding structures. Newer clips are composed of non-ferromagnetic materials, such as titanium, which are MRI compatible and produce fewer artifacts on CT.

Surgery for aneurysm clipping consists of performing a craniotomy. In addition, variable amounts of the anterior clinoid process may be resected in order to access paraclinoid aneurysms (Fig. 12.11). Deeply positioned aneurysms can be difficult to attain for clipping, which can result in aneurysm remnants. Incomplete clipping can present as increased hemorrhage shortly after clipping of ruptured aneurysms, for example, and can be addressed by endovascular embolization (Fig. 12.12). Although the brain can be retracted in order to maximize the field of view and access for centrally located aneurysms, vascular injury can result. Likewise, vessels adjacent to aneurysms that have poor visibility can be inadver-

tently clipped, such as the recurrent artery of Heubner, which can result in caudate infarcts (Fig. 12.13).

Vasospasm is a significant source of morbidity in patients with ruptured cerebral aneurysms and typically manifests 7–10 days after the episode of subarachnoid hemorrhage. Transcranial Doppler ultrasound is routinely used to assess for cerebral vasospasm, but the modality has limited sensitivity and specificity. CTA is also commonly implemented for the detection of cerebral vasospasm following subarachnoid hemorrhage and may demonstrate multifocal steno-occlusive lesions and areas of hemorrhage (Fig. 12.14). In addition, CT perfusion can be performed concurrently to provide insight into the extent of cerebral ischemia resulting from vasospasm. Unfortunately, streak artifact from the aneurysm clip can limit the assessment of the adjacent vasculature. Ultimately, catheter-based angiography has been considered to be the historical gold standard to diagnose vasospasm.

The incidence of recurrent aneurysms after complete clipping is approximately is low, but this complication can lead to subarachnoid hemorrhage and requires repeat clipping or endovascular intervention. It is also important to carefully search for new aneurysms on postoperative scans, since the annual rate of de novo aneurysm formation is about 0.9%. These occur on average at about 10 years after surgery. Thus, long-term angiographic follow-up is warranted in patients with clipped aneurysms.

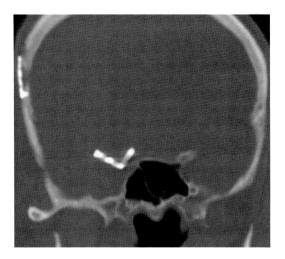

Fig. 12.11 Anterior clinoid process resection. Coronal CT image shows absence of the right anterior clinoid process and a right curved-tip aneurysm clip

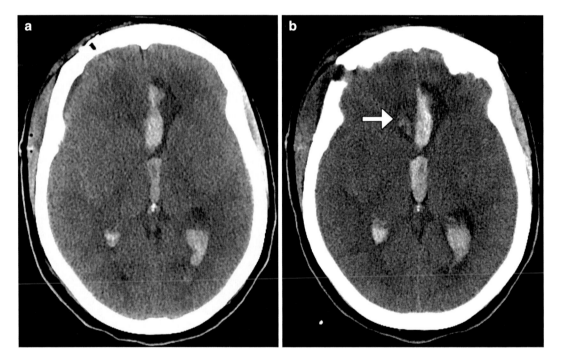

Fig. 12.12 Incomplete aneurysm clipping. Axial CT image at initial presentation (**a**) shows hemorrhage into the left frontal lobe (*arrow*) and in the ventricular system due to aneurysm rupture. Axial CT image obtained shortly after anterior communicating artery aneurysm clipping (**b**) shows new hemorrhage in the right frontal lobe. Digital subtraction angiogram (**c**) shows residual filling of the aneurysm sac (*encircled*) adjacent to the clip. The residual aneurysm sac was then embolized (**d**)

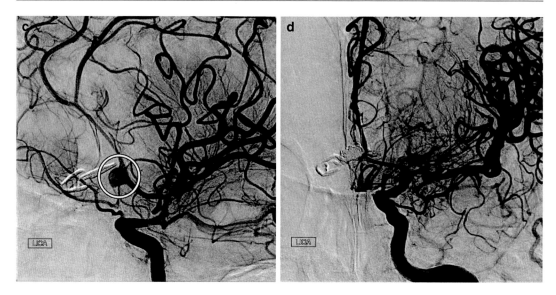

Fig. 12.12 (continued)

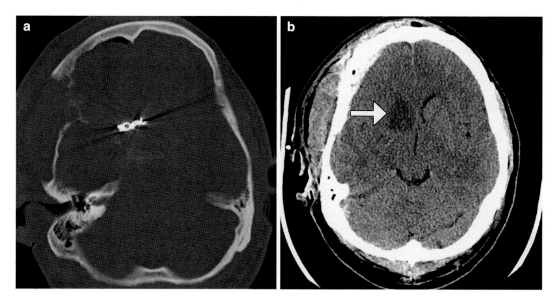

Fig. 12.13 Adjacent vessel clipping. Axial CT images (**a, b**) show an anterior communicating artery clip and a recent right caudate infarct (*arrow*) due to recurrent artery of Heubner compromise

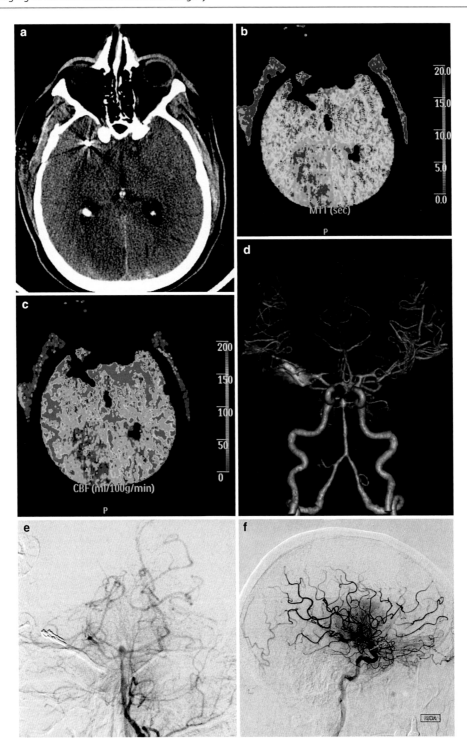

Fig. 12.14 Vasospasm. Axial CT image (**a**) obtained 1 week after clipping of a ruptured cerebral aneurysm shows areas of hypoattenuation in multiple vascular territories and scattered subarachnoid hemorrhage. The MTT (**b**) and CBF (**c**) maps show perfusion deficits in the bilateral anterior cerebral artery and right posterior cerebral artery territories. The CTA (**d**) and digital subtraction angiography images (**e, f**) show severe vasospasm in the anterior and posterior cerebral vessels, with relatively less pronounced involvement of the middle cerebral artery territories

12.1.5 Vascular Malformation Surgery

When possible, microsurgical resection is the optimal treatment option for arteriovenous malformations and cavernous malformations. While the nidus of the arteriovenous malformation represents the target of resection, the remaining draining vein can be clipped for hemostasis (Fig. 12.15). However, proximal ligation of the supplying arteries alone can make subsequent embolization more difficult and may rapidly lead to revascularization. For inoperable arteriovenous malformations that require treatment, stereotactic radiosurgery is an alternative. This treatment essentially results in thrombosis of the malformation. Further, sometimes radiation necrosis can result, which may appear as a peripherally enhancing lesion with surrounding vasogenic edema (Fig. 12.16).

With respect to cavernous malformations, developmental venous anomalies are often incidental findings that are not generally considered targets for treatment. However, seizure outcome after resection of cavernous malformations is better when surrounding hemosiderin-stained brain also is removed, although this can be challenging when critical structures are involved (Fig. 12.17).

Head and neck lymphatic malformations are often transspatial and are often not amenable to complete surgical resection. However, when lymphatic malformations compromise critical structures, such as the airway, partial resection may be performed. MRI is a suitable modality for accurate delineation of the residual tumor, which is useful for planning subsequent additional surgery or sclerotherapy if needed (Fig. 12.18). Obtaining up-to-date imaging is particularly relevant since the lesions often evolve spontaneously, with new and enlarging components.

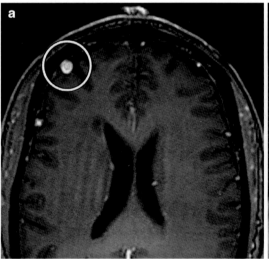
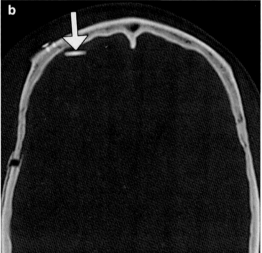

Fig 12.15 Arteriovenous malformation resection. The patient has a history of a right frontal lobe arteriovenous malformation. Preoperative axial post-contrast T1-weighted MRI (**a**) shows an enlarged draining right cortical vein (*encircled*). Postoperative axial CT image (**b**) shows a Weck clip (*arrow*) used to ligate the vein during surgery

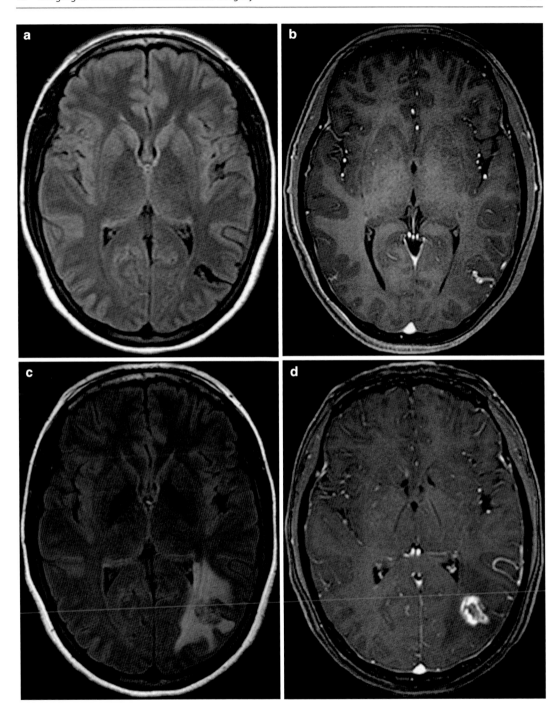

Fig 12.16 Arteriovenous malformation stereotactic radiosurgery with radiation necrosis. Pretreatment axial FLAIR (**a**) and post-contrast T1-weighted (**b**) MR images show a left temporo-occipital nidus. Posttreatment FLAIR (**c**) and post-contrast T1-weighted (**d**) MR images show interval development of extensive vasogenic edema surrounding a peripherally enhancing lesion due to radiation necrosis at the site of the arteriovenous malformation, which is no longer apparent

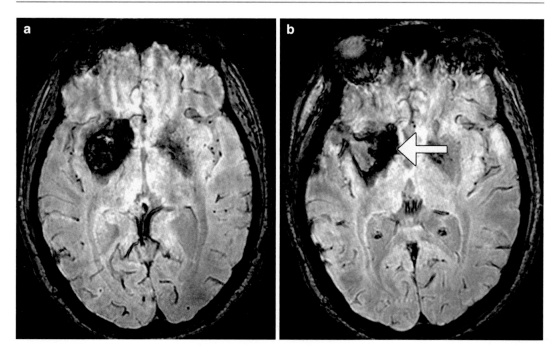

Fig. 12.17 Residual hemosiderin staining after cavernous malformation surgery. Preoperative SWI MRI (**a**) shows a large right basal ganglia cavernous malformation. Postoperative SWI MRI (**b**) shows that the bulk of the cavernous malformation is no longer present, but there is abundant peripheral hemosiderin staining that remains (*arrow*)

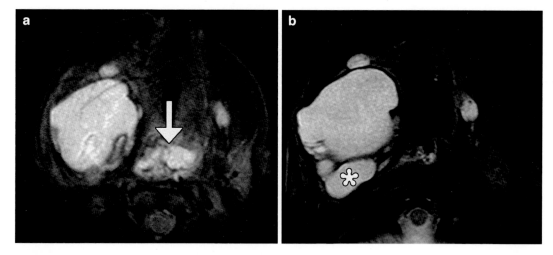

Fig. 12.18 Partial resection of lymphatic malformation. Preoperative axial T2-weighted MRI (**a**) shows a transspatial macrocystic lesion with a component that obstructs the upper airway (*arrow*). Postoperative axial T2-weighted MRI (**b**) shows successful resection of the component of the lymphatic malformation that compromised the airway but interval appearance of an adjacent cystic component (*)

12.1.6 Microvascular Decompression/Jannetta Procedure

12.1.6.1 Discussion

Microvascular decompression can be used to effectively treat vascular loop syndromes, such as trigeminal neuralgia and glossopharyngeal neuralgia (Figs. 12.19, 12.20, and 12.21). The technique essentially consists of interposing Teflon between the affected nerve and the offending vessel. The concept behind this procedure is that the Teflon distances and redirects the transmitted pulsation of the adjacent artery away from the nerve. Teflon is hyperattenuating on CT and low signal intensity on all MRI sequences. High-resolution T2-weighted MRI sequences are particularly useful for analyzing the position of the pledgets and altered anatomy, which often entails distortion of the nerve course. During the early postoperative period, reversible elevated T2 signal and restricted diffusion is often observed in the ipsilateral pons after trigeminal decompression and does not necessarily indicate infarction. Perhaps the most common complication of microvascular decompression is recurrent symptoms related to suboptimal pledget positioning (Fig. 12.22). For example, in patients with persistent hemifacial spasm after microvascular decompression, residual vascular compression is most commonly encountered proximal to the pledget, along the attached segment of the nerve. Hearing loss is a more unusual complication that can result from Teflon migration or the use of excess Teflon that compresses cranial nerve 8 within the internal auditory canal (Fig. 12.23). Granulomas can occasionally form in reaction to the presence of Teflon, which forms a mass that has low T2 signal and enhances (Fig. 12.24).

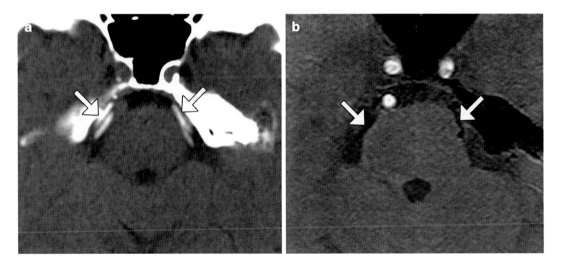

Fig. 12.19 Microvascular decompression for trigeminal neuralgia. Axial CT (**a**) and 3D time-of-flight MRA (**b**) show Teflon pledgets in the region of the bilateral trigeminal nerve root entry zones (*arrows*)

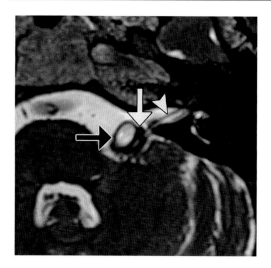

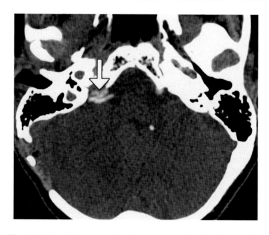

Fig. 12.21 Microvascular decompression for glossopharyngeal neuralgia. Axial CT image shows pledgets (*arrow*) used to isolate the right glossopharyngeal nerve root entry zone from surrounding vessels

Fig. 12.20 Microvascular decompression for hemifacial spasm. Axial CISS MRI shows Teflon (*white arrow*) interposed between the left facial nerve (*arrowhead*) and the enlarged, tortuous basilar artery (*black arrow*)

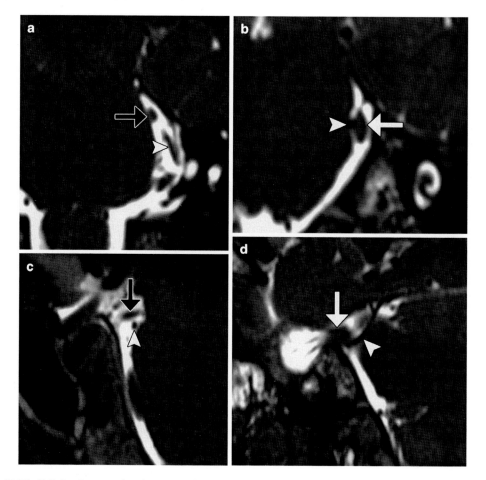

Fig. 12.22 Failed microvascular decompression. The patient presented with persistent symptoms of trigeminal neuralgia following attempted decompression. Coronal (**a, b**) and sagittal (**c, d**) CISS (thin section) MR images show that the pledget (*black arrows*) is positioned superior to the superior cerebellar artery (*arrowheads*), which directly contacts the left trigeminal nerve (*white arrows*)

Fig. 12.23 Cochlear nerve compression after microvascular decompression. The patient presented with hearing loss after microvascular decompression via Teflon injection for hemifacial spasm. Axial CT image shows a large amount of Teflon in the left cerebellopontine angle, which enters the internal auditory canal (*arrow*), presumably compressing the cranial nerve 8

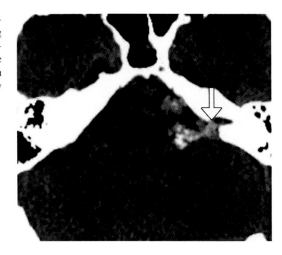

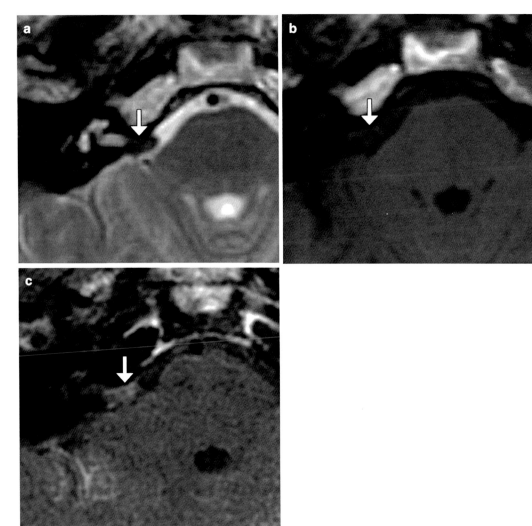

Fig. 12.24 Teflon granuloma. Axial T2-weighted MRI (**a**) shows a globular hypointense lesion in the right cerebellopontine angle cistern (*arrow*). Axial pre- (**b**) and post-contrast T1-weighted (**c**) MR images show corresponding mild enhancement of the lesion (*arrows*)

12.1.7 Carotid Endarterectomy

12.1.7.1 Discussion

Carotid endarterectomy (CEA) is considered the treatment of choice for symptomatic and asymptomatic patients with high-grade carotid artery stenosis. In order to appropriately interpret imaging studies obtained following CEA, it is helpful to be familiar with the surgical techniques involved.

CEA can be performed through an incision made anterior to the sternocleidomastoid and ligation of the facial vein in order to expose the carotid bifurcation and clamping of the carotid artery distal to the endarterectomy. Consequently, a small hematoma within or adjacent to the sternocleidomastoid and mild circumferential narrowing of the carotid artery resulting from clamp placement during surgery can be appreciated on follow-up CT (Fig. 12.25). These findings are usually self-limited.

CEA involves opening the carotid artery, removing the plaque and associated endothelium, and suturing the vessel wall closed with or without an enlargement patch. The patch is usually composed of Dacron, which is not readily visible on CT, but can appear as a thin hyperechoic mesh on ultrasound (Fig. 12.26). Alternatively, the section of carotid artery that is resected can be reconstructed using a saphenous vein graft. This has a distinct patulous or bulbous appearance on imaging (Fig. 12.27).

Complications related to CEA include localized intimal flap or dissection, reperfusion syndrome, patch infection, restenosis, cerebral infarction, and cranial nerve injury, usually facial and hypoglossal (Figs. 12.28, 12.29, 12.30, 12.31, 12.32, and 12.33).

Wound infection following carotid endarterectomy occurs in about 2% of cases. *Staphylococcus* species are the most common causative organisms. Patients typically present with wound swelling, drainage, and fever. On imaging, abscess appears as a fluid collection that abuts the surgical site. Characteristic rim enhancement and cellulitis are often present. There may also be debris, septations, and draining sinus that extends from the operative bed to the incision. Wound abscesses usually resolve with antibiotics and debridement. However, periarterial abscess or patch infection may predispose to dehiscence of the suture line, resulting in pseudoaneurysm formation.

Hyperperfusion or reperfusion syndrome is an unusual complication of carotid endarterectomy or carotid artery stenting, occurring in 0.3–1.2% of cases. A possible etiology for this condition is impaired cerebrovascular autoregulation. Predisposing factors include severe underlying cerebrovascular disease, diabetes mellitus, longstanding hypertension, prolonged cross clamping during endarterectomy, and a greater than 100% increase in the degree of reestablished cerebral blood flow, which is usually associated with greater than 90% carotid artery stenosis. Patients may present with headaches, seizures, focal neurological deficits, or confusion within several days after surgery. Patients may recover completely if the diagnosis is made promptly. However, in some series, there is a mortality rate of up to 50%. The diagnosis of cerebral hyperperfusion syndrome can be suggested on CT in the proper setting by noting the presence of edema, often in the watershed zones ipsilateral to the side of surgery. On MRI, focal ipsilateral vasogenic edema is apparent. Diffusion-weighted imaging and apparent diffusion coefficient maps help confirm the presence of vasogenic edema. On MRA, prominent vessels on the affected side may be apparent. Similarly, perfusion-weighted imaging can depict the relative increased flow to the affected side. The finding of hemorrhage portends a poor prognosis. Imaging can help identify hyperperfusion syndrome before serious sequelae result. Differential considerations for the imaging appearance of cerebral hyperperfusion syndrome include hypertensive encephalopathy, cyclosporine toxicity, and eclampsia. The lack of restricted diffusion helps exclude cerebral ischemia.

Recurrent stenosis after carotid endarterectomy occurs at the rate of about 1% per year. This complication is the main limitation of carotid endarterectomy and predisposes to cerebrovascular ischemia. Acute thrombotic occlusion is much less common and is a potentially devastating complication that can result in cerebral infection. Conventional carotid end-

arterectomy with patch angioplasty and the use of lipid-lowering pharmaceuticals are associated with lower rates of restenosis. Risk factors for restenosis include female gender and renal failure. CTA, MRA, and Doppler ultrasound are all appropriate for evaluation of suspected restenosis or occlusion after carotid endarterectomy. Each of these modalities has advantages and disadvantages. CTA with reformats, especially the curved planar reformats, is useful for studying stenoses. In the setting of carotid endarterectomy with patching, the internal carotid artery velocities on Doppler ultrasound must be interpreted with caution, since these are normally higher than in the nonoperated counterparts. MRA is best suited for identifying pseudo-occlusions.

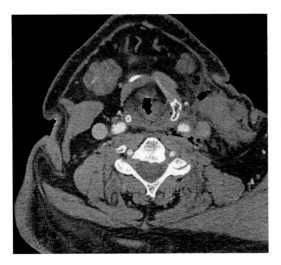

Fig. 12.25 Expected carotid endarterectomy early postoperative changes. Axial contrast CT after recent CEA demonstrates several foci of air scattered within and adjacent to the surgical bed, left sternocleidomastoid swelling, and edema in the fat planes

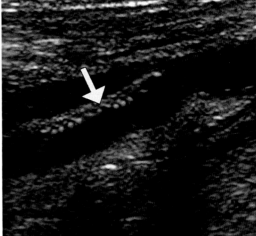

Fig. 12.26 Patch endarterectomy ultrasound image shows the echogenic Dacron patch (*arrow*) in the proximal internal carotid artery

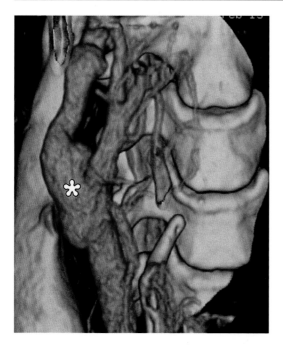

Fig. 12.27 Endarterectomy with saphenous vein graft. 3D CT image shows a patulous reconstructed right carotid bifurcation (*)

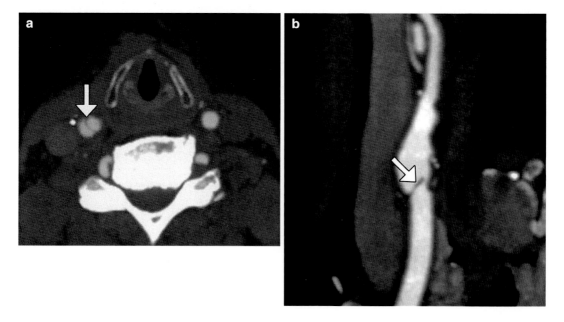

Fig. 12.28 Localized intimal flap. Axial (**a**) and curved planar reformatted (**b**) CT images show a linear filling defect (*arrows*) at the junction of the endarterectomy patch and native carotid artery

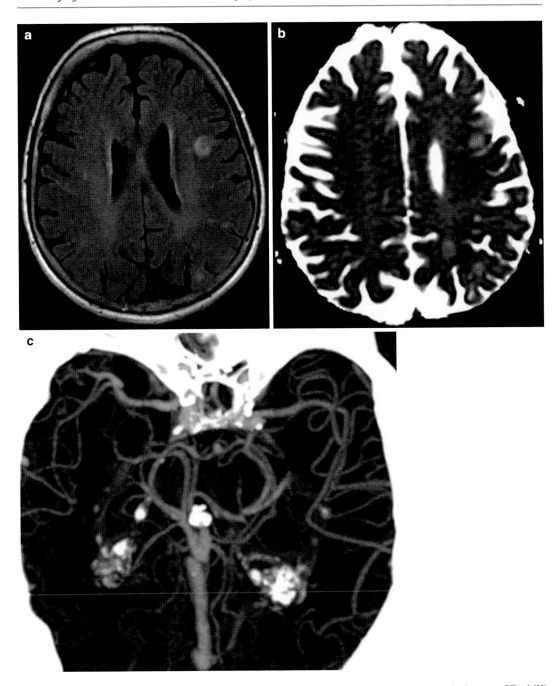

Fig. 12.29 Reperfusion syndrome. The patient presented with acute onset of seizures 1 week status post left carotid endarterectomy . Axial FLAIR MRI (**a**) and ADC map (**b**) show areas of high T2 signal with elevated diffusivity in the left cerebral hemisphere watershed zones. CTA MIP image (**c**) shows asymmetrically prominent left middle cerebral artery branches diffusely

Fig. 12.30 Patch infection. The patient presented with fever, swelling, and purulent drainage from the left carotid endarterectomy incision site. Axial CT image shows a rim-enhancing fluid collection (*arrow*) surrounding the left carotid artery surgical bed

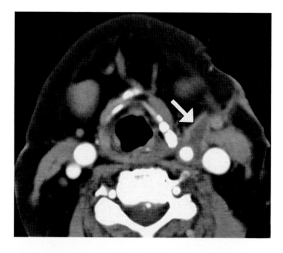

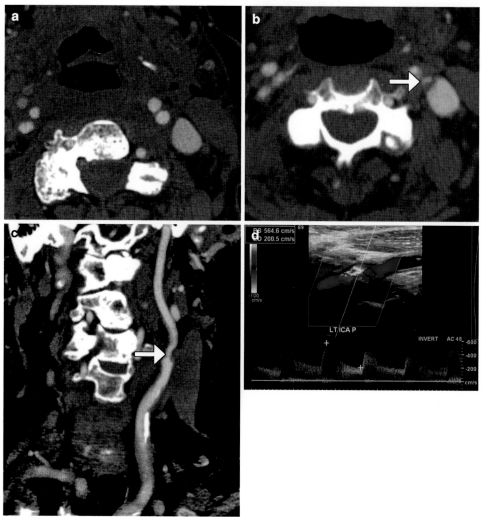

Fig. 12.31 Carotid artery restenosis. Initial postoperative axial CTA image (**a**) shows a patent proximal left internal carotid artery. Axial (**b**) and curved planar reformatted (**c**) CTA images obtained 6 months later now show focal high-grade stenosis at the origin of the left internal carotid artery due to low-density plaque at the site of reanastomosis (*arrows*). Doppler ultrasound (**d**) confirms the presence of high-grade stenosis of the proximal internal carotid artery with turbulent flow and velocities surpassing 500 cm/s

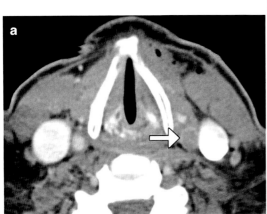

Fig. 12.32 Post-endarterectomy carotid artery occlusion and cerebral infarction. Delayed phase axial CTA image (**a**) shows occlusion of the CCA at the site of recent CEA (*arrow*). The diffusion-weighted image (**b**) shows an associated left internal capsule/insula infarction (*arrow*)

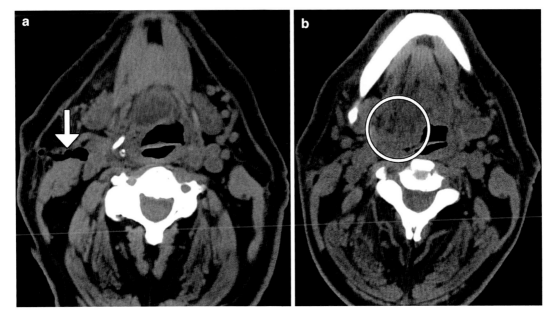

Fig. 12.33 Cranial nerve injury. The patient presented with right cranial nerve XII deficit after right internal carotid endarterectomy. Initial postoperative axial CT image (**a**) shows that the endarterectomy was performed at the expected level of the right hypoglossal nerve (*arrow*). A subsequent axial CT image (**b**) shows prolapse and fatty infiltration of the right hemi-tongue (*encircled*)

12.1.8 Carotid Body Stimulation

12.1.8.1 Discussion

Electrical stimulation of the carotid sinus can be used to treat systemic hypertension that is unresponsive to medical therapy. The phenomenon is effectuated by initiating the baroreceptor reflex and decreasing sympathetic tone. Implanted carotid sinus stimulation systems comprise a pulse generator and bilateral perivascular carotid sinus leads (Fig. 12.34). Insertion of these devices does not appear to cause carotid artery injury or other major side effects.

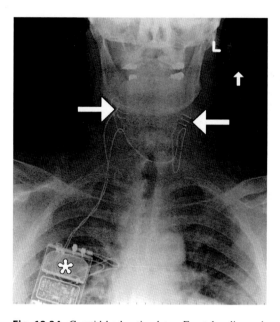

Fig. 12.34 Carotid body stimulator. Frontal radiograph shows a Rheos device with bilateral carotid sinus electrodes (*arrows*) and pulse generator in the right chest subcutaneous tissues (*)

12.1.9 Adjustable Vascular Clamp

12.1.9.1 Discussion

Adjustable vascular clamps were first introduced in the 1950s for treating carotid system aneurysms. Several varieties of metallic extracranial carotid vascular clamps have been developed, including the Selverstone, Crutchfield, Poppen-Blaylock, Salibi, and Kindt. The principle behind such vascular clamps is to reduce blood flow and to promote clotting of the aneurysm. If collateral circulation via the circle of Willis is inadequate, the clamps can be loosened. Gradual, graded occlusion of the carotids would yield better results than immediate occlusion. Over time, however, carotid revascularization can occur through the clamp and regular follow-up is recommended. On imaging, the clamps are recognized as rectangle-shaped metallic parts with central openings of variable sizes (Fig. 12.35). The lumen distal to the clamp becomes diffusely narrowed and usually remains as such even after the clamp is removed.

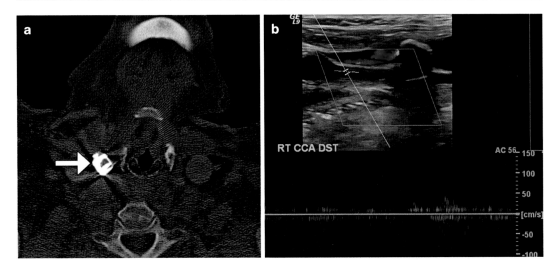

Fig. 12.35 Selverstone clamp. The patient has a history of right carotid body paraganglioma status post radiation and right common carotid artery aneurysm status post application of vascular clamp. Axial CT image (**a**) dem- onstrates a right common carotid artery clamp (*arrow*). Doppler ultrasound (**b**) shows paucity of flow in the common carotid artery distal to the clamp

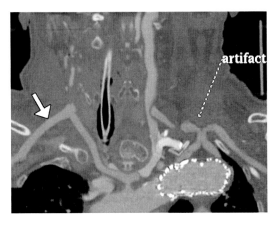

Fig. 12.36 Aberrant right subclavian artery reconstruc- tion. Curved planar reformatted image shows a right axil- lary to right common carotid artery bypass (*arrow*) with retrograde opacification of the proximal axillary and distal right subclavian arteries. The proximal right subclavian artery has been sacrificed. There is also a left common carotid to subclavian artery bypass and an aortic endo- graft. There is artifactual duplication of the proximal left subclavian artery

12.1.10 Reconstruction of the Great Vessels

12.1.10.1 Discussion

Reconstruction of the great vessels may be per- formed for treatment of steno-occlusive lesions of congenital aberrations. The surgical maneu- vers can be complicated and involve reimplanta- tion of normal vessels onto others (Fig. 12.36) and/or the use of bypass grafts, such as collagen- impregnated Dacron and polytetrafluoroethylene (Figs. 12.37 and 12.38), each with different imaging appearing. Postoperative MRA, CTA, Doppler ultrasound, or catheter angiography can be used to evaluate suspected restenosis or occlu- sion (Fig. 12.39).

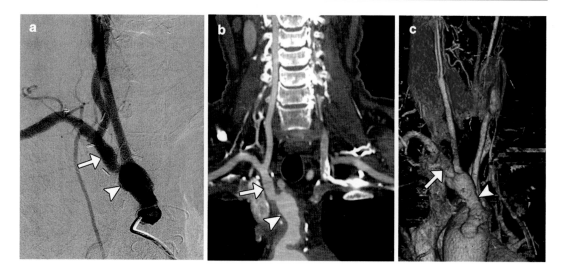

Fig. 12.37 Dacron graft. The patient has a history of symptomatic right common carotid and innominate artery occlusive disease. The patient is status post recent aorta to right common carotid/right subclavian artery bypass from the ascending aorta utilizing a 10 mm Hemashield graft. The innominate artery underwent endarterectomy and end-to-end anastomosis with the 10 mm Hemashield, which in turn was anastomosed to the ascending aorta, also end to end. Catheter angiogram (**a**) shows a widely patent Hemashield graft (*arrow*) and distal vessels (*arrowhead*). CT angiography curved vessel trace (**b**) and 3D volume rendering (**c**) show patency of the aorta to right common carotid bypass components. The Hemashield graft (*arrowheads*) is a short bulbous segment connected to the stump of the innominate artery (*arrows*)

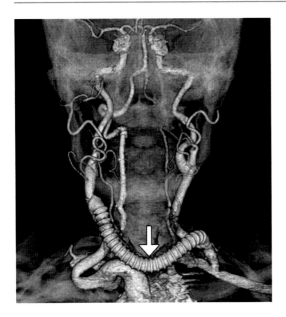

Fig. 12.38 Debranching of cerebral vessels, right-to-left common carotid artery crossover bypass, and left common carotid artery transposition to the left subclavian artery for treatment of thoracoabdominal aortic dissection. The 3D CTA reformatted image shows the crossover polytetrafluoroethylene bypass graft (*arrow*)

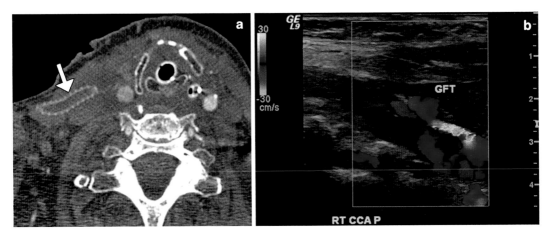

Fig. 12.39 Thrombosed graft. The patient is status post aortic repair and subclavian injury followed by placement of a right carotid to axillary bypass graft with 6 mm externally supported polytetrafluoroethylene. Axial CTA image (**a**) shows lack of enhancement within the artificial graft (*arrow*), which is suggestive of thrombosis. There is also poor opacification of the distal right common carotid artery. Doppler ultrasound (**b**) of the distal graft anastomosis site reveals paucity of flow through the graft (*GFT*)

12.2 Endovascular Surgery

12.2.1 General Imaging Considerations Following Endovascular Cerebrovascular Procedures

Endovascular cerebrovascular procedures include endovascular reconstruction or deconstruction for cerebrovascular occlusive disease or active bleeding using stents or embolic material; embolization of tumors, aneurysms, or vascular malformations either preoperatively or for treatment; and mechanical or chemical thrombolysis for acute ischemic stroke or vasospasm. Materials that are typically used during neuroendovascular procedures include metal containing devices, such as coils, plugs, and stents, liquid embolic agents, balloons, and particles. Certain metals contained in some of these endovascular treatment modalities create substantial streak artifact on CT, rendering imaging less sensitive to vascular assessment. Most intracranial endovascular devices create relatively less artifact on MRI compared to CT. For example, embolic coils used in aneurysm are predominantly made of platinum. These have only mild susceptibility effect on MRI/MRA. Indeed, MRA is an effective means to assess small degrees of aneurysm recurrence following coil embolization (Fig. 12.40). Most intracranial stents have relatively low mass, but still produce susceptibility artifacts on MRI, giving the corresponding vessel's intraluminal diameter a false appearance of being narrowed (Fig. 12.41). Liquid embolic agents, such as Onyx, generally produce a signal void on MRA, T1-, and T2-weighted MRI without significant obscuration of adjacent vasculature (Fig. 12.42). However, Onyx HD500 used for treating aneurysms is associated with more susceptibility effect compared to Onyx used for arteriovenous malformation embolization, which can overestimate the degree of stenosis on MRA (Fig. 12.43).

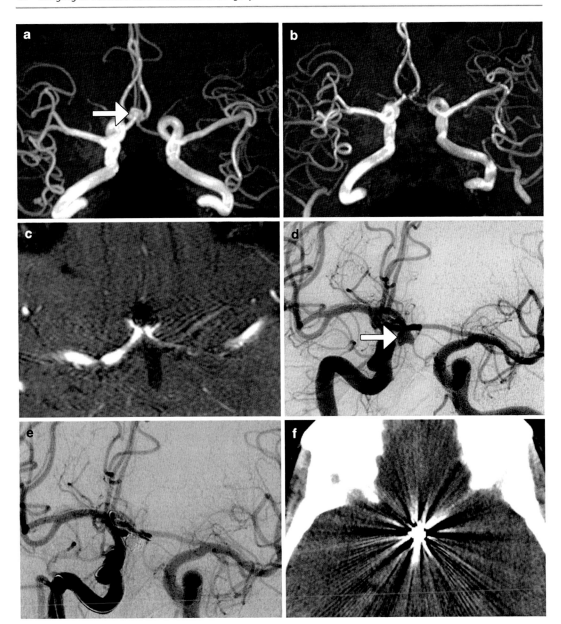

Fig. 12.40 Embolic coil occlusion. MRA before (**a**) and after (**b**, **c**) the anterior communicating artery aneurysm (*arrows*) demonstrate complete occlusion of the aneurysm, as demonstrated on pre- and post-embolization digital subtraction arteriograms (**d**, **e**). Axial CT image (**f**) following aneurysm embolization demonstrates substantial streak artifact which precludes evaluation for early recurrence as opposed to the MRA, which has negligible artifact, allowing for satisfactory evaluation of potential recurrence

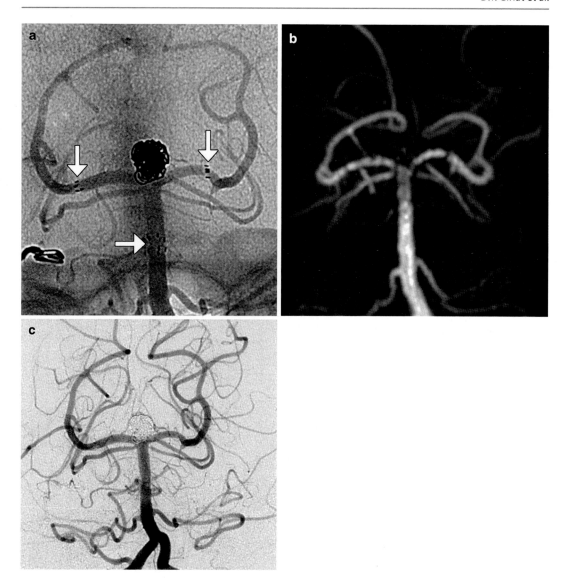

Fig. 12.41 Stents. Unsubtracted angiographic image (**a**) following Y-shaped stent-assisted coiling of a basilar tip aneurysm demonstrates the proximal and distal markers (*arrows*) of the stents as well as coils within the aneurysm. MRA following the procedure (**b**) demonstrates occlusion of the aneurysm with artifact giving a false impression of stenosis along the stent despite lack of evidence for this on digital subtraction angiography (**c**)

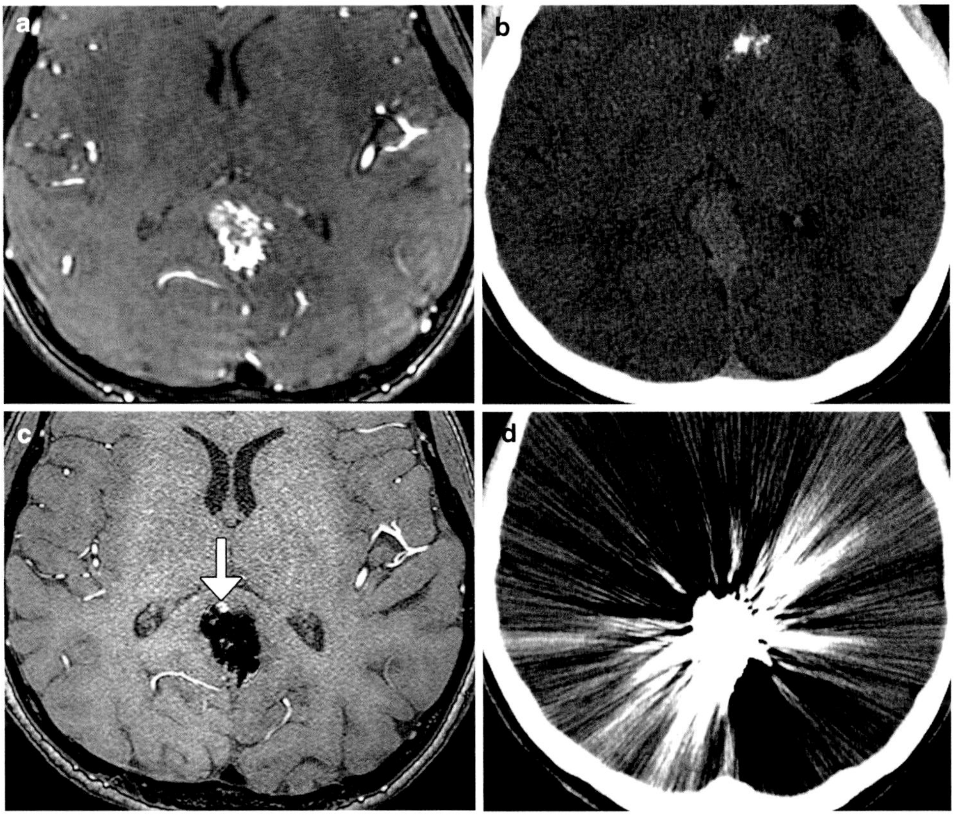

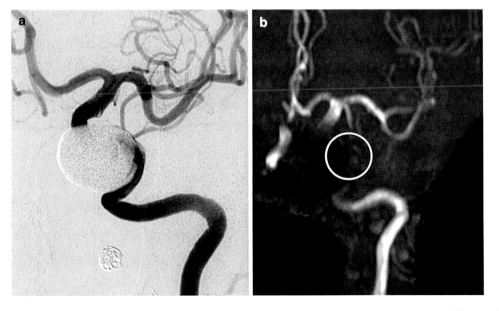

Fig. 12.42 Onyx liquid embolization. Time-of-flight MRA and CT before (**a, b**) and after (**c, d**) embolization of a posterior cingulate gyrus arteriovenous malformation using Onyx. Note that the embolic material creates signifi-cant artifact on CT preventing adequate evaluation, whereas time-of-flight MRA has the ability to detect a residual component of the arteriovenous malformation (*arrow*)

Fig. 12.43 Onyx HD500. Digital subtraction angiogra-phy (**a**) after embolization of a giant aneurysm of the left internal carotid artery cavernous segment demonstrates patency of adjacent vessels, while susceptibility artifact on MRA (**b**) obscures the surrounding vessels (*encircled*)

12.2.2 Endovascular Treatment for Aneurysms

Endovascular occlusion of cerebral aneurysms can be achieved via coil embolization, liquid embolic embolization, or flow-diverting stents (Figs. 12.40, 12.41, 12.43, and 12.44). The number of coils utilized depends on the size of the lesion and the type of coil. For example, fewer hydrogel coils are required than bare metal coils for comparable aneurysm sizes. Stents are sometimes used to support the coils, especially for wide-necked and fusiform aneurysms. Flow-diverting stents, such as the Pipeline and Silk devices, are an option for treating large, wide-necked, or otherwise untreatable aneurysms. The devices provide 30–35% metal coverage of the inner surface of the target vessel with a pore size of 0.02–0.05 mm. The tube mesh implants are believed to achieve their results via functional reconstruction of the parent artery with rerouting of blood flow away from the aneurysm while preserving flow to branch vessels. Although aneurysm opacification is often observed on angiography during the early postoperative period, complete occlusion is achieved in the majority of treated aneurysms by 6 months. Protocols for follow-up imaging after aneurysm coil embolization vary among institutions and include either conventional angiography, CTA, MRA, or a combination of these.

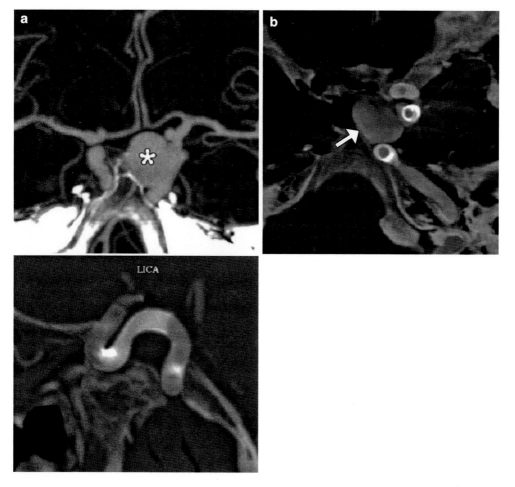

Fig. 12.44 Flow-diverting stent. Preoperative CTA image (**a**) shows a large, wide-necked left supraclinoid internal carotid artery aneurysm (*). CTA obtained at 2 months after Pipeline stent insertion (**b**) shows residual filling of the aneurysm (*arrow*). CTA image obtained 12 months after Pipeline stent insertion (**c**) shows obliteration of the aneurysm

12.2.3 Endovascular Embolization of Arteriovenous Malformations and Fistulas

Liquid embolization agents, such as n-butyl cyanoacrylate, Onyx, and particles, such as polyvinyl alcohol (PVA), are commonly used to treat arteriovenous malformations and fistulas, sometimes in conjunction with coils (Fig. 12.45). Liquid embolic agents that are not inherently radiopaque are often mixed with tantalum powder in order to improve visibility during fluoroscopy. The embolic agent forms casts of the embolized vessel, which is visible on CT due to the tantalum powder and creates a signal void on MRI. The presence of tantalum powder within the liquid agents is responsible for the streak artifact on CT and may require catheter angiography for more definitive assessment. On the other hand, particles, such as PVA, used for embolization are not directly apparent on imaging. In the past, arteriovenous malformations were sometimes treated with Silastic beads, which appear as tiny spherical hyperattenuating structures measuring 1–5 mm in diameter (Fig. 12.46). Clinical improvement could be achieved even without occlusion of symptomatic arteriovenous malformation due to reduction of cerebral steal phenomenon. Furthermore, remaining portions of the malformation can sometimes spontaneously thrombose after treatment and not require further intervention. Otherwise, surgical resection is often performed after partial embolization.

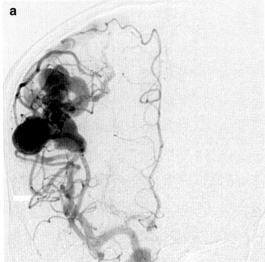

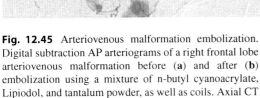

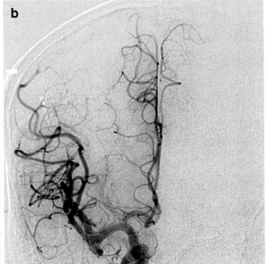

Fig. 12.45 Arteriovenous malformation embolization. Digital subtraction AP arteriograms of a right frontal lobe arteriovenous malformation before (**a**) and after (**b**) embolization using a mixture of n-butyl cyanoacrylate, Lipiodol, and tantalum powder, as well as coils. Axial CT images following the embolization display streak artifact related to the tantalum powder and coils used (**c**) and thrombosis of a large intranidal venous structure (**d**). The AVM did not recur following embolization

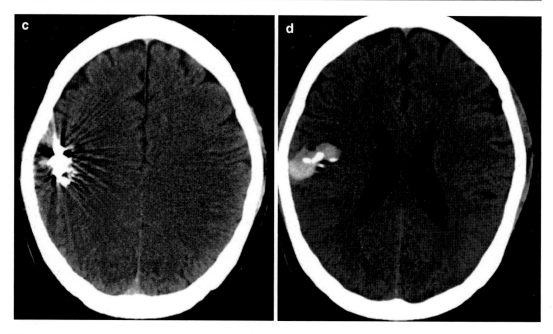

Fig. 12.45 (continued)

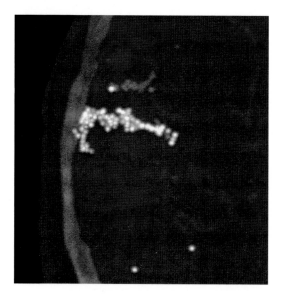

Fig. 12.46 Silastic bead embolization. Axial MIP image shows spherical hyperattenuating foci within an arteriovenous malformation treated many years before

12.2.4 Endovascular Deconstructive Treatment for Vessel Sacrifice

Vessel sacrifice is an accepted method for treatment of cerebrovascular lesions including carotid blowout, aneurysms, dissections, epistaxis, dissection, or preoperatively to facilitate tumor resection. Occlusive materials may include but are not limited to detachable balloons, coils, particles, plugs, or liquid embolic material. When these involve the carotid or vertebral artery, a test occlusion often precedes the vessel sacrifice (balloon test occlusion). Post-procedural findings include identification of the embolic material within the sacrificed vessel. In particular, intra-

vascular detachable balloons have been used to treat intracranial aneurysms, often in conjunction with coil embolization. Detachable balloons are generally used to achieve permanent occlusion. Balloons are usually composed of silicone or latex and can be filled with contrast material in order to increase conspicuity on imaging (Fig. 12.47). Vascular plugs can be used successfully for permanent occlusion of head and neck vessels. Amplatzer vascular plugs, for example, are composed of self-expandable nitinol mesh with one or more lobes and radiopaque platinum markers at each end (Fig. 12.48). Major complications are uncommon and include cerebral infarction, blindness, and cranial nerve palsies.

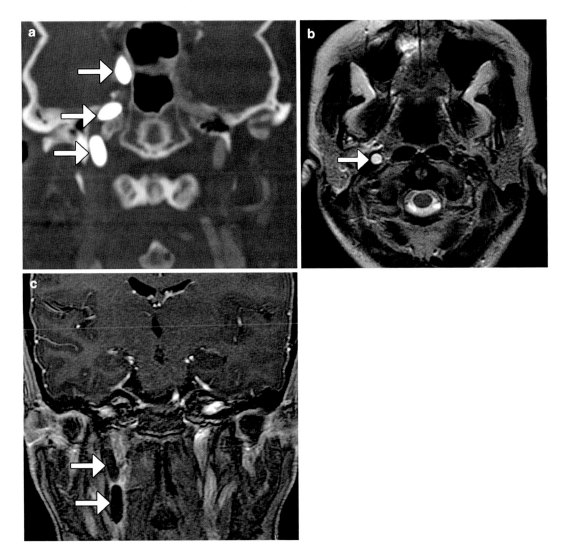

Fig. 12.47 Detachable balloons. CT image (**a**) shows multiple Silastic balloons within the right internal carotid artery (*arrows*). The balloons appear as a high T2 signal (**b**) and low T1 signal (**c**) filling defects in the carotid artery (*arrows*)

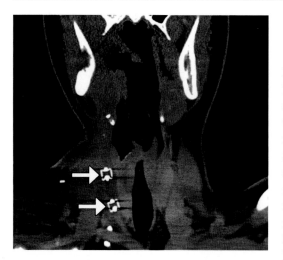

Fig. 12.48 Vascular plugs. Lateral radiograph (**a**) and curved planar reformatted CTA image (**b**) show an Amplatzer plugs (*arrows*) within the right common carotid artery

12.2.5 Preoperative Embolization of Neoplasms

Preoperative embolization of intracranial vascular neoplasms typically uses particles and occasionally liquid embolic material or coils with the aim to occlude vessels within the tumor or immediately proximal to the vascular neoplasm. Since such patients often go to surgery shortly after the embolization, they do not undergo imaging unless symptomatic or for presurgical planning. Possible post-procedural complications include thromboembolic events and intratumoral hemorrhage as well as parent vessel dissection. However, the effects of particle embolization can be apparent. For example, absence of a contrast blush or enhancement due to tumor necrosis indicates successful treatment (Fig. 12.49). Furthermore, restricted diffusion can appear in the embolized tumors due to infarction.

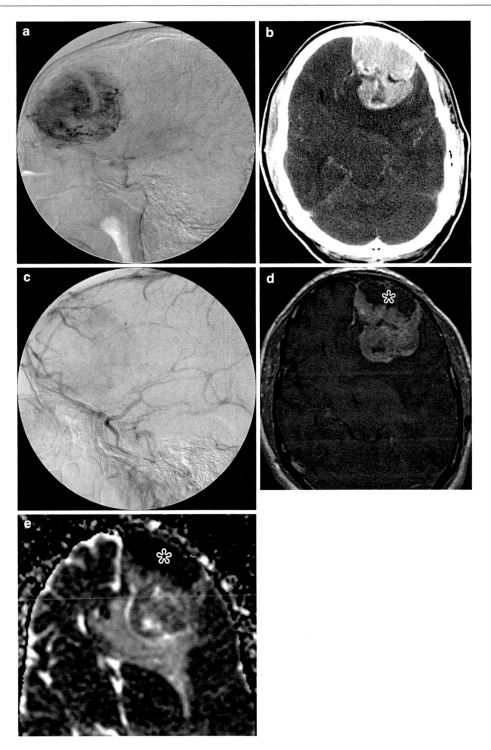

Fig. 12.49 Tumor embolization. The left frontal meningioma underwent PVA particle embolization prior to surgical resection. Pre-embolization DSA image (**a**) shows a strong tumor blush. The corresponding CT with contrast (**b**) shows a large, early homogeneously enhancing left frontal extra-axial mass. Following microparticle embolization of the feeding vessels, there is no longer a tumor blush (**c**). Post-embolization contrast-enhanced T1-weighted MRI (**d**) and ADC map (**e**) images obtained within 24 h of the procedure show a large area of nonenhancement with corresponding restricted diffusion within the meningioma (*), which represents embolization-induced tumor infarction

12.2.6 Endovascular Sclerotherapy for Head and Neck Lymphatic Malformations

Percutaneous sclerotherapy is a minimally invasive means to treat low-flow vascular malformations in the head and neck in which sclerosing agents such as bleomycin, sodium tetradecyl sulfate, and alcohol, among other agents are infused directly into the lesion. Imaging following sclerotherapy for a low-flow vascular malformation of the head and neck is used to identify lesional shrinkage, decreased enhancement, and intralesional fibrosis (Fig. 12.50). MRI is a suitable modality for evaluating treatment response following sclerotherapy in the deep soft tissues, due to the lack of ionizing radiation, excellent soft tissue contrast resolution, and multiplanar

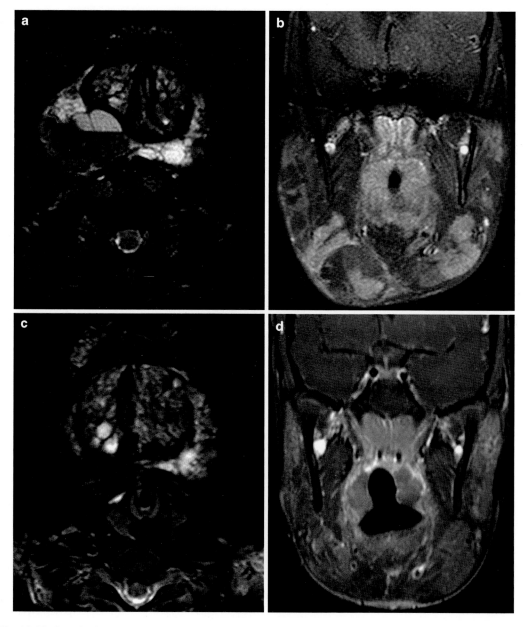

Fig. 12.50 Lymphatic malformation sclerotherapy. STIR and post-contrast fat-suppressed T1-weighted MRI images before (**a**, **b**) and after (**c**, **d**) percutaneous sclero-therapy using sodium tetradecyl sulfate demonstrate involution of the right facial lymphatic malformation

capabilities. MRI is also useful for planning subsequent treatments, if needed.

12.2.7 Endovascular Reconstructive Treatment for Acute Ischemic Stroke Using Intra-arterial Thrombolysis or Embolectomy

Various catheter-based devices and techniques have been devised for clot removal from the cerebral arteries. Some of these include the use of a snare, the alligator retrieval system, the Phenox clot retriever, the Merci catheter, and the Penumbra and stent retrievers among others (Fig. 12.51). Angiographic imaging can confirm successful recanalization following mechanical thrombectomy or intra-arterial thrombolysis

(Fig. 12.52). Following successful embolectomy or thrombolysis, patients are at risk for reperfusion hemorrhage, which occurs in an estimated 5–10% of patients. Edema due to infarction peaks at approximately 72 h following the procedure, whereas edema due to hemorrhage may take a week to reach its peak. Patients are at risk for herniation during this time. Imaging can be used to evaluate the extent of infarction, reperfusion edema, and hemorrhage. Potential complications from embolectomy that can be visible on cerebrovascular imaging include intraprocedural hemorrhage, vessel rupture, and vessel dissection. Potentially confounding is the frequently encountered extravasation of contrast into areas where there has been breakdown of the blood-brain barrier. Residual contrast staining from the procedure due to blood-brain barrier leakage in infarcted

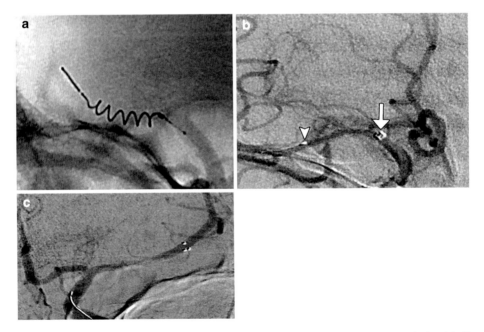

Fig. 12.51 Mechanical thrombectomy devices. Angiographic images of the Merci retriever device (**a**); Penumbra device, with catheter tip (*arrow*) and separator tip (*arrowhead*) (**b**); and Solitaire stent retriever device (**c**)

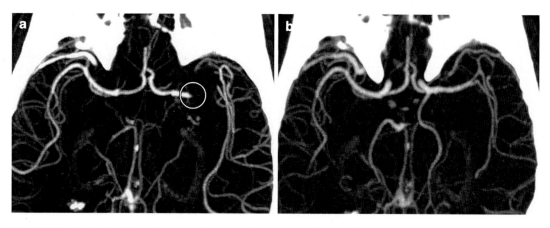

Fig. 12.52 Mechanical thrombectomy. Pre-procedure axial CTA MIP image (**a**) shows complete occlusion of the left distal M1 (*encircled*). Post-procedure CTA MIP image (**b**) shows interval patency of the left M1 with minimal residual irregularity

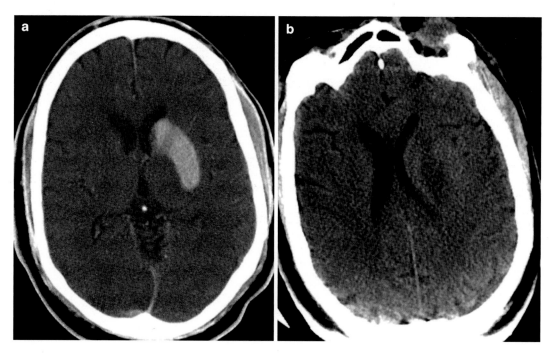

Fig. 12.53 Retained contrast in infarcted parenchyma. Axial CT image obtained 18 h following embolectomy (**a**) shows hyperattenuation within the left basal ganglia. Axial CT image obtained 24 h later (**b**) shows that the hyperattenuation has nearly cleared and instead there is hypoattenuation due to edema from infarction in the left basal ganglia

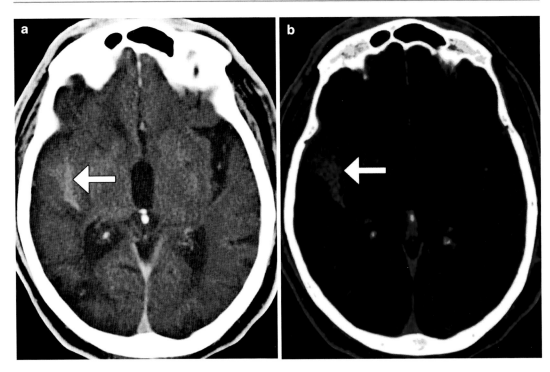

Fig. 12.54 Retained contrast and dual energy CT. Axial (**a**) CT image at 120 keV obtained after mechanical thrombectomy shows a hyperattenuating area in the right insula (*arrow*). The corresponding iodine overlay image (**b**) confirms the presence of contrast (Courtesy of Rajiv Gupta, M.D., Ph.D.)

parenchyma can resemble hemorrhagic transformation (Fig. 12.53). Dual energy CT with iodine overlay maps can help distinguish the two possibilities if necessary (Fig. 12.54).

12.2.8 Endovascular Reconstruction for Intracranial Cerebrovascular Steno-occlusive Lesions

Treatment for intracranial cerebrovascular occlusive disease includes angioplasty with stent placement or angioplasty without stent placement. These patients receive antiplatelet treatment following the procedure and are usually also anticoagulated in the first 24 h. The intent of the treatment is not to achieve 100% luminal diameter, but to achieve adequate improvement in flow. Therefore, comparison of posttreatment luminal diameter to pretreatment luminal diameter is appropriate. Postoperative imaging can be used to determine if the vessel diameter improves and if it does, that it is sustained and associated with improvement in cerebrovascular perfusion. Typical posttreatment imaging may include MR angiography, conventional angiography, and CT angiography. Conventional angiography is the gold-standard imaging assessment for such lesions. Otherwise, MR angiography, CT angiography, MR perfusion, SPECT, and CT perfusion are powerful noninvasive means to assess posttreatment effects. In par-

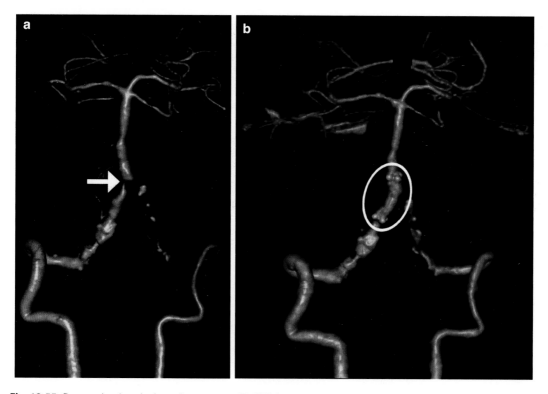

Fig. 12.55 Stent-assisted angioplasty. Pretreatment 3D CTA image (**a**) shows critical stenosis at the right distal vertebral artery (*arrow*). Posttreatment 3D CT image (**b**) shows interval patency of the vessel with a stent in position (*encircled*)

ticular, 3D reconstructions can provide as helpful overview of the vessels (Fig. 12.55). The standard method for characterizing intracranial stenosis is based on the WASID criteria, whereby percent stenosis = [(1 − (vessel diameter at the stenosis/normal vessel diameter))] × 100%.

12.2.9 Angioplasty and Intra-arterial Spasmolysis for Vasospasm

For symptomatic vasospasm refractory to hemodynamic therapy, endovascular techniques, such as balloon angioplasty and intra-arterial spasmolysis with papaverine or nimodipine, may be considered in order to improve cerebral perfusion. Following successful angioplasty or spasmolysis for vasospasm, imaging with CTA or MRA may be used to characterize the extent of infarction, improvement in cerebral perfusion, and luminal diameter of the affected vessels (Fig. 12.56). Otherwise, transcranial Doppler ultrasound is a convenient modality for assessing the degree of vasospasm due to its availability at the bedside.

12.2.10 Endovascular Stent Reconstructive Treatment for Extracranial Cerebrovascular Occlusive Disease

Carotid artery stenting is mainly reserved for patients with symptomatic carotid stenosis greater than 50% or asymptomatic stenosis greater than 70% by NASCET criteria who are otherwise poor surgical candidates for endarterectomy. The procedure consists of endovascular placement of a flexible, self-expanding stent following angioplasty of the affected vessel and use of a distal protection device. Imaging following stent placement may be performed in order to determine if the luminal diameter following angioplasty and stent placement has improved. The standard methods for assessing stenosis at the carotid bifurcation use NASCET or ECAS criteria. Methods used to assess luminal diameter include carotid duplex ultrasound conventional angiography, MRA, and CTA (Fig. 12.57). The morphology of the stent can vary considerably depending on the design and amount of atherosclerotic disease in the vessel. For example, stents can be straight or tapered. Tapered stents can have a conical design, in which

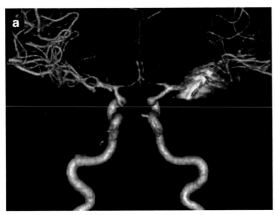 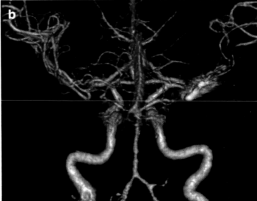

Fig. 12.56 Spasmolysis. This patient developed symptomatic vasospasm involving the left middle cerebral artery after aneurysm clipping, which was documented on CTA (**a**). Following angioplasty of the proximal anterior cerebral arteries with intra-arterial pharmacologic spasmolysis using calcium channel blockers, there was significant and sustained improvement in the diameter of the anterior cerebral arteries (**b**)

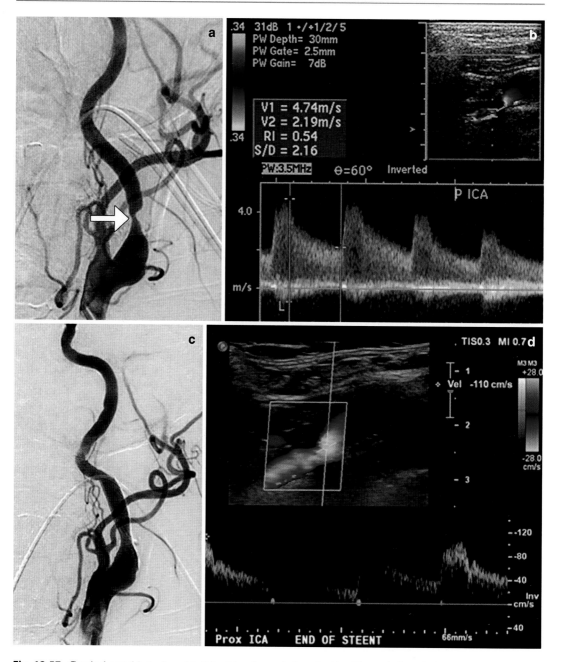

Fig. 12.57 Cervical carotid stenting. Digital subtraction angiography (DSA) color duplex ultrasound before and after angioplasty and stent placement for high-grade stenosis in a patient who had symptomatic stenosis. Both DSA and color duplex arteriography demonstrate the stenosis with high flow velocities on the carotid duplex scan before (**a**, **b**) with resolution of the stenosis immediately after (**c**) and 1 month following stent placement (**d**). Carotid duplex ultrasound is a noninvasive means to evaluate carotid stent placement for carotid bifurcation stenosis

there is gradual decrease in caliber of the stent from proximal to distal, versus shoulder-tapered, in which there is an abrupt change in caliber in the midportion of the stent. Atherosclerotic plaque can produce a waist in the stent. A residual waist of less than 20% of the lumen diameter is considered acceptable. Following the deployment of stents for reconstruction, there are expected artifacts that affect the imaging appearance of the treated vessel for extracranial carotid disease or carotid blowout disease.

12.2.11 Endovascular Reconstructive Treatment for Active Extracranial Hemorrhage or Pseudoaneurysm

Endovascular reconstructive treatment is currently performed using covered stents or a combination of stents and embolic material. Covered stents are deployed in circumstances where a

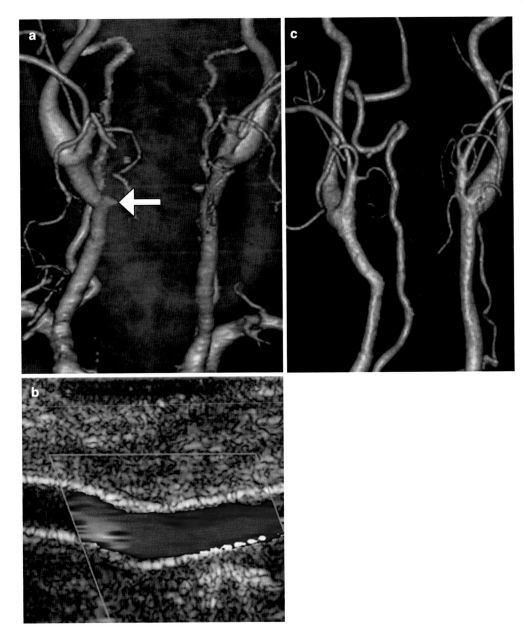

Fig. 12.58 Covered stent. CTA (**a**) shows a pseudoaneurysm along the midportion of the right common carotid artery (*arrow*). Following placement of a covered stent, the aneurysm is no longer identified on follow-up carotid duplex ultrasound (**b**) and CT angiography (**c**)

patient has had a carotid blowout due to open communication of the parent artery with the airway or skin surface (Fig. 12.58) and it is felt that the patient would be unable to tolerate parent vessel sacrifice without high risk for neurologic deficit. Posttreatment imaging may be performed in order to assess luminal patency and intracranial events. Methods used to assess luminal diameter include carotid duplex ultrasound conventional angiography, MRA, and CTA. Patients who receive covered stents are at risk for devel-

oping blood flow around the stent or endoleak, which may result in rehemorrhage, as well as infection in the form of septic emboli with brain abscess formation.

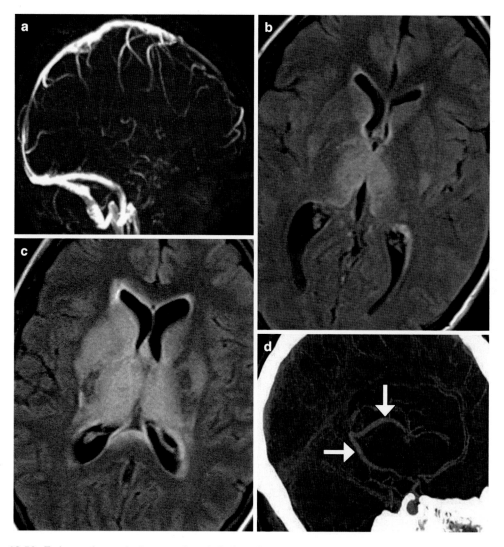

Fig. 12.59 Endovascular cerebral venous thrombolysis. The MR venogram (**a**) shows thrombosis of the internal cerebral veins, straight sinus, and basal vein of Rosenthal. The T2-FLAIR MRI (**b**) demonstrates associated edema within the bilateral thalami and to a lesser extent in the basal ganglia. The patient deteriorated and the degree of edema worsened as depicted on the T2- FLAIR MRI 24 h later despite anticoagulation (**c**). The patient underwent embolectomy using penumbra device, and recanalization of the previously thrombosed vessels (*arrows*) was achieved, as demonstrated on the follow-up CT venography (**d**) and the edema regressed on the T2- FLAIR MRI (**e**). Susceptibility-weighted imaging (**f**) demonstrates a few microhemorrhages within the thalami

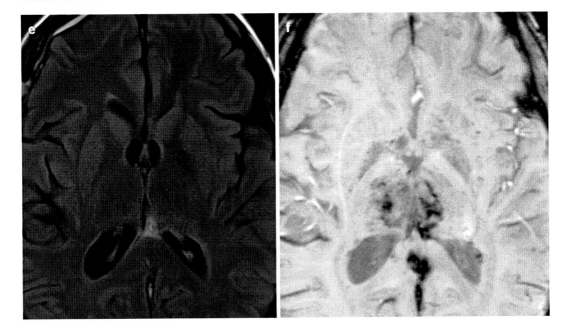

Fig. 12.59 (continued)

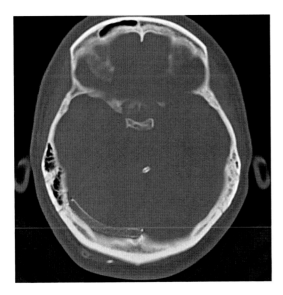

Fig. 12.60 Transverse sinus stent. Axial CT image shows a stent in the right transverse sinus

12.2.12 Endovascular Treatment for Intracranial Venous Stenosis and Occlusion

Endovascular treatment for symptomatic internal cerebral vein thrombosis or dural sinus thrombosis may include fibrinolytic infusion and mechanical embolectomy. Imaging typically demonstrates resolution of cerebral edema following successful therapy (Fig. 12.59). Alternatively, venous sinus stenting can be performed to treat stenoses that are unresponsive to medical therapy, most commonly in the transverse sinus (Fig. 12.60). The procedure can be performed for restoring patency of transverse sinuses in patients with idiopathic intracranial hypertension. Stenting is most appropriate if a pressure gradient of more than 10 mmHg exists across a stenosis. Either self-expandable or balloon-expandable stents can be used. The most common complications include in-stent thrombosis, headache, and hearing loss.

12.2.13 Complications Related to Endovascular Procedures

Access Site Complications. Non-neurologic complications related to head and neck endovascular interventions are uncommon, occurring in 0.14% of cases who undergo femoral artery

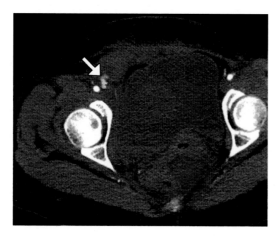

Fig. 12.61 Access site hemorrhage. The patient experienced dropping hematocrit after carotid artery stenting. Axial CTA image showsright groin and pelvic hemorrhage and a right femoral arterypseudoaneurysm (*arrow*)

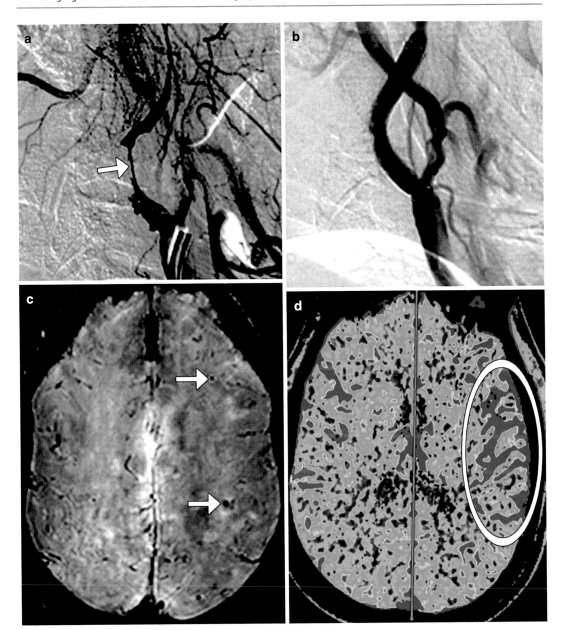

Fig. 12.62 Hyperperfusion syndrome. The initial digital subtraction arteriography (**a**) demonstrates a long-segment high-grade stenosis (*arrow*). Following the stent placement, the left internal carotid artery dilated to its normal diameter (**b**). Although the patient was doing well initially, the patient experiences seizure following the procedure, as well as right hemiparesis and aphasia. Susceptibility-weighted imaging (**c**) demonstrates punctate left cerebral hemisphere microhemorrhages (*arrows*). CT perfusion cerebral blood flow map (**d**) demonstrates relatively higher blood flow to the left hemisphere (*encircled*)

access. Such complications include femoral abscess, occlusions of the femoral artery with leg ischemia, dissection and pseudoaneurysm formation, retroperitoneal hemorrhage requiring transfusion, or a combination of these. CT/CTA is a reasonable option for evaluating patients with suspect vascular compromise and hemorrhage in the emergent setting (Fig. 12.61).

Cerebral Hyperperfusion Syndrome. Cerebral hyperperfusion syndrome classically occurs within the first few days following carotid artery revascularization for severe stenosis. Patients present with severe headache or neurologic deficits. It is often accompanied by seizures and may result in intracranial hemorrhage. In general, patients with severe stenosis have chronic maximal dilation of the intracranial vasculature, which

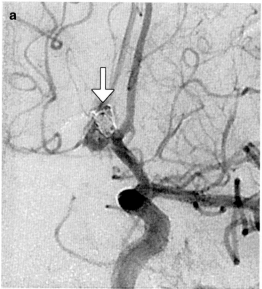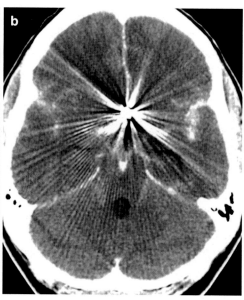

Fig. 12.63 Intraprocedural aneurysm rupture. Digital subtraction angiography (**a**) shows aneurysm rupture as evidenced by contrast extruding beyond the confines of the aneurysm (*arrow*), which was treated by immediate

deployment of a balloon and continued embolization using coils. CT obtained immediately following the procedure (**b**) demonstrates scattered subarachnoid hemorrhage, which was not present before the procedure

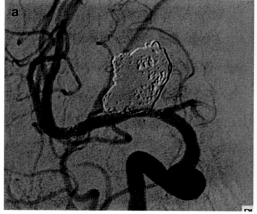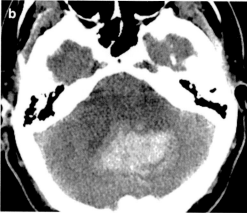

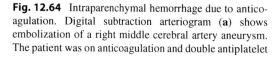

Fig. 12.64 Intraparenchymal hemorrhage due to anticoagulation. Digital subtraction arteriogram (**a**) shows embolization of a right middle cerebral artery aneurysm. The patient was on anticoagulation and double antiplatelet

treatment during the procedure, and 16 h following embolization, the patient suddenly deteriorated due to a remote hemorrhage in the cerebellum, as shown on CT (**b**)

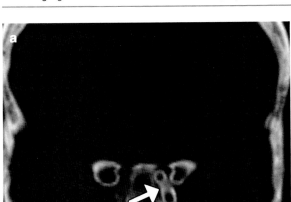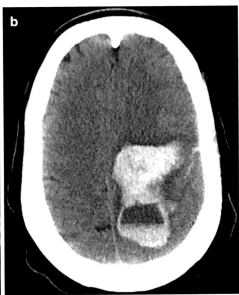

Fig. 12.65 Intracranial hemorrhage complicating flow diversion. The patient presented with right-sided weakness after treatment of a left cavernous carotid aneurysm. The coronal CT image (**a**) shows a left intracranial artery Pipeline stent (*arrow*). The axial CTA image (**b**) shows a large left frontoparietal hematoma with a hematocrit level

does not immediately reverse at the time of reperfusion by stenting. This results in a hyperperfusion phenomenon. Imaging can be performed to evaluate for associated hemorrhage, and the diagnosis is supported by the finding of increased perfusion ipsilateral to the stented vessel (Fig. 12.62).

Intracranial Hemorrhage. Hemorrhagic complications may include intraprocedural aneurysm rupture (Fig. 12.63), intraparenchymal hemorrhage related to anticoagulation and/or antiplatelet treatment (Fig. 12.64), and hyperperfusion syndrome with revascularization procedures, as mentioned before. Furthermore, delayed ipsilateral intraparenchymal hemorrhage has been described as a potential complication following flow diversion of anterior circulation aneurysms, perhaps due to decreased arterial wall compli-

ance and altered Windkessel effect. The intraparenchymal hemorrhages in such cases can be large and contain hematocrit levels (Fig 12.65), since the patients are typically anticoagulated. CT tends to be the modality of choice for evaluating post-procedure hemorrhage, even if metal artifact may degrade the images in some cases.

Stent Steno-occlusive Disease. Patency of the stent can be evaluated using MRA, CTA, or Doppler ultrasound. Velocity criteria for extracranial internal carotid artery stents have been proposed as follows:

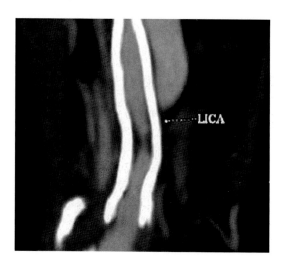

Fig. 12.66 Intimal hyperplasia. Curved planar reformatted CTA image shows thin, low attenuation material within the stent lumen

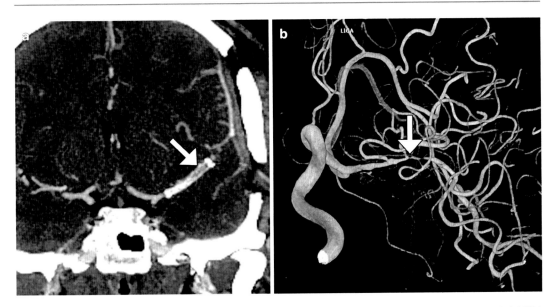

Fig. 12.67 Stent stenosis. Coronal CTA image (**a**) shows a filling defect (*arrow*) in the distal portion of the left MCA stent. Catheter angiography 3D reconstruction (**b**) confirms a severe, near-critical stenosis in the stent (*arrow*)

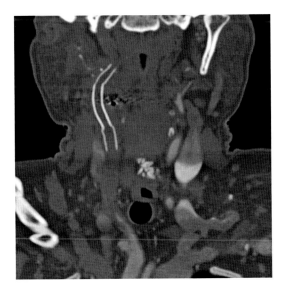

Fig. 12.68   Stent occlusion. Delayed curved planar reformatted CTA image shows complete lack of opacification of the left internal carotid stent

- Residual stenosis ≥20%: peak systolic velocity ≥150 cm/s and ICA/CCA ratio ≥2.15
- In-stent restenosis ≥50%: peak systolic velocity ≥220 cm/s and ICA/CCA ratio ≥2.7
- In-stent restenosis ≥80%: peak systolic velocity 340 cm/s and ICA/CCA ratio ≥4.15

Intimal hyperplasia is the process of endothelial regrowth after injury and can occur within the lumen of stents, usually with a thickness of 1 or 2 mm. However, intimal hyperplasia is sometimes more extensive and can lead to hemodynamically significant stenosis. On ultrasound, intimal hyperplasia is typically homogeneously hypoechoic, and on

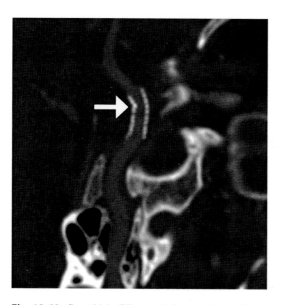

Fig. 12.69 Stent kink. CT curved planar reformat shows a focal angulation (*arrow*) in the lateral aspect of this curved supraclinoid internal carotid artery stent, which is otherwise intact

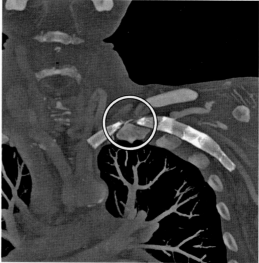

Fig. 12.70 Stent compression and fracture. Coronal CT MIP image demonstrates deformity and a gap between fragments of a subclavian artery stent at the thoracic outlet (*encircled*). The ends of the stent adjacent to the fracture are compressed

CT it appears as mural hypoattenuation (Fig. 12.66).

Significant stent restenosis is a fairly common complication, occurring in about 15% of cases within several months of the procedure. Restenosis is more likely with self-expandable stents than balloon-expandable stents. CTA can demonstrate filling defects in the lumen of the stent (Fig. 12.67). Catheter angioplasty is more sensitive and allows further treatment, such as angioplasty, to be performed.

Stent occlusion is a serious complication that can result from in-stent thrombosis. As before, several modalities can be used to evaluate this complication. CTA with delayed imaging can be helpful for differentiating high-grade stenosis versus occlusion (Fig. 12.68).

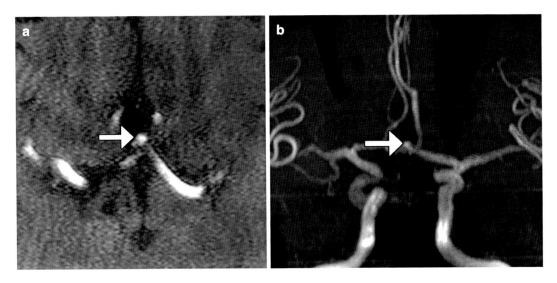

Fig. 12.71 Residual aneurysm. Time-of-flight MRA source (**a**) and MIP (**b**) images show flow into a small residual anterior communicating artery aneurysm neck (*arrows*) after coil embolization

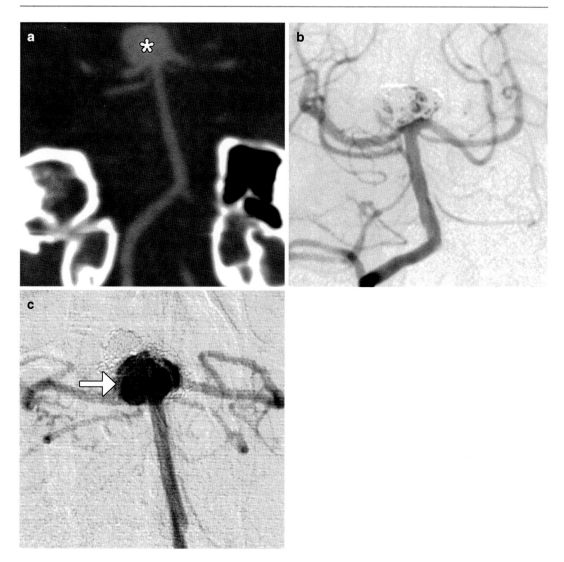

Fig. 12.72 Coil compaction. Pre-procedure CT angiography curved planar reformatted image (**a**) shows a large basilar tip aneurysm (*). Immediate post-embolization catheter angiogram (**b**) shows near-complete occlusion of the basilar tip aneurysm with metal coils. Follow-up digital subtraction angiogram (**c**) shows interval coil compaction with substantial aneurysm filling (*arrow*)

Mechanical Stent Failure. Mechanical stent failure can manifest as indentation, compression, kinking, and/or fracture (Figs. 12.69 and 12.70). Deformed stents can lead to vascular occlusion and/or embolization, which can be depicted on Doppler ultrasound and/or angiography imaging. This complication is less likely with self-expanding stents than with balloon-expanding stents. Treatment consists of inserting smaller caliber stents into the damaged stent lumen or retrieving the fractured device. Anatomy of the stented vessel plays an important role in stent deformity, such that this phenomenon tends to occur along curvatures, such as in the carotid siphon region. Flat-panel CT is reported to be more sensitive for depicting stent deformities than is digital subtraction angiography.

Residual and Recurrent Aneurysms. It can be challenging or even risky to completely obliterate

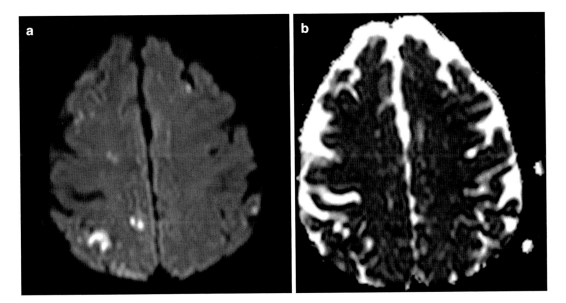

Fig. 12.73 Silent thromboembolic events. There are multiple foci of restricted diffusion shown on DWI (**a**) ADC map (**b**) obtained after recent coiling of a ruptured 6 mm anterior communicating artery aneurysm

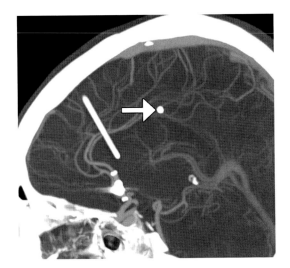

Fig. 12.74 Nontarget embolization. Sagittal CT image shows a coil in the distal anterior cerebral artery (*arrow*) from proximal stent-assisted aneurysm coiling

aneurysms via coil embolization, particularly in cases of aneurysm rupture. However, the presence of a small residual neck does not necessarily warrant further intervention, unless there is growth of the aneurysm. Thus, surveillance imaging via MRA is typically performed to ensure

stability of the aneurysm (Fig. 12.71). On the other hand, coil compaction is deemed to be the most common cause of aneurysm recurrence after embolization and is a process whereby aneurysm coil mass volume decreases over time and is more likely to occur after embolization of

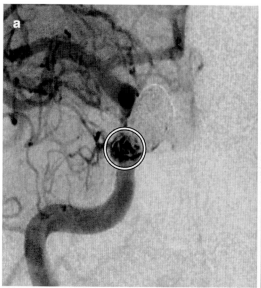 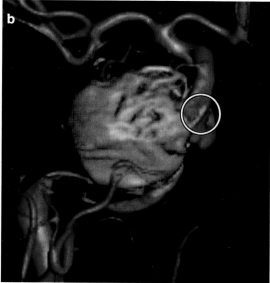

Fig. 12.75 Coil prolapse. Digital subtraction angiogram (**a**) and 3D angiogram in a different patient (**b**) depict loops of coils (*encircled*) that project from the coil masses

into the lumen of the adjacent vessel (ICAs). The prolapsed coils were not significantly flow limiting

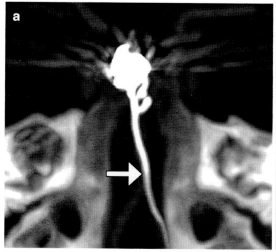 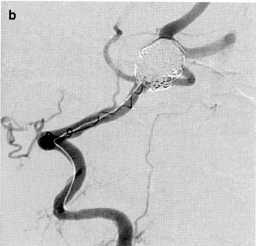

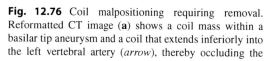

Fig. 12.76 Coil malpositioning requiring removal. Reformatted CT image (**a**) shows a coil mass within a basilar tip aneurysm and a coil that extends inferiorly into the left vertebral artery (*arrow*), thereby occluding the

vessel. Digital subtraction angiogram (**b**) shows attempted coil retrieval using the Merci device, which is wrapped around the coil

ruptured aneurysms as well. This process can be observed on serial imaging in which there is enlargement of the aneurysm sac from baseline (Fig 12.72).

Embolic Phenomena. Silent thromboembolic events associated with neurointerventional procedures are a relatively common occurrence, despite meticulous technique and systemic anticoagulation. This can occur due to the formation of thrombus associated with the devices used during the procedure or the introduction of intravascular air. Nevertheless, significant clinical consequences are rare. The lesions are typically small, often multifocal, and usually localize to the vascular territory of the vessel

being treated (Fig. 12.73). Distal migration of stents or coils can occur during or after the intervention and can also be associated with morbidity. However, immediate removal of the devices is often feasible and effective before clots form. Furthermore, anticoagulation can be helpful in maintaining blood flow. Beyond the immediate intraprocedural period, imaging via CTA can help localize the migrated hardware and assess for associated complications (Fig. 12.74).

Coil Malpositioning/Prolapse. Coils in excessively packed aneurysms can potentially prolapse through the aneurysms' neck into the parent vessels, particularly in cases of wide aneurysm necks

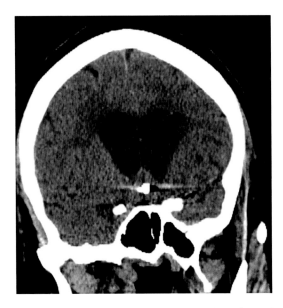

Fig. 12.77 Hydrocephalus after embolization. Coronal CT image shows disproportionate dilatation of the lateral ventricles following unruptured anterior communicating aneurysm embolization

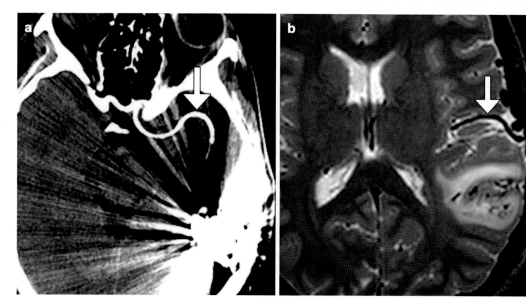

Fig. 12.78 Retained microcatheter. The patient underwent left temporal arteriovenous malformation embolization. Axial CT image (**a**) shows the serpiginous course of the intravascular catheter (*arrow*), which appears hyperattenuating due to the presence of concentrated embolic material retained in the lumen. The microcatheter (*arrow*) is hypointense on the T2-weighted MRI (**b**)

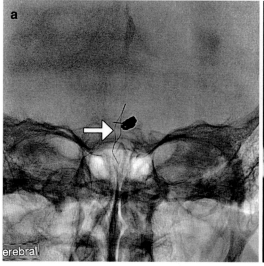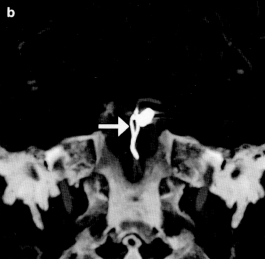

Fig. 12.79 Retained snare. The patient is status post coil embolization of a left superior cerebellar artery aneurysm with coil migration into the basilar artery and iatrogenic retained distal fragment of snare device within the distal basilar artery while attempting to retrieve the malpositioned coil. These materials were left in situ and the patient is treated with dual antiplatelet treatment to permit endothelialization until future follow-up, due to concern that further manipulation of this adherent fragment might have catastrophic consequences. Frontal spot image (**a**) at the end of the procedure shows a retained fragment of the snare device (*arrow*) in the basilar artery, adjacent to the coils projecting into the basilar artery. Coronal (**b**) CTA image shows the fractured snare (*arrow*) and embolization coils remain position, but the basilar artery and distal branches are patent

and partially thrombosed aneurysms. Prolapse of only a few coils is not necessarily flow limiting (Fig. 12.75). However, extension of greater lengths of coils into the parent vessels can predispose to significant thromboembolic events and may warrant removal (Fig. 12.76). A variety of devices can be used to remove the migrated coils, such as microsnares and the Merci retriever.

Hydrocephalus After Coil Embolization. Hydrocephalus commonly results from subarachnoid and intraventricular hemorrhage from ruptured aneurysms. Hydrocephalus can also occur following embolization of unruptured aneurysms, particularly with hydrogel coils. The mechanism by which hydrogel coils may induce hydrocephalus is not well understood. However, one possible etiology is that hydrogel coils undergo progressive expansion once exposed to the physiological environment and increase overall aneurysm filling. Another possibility is that it may be some-

how related to an exaggerated inflammatory response during aneurysm healing. MRI or CT can readily depict post-coiling hydrocephalus (Fig 12.77).

Retained Hardware. A potential complication of endovascular procedures involving embolization material is entrapment of the microcatheter. Imaging may be obtained to evaluate the extent and location of the entrapped microcatheter, which appears as hyperattenuating on CT and low signal intensity on MRI due to the retained embolization material (Fig. 12.78). If endovascular attempts fail to remove the microcatheters, these can be removed via microsurgical retrieval. Another more unusual situation is fragmentation and retention of a snare used to retrieve malpositioned coils (Fig. 12.79). Thus, it is useful to be familiar with the imaging appearance of various devices used, in case such situations are encountered in practice.

Further Reading

Vascular Surgery

Direct Extracranial-Intracranial Revascularization

Amin-Hanjani S (2011) Cerebral revascularization: extracranial-intracranial bypass. J Neurosurg Sci 55(2): 107–116

Fluri F, Engelter S, Lyrer P (2010) Extracranial-intracranial arterial bypass surgery for occlusive carotid artery disease. Cochrane Database Syst Rev (2):CD005953

Ginat DT, Smith ER, Robertson RL, Scott RM, Schaefer PW (2013) Imaging after direct and indirect extracranial-intracranial bypass surgery. AJR Am J Roentgenol 201(1):W124-W132

Indirect Extracranial-Intracranial Revascularization

Ginat DT, Smith ER, Robertson RL, Scott RM, Schaefer PW (2013) Imaging after direct and indirect extracranial-intracranial bypass surgery. AJR Am J Roentgenol 201(1):W124-W132

Houkin K, Ishikawa T, Yoshimoto T, Abe H (1997) Direct and indirect revascularization for moyamoya disease surgical techniques and peri-operative complications. Clin Neurol Neurosurg 99(Suppl 2):S142–S145

Irikura K, Miyasaka Y, Kurata A, Tanaka R, Yamada M, Kan S, Fujii K (2000) The effect of encephalo-myo-synangiosis on abnormal collateral vessels in childhood moyamoya disease. Neurol Res 22(4):341-346

Park JH, Yang SY, Chung YN, Kim JE, Kim SK, Han DH, Cho BK (2007) Modified encephaloduroarteriosynangiosis with bifrontal encephalogaleoperiosteal synangiosis for the treatment of pediatric moyamoya disease. Technical note. J Neurosurg 106(3 Suppl):237–242

Robertson RL, Burrows PE, Barnes PD, Robson CD, Poussaint TY, Scott RM (1997) Angiographic changes after pial synangiosis in childhood moyamoya disease. AJNR Am J Neuroradiol 18(5):837–845

Sekhar LN, Natarajan SK, Ellenbogen RG, Ghodke B (2008) Cerebral revascularization for ischemia, aneurysms, and cranial base tumors. Neurosurgery 62(6 Suppl 3):1373–1408; discussion 1408–1410

Shirane R, Yoshida Y, Takahashi T, Yoshimoto T (1997) Assessment of encephalo-galeo-myo-synangiosis with dural pedicle insertion in childhood moyamoya disease: characteristics of cerebral blood flow and oxygen metabolism. Clin Neurol Neurosurg 99(Suppl 2): S79–S85

Aneurysm and Hemostatic Ligation Clips

Bracchi M, Savoiardo M, Triulzi F, Daniele D, Grisoli M, Bradac GB, Agostinis C, Pelucchetti D, Scotti G (1993)

Superficial siderosis of the CNS: MR diagnosis and clinical findings. AJNR Am J Neuroradiol 14(1):227–236

el-Beltagy M, Muroi C, Roth P, Fandino J, Imhof HG, Yonekawa Y (2010) Recurrent intracranial aneurysms after successful neck clipping. World Neurosurg 74(4–5):472–477

Shellock FG, Tkach JA, Ruggieri PM, Masaryk TJ, Rasmussen PA (2003) Aneurysm clips: evaluation of magnetic field interactions and translational attraction by use of "long-bore" and "short-bore" 3.0-T MR imaging systems. AJNR Am J Neuroradiol 24(3): 463–471

Thielen KR, Nichols DA, Fulgham JR, Piepgras DG (1997) Endovascular treatment of cerebral aneurysms following incomplete clipping. J Neurosurg 87(2):184-189

Thornton J, Bashir Q, Aletich VA, Debrun GM, Ausman JI, Charbel FT (2000) What percentage of surgically clipped intracranial aneurysms have residual necks? Neurosurgery 46(6):1294–1298; discussion 1298–300

Tsutsumi K, Ueki K, Morita A, Usui M, Kirino T (2001) Risk of aneurysm recurrence in patients with clipped cerebral aneurysms: results of long-term follow-up angiography. Stroke 32(5):1191–1194

Yasui K, Kotani Y, Takeda Y, Minami A (2003) Migration of intracranial hemostatic clip into the lumbar spinal canal causing sacral radiculopathy: a case report. Spine (Phila Pa 1976) 28(24):E511-E514

Intracranial Aneurysm Muscle Wrap

Choudhari KA (2004) Wrapping and coating of cerebral aneurysms: history, evolution and surgical management after a re-bleed. Br J Neurosurg 18(3):259–267

Cohen-Gadol AA, Spencer DD, Harvey W (2004) Cushing and cerebrovascular surgery: part I, aneurysms. J Neurosurg 101(3):547–552

Onoue H, Abe T, Tashibu K, Suzuki T (1992) Two undesirable results of wrapping of an intracranial aneurysm. Neurosurg Rev 15(4):307–309

Vascular Malformation Surgery

Baumann CR, Schuknecht B, Lo Russo G, Cossu M, Citterio A, Andermann F, Siegel AM (2006) Seizure outcome after resection of cavernous malformations is better when surrounding hemosiderin-stained brain also is removed. Epilepsia 47(3):563-566.

Gross BA, Du R (2014) Diagnosis and treatment of vascular malformations of the brain Curr Treat Options Neurol 16(1):279

Watzinger F, Gössweiner S, Wagner A, Richling B, Millesi-Schobel G, Hollmann K (1997) Extensive facial vascular malformations and haemangiomas: a review of the literature and case reports. J Craniomaxillofac Surg 25(6):335-343

Microvascular Decompression/ Jannetta Procedure

Ali MJ, Gebarski S, Thompson BG (2004) Transient magnetic resonance imaging signal alterations in the brainstem after microvascular decompression for trigeminal neuralgia: case report. Neurosurgery 55(4):987

Capelle HH, Brandis A, Tschan CA, Krauss JK (2010) Treatment of recurrent trigeminal neuralgia due to Teflon granuloma. J Headache Pain 11(4):339-344.

Dannenbaum M, Lega BC, Suki D, Harper RL, Yoshor D (2008) Microvascular decompression for hemifacial spasm: long-term results from 114 operations performed without neurophysiological monitoring. J Neurosurg 109(3):410–415

Hitotsumatsu T, Matsushima T, Inoue T (2003) Microvascular decompression for treatment of trigeminal neuralgia, hemifacial spasm, and glossopharyngeal neuralgia: three surgical approach variations: technical note. Neurosurgery 53(6):1436–1441; discussion 1442–1443

Hughes MA, Branstetter BF, Taylor CT, Fakhran S, Delfyett WT, Frederickson AM, Sekula RF Jr. (2015) MRI findings in patients with a history of failed prior microvascular decompression for hemifacial spasm: how to image and where to look. AJNR Am J Neuroradiol 36(4):768-773

Jawahar A, Kondziolka D, Kanal E, Bissonette DJ, Lunsford LD (2001) Imaging the trigeminal nerve and pons before and after surgical intervention for trigeminal neuralgia. Neurosurgery 48(1):101–106; discussion 106–107

McLaughlin MR, Jannetta PJ, Clyde BL, Subach BR, Comey CH, Resnick DK (1999) Microvascular decompression of cranial nerves: lessons learned after 4400 operations. J Neurosurg 90(1):1–8

Carotid Endarterectomy

Back MR, Rogers GA, Wilson JS, Johnson BL, Shames ML, Bandyk DF (2003) Magnetic resonance angiography minimizes need for arteriography after inadequate carotid duplex ultrasound scanning. J Vasc Surg 38(3):422–430; discussion 431

Crawford RS, Chung TK, Hodgman T, Pedraza JD, Corey M, Cambria RP (2007) Restenosis after eversion vs patch closure carotid endarterectomy. J Vasc Surg 46(1):41–48

D'Angelo V, Catapano G, Bozzini V, Catapano D, De Vivo P, Ciritella P, Parlatore L (1999) Cerebrovascular reactivity before and after carotid endarterectomy. Surg Neurol 51(3):321–326

Diaz FG, Ausman JI, Malik GM (1988) Pitfalls during carotid endarterectomy. Acta Neurochir 91(3–4):87–94

Goode SD, Altaf N, Auer DP, MacSweeney ST (2009) Carotid endarterectomy improves cerebrovascular reserve capacity preferentially in patients with preoperative impairment as indicated by asymmetric BOLD response to hypercapnia. Eur J Vasc Endovasc Surg 38(5):546–551

Goodney PP, Nolan BW, Eldrup-Jorgensen J, Likosky DS, Cronenwett JL, Vascular Study Group of Northern New England (2010) Restenosis after carotid endarterectomy in a multicenter regional registry. J Vasc Surg 52(4):897–904, 905.e1–905.e2; discussion 904–905

Karapanayiotides T, Meuli R, Devuyst G, Piechowski-Jozwiak B, Dewarrat A, Ruchat P, Von Segesser L, Bogousslavsky J (2005) Postcarotid endarterectomy hyperperfusion or reperfusion syndrome. Stroke 36(1):21–26

Link J, Müller-Hülsbeck S, Grabener M, Stock U, Brossmann J, Heller M (1995) CT angiography in the follow-up after carotid endarterectomy. Rofo 163(3):215–218

Loftus CM, Biller J, Godersky JC, Adams HP, Yamada T, Edwards PS (1988) Carotid endarterectomy in symptomatic elderly patients. Neurosurgery 22(4):676–680

Naylor AR, Merrick MV, Sandercock PA, Gillespie I, Allen P, Griffin TM, Ruckley CV (1993) Serial imaging of the carotid bifurcation and cerebrovascular reserve after carotid endarterectomy. Br J Surg 80(10):1278–1282

Roth SM, Back MR, Bandyk DF, Avino AJ, Riley V, Johnson BL (1999) A rational algorithm for duplex scan surveillance after carotid endarterectomy. J Vasc Surg 30(3):453–460

van Mook WN, Rennenberg RJ, Schurink GW, van Oostenbrugge RJ, Mess WH, Hofman PA, de Leeuw PW (2005) Cerebral hyperperfusion syndrome. Lancet Neurol 4(12):877–888

Carotid Body Stimulation

Sanchez LA, Illig K, Levy M, Jaff M, Trachiotis G, Shanley C, Irwin E, Jim J, Rossing M, Kieval R (2010) Implantable carotid sinus stimulator for the treatment of resistant hypertension: local effects on carotid artery morphology. Ann Vasc Surg 24(2):178–184

Adjustable Vascular Clamp

Helm GA, Simmons NE, diPierro CD, Kassell NF (1993) Carotid artery revascularization following Crutchfield clamp placement. Report of two cases. J Neurosurg 79(5):779–781

Mount LA (1959) Results of treatment of intracranial aneurysms using the Selverstone clamp. J Neurosurg 16:611–618

Teitelbaum GP, Lin MC, Watanabe AT, Norfray JF, Young TI, Bradley WG Jr (1990) Ferromagnetism and MR imaging: safety of carotid vascular clamps. AJNR Am J Neuroradiol 11(2):267–272

Reconstruction of the Great Vessels

Atkin GK, Grieve PP, Vattipally VR, Ravikumar KH, Das SK (2007) The surgical management of aortic root vessel anomalies presenting in adults. Ann Vasc Surg 21(4):525–534

Backer CL, Hillman N, Mavroudis C, Holinger LD (2002) Resection of Kommerell's diverticulum and left subclavian artery transfer for recurrent symptoms after vascular ring division. Eur J Cardiothorac Surg 22(1): 64–69

Chen CL (1990) Repair of right aortic arch with aberrant left subclavian artery and left ligamentum arteriosum. J Pediatr Surg 25(7):795–796

Criado FJ, Queral LA (1995) Carotid-axillary artery bypass: a ten-year experience. J Vasc Surg 22(6):717–722; discussion 722–723

Meyer FB, Windschitl WL (1998) Repair of carotid endarterectomy with a collagen-impregnated fabric graft. J Neurosurg 88(4):647–649

Rich NM, Collins GJ Jr, Hobson RW 2nd, Andersen CA, McDonald PT (1977) Carotid-axillary bypass: clinical and experimental evaluation. Am J Surg 134(6): 805–808

Sundaram B, Quint LE, Patel HJ, Deeb GM (2007) CT findings following thoracic aortic surgery. Radiographics 27(6):1583–1594

Endovascular Surgery

General Imaging Considerations Following Endovascular Cerebrovascular Procedures

Anzalone N, Righi C, Simionato F, Scomazzoni F, Pagani G, Calori G, Santino P, Scotti G (2000) Three-dimensional time-of-flight MR angiography in the evaluation of intracranial aneurysms treated with Guglielmi detachable coils. AJNR Am J Neuroradiol 21(4):746–752

Hartman J, Nguyen T, Larsen D, Teitelbaum GP (1997) MR artifacts, heat production, and ferromagnetism of Guglielmi detachable coils. AJNR Am J Neuroradiol 18(3):497–501

Jiang L, He ZH, Zhang XD, Lin B, Yin XH, Sun XC (2011) Value of noninvasive imaging in follow-up of intracranial aneurysm. Acta Neurochir Suppl 110(Pt 2):227–232

Endovascular Treatment for Aneurysms

Cognard C, Weill A, Spelle L et al. (1999) Long-term angiographic follow-up of 169 intracranial berry aneurysms occluded with detachable coils. Radiology 212:348–356

Cruz JP, Chow M, O'Kelly C, Marotta B, Spears J, Montanera W, Fiorella D, Marotta T (2012) Delayed ipsilateral parenchymal hemorrhage following flow diversion for the treatment of anterior circulation aneurysms. AJNR Am J Neuroradiol 33(4): 603–608

de Barros Faria M, Castro RN, Lundquist J, Scrivano E, Ceratto R, Ferrario A, Lylyk P (2011) The role of the pipeline embolization device for the treatment of dissecting intracranial aneurysms. AJNR Am J Neuroradiol 32(11):2192–2195

Deutschmann HA, Wehrschuetz M, Augustin M, Niederkorn K, Klein GE (2012) Long-term follow-up after treatment of intracranial aneurysms with the Pipeline embolization device: results from a single center. AJNR Am J Neuroradiol 33(3):481–486

Kurre W, Berkefeld J (2008) Materials and techniques for coiling of cerebral aneurysms: how much scientific evidence do we have? Neuroradiology 50(11):909–927

Nelson PK, Lylyk P, Szikora I, Wetzel SG, Wanke I, Fiorella D (2011) The pipeline embolization device for the intracranial treatment of aneurysms trial. AJNR Am J Neuroradiol 32(1):34–40

Sprengers ME, Schaafsma J, van Rooij WJ, Sluzewski M, Rinkel GJ, Velthuis BK, van Rijn JC, Majoie CB (2008) Stability of intracranial aneurysms adequately occluded 6 months after coiling: a 3 T MR angiography multicenter long-term follow-up study. AJNR Am J Neuroradiol 29(9):1768–1774

van Rooij WJ, Sluzewski M (2007) Coiling of very large and giant basilar tip aneurysms: midterm clinical and angiographic results. AJNR Am J Neuroradiol 28(7):1405–1408

Endovascular Embolization of Arteriovenous Malformations and Fistulas

Gailloud P (2005) Endovascular treatment of cerebral arteriovenous malformations. Tech Vasc Interv Radiol 8(3):118–128

Yuki I, Kim RH, Duckwiler G, Jahan R, Tateshima S, Gonzalez N, Gorgulho A, Diaz JL, De Salles AA, Viñuela F (2010) Treatment of brain arteriovenous malformations with high-flow arteriovenous fistulas: risk and complications associated with endovascular embolization in multimodality treatment. Clinical article. J Neurosurg 113(4):715–722

Endovascular Deconstructive Treatment for Vessel Sacrifice

Hunter TB, Yoshino MT, Dzioba RB, Light RA, Berger WG (2004) Medical devices of the head, neck, and spine. Radiographics 24(1):257–285

Macht S, Mathys C, Schipper J, Turowski B (2012) Initial experiences with the Amplatzer vascular plug 4 for permanent occlusion of the internal carotid artery in the skull base in patients with head and neck tumors. Neuroradiology 54:61–64

Nelson PK, Levy DI (2001) Balloon-assisted coil embolization of wide-necked aneurysms of the internal carotid artery: medium-term angiographic and clinical follow-up in 22 patients. AJNR Am J Neuroradiol 22(1): 19–26

Preoperative Embolization of Neoplasms

Ashour R, Aziz-Sultan A (2014) Preoperative tumor embolization. Neurosurg Clin N Am 25(3):607–617

Raper DM, Starke RM, Henderson F Jr, Ding D, Simon S, Evans AJ, Jane JA Sr, Liu KC (2014) Preoperative embolization of intracranial meningiomas: efficacy, technical considerations, and complications. AJNR Am J Neuroradiol 35(9):1798–1804

Endovascular Sclerotherapy for Head and Neck Lymphatic Malformations

Deveikis JP (2005) Percutaneous ethanol sclerotherapy for vascular malformations in the head and neck. Arch Facial Plast Surg 7(5):322–325

Jeong HS, Baek CH, Son YI, Kim TW, Lee BB, Byun HS (2006) Treatment for extracranial arteriovenous malformations of the head and neck. Acta Otolaryngol 126(3):295–300

Rimon U, Garniek A, Galili Y, Golan G, Bensaid P, Morag B (2004) Ethanol sclerotherapy of peripheral venous malformations. Eur J Radiol 52(3):283–287

Endovascular Reconstruction for Intracranial Cerebrovascular Steno-occlusive Lesions

Bose A, Henkes H, Alfke K, Reith W et al (2008) Penumbra phase 1 stroke trial investigators. The penumbra system: a mechanical device for the treatment of acute stroke due to thromboembolism. AJNR Am J Neuroradiol 29(7):1409–1413

González A, Mayol A, Martínez E, González-Marcos JR, Gil-Peralta A (2007) Mechanical thrombectomy with snare in patients with acute ischemic stroke. Neuroradiology 49(4):365–372

Kim D, Jahan R, Starkman S, Abolian A et al (2006) Endovascular mechanical clot retrieval in a broad ischemic stroke cohort. AJNR Am J Neuroradiol 27(10):2048–2052

Lee R, Lui WM, Cheung RT, Leung GK, Chan KH (2007) Mechanical thrombectomy in acute proximal middle cerebral artery thrombosis with the alligator retrieval device. Cerebrovasc Dis 23(1):69–71

Lutsep HL (2008) Mechanical endovascular recanalization therapies. Curr Opin Neurol 21(1):70–75

Smith WS, Sung G, Saver J, Budzik R et al (2008) Mechanical thrombectomy for acute ischemic stroke: final results of the multi MERCI trial. Stroke 39(4):1205–1212

Stead LG, Gilmore RM, Bellolio MF, Rabinstein AA, Decker WW (2008) Percutaneous clot removal devices in acute ischemic stroke: a systematic review and meta-analysis. Arch Neurol 65(8):1024–1030

Angioplasty and Intra-arterial Spasmolysis for Vasospasm

American Society of Interventional and Therapeutic Neuroradiology (2001) Mechanical and pharmacologic treatment of vasospasm. AJNR Am J Neuroradiol 22(8 Suppl):S26-S27

Hänggi D, Turowski B, Beseoglu K, Yong M, Steiger HJ (2008) Intra-arterial nimodipine for severe cerebral vasospasm after aneurysmal subarachnoid hemorrhage: influence on clinical course and cerebral perfusion AJNR Am J Neuroradiol 29(6):1053-1060

Smith TP, Enterline DS (2000) Endovascular treatment of cerebral vasospasm. J Vasc Interv Radiol 11(5):547-559

Vajkoczy P, Horn P, Bauhuf C, Munch E, Hubner U, Ing D, Thome C, Poeckler-Schoeninger C, Roth H, Schmiedek P (2001) Effect of intra-arterial papaverine on regional cerebral blood flow in hemodynamically relevant cerebral vasospasm. Stroke 32(2):498-505

Endovascular Stent Reconstructive Treatment for Extracranial Cerebrovascular Occlusive Disease

Benndorf G, Campi A, Schneider GH, Wellnhofer E, Unterberg A (2001) Overlapping stents for treatment of a dissecting carotid artery aneurysm. J Endovasc Ther 8(6):566–570

Benndorf G, Herbon U, Sollmann WP, Campi A (2001) Treatment of a ruptured dissecting vertebral artery aneurysm with double stent placement: case report. AJNR Am J Neuroradiol 22(10):1844–1848

Brown KE, Usman A, Kibbe MR, Morasch MD, Matsumura JS, Pearce WH, Amaranto DJ, Eskandari MK (2009) Carotid stenting using tapered and nontapered stents: associated neurological complications and restenosis rates. Ann Vasc Surg 23(4):439–445

Chimowitz MI, Lynn MJ, Derdeyn CP, Turan TN, Fiorella D, Lane BF, Janis LS, Lutsep HL, Barnwell SL, Waters MF, Hoh BL, Hourihane JM, Levy EI, Alexandrov AV, Harrigan MR, Chiu D, Klucznik RP, Clark JM, McDougall CG, Johnson MD, Pride GL Jr, Torbey MT, Zaidat OO, Rumboldt Z, Cloft HJ, SAMMPRIS Trial Investigators (2011) Stenting versus aggressive medical therapy for intracranial arterial stenosis. N Engl J Med 365(11):993–1003

de Donato G, Setacci C, Deloose K, Peeters P, Cremonesi A, Bosiers M (2008) Long-term results of carotid artery stenting. J Vasc Surg 48(6):1431–1440; discussion 1440–1441

Ebrahimi N, Claus B, Lee CY, Biondi A, Benndorf G (2007) Stent conformity in curved vascular models with simulated aneurysm necks using flat-panel CT: an in vitro study. AJNR Am J Neuroradiol 28(5): 823–829

Gröschel K, Schnaudigel S, Pilgram SM, Wasser K, Kastrup A (2009) A systematic review on outcome after stenting for intracranial atherosclerosis. Stroke 40(5):e340–e347

Fifi JT, Meyers PM, Lavine SD, Cox V, Silverberg L, Mangla S, Pile-Spellman J (2009) Complications of modern diagnostic cerebral angiography in an academic medical center. J Vasc Interv Radiol 20(4):442-447

Jou LD, Mawad ME (2011) Hemodynamic effect of neuroform stent on intimal hyperplasia and thrombus formation in a carotid aneurysm. Med Eng Phys 33(5):573–580

Kim SR, Baik MW, Yoo SH, Park IS, Kim SD, Kim MC (2007) Stent fracture and restenosis after placement of a drug-eluting device in the vertebral artery origin and treatment with the stent-in-stent technique. Report of two cases. J Neurosurg 106(5):907–911

Kirsch EC, Khangure MS, van Schie GP, Lawrence-Brown MM, Stewart-Wynne EG, McAuliffe W (2001) Carotid arterial stent placement: results and follow-up in 53 patients. Radiology 220(3):737–744

Kitchens C, Jordan W Jr, Wirthlin D (2002) Whitley D . Vascular complications arising from maldeployed stents. Vasc Endovascular Surg 36(2):145-154

Lal BK, Hobson RW 2nd, Tofighi B, Kapadia I, Cuadra S, Jamil Z (2008) Duplex ultrasound velocity criteria for the stented carotid artery. J Vasc Surg 47(1):63–73

Lee CE, Shaiful AY, Hanif H (2009) Subclavian artery stent fracture. Med J Malaysia 64(4):330–332

Lövblad KO, Yilmaz H, Chouiter A, San Millan Ruiz D, Abdo G, Bijlenga P, de Tribolet N, Ruefenacht DA (2006) Intracranial aneurysm stenting: follow-up with MR angiography. J Magn Reson Imaging 24(2): 418–422

Schillinger M, Dick P, Wiest G, Gentzsch S, Sabeti S, Haumer M, Willfort A, Nasel C, Wober C, Zeitlhofer J, Minar E (2006) Covered versus bare self-expanding stents for endovascular treatment of carotid artery stenosis: a stopped randomized trial. J Endovasc Ther 13(3):312–319

Watarai H, Kaku Y, Yamada M, Kokuzawa J, Tanaka T, Andoh T, Iwama T (2009) Follow-up study on in-stent thrombosis after carotid stenting using multidetector CT angiography. Neuroradiology 51(4):243–251

Endovascular Reconstructive Treatment for Active Extracranial Hemorrhage or Pseudoaneurysm

Gupta R, Thomas AJ, Masih A, Horowitz MB (2008) Treatment of extracranial carotid artery pseudoaneurysms with stent grafts: case series. J Neuroimaging 18(2):180-183

Seward CJ, Dumont TM, Levy EI (2015) Endovascular therapy of extracranial carotid artery pseudoaneurysms: case series and literature review. J Neurointerv Surg 7(9):682-689

Endovascular Treatment for Intracranial Venous Stenosis and Occlusion

Arac A, Lee M, Steinberg GK, Marcellus M, Marks MP (2009) Efficacy of endovascular stenting in dural venous sinus stenosis for the treatment of idiopathic intracranial hypertension. Neurosurg Focus 27(5): E14

Bussière M, Falero R, Nicolle D, Proulx A, Patel V, Pelz D (2010) Unilateral transverse sinus stenting of patients with idiopathic intracranial hypertension. AJNR Am J Neuroradiol 31(4):645–650

Formaglio M, Catenoix H, Tahon F, Mauguière F, Vighetto A, Turjman F (2010) Stenting of a cerebral venous thrombosis. J Neuroradiol 37(3):182-184

Starke RM, Wang T, Ding D, Durst CR, Crowley RW, Chalouhi N, Hasan DM, Dumont AS, Jabbour P, Liu KC (2015) Endovascular treatment of venous sinus stenosis in idiopathic intracranial hypertension: complications, neurological outcomes, and radiographic results. Scientific World Journal 2015:140408

Philips MF, Bagley LJ, Sinson GP, Raps EC, Galetta SL, Zager EL, Hurst RW (1999) Endovascular thrombolysis for symptomatic cerebral venous thrombosis. J Neurosurg 90(1):65-71

Complications Related to Endovascular Procedures

Carli DF, Sluzewski M, Beute GN, van Rooij WJ (2010) Complications of particle embolization of meningiomas: frequency, risk factors, and outcome. AJNR Am J Neuroradiol 31(1):152–154

Fanning NF, Willinsky RA, ter Brugge KG (2008) Wall enhancement, edema, and hydrocephalus after endovascular coil occlusion of intradural cerebral aneurysms. J Neurosurg 108(6):1074-1086

Haw CS, ter Brugge K, Willinsky R, Tomlinson G (2006) Complications of embolization of arteriovenous malformations of the brain. J Neurosurg 104(2):226–232

Jayaraman MV, Marcellus ML, Hamilton S, Do HM, Campbell D, Chang SD, Steinberg GK, Marks MP (2008) Neurologic complications of arteriovenous malformation embolization using liquid embolic agents. AJNR Am J Neuroradiol 29(2):242–246

Marchan EM, Sekula RF Jr, Ku A, Williams R, O'Neill BR, Wilberger JE, Quigley MR (2008) Hydrogel coil-related delayed hydrocephalus in patients with unruptured aneurysms. J Neurosurg 109(2):186-190

Phatouros CC, McConachie NS, Jaspan T (1999) Postprocedure migration of Guglielmi detachable coils and mechanical detachable spirals. Neuroradiology 41(5):324–327

Rordorf G, Bellon RJ, Budzik RE Jr, Farkas J, Reinking GF, Pergolizzi RS, Ezzeddine M, Norbash AM, Gonzalez RG, Putman CM (2001) Silent thromboembolic events associated with the treatment of unruptured cerebral aneurysms by use of Guglielmi detachable coils: prospective study applying diffusion-weighted imaging. AJNR Am J Neuroradiol 22(1):5-10

Teksam M, McKinney A, Truwit CL (2004) A retained neurointerventional microcatheter fragment in the anterior communicating artery aneurysm in multislice computed tomography angiography. Acta Radiol 45(3):340–343

Turek G, Kochanowicz J, Lewszuk A, Lyson T, Zielinska-Turek J, Chwiesko J, Mariak Z (2015) Early surgical removal of migrated coil/stent after failed embolization of intracranial aneurysm. J Neurosurg 123(4):841-847 van Rooij WJ, Sprengers ME, Sluzewski M, Beute GN (2007)Intracranial aneurysms that repeatedly reopen over time after coiling: imaging characteristics and treatment outcome. Neuroradiology 49(4):343–349

Vora N, Thomas A, Germanwala A, Jovin T, Horowitz M (2008)Retrieval of a displaced detachable coil and intracranial stent with an L5 merci retriever during endovascular embolization of an intracranial aneurysm. J Neuroimaging 18(1):81–84

Walcott BP, Gerrard JL, Nogueira RG, Nahed BV, Terry AR, Ogilvy CS (2011) Microsurgical retrieval of an endovascular microcatheter trapped during Onyx embolization of a cerebral arteriovenous malformation. J Neurointerv Surg 3(1):77-79

Yu SC, Boet R, Wong GK, Lam WW, Poon WS (2004) Postembolization hemorrhage of a large and necrotic meningioma. AJNR Am J Neuroradiol 25(3): 506–508

Zoarski GH, Bear HM, Clouston JC, Ragheb J (1997) Endovascular extraction of malpositioned fibered platinum microcoils from the aneurysm sac during endovascular therapy. AJNR Am J Neuroradiol 18(4):691-695

Zoarski GH, Lilly MP, Sperling JS, Mathis JM (1999) Surgically confirmed incorporation of a chronically retained neurointerventional microcatheter in the carotid artery. AJNR Am J Neuroradiol 20(1): 177–178

Index

A

ABIs. *See* Auditory brainstem implants (ABIs)
Absorbable hemostatic agents
    description, 149
    gelatin foam, 149, 151
    gelatin-thrombin matrix, 149, 152
    oxidized regenerated cellulose, 149, 150
    retained cottonoid, 149, 153
    Surgicel, 149, 150
    surgifoam, 149, 151
    types, 149
Adjacent segment disease, 601
Amygdalohippocampectomy, 249–250
Aneurysm clips
    anterior clinoid process resection, 636, 637
    description, 636
    recurrence, 636, 656
    right supraclinoid, 683
    straight-tip, 636, 673
Anterior craniofacial resection
    bone graft reconstruction, 311, 314–315
    cerebral infarction, 311, 315
    encephalocele, 312, 317
    intraparenchymal abscess, 312, 316
    mesh reconstruction, 311, 314
    pericranial flap, 311–314
    radiation necrosis, 312, 317
    rectus muscle injury, 312, 317
    scalp abscess, 311, 315
    skull base reconstruction, 311, 312
    SNUC, 311, 314
    squamous cell carcinoma, 312, 316
Anterior temporal lobectomy
    choroid plexus changes, 245, 246
    description, 244–245
    dominant hemisphere, 244, 245
    gliosis, 245, 247
    nondominant hemisphere, 244, 245
    optic pathway changes, 245, 247
    posterior cerebral artery territory infarction, 245, 248
Arachnoiditis
    arachnoiditis ossificans, 592
    "empty sac" sign, 591

    nerve root clumping, 591
    postoperative, 591–592
Artificial bypass grafts
    carotid-axillary/carotid-subclavian artery bypass, 653, 654
    Dacron graft, 646, 654
    thrombosed polytetrafluoroethylene graft, 653, 655
Atresiaplasty
    preoperative axial, 357, 362
    recurrent cholesteatoma, 357, 358
Auditory brainstem implants (ABIs)
    cochlear implants, 407
    neuro fibromatosis type 2, 407
    suboptimal production, 407
Auricular reconstruction
    porous polyethylene, 355
    rib graft, 354
Auriculectomy
    auricular reconstruction, rib graft, 354, 355
    flap reconstruction, 396
Autocranioplasty
    bone flaps, 139
    frontal radiograph and axial CT image, 139

B

Bone-anchored hearing aid (BAHA)
    aural atresia, 352, 357
    intracranial abscess, 351
Bone flap resorption, 176
Box osteotomy, 148
Brachytherapy
    imaging, 517
    rods, 517
    seeds, brain tumors
        I-125 interstitial radiation, 214
        radioactive isotopes, 214
BrainGate. *See* Neural interface system
Brain imaging
    neurodegenerative, neuropsychiatric and epilepsy surgery
        anterior temporal lobectomy, 244–248
        callosotomy (*see* Callosotomy)

Brain imaging (cont.)
  cingulotomy, 220–221
  corticectomy, 238, 239
  DBS, 238, 239
  DBS (*see* Deep brain stimulation (DBS))
  epidural motor cortex stimulator, 230
  limbic leucotomy, 222–224
  microcatheter subthalamic infusion, 232
  neural interface system, 231
  pallidotomy, 219
  prefrontal lobotomy, 217–218
  seizure monitoring electrodes and neuropace,
      232–237
  selective amygdalohippocampectomy, 249–250
  subcaudate tractotomy, 222–223
  thalamotomy, 225
Brain tumors
  brachytherapy seeds, 214
  chemotheraphy wafers, 213
  intraoperative MRI
    brain shift, 183, 184
    hyperacute hemorrhage and hemostatic material,
        183, 186
    laser ablation, 183, 186
    transient swelling, after laser ablation, 183, 187
    tumor progression, after laser ablation, 184, 188
    tumor resection and contrast leakage, 183, 185
  Ommaya reservoirs, 208–212
  resection cavities
    evolution, 191, 192
    granulation tissue, 201, 202
    GRE/SWI sequences, 197
    hypertrophic olivary degeneration, 193, 196
    lesion enhancement, 201
    metastatic glioblastoma, in spinal canal, 201, 207
    operative bed hemorrhage, 197, 198
    perioperative infarct, 201–203
    peri-resection infarction, 193, 194
    radiation necrosis, 201, 206
    retraction-induced vasogenic edema, 193, 195
    superficial siderosis, 197, 200
    surgical cavity, blood products, 191–192
    tumor progression, 201, 204–205
    wounded tumor, 197, 199
  stereotactic brain biopsy
    blood products, 189
    cavity marker, 189
    expected biopsy path enhancement, 189, 190
    tumor seeding, 189, 190
Burr holes
  craniostomy, 126
  description, 126
  enhancement, 126, 127

C

Calcified VP shunt catheter
  pericatheter dystrophic calcifications, 299
  radiographs, 299
Caldwell-Luc procedure
  chronic recurrent sinusitis, 83

  description, 83
  left anterior maxillary sinus wall, 83
  nasoantral, 83
Callosotomy
  description, 242
  microstructural changes, 242
  partial, 242, 243
  via laser ablation, 242, 244
Canaloplasty and meatoplasty, 356
Carotid endarterectomy (CEA)
  carotid artery restenosis, 650
  clamp deformity, 646
  conventional carotid endarterectomy, 647
  cranial nerve injury, 646, 651
  description, 646
  expected early postoperative changes, 647
  hyperperfusion/reperfusion syndrome, 646
  internal carotid artery velocities, 647
  localized intimal flap, 646, 648
  patch endarterectomy, 647
  patch infection, 646, 650
  post-endarterectomy carotid artery
      occlusion, 651
  recurrent stenosis, 647
  reperfusion syndrome, 646, 649
  saphenous vein graft, 646, 648
  wound infection, 646
Cerebrospinal fluid shunts, drains and diversion
    techniques
  atypical ventricular shunts, 267–268
  complications
    calcified VP shunt catheter, 299
    Chiari decompression (*see* Chiari decompression
        complications)
    corpus callosum changes, 282
    CSF leakage syndrome (*see* CSF leakage
        syndrome)
    hyperostosis, 287, 288
    intracranial hypotension, 287
    intraparenchymal pericatheter cysts and interstitial
        CSF, 295
    intraventricular fat migration, 284
    isolated ventricle (*see* Isolated/trapped ventricle)
    MRI-induced programmable valve setting
        alteration, 285
    shunt-associated infections, 289–291
    shunt-associated intracranial hemorrhage and
        gliosis, 283–284
    shunt fracture and retained fragments, 294
    shunt malposition and migration, 292–293
    slit ventricle syndrome (*see* Slit ventricle
        syndrome)
    tumor seeding, 298
    VP shunt pseudocysts, 260–266
  cystoperitoneal and cystoventriculostomy shunts
    internal drainage, arachnoid cysts, 272
    ventriculoperitoneal shunt placement, 272
  decompression, Chiari malformation
    cine phase-contrast, 277
    posterior fossa decompression, 306
    suboccipital craniectomy, 300

endoscopic choroid plexus fulguration (*see* Choroid plexus fulguration)
endoscopic septum pellucidum and cyst fenestration
    postoperative MRI, 278
    preoperative T2 MRI, 279
    ventricular system, 278, 279
EVD (*see* External ventricular drains (EVD))
lumboperitoneal shunt (*see* Lumboperitoneal shunting)
subdural-peritoneal shunt, 271
syringosubarachnoid and syringopleural shunts, 274–275
third ventriculostomy
    defect, Liliequist's membrane, 277
    endoscopic fenestration, 277
    hemodynamic changes, 277
Torkildsen shunt (*see* Torkildsen shunt)
VP shunts (*see* Ventriculoperitoneal (VP) shunts)
Cheek and nasolabial fold augmentation
    anterior face and calcium hydroxylapatite injection, 7, 9
    anterior face and hyaluronic acid augmentation, 7, 10
    collagen injection, 7, 11
    coral implants, 7, 8
    heterotopic ossification, 7, 17
    HIV lipoatrophy, 7
    hyaluronic acid eyelid migration, 7, 17
    implant
        abscess, 7, 14
        bone erosion and maxillary sinus penetration, 7, 17
        seroma, 7, 13
    inflammation, 7, 16
    injectable silicone
        granulomas, 7, 16
        scars, 7, 16
    liquid silicone injection, acne scar treatment, 7, 8
    osteomyelitis, 7, 15
    polyacrylamide gel polymer treatment, 7, 12
    polytetrafluoroethylene filler, 7, 9
    silicone implant and calcium hydroxylapatite, 7, 8, 12
Cheiloplasty *see* Lip reconstruction
Chemotherapy wafers
    carmustine, 213
    Gliadel, 213
    tumor recurrence, 213
Chiari decompression complications
    arachnoid cyst formation and cerebellar ptosis, 272
    pseudomeningoceles, 300
Choroid plexus fulguration
    dilatation, lateral ventricle, 280, 281
    hydrocephalus, 280
    tumor resection, 281
Cingulotomy, 220–221
Cochlear implants
    complications
        facial nerve, 398, 400
        implant extrusion, 402, 404
        incomplete insertion, 402

        lateral malpositioning, 403, 404
        medial malpositioning, 402, 403
        perilymphatic fistula, 400, 402
        receiver-stimulator skull erosion, 402
    components, 398, 399
    insertion, cochlear drill out, 400
Coil embolization, endovascular surgery
    aneurysm coiling, 660, 686, 687
    angiography, pipeline stent insertion, 660
    compaction, 685, 687
    detachable coil, 663
    migration, 688, 689
    nontarget embolization, 686, 688
    prolapse, 688
    retained catheter fragment, 689, 688
    retained snare, 689, 688
    stent-assisted coiling, 658, 660
    vertebral artery embolization, 663, 670, 671, 687
Conjunctivodacryocystorhinostomy (CDCR), 43, 44
Coronoidectomy, 436–437
Corpectomy
    anterior slippage, expandable cage, 536
    bone graft reconstruction, 533
    dislocated bone grafts, 536
    expandable cage, 535, 536
    expandable cage subsidence, 535
    Harms cage, 533, 534
    stackable carbon fiber reconstruction, 535
Corpus callosum changes, shunt catheterization
    injury, 282
    scalloping deformity, 282
    swelling, 282
Corticectomy
    description, 238
    residual lesions, 238, 239
    tuberous sclerosis and intractable seizures, 238
Cranial vault encephalocele repair
    description, 146
    occipital encephalocele resection, 146
    preoperative sagittal, 147
Cranial vault surgical remodeling
    Barrel stave osteotomies, 142, 143
    calcium phosphate cement, 142, 145
    correction cranioplasty and orbitofrontal advancement, 142–144
    description, 142
    endoscopic strip craniectomy, 142, 145
    orbitofrontal advancement surgery, onlay cement, 142, 144
    posterior cranial vault distraction, 142, 144
Craniectomy, 140–141
Cranioplasty
    hydroxyapatite cement, 132, 134
    intraoperatively fashioned acrylic, 133
    Porex, 132, 136–137
    preformed acrylic, 132, 134
    split-thickness bone graft, 132, 138
    synthetic bone grafts, 132
    synthetic HTR bone graft, 132, 137
    titanium mesh, 132, 135
    titanium plate, 132, 136

Craniotomy
  complications, 128
  description, 128
  dural enhancement and bone flap granulation tissue, 128, 130
  fixation wires, 128, 130
  hemicraniotomy, 128
  hinge craniotomy, 128, 130
  imaging appearance, 128
  intracranial air, 128
  micro fixation plates, 128, 129
  postoperative pneumocephalus, 128, 131
  skin staples, 128, 129
  standard types, 128
  temporalis muscle swelling, 128, 131
CSF leakage syndrome
  description, 297
  lower chest, 297
  lumboperitoneal shunt placement, 276
Cyst decompression, 435
Cystic craniopharyngiomas
  drainage, 318, 319
  fenestration, 318
  infection, 318, 320
  postoperative cyst growth, 318, 319

D
Dacryocystorhinostomy and nasolacrimal duct stents
  CDCR, 43, 44
  dacryocystogram patency, 43–44
  description, 43
  pneumo-orbit with Jones tube, 43, 44
Decompression, spine
  cordectomy, 537
  corpectomy, 524, 533, 535–537, 550
  facetectomy, 524, 529
  laminectomy, 526–528
  laminoplasty, 532
  laminotomy and foraminotomy, 525
  microdiscectomy, 530–531
  vertebrectomy, 524, 533–536
Deep brain stimulation (DBS)
  brain stimulator insertion infarct, 226, 229
  electrode migration, 226, 228
  subthalamic nucleus stimulation, 226
  ventralis caudalis nucleus stimulator, 226, 227
Detachable balloon embolization, 663
Duraplasty and sealant agents
  collagen matrix, 154, 155
  complications, 154
  description, 154
  photograph, suturable DuraGen, 155
  polytetrafluoroethylene (Gore-Tex), 154, 156
Dysthyroid orbitopathy
  description, 41
  medial and lateral orbital wall decompression, 41
  orbital rim augmentation, 41, 42
  paranasal sinus obstruction, 41, 42
  transnasal endoscopic approach, 41

E
Ear and temporal bone imaging
  atresiaplasty, 357–358
  auricular reconstruction, 354–355
  auriculectomy, 353–354
  BAHA device, 352
  canaloplasty and meatoplasty, 356
  cochlear implants (see Cochlear implants)
  endolymphatic sac decompression and shunting, 409
  eustachian tube occlusion procedures, 384–385
  incus interposition, 367, 368
  labyrinthectomy, 410–411
  lateral temporal bone resection, 353, 395, 397
  mastoidectomy (see Mastoidectomy)
  myringotomy and tympanostomy tubes, 359–360
  ossicular prosthesis, 378–382
  PORP, TORP and VORP, 369–373
  repair, perilymphatic fistula, 408
  stapedectomy, stapedotomy and stapes prosthesis
    malleus grip prosthesis, 374, 376
      Robinson bucket handle prosthesis, 375
      Schuknecht teflon wire stapes prosthesis, 374, 375
      smart nitinol wire, 374, 375
      susceptibility artifact, 374, 377
  superior semicircular canal dehiscence repair, 413
  transcanal atticotomy, 382
  tube drainage, cholesterol cysts, 414–415
  vestibular nerve sectioning, 412
Effusions, 166, 167
Eminectomy and meniscalplication, 441
Endolymphatic sac decompression and shunting, 409
Endovascular surgery
  coil embolization (see Coil embolization, endovascular surgery)
  detachable balloon embolization, 663
  extracranial carotid artery stents (see Extracranial carotid artery stents)
  intracranial arterial stents (see Intracranial arterial stents)
  liquid agent and particle embolization
    arteriovenous malformations, 661–662
    incomplete embolization, 636, 637
    left frontal meningioma, 665
    onyx embolization, 665
    retained catheter fragment, 661
    Silastic beads, 661, 662
    tantalum powder, 661
  mechanical stent failure
    flat-panel CT, 686
    fracture, 683, 686
    stent kink, 683, 686
  mechanical thrombectomy (see Thrombectomy, mechanical)
  percutaneous sclerotherapy, 666–667
  vascular plugs, 663, 664
  venous sinus stents, 676, 677
Epidural motor cortex stimulator, 230
Eustachian tube occlusion
  catheter migration, 384, 385
  hydroxyapatite injection, 384
  teflon injection, 384, 385

EVD (*see* External ventricular drains (EVD)
Expanded polytetrafluoroethylene (ePTFE), 35
External brain herniation, 175
External ethmoidectomy, 84
External ventricular drains (EVD), 259, 261
Extracranial carotid artery stents
   cervical, 672
   complications, 677, 684
   description, 673
   intimal hyperplasia, 681, 683
   stent occlusion, 682, 684
Extracranial-intracranial revascularization, vascular
      surgery
   direct
      MCA-STA bypass, 628
      occlusion, 627, 629
      saphenous vein graft, 627, 628
   indirect
      ADC maps, 631
      angiography, 631
      cerebral infarction, 631, 646
      encephaloduroarteriosynangiosis/pial synangiosis,
         631, 633
      encephaloduromyosynangiosis, 631, 633
      multiple burr holes, 631

F
Facetectomy
   partial, 529
   total, 529
Facial cosmetic surgery
   augmentation
      cheek and nasolabial fold, 7–17
      chin and jaw, 26–28
      forehead, 5–6
      lip, 25
   materials and imaging features
      complications, 1
      fillers and injectables, 1, 4
      implants and grafts, 1, 3
      photographs, facial implants, 1, 2
   rhinoplasty, 18–24
Facial reanimation
   free gracilis muscle transfer, 472
   SOOF lift, 472–475
   temporalis muscle transposition, 472–475
   temporoparietal fascia, 473, 474
   tensor fascia lata graft implantation, 472, 473
Failed back surgery syndrome (FBSS)
   adjacent segment disease, 601
   arachnoiditis, 591–592
   causes, 582
   deformity
      flat-back syndrome, 558, 602
      pedicle subtraction osteotomy, 602
      wedge osteotomy, 602
   description, 582
   epidural hematoma
      laminectomy, 588
      spinal canal stenosis, 588

gossypiboma, 600–601
hardware
   displacement, 583
   interbody fusion device retropulsion, 584
   lucency, 585
   malpositioning, 583, 584
   pseudarthrosis, 585
   rod displacement, 583
   transsacral interbody fusion, 585
infection
   discitis/osteomyelitis, 589
   epidural abscess, 547
   hardware removal, 589, 590
   retroperitoneal abscess, 559, 566
   Staphylococcus aureus, 589
intradural inclusion cyst
   formation, 591
   ovoid cystic mass, 597
neuritis
   left lower extremity weakness, 591
   MRI, 591
pseudomeningocele and CSF leak
   CT myelogram, 583, 587
   management, 587
   pseudomeningocele, 587
residual/recurrent disc material *vs.* epidural scar
   epidural fibrosis, 591, 593
   sequestered disc fragment, 594
residual/recurrent tumors, 596–597
retained bone fragments, 599
retained drill bit
   broken drill bit fragment, 599, 603
   CT, 599
synovial cyst
   de novo synovial cyst, 595
   puncture and aspiration, 595
FBSS. *See* Failed back surgery syndrome (FBSS)
FESS. *See* Functional endoscopic sinus surgery (FESS)
Flat-back syndrome, 602
Forehead augmentation
   description, 5
   lateral brow augmentation, 5, 6
   mid-forehead
      calcium hydroxylapatite, 5
      polytetrafluoroethylene, 5
Free flap reconstruction
   complications, 123
   description, 123
   Latissimus dorsi muscle, 123, 124
   omental, 123, 125
Frontalis suspension ptosis repair, 35
Frontal sinus cranialization, 100
Frontal sinus trephination, 101
Functional endoscopic sinus surgery (FESS)
   anterior, cerebral artery pseudoaneurysm, 91
   bolgerization, 85
   CSF leak, 89
   description, 84
   draf type I, II and III frontal sinusectomy,
      85–88
   empty nose syndrome, 96

Functional endoscopic sinus surgery (FESS) (*cont.*)
   encephaloceles
      and intraparenchymal hemorrhage, 89
      meningoceles, 89
   ethmoid artery injury, 91
   intraorbital complications, 90
   lateralized middle turbinate, 95
   medialized lamina papyracea, 92
   middle turbinectomy, 84, 85
   mucocele, 94
   mucosal inflammation, 93
   nasoantral window, 85, 88
   optic nerve injury, 90
   orbital injury, 90
   osteoneogenesis, 95
   pattern, ostiomeatal unit, 84, 85
   posterior drainage pathway, 85, 86
   recurrent polyposis, 94
   retained surgical packing, 88
   sphenoidotomy, 85
   surgical packing material, 88
   uncinectomy, 84

G
GAD. *See* Glutamic acid decarboxylase (GAD)
Genioplasty
   combined osteotomy and porous polyethylene,
      424, 425
   coronal and CT images lengthening,
      423, 424
   shortening, 3D CT image, 424
   silicone, 424, 425
Glaucoma surgery
   Ahmed valve, 47, 48
   Baerveldt shunt, 47
   blebs, 47, 49
   description, 47
   Ex-PRESS glaucoma shunt, 47, 50
   glaucoma valve, photo, 48
   hemorrhagic suprachoroidal detachments,
      47, 49
   orbital cellulitis, 47, 49
   valves drainage, maxillary sinus, 48
GliaSite radiation therapy system, 215–216
Glossectomy and mouth floor reconstruction
   marginal mandibulectomy, 477
   minimal tongue excision and primary closure, 476
   partial glossectomy, 476
   pharyngocutaneous fistula, 493
   sialocele, 476, 478
   squamous cell carcinoma recurrence, 478
   submandibular gland, 476, 479
   total glossectomy, 477
Glutamic acid decarboxylase (GAD), 232
Gossypiboma. *See also* Retained surgical packing
   description, 600
   lumbar stenosis, 600
   MRI, 600–601

H
Halo and traction devices
   Gardner-Wells device, 538
   halo vest, 538
Harrington, Knodt and Luque rods
   dislocation, 556
   flat-back syndrome, 556
   frontal radiographs, 556
   rod fracture, 556, 557
Hemicraniectomy, 125, 137, 140, 156
Hemispherectomy
   anatomical, 251, 252
   description, 251
   functional, 251
Hemorrhage and hematomas
   adjacent epidural, 162
   adjacent intraparenchymal, 162, 163
   asymptomatic, 162
   regional subdural, 162, 163
   remote cerebellar hemorrhage, 162, 164
   skull flap, subjacent to, 162, 165
   subgaleal, 162
Hydrogel expander, 65
Hygromas, 166
Hyperostosis
   calvarial, 288
   dural, 300
   imaging, 287

I
IMF. *See* Intermaxillary fixation (IMF)
Implantable bone stimulators
   description, 542
   frontal and lateral, 542
Incus interposition
   dislocation, 367, 368
   osteonecrosis, 367, 368
Inferior turbinate outfracture and reduction, 79
Intermaxillary fixation (IMF), 432
Intracranial aneurysm muscle wrap
   growing left P1 segment aneurysm, 635
   temporalis muscle, 631, 632
Intracranial arterial stents
   CT angiography, 670, 673
   stent stenosis, 682, 684
Intracranial hypotension, chronic overshunting
   diffuse thickening and avid enhancement,
      meninges, 287
   symptom, 287
Intraocular lens (IOL)
   cataracts, 56
   components, 56
   implant dislocation, 56, 57
   implant dystrophic calcifications, 56, 57
   posterior chamber, 56
Intraocular silicone injection, 59–60
Intraparenchymal pressure monitor, 157
Intrathecal spinal infusion pump

Baclofen pump components, 604
metastatic disease, 603
spinal hypotension syndrome, 603, 604
Intraventricular fat migration, 284
IOL. *See* Intraocular lens (IOL)
Isolated/trapped ventricle
asymmetric ventricles, 286
obstruction level, 286
right lateral ventricle collapse, 283

J
Jannetta procedure. *See* Microvascular decompression
Jaw augmentation
chin augmentation
"button" bone graft, 26
silicone implant, 26
chin implant
bone erosion, 26, 28
bone formation, 26, 28
and prejowl porous polyethylene implant, 26, 27
seroma, 26, 28
combined bone and silicone chin implant, 26, 27
lateral/mandibular angle implants, 26, 28
prejowl implant migration, 26, 27
Jones tube, 43, 44

K
Keratoprostheses
complications, 55
description, 55
Kpro type 1 and II device, 55

L
Labyrinthectomy
chemical, 410
transcanal, 410, 411
transmastoid, 410
Laminectomy
bilateral, 526
and duraplasty, 527
hemilaminectomy/unilateral, 526
infarct, 526, 528
spinal cord laceration, 537
Laminoplasty
partial osteotomy, 532
unilateral right-sided titanium lamina prosthesis, 532
Laminotomy and foraminotomy
artificially widening L5–S1 neural foramen, 525
thinning, 525
Laryngeal stents, 499
Laryngectomy
abscess, pseudoaneurysm, 494
anastomotic leak, 493
angiolytic laser cordectomy, 488
aortic graft, 488, 493
contrast-enhanced CT, 493

granulation tissue, 493
horizontal, 490, 492
infected leak, 493
postoperative laryngocele, 494
recurrent tumor, 493
supracricoid, 490, 492
total laryngectomy, 477, 491, 493
total pharyngolaryngectomy, 491
types, 488, 492
vertical partial laryngectomy, 489, 492
Laryngoplasty and vocal fold injection
cartilage graft, 500, 501
"classical" laryngoplasty, 501
excess medialization, 500, 501
fat injection, 503
hyaluronic acid, 501, 503
hydroxyapatite prostheses, 500, 501
insufficient medialization, 505
material extrusion, 504
material supraglottic migration, 505
medialization laryngoplasty, 500
micronized acellular human dermis, 504
montgomery prosthesis, 500, 505
polytetrafluoroethylene, medialization laryngoplasty, 500, 502
teflon granuloma, 501, 504
types, agents, 501
vocal fold augmentation, injectable calcium hydroxylapatite, 502
Lateral temporal bone resection
description, 395, 397
tumor recurrence, 395, 397
type I, 395, 397
type II, 395, 397
type III, 395, 397
type IV, 395, 397
Leucotomy. *See* Prefrontal lobotomy
Limbic leucotomy, 222–224
Lip augmentation
calcium hydroxylapatite, 25
complications, 25
polytetrafluoroethylene implants, 25
Lip reconstruction
closure techniques, 453
perioral myocutaneous flap, 453, 454
radial forearm free flap, 457
Lumboperitoneal shunting
description, 276
gravity-actuated horizontal-vertical valve system, 276
programmable valve, 276
pseudotumor cerebri and CSF rhinorrhea, 276

M
Mandible fractures
external fixation, 432, 433
IMF, 432
maxillomandibular, Erich arch bars, 432
open reduction, 432, 433

Mandible surgery
   core excision and enucleation
      biopsy, 434
      brown tumor, mandible, 434
   coronoidectomy, 436
   cyst decompression, 435
   distraction, mandibular, 426–427
   eminectomy and meniscalplication, 441
   fixation, mandible fractures, 432–433
   genioplasty (see Genioplasty)
   mandibular angle augmentation, 425
   mandibulectomy and mandibular reconstruction,
      438–440
   mandibulotomy, 433
   osteotomy
      sagittal split, 423
      vertical ramus, 421–422
Mandibular angle augmentation, 425
Mandibular distraction
   curvilinear distraction device, 426, 427
   mature osteogenesis, 426, 431
   single-vector distraction device, 426
   transport distraction device, 427
Mandibulectomy and mandibular reconstruction
   condylectomy, 438, 439
   and condylectomy, condylar prosthesis,
      438, 439
   devitalized fibular graft, 438, 439
   graft, abscess, 428, 430
   hardware fracture, 438, 440
   marginal mandibulectomy, 438
   segmental mandibulectomy, 438
   TMJ dislocation and accelerated arthritis,
      440, 446
   tumor recurrence, 434, 438, 440
Mandibulotomy, 433
Marcus Gunn jaw-winking syndrome, 35
Mastoidectomy
   complications
      CSF leak and encephalocele, 389, 413
      encephalocele, 389, 394
      extratemporal cholesteatoma recurrence/inclusion
         cyst, 389, 391
      facial nerve dehiscence, 392
      facial nerve injury and reparative neuroma,
         389, 393
      graft resorption, 384, 389
      granulation tissue, 389, 390
      labyrinthitis ossificans, 398
      mucosalized mastoid bowl, 386, 387, 394
      recurrent cholesteatoma, 389, 391
      repair, tegmen, 389, 394
   and mastoid obliteration
      bone dust, 388
      canal-wall-down, 398
      canal-wall-up, 398
      drainage tubes, 414
      fat graft, 387
      radical, 386, 387
      simple/partial, 357, 386

Maxillary swing
   description, 110
   nasopharyngeal carcinoma, 110
   recurrent tumor, 110, 111
Maxillectomy and palatectomy
   antibiotic-impregnated beads, 104, 109
   flap reconstruction, tumor recurrence, 104, 109
   foreign body reaction, 104, 109
   obturator, 104, 105
   osteomyocutaneous flap reconstruction, 104, 107
   partial and total, 104, 105
   postoperative dacryocystocele, 104, 109
   postoperative pterygopalatine fossa, 104, 108
   radial forearm, 104, 106
Meningogaleal complex, 140–141
Microcatheter subthalamic infusion, 232
Microdiscectomy
   description, 530
   left ligamentum flavum absence, 530
   surgicel mimicking disc sequestration, 531
Microvascular decompression
   cranial nerve 8 compression, 643, 645
   failed, 644
   glossopharyngeal neuralgia, 643, 644
   hemifacial spasm, 643–645
   Teflon, 643–645
   trigeminal neuralgia, 643, 644
Middle cranial fossa
   reconstruction
      fat and bone grafts, 336, 337
      myocutaneous flap, 336, 337
      titanium mesh and bone graft, 336
   temporal lobe encephalomalacia, 336
   vestibular schwannoma resection, 338–347
Mohs micrographic surgery, 122
Montgomery® laryngeal stent®, 499
Montgomery® salivary bypass tube®, 498
Myringoplasty and tympanoplasty
   graft cholesteatoma, 359, 361
   tubes
      extrusion, tympanostomy tube, 360
      medial dislocation, 360
      metal grommet, 359
      plastic grommet, 359
      plastic shaft tympanostomy tube, 360
   type description, 365, 366
   type I
      cartilage graft, 361, 363
      silastic implant, 363
      temporalis fascia, 361, 362
   type II, 363
   type III
      stapes columella, 364, 365
      tympanoplasty, minor columella, 364, 365
   type IV, 364, 366

N
Nasal packing, 80
Nasal septal button prosthesis, 78

Neck dissection
   abscess, 461, 467
   extended, 461, 463–464
   lymphocele, 461, 467
   modified radical, 461, 464
   neuropathic joint, 461, 468
   osteomyelitis, 461, 467
   pectoralis rotational flap, radical, 464
   postoperative imaging, 461
   selective, 461–463
   tongue atrophy, 461, 464
   types, 461–463
Neck imaging
   arytenoidectomy, 507
   brachytherapy, 517
   facial reanimation (*see* Facial reanimation)
   glossectomy and mouth floor reconstruction,
      476–478
   laryngeal framework reconstruction
      hematomas, 508
      miniplates, 508
      panorex and 3D CT, 508
   laryngeal stents, 499
   laryngectomy, 488–494
   laryngoplasty and vocal fold injection (*see*
      Laryngoplasty and vocal fold injection)
   lip reconstruction (*see* Lip reconstruction)
   montgomery T-tubes, 497
   neck dissection, 461–468
   neck exploration and parathyroidectomy
      failed, 514, 516
      parathyroid gland autotransplantation, 514
      recurrent parathyroid adenoma, 470
   parotidectomy, 469, 470, 473, 474
   reconstruction flaps (*see* Reconstruction flaps)
   salivary bypass stent, 498
   salivary duct stenting
      sialendoscopic extraction, 471
      submandibular duct stent, 471
   Sistrunk procedure (*see* Sistrunk procedure)
   thyroidectomy, 512–515
   tonsillectomy and adenoidectomy, 480–483
   tracheoesophageal puncture and voice prostheses,
      495–496
   vagal nerve stimulator, 518
Neural interface system, 231

O
Ommaya reservoirs
   catheter-associated cyst, 208, 212
   catheter infection, 208, 210
   components, 208, 209
   description, 208
   infection, 208
   methotrexate extravasation, 208, 211
Orbital exenteration
   description, 66
   and facial implant, 66
   graft necrosis, 66, 68

   with implant, 66, 68
   maxillectomy and flap reconstruction, 66, 67
   radiation-induced osteosarcoma, 66, 69
   radical, 66, 68
   tumor recurrence, 66, 69
Orbital radiation therapy fiducial markers, 70
Orbital tissue expanders, 65
Orbital wall reconstruction and augmentation
   bone graft, 36
   cerebrospinal fluid leak., 36, 40
   hematic cyst, 36, 39
   infection, 36, 38
   inferiorly positioned mesh, 36, 39
   medial canthus stabilization device, 36, 38
   mesh deformity, 36, 39
   mucocele, 36, 40
   nasolacrimal duct obstruction, 36, 40
   porous polyethylene implant, 37
   porous structure, 36
   rectus muscle impingement, 40
   silicon implant, 36
   titanium mesh, 36, 37
   wedge implant designs, 36, 38
Orbit imaging
   dacryocystorhinostomy and nasolacrimal duct stents,
      43–44
   decompression (*see* Dysthyroid orbitopathy)
   enucleation, evisceration and globe prostheses
      components, 61
      description, 61
      globe implant exposure, 61, 64
      globe implant rotation and inflammation,
         61, 63
      hollow glass globe implant, 61
      hydroxyapatite prosthesis, 61
      orbital augmentation beads, 61, 63
      orbital augmentation with silicone implant,
         61, 63
      porous polyethylene implant, 61, 62
      scleral cover shell, 61, 63
      silicone implant, 61, 62
   eyelid weights
      complications, 31
      facial nerve deficit, 31
      left cranial nerve VII palsy, 31, 32
   frontalis suspension ptosis repair, 35
   glaucoma surgery, 47–50
   intraocular silicone injection, 59–60
   IOL implants (*see* Intraocular lens (IOL))
   keratoprostheses, 55
   orbital radiation therapy fiducial markers, 70
   palpebral spring
      description, 33
      eyelid, 33–34
   scleral buckles, 51–54
   strabismus surgery, 45–46
   subretinal gas/anterior chamber migration, 58
   surgical aphakia, 58
   tissue expanders, 65
   wall reconstruction and augmentation, 36–40

Ossicular prosthesis complications
  detachment, stapes prosthesis, 378, 379
  dislocated
    PORP, 378, 380
    TORP, 378, 381
  extruded TORP, 378, 381
  lateralized stapes prosthesis, 379
  migration, PORP and TORP, 378
  perilymphatic fistula, 378
  prosthesis fracture, 382
  recurrent cholesteatoma, TORP, 378, 381
  stapes prosthesis, 378
  tympanic membrane dehiscence, 378, 382
  vestibular perforation, 378
Osteoplastic flap, frontal sinus obliteration
  cosmetic deformity, 97, 99
  description, 97
  expected appearance, 97
  extruded packing material, 97, 99
  frontal sinus obliteration, 97, 98
  retained secretions, 97, 98
Osteotomy
  sagittal split, 423
  vertical ramus
    muscle atrophy, 421, 422
    TMJ dysfunction, 421, 422

P
Pallidotomy, 219
Paranasal sinuses and nasal cavity
  Caldwell-Luc procedure, 83
  decompression and drainage, 102
  enucleation and ostectomy, 102, 103
  external ethmoidectomy, 84
  FESS (see Functional endoscopic sinus surgery
      (FESS))
  frontal sinus cranialization, 100
  frontal sinus trephination, 101
  inferior turbinate outfracture and reduction, 79
  maxillary swing, 110–111
  maxillectomy and palatectomy, 104–109
  nasal packing, 80
  nasal septal button prosthesis, 78
  osteoplastic flap, frontal sinus obliteration, 97–99
  paranasal sinus stents, 101
  posttraumatic rhinoplasty, 75–76
  residual/recurrent lesion, 102, 103
  rhinectomy, 81
  septoplasty, 77–78
  sinus lift procedure, 82
Paranasal sinus stents, 101
Parotidectomy
  facial nerve sacrifice, 470, 473
  parotid pleomorphic adenoma recurrence,
      469, 470
  partial superficial, 469
  skin cancers and chronic inflammatory diseases, 469
  superficial parotidectomy, graft reconstruction, 469
  total parotidectomy, 469, 470

Partial ossicular reconstruction prosthesis (PORP)
  Applebaum, 371, 372
  Black oval-top, 372, 381
  dislocated, 380, 381
  migration, TORP, 378
  stapes, 378
  tympanic membrane, 378, 379
Percutaneous sclerotherapy
  alcohol sclerotherapy, 666
  MRI, 666–667
  surgical resection, 665
Percutaneous spine treatments
  adjacent level vertebral body fracture,
      kyphoplasty, 609
  cement extravasation
    degenerative changes, 609
    disc space cement leakage, 609, 611
    paravertebral extravasation, 609, 611
    spinal canal cement leakage, 611
  cement intravasation and embolism
    chest imaging, 609
    pulmonary embolism, 612
  fusion
    homogeneously hyperdense material, 593
    OptiMesh, 614
  percutaneous perineural cyst decompression, 616
  sacroplasty, 524, 613
  vertebral augmentation (see Vertebral
      augmentation)
Perilymphatic fistula repair, 408
Pneumatic retinopexy, 58
PORP. See Partial ossicular reconstruction prosthesis
    (PORP)
Posttraumatic rhinoplasty
  cortical bone reconstruction, 75, 76
  description, 75
  nasal bone fracture reconstruction,
      75, 76
Prefrontal lobotomy, 217–218
Pseudoaneurysm, 169
Pseudomeningoceles, 168

R
Reconstruction flaps
  aerodigestive track, 453, 458
  colonic interposition, 457, 458
  complications, 454
  facial soft-tissue defects, 453
  fasciocutaneous rotation advancement flap,
      454, 455, 458
  gastric transposition, 457
  myocutaneous
    flap neopharynx, 457, 459
    free flap, 453, 456, 457
    rotational flap, 456
  osteomyocutaneous
    and bone grafts, 453
    flap, 453, 454, 456
  pectoralis major muscle flap, 453

rugal folds and haustra, 453
temporalis flap, 455
tissue flaps types, 454
tumor recurrence, 459
types, 453, 454, 458
Retained surgical packing, 88
Rhinectomy, 81
Rhinoplasty
cellulitis, 18, 22
cranial nerve V2 injury, 18, 23
description, 18
dorsal augmentation, bone, 18, 19
filler, 18, 21
fistula implant, 18, 21
frontal radiograph, 18, 23
implant abscess, 18, 22
implant extrusion, 18, 22
lateral osteotomy, 18
nasal cavity, turbulent, 18, 24
nasal obstruction, 18, 23
open rhinoplasty, 18
polytetrafluoroethylene implant, 18, 21
retained foreign body, 18, 21
silicone dorsal tip and columellar nasal implant,
    18, 20
tip augmentation, bone, 18

S
Sacroplasty
cement, bilateral sacral ala, 613
complications, 613
description, 613
Scalp and cranium imaging
absorbable hemostatic agents, 149–153
air leak, 160, 161
autocranioplasty, 139
bone flap resorption, 176
box osteotomy, 148
Burr holes, 126, 127
cranial vault
    encephalocele repair, 146–147
    surgical remodeling, 142–145
craniectomy, meningogaleal complex and
    suboccipital craniectomy, 140–141
cranioplasty (see Cranioplasty)
craniotomy (see Craniotomy)
duraplasty and sealant agents, 154–156
effusions, 166, 167
entered orbit, 160
external brain herniation, 175
free flap reconstruction, 123–125
frontal sinus, entered, 160
hemorrhage and hematomas, 162–165
hygromas, 166
infection
    cranioplasty prosthesis, 170, 172
    craniotomy bed, 170–172
intracranial pressure monitor, 157
Mohs micrographic surgery and skin grafting, 122

occipital nerve stimulator, 117–118
pseudomeningoceles, 168
rotational galeal flap scalp reconstruction, 123
scalp tissue expander, 119
scalp tumor recurrence, 125
subdural drainage catheters, 158
Sunken skin flap syndrome, 174
temporal fossa implant, 120–121
tension pneumocephalus, 159
textiloma, 173
Scalp tissue expander, 119
Scleral buckles
combined silicone rubber band and sponge, 51, 52
description, 51
hydrogel
    fragmentation and migration, 51, 54
    hydration and expansion, 51, 54
infected, 51, 53
silicone rubber encircling, 51–52
silicone sponge scleral buckle, 51, 52
tantalum clip, 51, 53
Seizure monitoring electrodes and neuropace
depth electrode, 232, 235
description, 232
electrode grids, 234
electrode strips, 233
foramen ovale electrodes, 232, 235
hematoma, 233, 236
infected electrodes, 233, 237
NeuroPace, 232, 236
Selective amygdalohippocampectomy
description, 249
visual pathway injury from laser ablation, 249, 250
Septoplasty
complications, 77
description, 77
nasal stents, 77, 78
septoplasty perforation, 77, 78
septum, nasal obstruction, 77
Shunt-associated intracranial hemorrhage and gliosis
predisposing factors, 283
subdural hemorrhage, 283, 284
ventriculomegaly and effacement, sulci, 296
Shunt catheter
associated infections
    cellulitis and subcutaneous abscesses, 289, 291
    intraperitoneal abscess, 291
    meningitis, 289
    ventriculitis, 289, 290
fracture and retained fragments
    detached intracranial shunt catheter
        fragment, 300
    migrated catheter fragments, 292, 297
    retained infected catheter fragment, 289
malposition and migration
    bowel perforation, 292, 293
    catheter tip projection, 292
    distal shunt catheter migration, 292
    laparotomy, 292
    retracted catheter, 292, 294

Silastic beads, 661, 662
Sinonasal undifferentiated carcinoma (SNUC),
        311, 314
Sinus lift procedure
    bone graft material, 82
    description, 82
    sinusitis and oroantral fistula, 82
Sistrunk procedure
    abscess, 487
    recurrent thyroglossal duct cyst, 486
    surgical defect, 486
Skin grafting, 122
Skull base and cerebellopontine angle imaging
    anterior craniofacial resection, 311–317
    cystic craniopharyngiomas, 318–320
    middle cranial fossa
        approach, 336
        reconstruction, 336–337
    vestibular schwannomas
        radiosurgery, 348
        surgical approaches, 338–347
Slit ventricle syndrome, 287
SNUC. See Sinonasal undifferentiated carcinoma
        (SNUC)
Spinal cord stimulators
    cervical, 528, 547
    description, 605
    infected lead, 606
    thoracic, 605
Spine imaging
    categories, surgery, 523, 524
    decompression (see Decompression, spine)
    dynamic facet replacement
        posterior, 579
        TOPS, 579
    dynamic rods
        complications, 580
        Dynesys, 580
    dynamic stabilization and miscellaneous devices,
        567–572
    FBSS (see Failed back surgery syndrome (FBSS))
    intrathecal spinal infusion pump, 603–604
    nucleus pulposus replacement, 573
    percutaneous (see Percutaneous spine treatments)
    posterior dynamic stabilization devices
        Coflex, 574, 577
        DIAM, 574, 576
        dislocated coflex, 578
        interspinous spacers, 576, 578
        isobar, 574, 575
        X-Stop, 574
    spinal cord stimulators, 605–606
    stabilization and fusion (see Stabilization and fusion,
        spine)
    total disc replacement
        adjacent-level disc herniation, 567, 572
        advent cervical spine total disc prosthesis, 569
        ankylosis, 567, 571
        anterior migration, 570
        Charite lumbar spine total disc prosthesis, 569

        heterotopic ossification, 567, 571
        lateral view, lumbar spine, 570
        NUBAC, 573
        prestige cervical spine total disc prosthesis, 568
        radiolucent core, 567
        subsidence, 567
        vertebral fracture, 571
Stabilization and fusion, spine
    anterior fusion
        anterior cervical discectomy and
            fusion (ACDF), 547
        bone graft subsidence, 547, 549
        iatrogenic spinal cord transection, 547, 549
        infection, 547, 548
        lumbar spine, 547
    anterolateral fusion
        adjustable plate system, 550
        Kaneda device, 550
    bone graft materials
        allograft bone chips, 540
        autologous bone graft, 539
        composite Mozaik moldable morsels, 541
        DBX putty, bone crouton, 539, 541
        demineralized bone matrix, 539
        local vertebral body bone harvest, 540
        mature bone graft fusion, 540
        recombinant BMP-induced osteolysis, 541
    craniocervical fusion
        atlantoaxial fusion, 543
        hardware loosening, 546
        indications, 543
        occipital screw intracranial penetration, 545
        occipitocervical fusion, 543–546
        uncoiled sublaminar wire, 543, 544
        vertebral canal entry, 549
    halo and traction devices, 538
    Harrington, Knodt, and Luque rods, 556
    implantable bone stimulators, 542
    interbody fusion
        ALIF, 564, 566
        disadvantage, 561
        femoral ring allograft, 561
        PLIF, 563, 566
        stalif, 565, 566
        tapered LT-cage, 562
        threaded cage, 562
        threaded titanium pin, 566
        TLIF, 563, 566
        transsacral fusion, 565, 566
        XLIF, 564, 566
        Zero P, 547
    posterior fusion
        facet screws, 551, 555
        medial malpositioning, 551
        pedicle hooks, 555
        pedicle screws, 551–553
        wire fixation, 554
    screw fixation, dens fractures, 542
    VEPTR (see Vertical expandable prosthetic titanium
        rib (VEPTR))

vertebral stapling
   C-shaped staples, 559
   description, 559
Stereotactic brain biopsy
  blood products, 189
  cavity marker, 189
  expected biopsy path enhancement, 189, 190
  tumor seeding, 189, 190
Strabismus surgery
  description, 45
  morphology, 45
  postoperative
    infection, 45, 46
    rectus muscle rupture, 45
  rectus transposition, 45
  Y splitting, 45
Subcaudate tractotomy, 222–223
Subdural drainage catheters, 158
Subdural-peritoneal shunt
  chronic subdural hematomas, 271
  complications, 271
Suboccipital craniectomy, 140–141
Sunken skin flap syndrome, 174
Superior semicircular canal dehiscence repair, 413
Surgical aphakia, 58
Syringopleural shunt, 274–275
Syringosubarachnoid shunt, 274–275

T
Temporal fossa implant
  methyl methacrylate, 120, 121
  porous polyethylene, 120
  silicone, 120, 121
  soft tissue deficiency, 120
Temporomandibular joint (TMJ) surgery
  arthroplasty
    Lorenz prosthesis, 445
    prosthesis, 445
    synthes total joint prosthesis, 446
  costochondral graft reconstruction
    resorption, rib graft, 443
    rib graft degenerative disease and
      demineralization, 443
  discectomy, 442
  disc implant and prosthesis failure
    implant intracranial migration, 447, 448
    implant perforation, 448
    loosening and dislocation, 447
    pseudoarthrosis, 447, 449
    teflon granuloma, 448
  disc replacement implants
    silastic implant, 444
    types, 444
  hemiarthroplasty
    glenoid implant, 445
    ramus-condyle unit implant, 445
Tension pneumocephalus, 159
Textiloma, 173
Thalamotomy, 225

Thrombectomy, mechanical
  complication, 667
  contrast stain, 667
  CTA, 668
  hemorrhage and contrast stain, 667
  residual contrast staining, 667, 670
Thyroidectomy
  abscess, 513
  fluid collection, 513
  hemithyroidectomy, 511–513
  ipsilateral subtotal resection, 511
  I-131 total body scans, 512
  near-total thyroidectomy, 511, 512
  recurrent papillary thyroid carcinoma, 513
  right strap muscle resection, 512
  thyroglossal duct remnant, 512
  types, 511
  vocal cord paralysis, 513
Tissue expanders, 65
Tonsillectomy and adenoidectomy
  axial fat-suppressed T2 and T1, 480
  cine MRI, 480, 481
  flap reconstruction, 481
  indications, 480
  postoperative infection, 483
  recurrent enlargement, 481
  velopharyngeal insufficiency, 480, 482
Torkildsen shunt
  description, 269
  internal shunt, 269
Total ossicular reconstruction prosthesis (TORP)
  Black oval-top, 372
  cortical bone sculpted, 371
  dislocated, 378, 381
  extruded, 381
  Goldenberg, 371
  manubrium, malleus, 367, 369
  migration, PORP, 378
  ossicular chain reconstruction, 369
  recurrent cholesteatoma, 378, 381
Tracheoesophageal puncture and voice prostheses
  Blom-Singer voice prosthesis, 496
  "esophageal speech", 495
  migration, 495, 496
  provox voice prosthesis, 495
Transcanal atticotomy, 382
Transsphenoidal tumor resection
  approach, 321, 322
  bone remodeling, 321, 323
  complications
    carotid artery injury, 327, 330
    cerebrospinal fluid leak, 328, 333
    chiasmopexy, 328, 334
    fibrosis, 328, 335
    GRE and SWI, 327
    hematoma, 327, 329
    infection, 327, 332
    merocel migration and brainstem compression,
      327, 331
    optic chiasm ptosis, 328, 334

Transsphenoidal tumor resection (*cont.*)
  optic nerve ischemia, 328, 334
  pituitary stalk transection, 328, 333
  postoperative fibrosis, 328, 335
  sellar hematomas, 327
  sinus inflammation, 327, 332
  suprasellar fat graft, 327, 331
  suprasellar fat graft, 327, 331fat graft, 321, 323
  granulation tissue, 321, 325
  merocel packing, 321, 324
  metal debris, residual, 321, 322
  pedicled mucosal flap, 321, 324
  subtotal resection, 321, 326
  titanium mesh sellar reconstruction, 321, 325
  transventricular-transsphenoidal, 321, 323
Tube drainage, cholesterol cysts
  drained cholesterol cyst, 414, 415
  trans-sphenoidal, 414

V

Vagal nerve stimulator
  complication, 518
  fontal neck radiograph, 518
Vascular clamp
  metallic extracranial carotid, 652
  Selverstone clamp, 652, 653
Vascular plugs
  Amplatzer device, 663
  right extracranial vertebral artery, 663, 670
Vascular surgery
  aberrant right subclavian artery, left aortic arch
    hybrid procedures, 653
    reconstruction, 653
  adjustable vascular clamp, 652–653
  aneurysm clips (*see* Aneurysm clips)
  artificial bypass grafts, 653, 655
  carotid body stimulator, 652
  CEA (*see* Carotid endarterectomy (CEA))
  extracranial-intracranial revascularization (*see*
    Extracranial-intracranial revascularization,
    vascular surgery)
  intracranial aneurysm muscle wrap, 634–635
  microvascular decompression (*see* Microvascular
    decompression)
  right aortic arch repair, aberrant left
    subclavian artery, 653
Venous sinus stents
  self-expandable/balloon-expandable stents, 677, 684
  transverse sinus stent, 676, 677
Ventricular shunts
  aqueductoplasty and stenting, 279
  atrial, 267
  fourth, 286, 300, 302
  pleural, 267–268, 274
  vesical, 267

Ventriculoperitoneal (VP) shunts
  Codman Hakim programmable shunt valve, 264
  complications, 260
  delta 1.5 valve VP shunt, 263
  MRI, 264, 266
  normal nuclear medicine shunt study, 260, 296
  programmable valves, 260
  "shuntogram", 260
  shunt series, 260, 262
  strata valve programmable shunt, 264, 285
  valve performance level setting chart, 265
  ventriculoperitoneal shunt components, 265
Ventriculosubgaleal shunt, 268, 270
VEPTR. *See* Vertical expandable prosthetic titanium rib
    (VEPTR)
Vertebral augmentation
  increased vertebral body height, 610
  kyphoplasty/vertebroplasty, 609
  polymethylmethacrylate cement
    injection, 609
  skyphoplasty, 524, 609
Vertebrectomy
  partial, residual tumor, 596
  resection, thoracic vertebra, 611
Vertical expandable prosthetic titanium rib (VEPTR),
    560
Vestibular nerve sectioning, 412
Vestibular schwannomas
  radiosurgery, 348
  resection
    encephalocele, 339, 344
    endolymphatic sac fluid signal loss, 339, 345
    fat graft aseptic lipoid meningitis, 338, 343
    fat graft necrosis, 338, 342
    infarction, 339, 347
    labyrinthitis, 339, 345
    labyrinthitis ossificans, 339, 346
    mastoid entry and cerebrospinal fluid leak,
      339, 343
    middle cranial fossa approach, 338, 339
    pseudomeningocele, 339, 344
    residual schwannoma, 338, 341
    retrosigmoid approach, 338, 341
    translabyrinthine approach, 338, 340
    venous sinus thrombosis, 339, 347
    wound abscess, 339, 346
Vibrating ossicular prosthesis (VORP)
  conductive and mixed hearing loss, 351
  extracranial magnet, 351
  mastoidectomy, 386
VP shunts. *See* Ventriculoperitoneal (VP) shunts

W

Wallerian degeneration, 242, 249
Wounded tumor syndrome, 197, 199

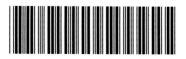